Sixth Edition

Advanced Fitness Assessment
and
Exercise Prescription

Vivian H. Heyward, PhD
University of New Mexico

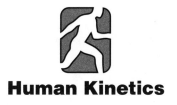

Human Kinetics

Library of Congress Cataloging-in-Publication Data

Heyward, Vivian H.
  Advanced fitness assessment and exercise prescription / Vivian H. Heyward. -- 6th ed.
    p. ; cm.
  Includes bibliographical references and index.
  ISBN-13: 978-0-7360-8659-2 (hard cover)
  ISBN-10: 0-7360-8659-5 (hard cover)
  1. Physical fitness--Testing. 2. Exercise tests. 3. Health. I. Title.
  [DNLM: 1. Physical Fitness--physiology. 2. Exercise Movement Techniques. 3. Exercise Test. QT 255 H622a 2010]
  GV436.H48 2010
  613.7--dc22
                    2009051573

ISBN-10: 0-7360-8659-5 (print)
ISBN-13: 978-0-7360-8659-2 (print)

Acquisitions Editors: Michael S. Bahrke, PhD, Roger W. Earle, and Amy N. Tocco; **Developmental Editors:** Jillian Evans and Kevin Matz; **Assistant Editors:** Martha Gullo and Steven Calderwood; **Copyeditor:** Joyce Sexton; **Indexer:** Michael Ferreira; **Permission Manager:** Dalene Reeder; **Graphic Designer:** Joe Buck; **Graphic Artists:** Denise Lowry and Yvonne Griffith; **Cover Designer:** Keith Blomberg; **Photographer (interior):** Sarah Ritz, except where otherwise noted. Figures 8.1, 8.2, and 8.12a-b © Human Kinetics; **Photo Production Manager:** Jason Allen; **Art Manager:** Kelly Hendren; **Assistant Art Manager:** Alan L. Wilborn; **Illustrators:** Craig Newsom and Alan L. Wilborn; **Printer:** Thomson-Shore, Inc.

We thank the Exercise Physiology Laboratory at the University of New Mexico, Albuquerque, New Mexico, for assistance in providing the location for the photo shoot for this book.

Printed in the United States of America   10   9   8   7   6   5   4   3

The paper in this book is certified under a sustainable forestry program.

Human Kinetics
Web site: www.HumanKinetics.com

United States: Human Kinetics, P.O. Box 5076, Champaign, IL 61825-5076
800-747-4457
email: humank@hkusa.com

Canada: Human Kinetics, 475 Devonshire Road Unit 100, Windsor, ON N8Y 2L5
800-465-7301 (in Canada only)
email: info@hkcanada.com

Europe: Human Kinetics, 107 Bradford Road, Stanningley, Leeds LS28 6AT, United Kingdom
+44 (0) 113 255 5665
email: hk@hkeurope.com

Australia: Human Kinetics, 57A Price Avenue, Lower Mitcham, South Australia 5062
08 8372 0999
e-mail: info@hkaustralia.com

New Zealand: Human Kinetics, P.O. Box 80, Torrens Park, South Australia 5062
0800 222 062
e-mail: info@hknewzealand.com

E4935

In memory of Mom—
for her gentle encouragement
and unwavering confidence in me.

Contents

Chapter 5   Designing Cardiorespiratory Exercise Programs   103

Chapter 6   Assessing Muscular Fitness   129

Chapter 7   Designing Resistance Training Programs   155

Chapter 8   Assessing Body Composition   189

Chapter 9   Designing Weight Management and Body Composition Programs   231

Chapter 10   Assessing Flexibility   265

Chapter 11   Designing Programs for Flexibility and Low Back Care   283

Chapter 12   Assessing Balance and Designing Balance Programs   297

Appendix A   Health and Fitness Appraisal   315

Appendix B   Cardiorespiratory Assessments   333

Preface

Advanced Fitness Assessment and Exercise Prescription, Sixth Edition is written primarily for exercise science students in advanced professional courses dealing with physical fitness appraisal and exercise prescription. This book is also a resource for exercise physiologists or personal trainers working in the public or private sector. Previous editions of this text have been adopted for course use by numerous universities and colleges and have been translated into Greek, Italian, Korean, Portuguese, and Spanish. Also, the sixth edition is now available as an electronic book, potentially allowing this book to reach a wider audience worldwide.

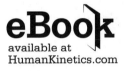

eBook
available at
HumanKinetics.com

This book provides exercise scientists with the knowledge and skills needed to assess the physical fitness of apparently healthy individuals rather than individuals who have suspected or documented cardiovascular disease. Since this text is not clinically oriented, it provides limited information on the etiology and pathophysiology of chronic diseases, on clinical exercise testing, and on exercise prescriptions for clinical populations. Exercise scientists working with clinical populations are encouraged to consult clinically oriented books that provide detailed information for exercise testing and prescriptions for these populations.

In its well-balanced approach to the assessment of physical fitness, *Advanced Fitness Assessment and Exercise Prescription* addresses five components:

- Cardiorespiratory endurance
- Muscular fitness
- Body weight and composition
- Flexibility
- Balance

This text is unique in its scope and in the depth of its content, organization, and approach to the subject matter. Introductory texts typically focus on field testing for evaluating physical fitness. Although this text includes some field tests, it emphasizes laboratory techniques for assessment. The scope and depth of information make this text an important resource for practitioners, especially those employed in health and fitness settings. Generally, the text is organized around physical fitness components, providing for each of them one chapter on assessment followed by one chapter on exercise prescription. The multidisciplinary approach of this text synthesizes concepts, principles, and theories based on research in exercise physiology, kinesiology, measurement, psychology, and nutrition. The result is a direct and clear-cut approach to physical fitness assessment and exercise prescription.

With the exception of the addition of a new chapter, "Assessing Balance and Designing Balance Programs," the scope and organization of the sixth edition of *Advanced Fitness Assessment and Exercise Prescription* are not substantially different from previous editions. The new chapter contains information dealing with assessment of balance and the design of exercise programs for improving balance.

Pedagogical tools include Key Questions at the beginning of each chapter and Key Points, Review Questions, and Key Terms at the end of each chapter. Each of the key terms is defined in the glossary at the back of the book. These tools will help you identify the key terms and concepts and test your knowledge and understanding of the material in each chapter.

Pertinent information from the latest edition (2010) of *ACSM's Guidelines for Exercise Testing and Prescription* is incorporated throughout the text. Updated phone numbers and Web sites for equipment manufacturers and suppliers are included. The following list highlights some of the changes in chapters of *Advanced Fitness Assessment and Exercise Prescription, Sixth Edition:*

Chapter 1

- Recent global and U.S. statistics on the prevalence of chronic diseases
- New research substantiating the link between physical activity and disease risk
- New physical activity recommendations from the U.S. government, the American Heart Association, and the American College of Sports Medicine (ACSM)
- Information about beneficial effects of physical activity on life expectancy

Chapter 2

- Updated information on automated sphygmomanometers
- Updated resources for measurement and interpretation of the electrocardiogram

Chapter 3

- Expanded information about psychological models related to behavior change
- Updated information about the certification and licensure of exercise professionals
- Comparison of selected professional certifications
- Use of technology to promote physical activity

Chapter 4

- Latest (2010) ACSM guidelines for exercise testing
- New equations for predicting maximum heart rate
- Recumbent stepper maximal exercise test protocol
- Use of the OMNI pictorial scales for ratings of perceived exertion during exercise

Chapter 5

- Latest (2010) ACSM guidelines for designing aerobic exercise programs
- Use of high-intensity interval training to improve $\dot{V}O_2$max

Chapter 6

- Use of handheld dynamometers for assessing isometric strength of muscle groups
- Updated guidelines for testing muscular fitness of children and older adults

Chapter 7

- Updated guidelines for developing resistance training programs for novice, intermediate, and advanced weightlifters
- Updated information on designing resistance training programs for children
- Use of whole-body vibration training to improve strength and reduce muscle soreness
- Use of stability balls and resistance bands to increase strength
- Updated information about functional training and core training
- Updated information about the effectiveness of supplements for increasing strength

Chapter 8

- Updated information about air displacement plethysmography and dual-energy X-ray absorptiometry as reference methods for body composition assessment
- Use of bioimpedance spectroscopy to estimate body composition
- Newly developed skinfold prediction equation for athletes
- Updated information on using anthropometric indices to classify disease risk

Chapter 9

- Updated statistics on the global prevalence of obesity in children and adults
- Use of high-intensity aerobic exercise for weight loss
- Updated information on weight loss diets, including OmniHeart diets
- Updated information on protein requirements for active individuals
- New guidelines from the ACSM and the American Dietetic Association for physical activity interventions for weight loss and weight gain

Chapter 10

- Updated information on ballistic stretching
- Validity of clinical tests for measuring hamstring flexibility

Chapter 11

- Updated guidelines for designing stretching programs
- Use of vibration training for improving flexibility
- Updated information about stretching and injury prevention
- New information from the North American Spine Society about exercises to prevent back pain

Chapter 12

- Factors affecting balance
- Guidelines for balance testing
- Field and laboratory tests for assessing balance
- Recommendations for designing balance training programs

Appendixes

- Updated Web sites for professional organizations
- OMNI pictorial scales for assessing ratings of perceived exertion of adults and children

These updates and additions provide a comprehensive approach to physical fitness appraisal and exercise prescription. I hope you will use *Advanced Fitness Assessment and Exercise Prescription, Sixth Edition,* to improve your knowledge, skill, and professional competence as an exercise scientist.

Acknowledgments

I have been authoring and publishing *Advanced Fitness Assessment and Exercise Prescription* since 1984. The first edition was titled *Designs for Fitness* and was published by Burgess Publishing Co. It was a softcover book having about 200 pages. My colleague, Dr. Swede Schoeller, took the photos for that edition, and my secretary at the university, Eileen Fletcher, typed the manuscript on her Smith-Corona.

The second edition was published by Human Kinetics Publishers in 1991. This edition was a hardcover book consisting of 350 pages. For this edition, my dear friend, Linda K. Gilkey, took the photos, and for the first time the manuscript was typed using a DOS word processing system by my secretary, Sandi Travis.

In 1998, the third edition was published by HK. The book grew in size from a 7" x 9" format to an 8" x 11" format. Once again, Linda K. Gilkey took the photos, and the computer graphics were done by Dr. Robert Roberts, Dr. Brent Ruby, and Dr. Peter Egan.

The fourth edition, published by HK in 2002, was 370 pages. My colleagues, Dr. Christine Mermier, Dr. Virginia Wilmerding, Dr. Len Kravitz, and Dr. Donna Lockner, shared their excellent ideas and expertise. My developmental editors, Elaine Mustain and Maggie Schwarzentraub, meticulously edited this edition.

In 2006, the fifth edition was released. For this edition, the total number of pages increased to 425, and HK updated all of the photos. Sarah Ritz did an excellent job organizing and taking these photos. My colleague, Dr. Dale Wagner, contributed the test question bank that accompanied this edition.

Finally, the sixth edition was released in May 2010. For the first time, this book was also published as an e-book. The book has expanded to 480 pages. Once again, I would like to acknowledge the contributions of my colleagues: Dr. Dale Wagner updated the test question bank, and Dr. Ann Gibson prepared the slides for the presentation package.

I am indebted to each individual who played a role in the metamorphosis and continued success of *Advanced Fitness Assessment and Exercise Prescription*.

Physical Activity, Health, and Chronic Disease

KEY QUESTIONS

- Are adults in the United States getting enough physical activity?
- What diseases are associated with a sedentary lifestyle, and what are the major risk factors for these diseases?
- What are the benefits of regular physical activity in terms of disease prevention, and how does physical activity improve health?
- How much physical activity is needed for improved health benefits?
- What kinds of physical activities are suitable for typical people, and how often should they exercise?

Although physical activity plays an important role in the prevention of chronic diseases, an alarming percentage of adults in the United States report no physical activity during leisure time. One of the national health objectives for the year 2010 is to increase to 30% the proportion of people aged 18 yr and older who regularly (preferably daily) engage in moderate physical activity at least 30 min per day (U.S. Department of Health and Human Services 2000a). According to a U.S. national survey from the Centers for Disease Control and Prevention (CDC 2005), less than half (49.1%) of the adults met this physical activity recommendation. Approximately 24% of the American population report no leisure-time physical activity. Generally, women (47.9%) are less likely to meet this recommendation than men (50.7%), and older (≥65 yr) adults are less likely (39.0%) to meet it than younger (18-24 yr) adults (59.6%) (American Heart Association 2008g).

Physical inactivity is not just a problem in the United States; it is a global issue. According to the World Health Organization (2002b), ~60% of the global population did not meet the daily minimum recommendation of 30 min of moderate-intensity physical activity. In 2003, only 37% of men and 25% of women in the United Kingdom met the government's physical activity guidelines (British Heart Foundation 2006). Also, the Canadian Fitness and Lifestyle Research Institute reported that 67% of Canadians (25-55 yr) were physically inactive (Public Health Agency of Canada 2009). Thus, as an exercise specialist, you face the challenge of educating and motivating your clients to incorporate physical activity as a regular part of their lifestyles.

This chapter deals with physical activity trends, risk factors associated with chronic diseases, the role of regular physical activity in disease prevention and health, and physical activity guidelines and recommendations for improved health. For definitions of terminology used in this chapter, see the glossary on page 411.

PHYSICAL ACTIVITY, HEALTH, AND DISEASE: AN OVERVIEW

Our increased reliance on technology has substantially lessened work-related physical activity, as well as the energy expenditure required for activities of daily living like cleaning the house, washing clothes and dishes, mowing the lawn, and traveling to work. What would have once required an hour of physical work now can be accomplished in just a few seconds by pushing a button or setting a dial. As a result, more time is available to pursue leisure activities. The unfortunate fact is, however, that many individuals do not engage in physical activity during their leisure time.

Although the human body is designed for movement and strenuous physical activity, exercise is not a part of the average lifestyle. One cannot expect the human body to function optimally and to remain healthy for extended periods if the body is abused or is not used as intended. Physical inactivity has led to a rise in chronic diseases. Some experts believe that physical inactivity is the most important public health problem in the 21st century (Blair 2009). Each year at least 1.9 million people die as a result of physical inactivity (Cavill, Kahlmeier, and Racioppi 2006). Data from the Aerobics Center Longitudinal Study (Blair 2009) indicated that low cardiorespiratory fitness accounts for substantially more deaths (16%) compared to other risk factors (i.e., obesity

2-3%; smoking 8-10%; high cholesterol 2-4%; diabetes 2-4%; and hypertension 8-16%). Individuals who do not exercise regularly are at greater risk than others of developing chronic diseases such as coronary heart disease, hypertension, hypercholesterolemia, cancer, obesity, and musculoskeletal disorders (see figure 1.1).

For years, exercise scientists and health and fitness professionals have maintained that regular physical activity is the best defense against the development of many diseases, disorders, and illnesses. The importance of regular physical activity in preventing disease and premature death and in maintaining a high quality of life received recognition in the first U.S. surgeon general's report on physical activity and health, in which physical activity was identified as a national health objective (U.S. Department of Health and Human Services 1996). This report identified physical inactivity as a serious nationwide health problem, provided clear-cut scientific evidence linking physical activity to numerous health benefits, presented demographic data describing physical activity patterns and trends in the U.S. population, and made physical activity recommendations for improved health. In 1995 the

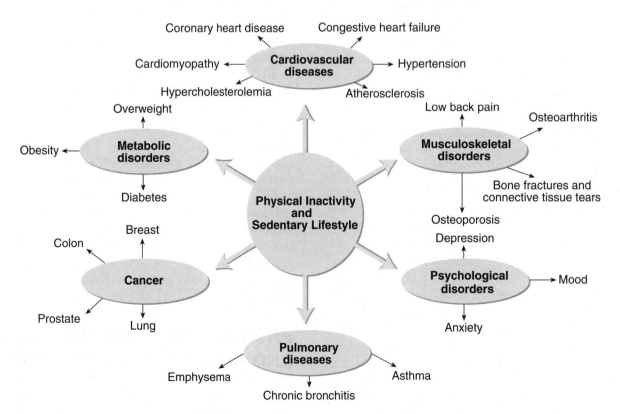

Figure 1.1 Role of physical activity and exercise in disease prevention and rehabilitation.

CDC and the American College of Sports Medicine (ACSM) recommended that every U.S. adult should accumulate 30 min or more of moderate-intensity physical activity on most, preferably all, days of the week (Pate et al. 1995).

Since 1995, new scientific evidence has increased our understanding of the benefits of physical activity for improved health and quality of life. In light of these findings, the ACSM and American Heart Association (AHA) updated physical activity recommendations for healthy adults and older adults (Haskell et al. 2007; Nelson et al. 2007). These recommendations address how much and what kind of physical activity are needed to promote health and reduce the risk of chronic disease in adults. Table 1.1 summarizes the ACSM and AHA physical activity recommendations for adults. The recommended amounts of physical activity are in addition to routine activities of daily living (ADL) such as cooking, shopping, and walking around the home or from the parking lot. The intensity of exercise is expressed in **metabolic equivalents (METs)**. A MET is the ratio of the person's working (exercising) metabolic rate to the resting metabolic rate. One MET is defined as the energy cost of sitting quietly. Moderate-intensity aerobic activity (3.0 to 6.0 METs or 5 to 6 on a 10-point perceived exertion scale) is operationally defined as activity that noticeably increases heart rate and lasts more than 10 min (e.g., brisk walking for 10 min). Vigorous-intensity activity (>6.0 METs or 7 to 8 on a 10-point perceived exertion scale) causes rapid breathing and increases heart rate substantially (e.g., jogging). For adults (18-64 yr) and older adults (≥65 yr), the ACSM and AHA recommend a minimum of 30 min of moderate-intensity aerobic activity 5 days per week, or 20 min of vigorous-intensity aerobic exercise 3 days per week. They also recommend moderate- to high-intensity (8- to 12-repetition maximum [RM] for adults and 10- to 15-RM for older adults) resistance training for a minimum of 2 nonconsecutive days per week. Balance and flexibility exercises are also suggested for older adults.

The U.S. Department of Health and Human Services released the 2008 "Physical Activity Guidelines for Americans" (Howley 2008). Table 1.2 summarizes these guidelines for children and adolescents (6-17 yr), adults (18-64 yr), and older adults (≥65 yr). The key message in these guidelines is that for substantial health benefits, adults should

Table 1.1 ACSM and AHA Physical Activity Recommendations

Population group	AEROBIC ACTIVITY[a]			MUSCLE-STRENGTHENING ACTIVITY			FLEXIBILITY OR BALANCE ACTIVITY
	Duration[b] (min/day)	Intensity	Frequency (days/wk)	Sets	Intensity and no. exercises	Frequency (days/wk)	
Healthy adults 18-64 yr	30	Moderate (3.0-6.0 METs)	Minimum 5	1	8-12 RM; 8-10 exercises for major muscle groups	≥2 nonconsecutive days	No specific recommendation
	20	Vigorous (>6.0 METs)	Minimum 3				
Older adults ≥65 yr	30	Moderate (5-6 on 10-pt. scale)	Minimum 5	1	10-15 RM; 8-10 exercises for major muscle groups	2 nonconsecutive days	For flexibility at least 2 days/wk for at least 10 min each day, including balance exercises for those at risk for falls
	20	Vigorous (7-8 on 10-pt. scale)	Minimum 3				

[a]Combinations of moderate and vigorous intensity may be performed to meet recommendation (e.g., jogging 20 min on 2 days and brisk walking on 2 other days).

[b]Multiple bouts of moderate-intensity activity, each lasting more than 10 min, can be accumulated to meet the minimum duration of 30 min.

Table 1.2 2008 Physical Activity Guidelines for Americans

Population group	AEROBIC ACTIVITIES			MUSCLE-STRENGTHENING ACTIVITIES			BONE-STRENGTHENING ACTIVITIES	FLEXIBILITY AND BALANCE ACTIVITIES
	Duration	Intensity[a]	Frequency	Sets	Intensity[a]	Frequency		
Children and adolescents 6-17 yr	≥60 min	Moderate and Vigorous	Daily 3 days/wk		Moderate to high	3 days/wk	3 days/wk	
Adults 18-64 yr								
Inactive	60-150 min/wk	Light (1.1-2.9 METs) to moderate (3.0-5.9 METs)		1	Light to moderate	1 day/wk		All adults should stretch to maintain flexibility for regular physical activity (PA) and activities of daily living (ADL)
Active	150-300 min/wk or 75-150 min/wk	Moderate (3.0-5.9 METs) or Vigorous (≥6.0 METs)		≥1	Moderate to high 8-12 RM	≥2 days/wk		
Highly active	>300 min/wk or >150 min/wk	Moderate (3.0-5.9 METs) or Vigorous (≥6.0 METs)		2-3	Moderate to high	≥2 days/wk		
Older adults ≥65 yr								
Inactive	150 min/wk	Light (RPE = 3-4) to moderate (RPE = 5-6)	5 days/wk	1	Light (RPE = 3-4) to moderate (RPE = 5-6)	2-3 days/wk		Older adults should stretch to maintain flexibility for regular PA and ADL. ≥3 days/wk balance
Active	150-300 min/wk or 75-150 min/wk	Moderate (RPE = 5-6) or Vigorous (RPE = 7-8)	≥3 days/wk	≥1	Moderate (RPE = 5-6) to high (RPE = 7-8) 8-12 RM	≥2 days/wk, nonconsecutive days		

[a]Intensity is expressed in METs and repetition maximums (RM) for adults; for older adults, intensity is expressed as a rating of perceived exertion (0-10 scale) and RM.

engage in aerobic exercise at least 150 min per week at a moderate intensity or 75 min per week at a vigorous intensity. In addition, adults and older adults should do muscle-strengthening activities at least 2 days per week. Children should do at least 60 min of physical activity every day. Most of the 60 min per day should be either moderate or vigorous aerobic activity and should include vigorous aerobic activities at least 3 days per week. Part of the 60 min or more of daily physical activity should be muscle-strengthening activities (at least 3 days a week) and bone-strengthening activities (at least 3 days a week).

Exercising 150 min/wk equates to expending approximately 1000 kcal·wk^{-1}. Participating in moderate-intensity physical activity on a daily basis reduces the risk of coronary heart disease by 50% and the risk of hypertension, diabetes, and colon cancer by 30% (U.S. Department of Health and Human Services 1996). Also, the risk of breast cancer decreases by 18% in women who walk briskly 1.25 to 2.5 hr/wk (McTiernan et al. 2003).

"Canada's Physical Activity Guide to Healthy Active Living" (Health Canada 2003) recommends accumulating 60 min of daily physical activity to stay healthy and participating in aerobic activities (4-7 days/wk), strength activities (2-4 days/wk), and flexibility activities (4-7 days/wk) to improve health. The duration of the activity depends on the intensity or effort: Perform light activities (e.g., walking or gardening) for 60 min, moderate activities (e.g., brisk walking or swimming) for 30 to 60 min, and vigorous activities (e.g., jogging or hockey) for 20 to 30 min.

Improvements in health benefits depend on the volume (i.e., combination of frequency, intensity, and duration) of physical activity. This is known as the **dose–response relationship** (Bouchard 2001; Canadian Society of Exercise Physiology 2003; Kesaniemi et al. 2001). Because of the dose–response relationship between physical activity and health, the ACSM and AHA physical activity recommendation states that "persons who wish to improve their personal fitness, reduce their risk for chronic diseases and disabilities, or prevent unhealthy weight gain will likely benefit by exceeding the minimum recommended amount of physical activity" (Haskell et al. 2007, p. 1431).

Figure 1.2 illustrates the general dose–response relationship between the volume of physical activity

---

Health Benefits of Physical Activity

Lower risk of

- premature death;
- coronary artery disease;
- stroke;
- type 2 diabetes and metabolic syndrome;
- high blood pressure;
- adverse blood lipid profile;
- colon, breast, lung, and endometrial cancers; and
- hip fractures.

Reduction of

- abdominal obesity and
- feelings of depression and anxiety.

Helps in

- weight loss, weight maintenance, and prevention of weight gain;
- prevention of falls and better functional health for older adults;
- improved cognitive function for older adults;
- increased bone density; and
- improved quality of sleep.

Data from U.S. Department of Health and Human Services, 2008, *Physical Activity Guidelines for Americans* (Washington, DC).

---

participation and selected health benefits that do not require a minimal threshold intensity for improvement like muscular strength and aerobic fitness. The volume of physical activity participation needed for the same degree of relative improvement (%) varies among health benefit indicators. For example, to improve triglycerides from 0% to 40% requires 250 kcal·wk^{-1} of physical activity compared to 1800 kcal·wk^{-1} for the same relative improvement (0% to 40%) in high-density lipoprotein (see figure 1.2). Additionally, you should note that too much physical activity, defined as engaging in 5 hr of structured high-intensity activity per week, may be associated with negative health consequences or overuse injuries. For extensive reviews of literature dealing with the dose–response relationship between physical activity and health, see *Medicine & Science in Sports & Exercise* (June 2001, Supplement).

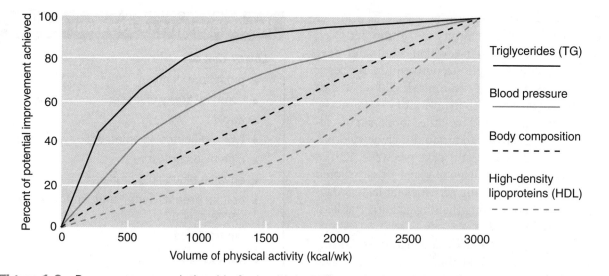

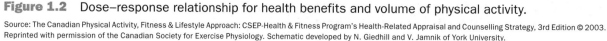

Figure 1.2 Dose–response relationship for health benefits and volume of physical activity.

Source: The Canadian Physical Activity, Fitness & Lifestyle Approach: CSEP-Health & Fitness Program's Health-Related Appraisal and Counselling Strategy, 3rd Edition © 2003. Reprinted with permission of the Canadian Society for Exercise Physiology. Schematic developed by N. Giedhill and V. Jamnik of York University.

Although the physical activity guideline—a minimum of 150 min per week of moderate-intensity aerobic activity—reduces disease risk, it may not be optimal for maintaining a healthy body weight. In 2002, the Institute of Medicine (IOM) recommended 60 min of daily moderate-intensity physical activity. In the IOM report, the expert panel stated that 30 min of daily physical activity is insufficient to maintain a healthy body weight and to fully reap the associated health benefits. The IOM recommendation addresses the amount of physical activity necessary to maintain a healthy body weight and to prevent unhealthful weight gain (Brooks et al. 2004). The IOM recommendation of 60 min of daily physical activity is consistent with recommendations for preventing weight gain

Examples of Moderate-Intensity and Vigorous-Intensity Aerobic Activities

This list provides several examples of moderate- and vigorous-intensity aerobic activities. Some activities can be performed at varied intensities. This list is not all-inclusive; examples are provided to help people make choices. For a detailed list of energy expenditures (METs) for conditioning exercises, sports, and recreational activities, see page 382. Generally, light activity is defined as <3.0 METs, moderate activity as 3.0 to 6.0 METs, and vigorous activity as >6.0 METs.

Moderate Intensity

- Walking briskly (3.0 mph [4.8 km·hr⁻¹] or faster, but not race walking)
- Water aerobics
- Bicycling slower than 10 mph (16 km·hr⁻¹)
- Tennis (doubles)
- Ballroom dancing
- General gardening

Vigorous Intensity

- Race walking, jogging, or running
- Swimming laps
- Tennis (singles)
- Aerobic dancing
- Bicycling 10 mph (16 km·hr⁻¹) or faster
- Jumping rope
- Heavy gardening (continuous digging or hoeing with heart rate increases)
- Hiking uphill or with a heavy backpack

Data from U.S. Department of Health and Human Services, 2008, *Physical Activity Guidelines for Americans* (Washington, DC).

made by other organizations (i.e., Health Canada, International Association for the Study of Obesity, and World Health Organization) (Brooks et al. 2004). The bottom line is that 150 min per week of moderate-intensity physical activity provides substantial health benefits but may be insufficient to prevent weight gain for many individuals. It is a good initial goal and a sufficient amount of activity to move individuals from a sedentary to a low physical activity level (Brooks et al. 2004). As individuals adopt regular physical activity and improve their lifestyle and fitness, they should increase the duration of daily physical activity to a level (60 min) that prevents weight gain and provides additional health benefits. This goal is especially important for individuals who have difficulty controlling their body weight (Blair, LaMonte, and Nichaman 2004; Lohman, Going, and Metcalfe 2004), and it is suf-

ficient to move individuals from a sedentary to an active physical activity level (Brooks et al. 2004).

The Exercise and Physical Activity Pyramid illustrates a balanced plan of physical activity and exercise to promote health and to improve physical fitness (see figure 1.3). You should encourage your clients to engage in physical activities around the home and workplace on a daily basis to establish a foundation (base of pyramid) for an active lifestyle. They should perform aerobic activities a minimum of 3 to 5 days/wk; they should do weight-resistance exercises and flexibility or balance exercises at least 2 days per week. Recreational sport activities (middle levels of pyramid) are recommended to add variety to the exercise plan. High-intensity training and competitive sport (top of pyramid) require a solid fitness base and proper preparation to prevent injury; most adults should engage in these activities sparingly.

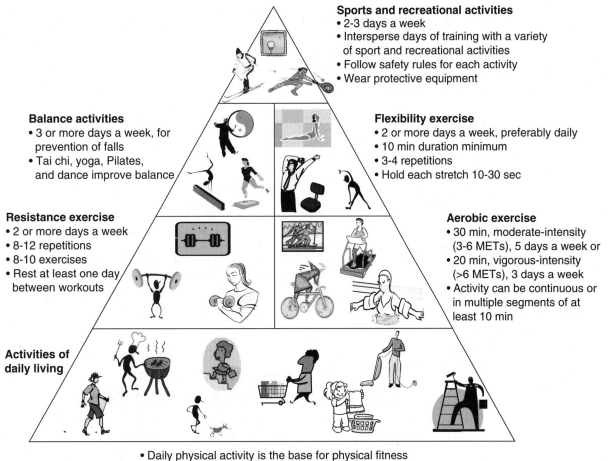

Sports and recreational activities
- 2-3 days a week
- Intersperse days of training with a variety of sport and recreational activities
- Follow safety rules for each activity
- Wear protective equipment

Balance activities
- 3 or more days a week, for prevention of falls
- Tai chi, yoga, Pilates, and dance improve balance

Flexibility exercise
- 2 or more days a week, preferably daily
- 10 min duration minimum
- 3-4 repetitions
- Hold each stretch 10-30 sec

Resistance exercise
- 2 or more days a week
- 8-12 repetitions
- 8-10 exercises
- Rest at least one day between workouts

Aerobic exercise
- 30 min, moderate-intensity (3-6 METs), 5 days a week or
- 20 min, vigorous-intensity (>6 METs), 3 days a week
- Activity can be continuous or in multiple segments of at least 10 min

Activities of daily living

- Daily physical activity is the base for physical fitness
- Try to be active for at least 30 min every day

Figure 1.3 The Exercise and Physical Activity Pyramid.

Adapted, by permission, from "Exercise and Activity Pyramid" Metropolitan Life Insurance Company, 1995.

CARDIOVASCULAR DISEASE

Cardiovascular disease (CVD) causes 17.5 million deaths worldwide each year, representing 30% of all global deaths (World Health Organization 2007). According to the World Health Organization (2007), over 80% of cardiovascular deaths occur in low- and middle-income countries. Cardiovascular disease is the principal cause of mortality in Europe, accounting for nearly half of all deaths (American Heart Association 2008d). In developing countries in Africa, Western Asia, and Southeastern Asia, 15% to 20% of the annual deaths are due to CVDs (American Heart Association 2001). The proportion of deaths from CVD ranges from 25% for Latin American countries to 45% for eastern Mediterranean countries (American Heart Association 2001). In 2005, diseases of the heart and blood vessels claimed the lives of 864,500 people in the United States alone. Cardiovascular disease accounted for 36.3% of deaths (one out of every three) in the United States. More than 80 million Americans have some form of CVD such as hypertension (73.6 million), coronary heart disease (16.8 million), and stroke (6.5 million) (American Heart Association 2008d).

One myth about CVD is that it is much more prevalent in men than in women. In 2006, the prevalence of CVD in women (34.9%) and men (37.6%) in the United States was similar (American Heart Association 2008d). Nearly 455,000 females die from CVD each year in the United States. Another misconception about CVD is that it afflicts only the older population. Although it is true that older people are at greater risk, over 60% of the people in the United States with CVD are less than 65 yr, and CVD ranks as the second-leading cause of death for children under age 15 (American Heart Association 2008d).

Coronary heart disease (CHD) accounts for more deaths worldwide than any other disease, with more than 7.6 million people dying in 2005 from CHD (World Health Organization 2007). Among American adults 20 yr of age or older, the estimated age-adjusted prevalence of CHD is higher for black men and women compared to Mexican American and white men and women (American Heart Association 2008d).

Coronary heart disease (CHD) is caused by a lack of blood supply to the heart muscle (myo-cardial ischemia), resulting from a progressive, degenerative disorder known as atherosclerosis. Atherosclerosis involves a buildup and deposition of fat and fibrous plaques in the intima, or inner lining, of the coronary arteries. These plaques restrict the blood flow to the myocardium and may produce angina pectoris, which is a temporary sensation of tightening and heavy pressure in the chest and shoulder region. A myocardial infarction, or heart attack, can occur if a blood clot, or thrombus, obstructs the coronary blood flow. In this case, blood flow through the coronary arteries is usually reduced by over 80%. The portion of the myocardium supplied by the obstructed artery dies and is replaced eventually with scar tissue.

Coronary Heart Disease Risk Factors

Epidemiological research indicates that many factors are associated with the risk of CHD. The greater the number and severity of risk factors, the greater the probability of CHD. The positive risk factors for CHD are

- age,
- family history,
- hypercholesterolemia,
- hypertension,
- use of tobacco,
- diabetes mellitus or prediabetes,
- overweight and obesity, and
- physical inactivity.

An increased level of high-density lipoprotein cholesterol or HDL-cholesterol (HDL-C) (>60 mg·dl^{-1}) in the blood decreases CHD risk. If the HDL-C is high, you should subtract one risk factor from the sum of the positive factors when assessing your client's CHD risk

Physical Activity and Coronary Heart Disease

Nearly 22% of all cases of CHD worldwide can be attributed to a lack of physical activity and a sedentary lifestyle (World Health Organization 2004a). As an exercise scientist, you must educate your clients about the benefits of physical activity and regular exercise for preventing CHD. Physically active people have lower incidences of myocardial infarction and mortality from CHD and tend to develop CHD at a later age compared to their sedentary counterparts (Berlin and Colditz 1990). Individuals who exercise regularly reduce their relative risk of developing CHD by a factor of 1.5 to 2.4 (American Heart Association 1999; Powell et al. 1987). Physical activity exerts its effect independently of smoking, hypertension, hypercholesterolemia, obesity, diabetes, and family history of CHD (Bouchard, Shephard, and Stephens 1994). Also, in a meta-analysis of studies dealing with the dose–response effects of physical activity and cardiorespiratory fitness on CVD and CHD risk, Williams (2001) reported that cardiorespiratory fitness and physical activity have significantly different relationships to CVD and CHD risk. Although physical fitness and physical activity each lower the risk of developing CVD and CHD, the reduction in relative risk was almost twice as great for cardiorespiratory fitness as for physical activity. These findings suggest that in addition to physical activity level, cardiorespiratory fitness level should be considered a potential risk factor for CHD (U.S. Department of Health and Human Services 2008).

HYPERTENSION

Hypertension, or high blood pressure, is a chronic, persistent elevation of blood pressure that is clinically defined as a systolic pressure ≥140 mmHg or a diastolic pressure ≥90 mmHg or as taking antihypertensive medicine. Prehypertension is a term used to describe individuals with a systolic pressure of 120 to 139 mmHg, a diastolic pressure of 80 to 89 mmHg, or both (Chobanian et al. 2003). About 62% of strokes and 49% of heart attacks are caused by hypertension (World Health Organization 2004a).

About 15% to 40% of the global adult population have hypertension. Generally, the average blood pressure of adults from European countries (England, Finland, Germany, Italy, and Spain) is higher than that of American and Canadian adults (Wolf-Maier et al. 2003). In England, approximately 35% of adult men and 28% of adult women are hypertensive (British Heart Foundation 2008). In comparison, the prevalence of hypertension is estimated to be 10% to 17% for adults in the eastern Mediterranean region, 4% to 12% for adults in India, 8% for people 15 yr and older in China, and 5% to 12% for adults in Africa (American Heart Association 2001).

In the United States, more than one out of three adults (33%) has high blood pressure, and 22% are prehypertensive (American Heart Association 2008c). Up to age 45 yr, the percentage of American men with hypertension (11% to 23%) is greater than that of women (6% to 18%). Between ages 45 and 54 yr, the prevalence of hypertension (37%) is similar for men and women. After age 55 yr, the percentage of women (55-84%) with high blood pressure is much higher than that of men (49-69%). Women with hypertension have a 3.5 times greater risk of developing CHD than do women with normal blood pressure. Also, the prevalence of high blood pressure for blacks in the United States (39-41%) is among the highest in the world and is substantially greater than that of American Indians or Alaskan Natives, Asians or Pacific Islanders, Mexican Americans, and whites in the United States (American Heart Association 2008c). Table 1.3 summarizes the risk factors associated with developing hypertension.

Epidemiological studies indicate an inverse relationship between the resting blood pressure and the level of physical activity in women and men (Fagard 1999). Regular physical activity prevents hypertension and lowers blood pressure in younger and older adults who are normotensive, prehypertensive, or hypertensive. Compared to what is seen in normotensive individuals, training-induced changes in resting systolic and diastolic blood pressures (5-7 mmHg) are greater for hypertensive individuals who participate in endurance exercise.

Exercise Prescription for Hypertension (Pescatello et al. 2004)

Mode: Primarily endurance activities supplemented by resistance exercises

Intensity: Moderate (40% to 60% $\dot{V}O_2R$)*

Duration: 30 min or more of continuous or accumulated physical activity per day

Frequency: Most, preferably all, days of the week

---

*$\dot{V}O_2R$ is the difference between the maximum and the resting rate of oxygen consumption. See "$\dot{V}O_2$ Reserve (MET) Method" on page 108 for more information.

Table 1.3 Summary of Factors Associated With Disease Risk

Factor	CHD	Diabetes	Hypertension	Hypercholesterolemia	Low back pain	Obesity	Osteoporosis	Cancer
Age	↑	↑	↑	↑	↑	↑	↑	↑
Gender	M > F[a]	F > M	F > M[b]	F > M[b]	F = M	F > M	F > M[b]	
Race	B, H > A, AI, W	AI, B, H > A, W	B > A, AI, H, W	B, H, W > A, AI		AI, B, H, W > A	A, W > AI, B, H	
Family history	↑	↑	↑	↑		↑	↑	↑
SES	↓	↓	↓	↓	↓	↓		↑
Alcohol use	↑		↑	↑			↑	↑
Smoking	↑		↑	↑			↑	↑
Nutrition								
Na intake			↑					
Ca intake, vitamin D							↓	
Fat and cholesterol intake	↑		↑	↑		↑		↑
CHO intake		↑						
Intake ≥ expenditure						↑		
Physical activity	↓	↓	↓	↓	↓	↓	↓	↓
Exercise amenorrhea							↑	
Flexibility					↓			
Muscular strength					↓		↓	
Skeletal frame size							↓	
Other diseases								
Anorexia nervosa							↑	
Diabetes	↑							
Hypertension	↑							
Hypercholesterolemia	↑							
Obesity and overweight	↑	↑	↑	↑	↑			↑

↑ = Direct relationship; as factor increases, risk increases.

↓ = Indirect relationship; as factor increases, risk decreases.

[a]Males (M) at higher risk than females (F) up to age 55 yr.

[b]Menopausal females at higher risk than males.

CHD = coronary heart disease; CHO = carbohydrate; A = Asian; AI = American Indian; B = black; H = Hispanic; W = white; Na = sodium; Ca = calcium; SES = socioeconomic status (reflects income and education levels).

However, even modest reductions in blood pressure (2-3 mmHg) by endurance or resistance exercise training decrease CHD risk by 5% to 9%, stroke risk by 8% to 14%, and all-cause mortality by 4% in the general population (Pescatello et al. 2004). In a position paper on exercise and hypertension (Pescatello et al. 2004), the ACSM endorsed the exercise prescription on page 9 to lower blood pressure in adults with hypertension.

HYPERCHOLESTEROLEMIA AND DYSLIPIDEMIA

Hypercholesterolemia, an elevation of total cholesterol (TC) in the blood, is associated with increased risk for CVD. Hypercholesterolemia is also referred to as hyperlipidemia, which is an increase in blood lipid levels; dyslipidemia refers to an abnormal blood lipid profile. Approximately 18% of strokes and 56% of heart attacks are caused by high blood cholesterol (World Health Organization 2002b). Over 106 million Americans age 20 yr and older have total blood cholesterol levels of 200 mg·dl^{-1} or higher. Of these, 37 million Americans have TC levels that are classified as high risk (>240 mg·dl^{-1}); more women (19 million) than men (17 million) have TC levels equaling or exceeding 240 mg·dl^{-1} (American Heart Association 2008b). Compared to those in Western countries, the average TC levels for adults in China, Japan, and Indonesia are uniformly lower (190-207 mg·dl^{-1}) (American Heart Association 2001). Risk factors for hypercholesterolemia are identified in table 1.3.

LDLs, HDLs, and TC

Cholesterol is a waxy, fatlike substance found in all animal products (meats, dairy products, and eggs). The body can make cholesterol in the liver and absorb cholesterol from the diet. Cholesterol is essential to the body and is used to build cell membranes, to produce sex hormones, and to form bile acids necessary for fat digestion. Lipoproteins are an essential part of the complex transport system that exchanges lipids among the liver, intestine, and peripheral tissues. Lipoproteins are classified by the thickness of the protein shell that surrounds the cholesterol. The four main classes of lipoproteins are chylomicron, derived from the intestinal absorption of triglycerides; very low-density lipoprotein (VLDL), made in the liver for the transport of triglycerides; low-density lipoprotein (LDL), a product of VLDL metabolism that serves as the primary transporter of cholesterol; and high-density lipoprotein (HDL), involved in the reverse transport of cholesterol to the liver. The molecules of LDL are larger than those of HDL and therefore precipitate in the plasma and are actively transported into the vascular walls. Excess LDL-cholesterol (LDL-C) stimulates the formation of plaque on the intima of the coronary arteries. Plaque formation reduces the cross-sectional area and obstructs blood flow in these arteries, eventually producing a myocardial infarction. Therefore, LDL-C values less than 100 mg·dl^{-1} are considered optimal for reducing CVD and CHD risk (National Cholesterol Education Program 2001). Over 30% of adult women and 32% of adult men in the United States have borderline high levels (≥130 mg·dl^{-1}) of LDL-C (American Heart Association 2008b).

The smaller HDL molecules are suspended in the plasma and protect the body by picking up excess cholesterol from the arterial walls and delivering it to the liver where it is metabolized. HDL-cholesterol (HDL-C) values less than 40 mg·dl^{-1} are associated with a higher risk of coronary heart disease. Approximately 7% to 13% of women and 15% to 28% of men in the United States have low HDL-C levels (American Heart Association 2008b).

Individuals with low HDL-C or high TC levels (dyslipidemia) have a greater risk of heart attack. Those with lower HDL-C (<37 mg·dl^{-1}) are at higher risk regardless of their TC level. This fact emphasizes the importance of screening for both TC and HDL-C in adults.

Physical Activity and Lipid Profiles

Regular physical activity, especially habitual aerobic exercise, positively affects lipid metabolism and lipid profiles (Durstine et al. 2002). Cross-sectional comparisons of lipid profiles in physically active and sedentary women and men suggest that physical fitness is inversely related to TC and the TC/HDL-C ratio (Despres and Lamarche 1994; Shoenhair and Wells 1995).

In a meta-analysis that examined the effects of aerobic exercise on lipids and lipoproteins in adult men, data from 49 randomized controlled trials were pooled for analysis. Results showed that aerobic exercise reduces TC (–2%), LDL-C (–3%), and

TG (–9%) and increases HDL-C (2%) in men 18 yr and older (Kelley and Kelley 2006). A 1% reduction in TC has been shown to reduce risk for CHD by 2%; likewise, a 1% reduction in HDL-C increases CHD risk by 2% to 3% (Gordon et al. 1989). However, for individuals with hyperlipidemia, lifestyle (e.g., healthy diet) or pharmagologic (e.g., statins) interventions, in addition to aerobic exercise, may be necessary for optimizing lipid and lipoprotein profiles (Durstine et al. 2002; Kelley and Kelley 2006).

Increases in HDL-C in response to aerobic exercise appear to be related to the training dose (interaction of the intensity, frequency, and duration of each exercise session and the length of the training period) and are less dramatic in women than in men. In an analysis of longitudinal and cross-sectional exercise studies, researchers concluded that 15 to 20 mi·wk^{-1} (24 to 32 km·wk^{-1}) of brisk walking or jogging (equivalent to 1200-2200 kcal of energy expenditure) decreases blood triglyceride levels by 5 to 38 mg·dl^{-1} and increases HDL-C by 2 to 8 mg·dl^{-1} (Durstine et al. 2002). In comparison, resistance training has no effect on blood triglyceride levels, and TC and LDL-C are lowered only when the training increases lean body mass and decreases relative body fat (Durstine et al. 2002). Also, resistance training has little or no effect on the HDL-C levels of men at risk for CHD.

TOBACCO

The World Health Organization (2008a) estimates that there are 1.3 billion smokers in the global population. In Great Britain, 25% of men and 23% of women ages 16 yr and older smoke cigarettes (British Heart Foundation 2008). In the United States, the prevalence of adults (18 yr and older) who smoke has declined by 50% since 1965. Approximately 18% of American women, 24% of American men, and 21.5% of Canadian adults are smokers (American Heart Association 2009; CDC 2007; Klein-Geltink, Choi, and Fry 2006). Globally, the prevalence of smoking is highest for men in Asian countries. About half of all men in Malaysia and Japan smoke, whereas in China, Cambodia, and Korea, 67% of men smoke (World Health Organization 2002c). While the prevalence of smoking is falling in well-developed countries, tobacco consumption is rising in developing countries by 3.4% per year (World Health Organization 2002c). Worldwide, one in five teenagers (13-15 yr) is a smoker. Also, the risk of death from CHD increases by 30% in those exposed to environmental tobacco smoke at home or at work (American Heart Association 2004).

Smoking is the largest preventable cause of disease and premature death. Cigarette smoking is linked to CHD, stroke, and chronic lung disease. It causes cancer of the lungs, larynx, esophagus, mouth, and bladder and is also associated with cancer of the cervix, pancreas, and kidneys (World Health Organization 2002c). Compared to non-smokers, smokers have more than twice the risk of heart attack. Cigarette smoking remains a major cause of stroke in the United States; there is a causal relationship between smoking and subclinical atherosclerosis (American Heart Association 2008h).

When individuals stop smoking, their risk of CHD declines rapidly, regardless of how long or how much they have smoked. One year after quitting, the risk of CHD decreases by 50%, and within 15 yr the relative risk of dying from CHD almost matches that of a longtime nonsmoker (American Heart Association 2004). Also the risk of stroke decreases steadily after smoking cessation; former smokers have the same risk as nonsmokers after 5 to 15 yr (American Heart Association 2008h).

DIABETES MELLITUS

There is a global diabetes epidemic. Over 180 million people worldwide have diabetes, and the World Health Organization (2008b) predicts that by 2030 this number is likely to more than double. At least 65% of people with diabetes mellitus die from some form of heart or blood vessel disease (American Heart Association 2008a). Also, diabetes is among the leading causes of kidney failure; 10% to 20% of people with diabetes die of kidney failure (World Health Organization 2008b).

Over 48 million adults in Europe and 17 million adults in the United States have diabetes, and the prevalence is increasing (American Heart Association 2008a; British Heart Foundation Health Promotion Research Group 2005). In 2006, the age-adjusted prevalence of diabetes for adults in the United States was 7.7% (American Heart Association 2008a). Compared to white adults in the United States, the prevalence of diabetes and impaired blood glucose levels for blacks, Hispanics, and American Indians is higher (American Heart Association 2008a). In fact, the prevalence of diabetes for American Indians and Alaskan Native adults (15.3%) is one of the highest in the world; 43.5% of American Indian men and 52.4% of American Indian women have diabetes (American Heart Association 2004).

Type 1, or **insulin-dependent diabetes mellitus (IDDM)**, usually occurs before age 30 but can develop at any age. Type 2, or **non-insulin-dependent diabetes mellitus (NIDDM)**, is more common; 90% to 95% of individuals with diabetes mellitus have type 2 diabetes (Kriska, Blair, and Pereira 1994). Risk factors for developing diabetes are presented in table 1.3. Healthy nutrition and increased physical activity can reduce the risk of diabetes by as much as 60% in high-risk individuals.

Research suggests that regular physical activity reduces one's risk of developing NIDDM through its association with weight loss and the effects of exercise on insulin sensitivity and glucose tolerance (Kelley and Goodpaster 1999; Kriska et al. 1994). Manson and colleagues (1991) reported that women who engaged in vigorous exercise at least once a week have a reduced risk of diabetes. The reduction in diabetes risk, however, appears to be associated with the frequency of exercise. The risk of diabetes decreased 23%, 38%, and 42%, respectively, in male physicians who exercised vigorously one time, two to four times, and five or more times a week (Manson et al. 1992). Vigorous exercise was defined as physical activity of sufficient duration to produce sweating. Specific guidelines for prescribing exercise programs for people who have type 1 and type 2 diabetes are available elsewhere (American College of Sports Medicine and American Diabetes Association 1997; Colberg 2001).

OBESITY AND OVERWEIGHT

In clinical guidelines established by the Obesity Education Initiative Task Force of the National Institutes of Health and National Heart, Lung, and Blood Institute (1998), **overweight** and **obesity** are classified using the **body mass index (BMI)** (weight [kg]/height squared [m^2]). Individuals with a BMI between 25 and 29.9 kg/m^2 are classified as overweight; those with a BMI of 30 kg/m^2 or more are classified as obese.

Using these definitions, the World Health Organization (2006) reported that more than 1.6 billion people worldwide are overweight and that at least 400 million overweight individuals are obese. The prevalence of obesity increases with the development of countries, as is seen in the data for undeveloped countries (1.8%), developing countries (4.8%), countries in transition (17.1%), and developed countries (20.4%) (World Health Organization 2001). In Indonesia, 12.5% of adults ages 25 to 64 are obese; and in Africa, 8.3% of men and 36% to 50% of women are obese (American Heart Association 2001). In 1995, only 8% to 12% of Chinese adults were overweight; projections indicate that by 2025, 37% of men and 40% of women in China will be overweight (American Heart Association 2008f).

In 2006, two out of every three adults in the United States were overweight or obese (BMI >25 kg/m^2), and one of every three adults was obese (BMI >30 kg/m^2). Regardless of ethnicity, the prevalence of obesity for American men is approximately 33%. Among American women, however, the prevalence of obesity is 33%, 42%, and 53%, respectively, for white, Hispanic, and black women (American Heart Association 2008f). Asian adults in the United States have a relatively lower prevalence of obesity (8.5%) compared to American Indians/Alaskan Native adults (38%) (American Heart Association 2008f).

Childhood obesity is also a global problem (see chapter 9, pp. 232-234). Overweight adolescents have a 70% chance of becoming overweight adults; this increases to 80% if one or both parents are overweight or obese (American Heart Association 2008f). A report from England in 2006 showed that 33% of boys and 35% of girls ages 2 to 15 yr were either overweight or obese (British Heart Foundation 2006). Similarly, in the United States, the prevalence of overweight and obesity in children and adolescents ages 2 to 19 yr was approximately 32% in 2006 (American Heart Association 2008f). The prevalence of overweight in children (6-11 yr) increased from 4% in 1971-1974 to 17.5% in 2001-2004. During this same time span, the prevalence of overweight in adolescents (12-19 yr) increased from 6% to 17%. Nearly 14% of preschool children (2-5 yr) are overweight (Ogden et al. 2006). In addition, studies show that another 16.5% of children and teens between the ages of 2 and 19 yr are considered at risk of being overweight (American Heart

Association 2008f). Table 1.3 summarizes factors associated with increased risk of obesity.

Excess body weight and fatness pose a threat to both the quality and quantity of one's life. Obese individuals have a shorter life expectancy and greater risks of CHD, hypercholesterolemia, hypertension, diabetes mellitus, certain cancers, and osteoarthritis (National Institutes of Health and National Heart, Lung, and Blood Institute 1998). Although obesity is strongly associated with CHD risk factors such as hypertension, glucose intolerance, and hyperlipidemia, the contribution of obesity to CHD appears to be independent of the influence of obesity on these risk factors. For a comprehensive report and roundtable discussion of the role of physical activity in the prevention and treatment of obesity and its comorbidities, see the November 1999 supplement to *Medicine & Science in Sports & Exercise*.

Obesity may be caused by genetic and environmental factors. Although studies suggest that genetic factors contribute to some of the variation in body fatness, there has been no substantial change in the genotype of the American population over the past 30 yr (Hill and Melanson 1999). Thus, the major cause of obesity in the United States may be linked to our environment. Over the past three decades, we have been exposed to an environment that strongly promotes not only the consumption of high-fat, energy-dense foods (increased energy intake) but also reliance on technology that discourages physical activity and reduces the amount of physical activity (decreased energy expenditure) needed for daily living (e.g., use of energy-saving devices and prepared foods) (Hill and Melanson 1999). As an exercise specialist, you play an impor-

tant role in combating this major health problem by encouraging a physically active lifestyle and by planning exercise programs and scientifically sound diets for your clients, in consultation with trained nutrition professionals. Restricting caloric intake and increasing caloric expenditure through physical activity and exercise are effective ways of reducing body weight and fatness while normalizing blood pressure and blood lipid profiles.

METABOLIC SYNDROME

Metabolic syndrome refers to a combination of CVD risk factors associated with hypertension, dyslipidemia, insulin resistance, and abdominal obesity. According to clinical criteria adopted by the National Cholesterol Education Program (2001), individuals with three or more CVD risk factors are classified as having metabolic syndrome (see table 1.4). Approximately 24% of adults in the United States have metabolic syndrome. Mexican American adults have a higher age-adjusted prevalence (32%) for metabolic syndrome compared to whites (24%), blacks (22%), and other ethnic groups (20%). Also, approximately 10% of adolescents (12-19 yr) in the United States have metabolic syndrome (American Heart Association 2008e). Metabolic syndrome increases the risk of developing CHD (by fourfold), CVD (by twofold), and diabetes (by five- to ninefold).

Age and BMI directly relate to metabolic syndrome (National Cholesterol Education Program 2001). The prevalence of this syndrome is higher (>40%) for older (>60 yr) adults than for younger (20-29 yr) adults (7%). Also, the prevalence of meta-

Table 1.4	Risk Factors for Metabolic Syndrome*
Risk factor	**Risk criteria**
Waist circumference	>102 cm (>40 in.) for men >88 cm (>35 in.) for women
Blood pressure (BP)	≥130 mmHg (systolic BP) or ≥85 mmHg (diastolic BP) or both
Fasting blood glucose	≥100 mg·dl^{-1} or ≥6.1 mmol·L^{-1}
Triglycerides	≥150 mg·dl^{-1} or ≥1.6 mmol·L^{-1}
High-density lipoprotein cholesterol (HDL-C)	<40 mg·dl^{-1} or <1.04 mmol·L^{-1} for men <50 mg·dl^{-1} or <1.29 mmol·L^{-1} for women

*Metabolic syndrome is defined as three or more risk factors.

National Cholesterol Education Program 2001

bolic syndrome is much higher for obese (BMI >30 kg/m²) individuals (~50%) than for normal-weight (BMI ≤25 kg/m²) individuals (6.2%). Lifestyle must be modified in order to manage metabolic syndrome. The combination of healthy nutrition and increased physical activity is an effective way to increase HDL-C and to reduce blood pressure, body weight, triglycerides, and blood glucose levels.

CANCER

Cancer is a leading cause of death worldwide, accounting for 7.9 million deaths in 2007. The main types of cancer leading to overall cancer mortality each year are lung (1.4 million/yr), stomach (866,000/yr), liver (653,000/yr), colon (677,000/yr), and breast (548,000/yr). The most frequent types of cancer worldwide among men are lung, stomach, liver, colorectal, esophagus, and prostate. For women, breast, lung, stomach, colorectal, and cervical cancer are more common. In high-income countries, tobacco use, alcohol use, and being overweight or obese are the primary causes of cancer, with tobacco use being the single most important risk factor. Other key risk factors include physical inactivity, low fruit and vegetable intake, air pollution, and sexually transmitted infections such as human immunodeficiency virus (HIV) and human papillomavirus (HPV) (World Health Organization 2008a).

Regular physical activity is associated with a 20% to 50% reduction of risk for uterine, colon, and breast cancers. There is strong evidence that physically active people have a significantly lower risk of colon cancer and breast cancer. However, moderate-intensity physical activity for 210 to 420 min/wk is needed to reduce risk of colon and breast cancer; 150 min/wk is not sufficient for providing this health benefit. The American Cancer Society (2006) recommends that adults engage in moderate-to-vigorous intensity physical activity for at least 30 min and preferably 45 to 60 min, 5 or more days per week. Children and adolescents are encouraged to engage in moderate to vigorous physical activity at least 60 min per day on at least 5 days per week. Additionally, maintaining a healthy body weight is important to reduce cancer risk (Thomson and Thompson 2008). Research also suggests that risk of endometrial cancer in women, prostate cancer in men, and lung cancer in men and women may be lower for physically active individuals compared to those who are inactive (Thune and Furberg 2001; U.S. Department of Health and Human Services 2008).

MUSCULOSKELETAL DISEASES AND DISORDERS

Diseases and disorders of the musculoskeletal system, such as osteoporosis, osteoarthritis, bone fractures, connective tissue tears, and low back syndrome, are also related to physical inactivity and a sedentary lifestyle. Osteoporosis is a disease characterized by the loss of bone mineral content and bone mineral density due to factors such as aging, amenorrhea, malnutrition, menopause, and physical inactivity (see table 1.3 for osteoporosis risk factors). Osteoporosis affects an estimated 75 million people in Europe, the United States, and Japan. Over 8 million women and 2 million men in the United States have osteoporosis (National Osteoporosis Foundation 2008). Approximately 30% of all postmenopausal women have osteoporosis in the United States and in Europe; at least 40% of these women will sustain one or more bone fractures due to this condition (International Osteoporosis Foundation 2009a).

Individuals with osteoporosis have bone mineral density values that are more than 2.5 standard deviations below the young adult mean value. Osteopenia, or low bone mineral mass, is a precursor to osteoporosis. More than one of every two adults aged 50 or older has either osteoporosis or osteopenia (National Osteoporosis Foundation 2004). Kanis and colleagues (2005) developed a free online tool, called FRAX, to identify an individual's 10 yr risk of developing osteoporosis and experiencing a hip fracture. FRAX can be accessed at www.shef.ac.uk/FRAX. To use this tool, the client answers 12 questions about age, height, weight, prior fracture history, parental history of hip fracture, smoking, long-term use of glucocorticoids, rheumatoid arthritis, and alcohol consumption. If available, the bone mineral density of the femoral neck may be included to better refine the accuracy of these estimations. This tool is becoming widely used in clinical settings around the world and has been integrated into the clinical guidelines for managing osteoporosis in the United Kingdom and the United States

(Lewiecki and Watts 2009). Versions of FRAX are also available for Austria, China, France, Germany, Italy, Japan, Spain, Sweden, Switzerland, and Turkey (International Osteoporosis Foundation 2009b).

Adequate calcium intake, vitamin D intake, and regular physical activity help counteract age-related bone loss. Epidemiological studies show that the incidence of bone fracture is lower in women with higher levels of physical activity. Although no data have demonstrated that exercise alone can prevent the loss of bone mass during and after menopause, the ACSM suggests the following exercise prescription to help counteract bone loss due to aging and to preserve bone health during adulthood (Kohrt et al. 2004).

Exercise Prescription for Bone Health (Kohrt et al. 2004)

Mode: Weight-bearing endurance activities (e.g., tennis, stair climbing, jogging, and walking with intermittent jogging), activities that involve jumping (e.g., volleyball and basketball), and resistance training

Intensity: Moderate to high in terms of bone-loading forces

Frequency: Three to five times per week for weight-bearing endurance activities; two to three times per week for resistance exercise

Duration: 30 to 60 min/day of a combination of weight-bearing endurance activities, activities that involve jumping, and resistance training that targets all major muscle groups

Peak bone mass is developed during childhood and adolescence and is a major factor associated with the risk of osteoporosis. Bone mass is higher in physically active children compared to less active children. Given that exercise-induced gains in bone mass during childhood and adolescence are maintained into adulthood, the ACSM recommends the following exercise prescription for developing peak bone mass in children and adolescents (Kohrt et al. 2004).

Low back pain afflicts millions of people each year. More than 80% of all low back problems are produced by muscular weakness or imbalance caused by a lack of physical activity (see table 1.3). If the muscles are not strong enough to support the vertebral column in proper alignment, poor posture

Exercise Prescription for Peak Bone Mass in Children and Adolescents (Kohrt et al. 2004)

Mode: Impact activities (e.g., gymnastics, plyometrics, and jumping), moderate-intensity resistance training, sports that involve running and jumping (e.g., soccer and basketball)

Intensity: High in terms of bone-loading forces; for resistance training, <60% 1-RM

Frequency: At least 3 days/wk

Duration: 10 to 20 min (twice a day may be more effective)

results and low back pain develops. Excessive weight, poor flexibility, and improper lifting habits also contribute to low back problems. While gender and age are associated with low back pain and are not modifiable risks, lifestyle behaviors such as smoking, physical inactivity, flexibility, and muscular strength and endurance are all modifiable risk factors that are related to low back pain (Albert et al. 2001).

Because the origin of low back problems is often functional rather than structural, in many cases the problem can be corrected through an exercise program designed to develop strength and flexibility in the appropriate muscle groups. Also, people who remain physically active throughout life retain more bone, ligament, and tendon strength and are therefore less prone to bone fractures and connective tissue tears (McGill 2002).

AGING

A sedentary lifestyle and lack of physical activity reduce life expectancy by predisposing the individual to aging-related diseases and by influencing the aging process itself. With aging there is a progressive loss of physiological and metabolic functions; however, biological aging may vary considerably among individuals due to variability in genetic and environmental factors that affect oxidative stress and inflammation. **Telomeres** are repeated DNA sequences that determine the structure and function of chromosomes. With aging and diseases associated with increased oxidative stress (e.g., CHD, diabetes mellitus, osteoporosis, and heart failure), telomere length decreases. A study, comparing the telomere length of normal, healthy twins, showed that the telomere length of leukocytes is positively associated with leisure-time physical activity levels. The longer telomere length observed in more physically active individuals could not be explained by age, gender, BMI, smoking, socioeconomic status, or physical activity at work (Cherkas et al. 2008).

Although long-term prospective studies are needed for a full understanding of the antiaging effects of regular exercise, this finding suggests that exercise scientists should promote the potential benefits of leisure-time physical activity in retarding the aging process and diminishing the risk of aging-related diseases.

KEY POINTS

- Less than 50% of all Americans meet the recommended amount of physical activity needed for health benefits.

- Major chronic diseases associated with a lack of physical activity are CVDs, diabetes, obesity, and musculoskeletal disorders.

- Cardiovascular diseases are responsible for 36% of all deaths in the United States and nearly 50% of all deaths in Europeans.

- The positive risk factors for CHD are age, family history, hypercholesterolemia, hypertension, cigarette smoking, glucose intolerance, obesity, and physical inactivity.

- The prevalence of obesity is on the rise, especially in developed countries; in the United States, two of every three adults and more than one of every three adolescents and children are overweight or obese.

- Metabolic syndrome is a combination of three or more CVD risk factors.

- Osteoporosis and low back syndrome are musculoskeletal disorders afflicting millions of people each year.

- FRAX is an online tool that can be used to assess your client's 10 yr risk of developing osteoporosis and of having a hip fracture.

- To benefit health and prevent disease, every adult should accumulate a minimum of 150 min/wk of moderate-intensity physical activity or 75 min/wk of vigorous-intensity physical activity. For additional health benefits, increase physical activity to 300 min/wk and 150 min/wk, respectively, for moderate- and vigorous-intensity exercise.

KEY TERMS

Learn the definition for each of the following key terms. Definitions of key terms can be found in the glossary on page 411.

angina pectoris	hypercholesterolemia	osteopenia
atherosclerosis	hyperlipidemia	osteoporosis
body mass index (BMI)	hypertension	overweight
cardiovascular disease (CVD)	LDL-cholesterol (LDL-C)	prehypertension
cholesterol	lipoprotein	telomeres
chylomicron	low back pain	total cholesterol (TC)
coronary heart disease (CHD)	low-density lipoprotein (LDL)	type 1 diabetes or insulin-dependent diabetes mellitus (IDDM)
dose–response relationship	metabolic equivalents (METs)	
dyslipidemia	metabolic syndrome	type 2 diabetes or non-insulin-dependent diabetes mellitus (NIDDM)
HDL-cholesterol (HDL-C)	myocardial infarction	
high blood pressure	myocardial ischemia	very low-density lipoprotein (VLDL)
high-density lipoprotein	obesity	

REVIEW QUESTIONS

In addition to being able to define each of the key terms just listed, test your knowledge and understanding of the material by answering the following review questions.

1. What percentage of the American population does not get the recommended amount of physical activity for health benefits?

2. What is the recommended minimum amount of daily physical activity for health?

3. Give examples of moderate physical activity.

4. What percentage of Americans have some form of CVD?

5. Name four types of CVD. Which is most prevalent?

6. Explain the etiology of CHD.

7. Identify the positive and negative risk factors for CHD.

8. Explain how regular physical activity affects each of the CHD risk factors, as well as overall CHD risk.

9. Define obesity and overweight relative to BMI.

10. What types of exercise are effective for counteracting bone loss due to aging?

11. Explain the relationship between physical inactivity and low back pain.

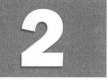
Preliminary Health Screening and Risk Classification

KEY QUESTIONS

1 ■ What are the major components of the health evaluation, and how is this information used to screen clients for exercise testing and participation?

2 ■ What factors do I need to focus on when evaluating the client's medical history and lifestyle characteristics?

3 ■ How is the client's disease risk classified?

4 ■ Do all clients need a physical examination and medical clearance from their physician before taking an exercise test?

5 ■ What are the standards for classifying blood cholesterol levels?

6 ■ How is blood pressure measured and evaluated? Are automated blood pressure devices accurate?

7 ■ How is heart rate measured? Are heart rate monitors accurate?

8 ■ What is an ECG, and does every client need to have one before taking an exercise test?

9 ■ Is it safe to give a graded exercise test to all clients? When does a physician need to be present?

10 ■ What are the major components of the lifestyle evaluation, and how can this information be used?

11 ■ What are the purposes of informed consent?

Before assessing your client's physical fitness profile, it is important to classify the person's health status and lifestyle. You will use information from the initial health and lifestyle evaluations to screen clients for physical fitness testing. You also will use this information to identify individuals with medical contraindications to exercise, with disease symptoms and risk factors, and with special needs.

This chapter discusses the components of a comprehensive health evaluation, including a coronary risk factor profile, medical history questionnaire, lifestyle evaluation, and informed consent. It also presents guidelines and standards for classifying blood cholesterol levels, blood pressures, and disease risk, along with techniques and procedures for measuring heart rate and blood pressure at rest and during exercise and for conducting a resting 12-lead electrocardiogram (ECG).

PRELIMINARY HEALTH EVALUATION

The purpose of the health evaluation is to detect the presence of disease and to assess the initial disease risk classification of your clients. The components of a comprehensive health evaluation are listed in table 2.1. To evaluate the client's health status, information from questionnaires and data from clinical tests are analyzed. Minimally, for pretest health screening of clients for exercise testing and exercise program participation, you should

- administer the Physical Activity Readiness Questionnaire (PAR-Q),
- identify signs and symptoms of diseases,
- analyze the coronary risk profile, and
- classify the disease risk of your clients.

Step-by-step procedures for conducting a comprehensive health evaluation are listed in "Procedures for Comprehensive Pretest Health Screening" on page 21.

Questionnaires and Screening Forms

Appendix A provides questionnaires and forms that may be used to obtain information for the preliminary health screening and evaluation of your clients. The client should complete the PAR-Q, medical history questionnaire, lifestyle evaluation,

and the informed consent form. You will interview your client to gather information about signs and symptoms of disease, analyze your client's coronary heart disease (CHD) risk factors, and determine your client's disease risk classification. For some clients, it may be necessary to obtain a medical clearance from their physician.

Physical Activity Readiness Questionnaire

The PAR-Q has seven questions designed to identify individuals who need medical clearance from their physicians before taking any physical fitness tests or starting an exercise program (see appendix A.1, "Physical Activity Readiness Questionnaire (PAR-Q)," p. 316). If clients answer "yes" to any of these questions, they should be referred to their physicians to obtain medical clearance before engaging in physical activity. Also, older clients and those who are not used to regular physical activity should always check with their physicians before starting an exercise program.

Table 2.1 Components of a Comprehensive Health Evaluation	
Component	**Purpose**
QUESTIONNAIRES OR SCREENING FORMS	
PAR-Q	To determine client's readiness for physical activity
Signs and symptoms of disease and medical clearance	To identify individuals in need of medical referral and to obtain evidence of physician approval for exercise testing and participation
Coronary risk factor analysis	To determine the number of coronary heart disease risk factors for client
Disease risk classification	To categorize clients as low, moderate, or high risk
Medical history	To review client's past and present personal and family health history, focusing on conditions requiring medical referral and clearance
Lifestyle evaluation	To obtain information about the client's living habits
Informed consent	To explain the purpose, risks, and benefits of physical fitness tests and to obtain client's consent for participation in these tests
CLINICAL TESTS	
Physical examination	To detect signs and symptoms of disease
Blood chemistry profile	To determine if client has normal values for selected blood values; values of blood cholesterol are used in the coronary risk factor analysis
Blood pressure assessment	To determine if client is hypertensive; these values are also used in the coronary risk factor analysis
12-lead electrocardiogram	To evaluate cardiac function and detect cardiac abnormalities that are contraindications to exercise
Graded exercise test	To assess functional aerobic capacity and to detect cardiac abnormalities due to exercise stress
Additional laboratory tests (e.g., angiograms, echocardiograms, pulmonary tests)	To provide a more in-depth assessment of clients' health status, particularly those with known disease

Procedures for Comprehensive Pretest Health Screening

Here are step-by-step procedures you should follow when conducting a comprehensive health evaluation:

- Greet the client.
- Explain the purpose of the health evaluation and lifestyle evaluation.
- Obtain the client's informed consent for health screening.
- Administer and evaluate the PAR-Q; refer client to physician if needed.
- Administer and evaluate client's medical history, focusing on signs, symptoms, and diseases; refer client to physician if needed.
- Evaluate client's lifestyle profile.
- Evaluate and classify the client's cholesterol and lipoprotein levels if test results are available.
- Measure and classify the client's resting blood pressure and heart rate.
- Assess the client's coronary risk factors.
- Classify the client's disease risk.
- Evaluate the client's blood chemistry profile if test results are available.

If so requested by the client's physician, you may do the following:

- Explain the purpose of and answer any questions about the 12-lead resting ECG and graded exercise test (GXT).
- Obtain the client's informed consent for these tests.
- Prepare the client and administer the 12-lead resting ECG.
- Have a physician interpret the results of the 12-lead resting ECG.
- Use the client's disease risk classification to determine whether a maximal or submaximal GXT should be administered and whether a physician needs to be present during this test.
- Assess the client's resting blood pressure and heart rate.
- Administer the GXT.
- Assess and classify the client's functional aerobic capacity.

Medical History Questionnaire

You should require your clients to complete a comprehensive medical history questionnaire that includes questions concerning personal and family health history (appendix A.2, "Medical History Questionnaire," p. 318). Use the questionnaire to

- examine the client's record of personal illnesses, surgeries, and hospitalizations (section A); past 3 years
- assess previous medical diagnoses and signs and symptoms of disease that have occurred within the past year or are currently present (section B); and
- analyze your client's family history of diabetes, heart disease, stroke, and hypertension (section C).

Also, when reviewing the medical history, you should carefully focus on conditions that require medical referral (see "Absolute and Relative Contraindications to Exercise Testing" [Gibbons et al. 2002] on p. 22). If any of these conditions are noted, refer your client to a physician for a physical examination and medical clearance prior to exercise testing or starting an exercise program. Some individuals have medical conditions and risk factors that outweigh the potential benefits of exercise testing. You should not administer an exercise test to individuals with absolute contraindications unless their physician orders an exercise test. Individuals with relative contraindications may be tested if the potential benefit from exercise testing outweighs the relative risk of testing. In some cases, individuals who are asymptomatic at rest can be tested using low-level endpoints. It is also important to note the types of medication being used by the client. Drugs such as digitalis, beta-blockers, bronchodilators, vasodilators, diuretics, and insulin may alter the individual's heart rate, blood pressure, ECG, and exercise capacity. If your client reports a medical condition or drug that is unfamiliar to you, be certain to consult medical references or a physician to obtain more information before conducting any exercise tests or allowing the client to participate in an exercise program.

Signs and Symptoms of Disease and Medical Clearance

As part of the pretest health screening, you should ask your clients if they have any of the conditions or symptoms listed in appendix A.3, "Checklist for Signs and Symptoms of Disease," page 320. Feel free to reproduce and use this checklist.

Clients with any of the signs or symptoms on the checklist should be referred to their physician to obtain a signed medical clearance prior to any exercise testing or participation. The Physical Activity Readiness Medical Examination (PARmed-X) was designed for this purpose. The PARmed-X is a physical activity-specific checklist (see appendix A.4, p. 322) that is used by the physician to assess and convey medical clearance for physical activity participation or to make a referral to a medically supervised exercise program for individuals who answered "yes" to one of the questions in the Physical Activity Readiness Questionnaire (PAR-Q). For definitions of specific medical terms used, refer to the glossary (p. 411).

Coronary Risk Factor Analysis

To assess your client's coronary risk profile, evaluate each item in table 2.2 carefully. Guidelines for classification of blood pressure and blood cholesterol levels in adults are presented in tables 2.3 and 2.4, respectively. If your client's high-density lipoprotein cholesterol (HDL-C) equals or exceeds 60 mg·dl^{-1},

---

Absolute and Relative Contraindications to Exercise Testing[a]

Absolute Contraindications

1. Acute myocardial infarction (within 2 days) or other acute cardiac event
2. Unstable angina
3. Uncontrolled cardiac arrhythmias causing symptoms or hemodynamic compromise
4. Uncontrolled symptomatic heart failure
5. Symptomatic severe aortic stenosis
6. Suspected or known dissecting aneurysm
7. Acute myocarditis or pericarditis
8. Acute pulmonary embolus or pulmonary infarction
9. Acute systemic infection, accompanied by fever, body aches, or swollen lymph glands

Relative Contraindications

1. Left main coronary stenosis
2. Moderate stenotic valvular heart disease
3. Known electrolyte abnormalities (hypokalemia, hypomagnesemia)
4. Severe arterial hypertension; resting diastolic blood pressure >110 mmHg or resting systolic blood pressure >200 mmHg or both
5. Tachydysrhythmias or bradydysrhythmias
6. Hypertrophic cardiomyopathy and other forms of outflow tract obstruction
7. High-degree atrioventricular block
8. Ventricular aneurysm
9. Chronic infectious disease (e.g., mononucleosis, acquired immune deficiency syndrome [AIDS], hepatitis)
10. Uncontrolled metabolic disease (e.g., diabetes, thyrotoxicosis, or myxedema)
11. Mental or physical impairment leading to inability to exercise adequately

[a]For definitions of specific medical terms, refer to the glossary on page 411.

From Gibbons, R.J. et al. 2002. ACC/AHA 2002 Guideline update for exercise testing. A report of the American College of Cardiology/American Heart Association Task Force on Practice Guidelines (Committee on Exercise Testing). American College of Cardiology Web site. www.acc.org/qualityandscience/clinical/guidelines/exercise/exercise_clean.pdf.

Table 2.2 Coronary Heart Disease Risk Factors

Positive risk factors	Criteria
1. Family history	Myocardial infarction, coronary revascularization, or sudden death before 55 yr of age in father or other first-degree male relative (brother or son) or before 65 yr of age in mother or other first-degree female relative (sister or daughter)
2. Cigarette smoking	Current cigarette smoking, or smoking cessation within previous 6 mo
3. Hypertension	Systolic BP ≥140 mmHg or diastolic BP ≥90 mmHg measured on two separate occasions, or individual taking antihypertensive medication
4. Dyslipidemia	TC ≥200 mg·dl⁻¹, or HDL-C <40 mg·dl⁻¹, or LDL-C ≥130 mg·dl⁻¹, or on lipid-lowering medication
5. Impaired fasting glucose	Fasting blood glucose ≥110 mg·dl⁻¹, measured on two separate occasions
6. Obesity	Body mass index ≥30 kg/m² or waist circumference >102 cm (40 in.) for men and >88 cm (35 in.) for women
7. Physical inactivity	Not participating in regular exercise program or not meeting the minimum physical activity recommendations from the ACSM and AHA (accumulating 150 min/wk or more of moderate-intensity aerobic exercise)

Negative risk factor[a]	
High HDL-C	Serum HDL-C ≥60 mg·dl⁻¹

[a]If HDL-C is high, subtract one risk factor from the sum of the positive risk factors.

Data from National Cholesterol Education Program Committee, 2001, "Executive Summary of the Third Report of the National Cholesterol Education Program (NCEP) Expert Panel on Detection, Evaluation, and Treatment of High Blood Cholesterol in Adults (Adult Treatment Panel III)," *Journal of the American Medical Association* 285(19): 2486–2497.

Table 2.3 Classification of Blood Pressure for Adults 18 yr or Older[a]

Systolic BP (mmHg)[b]	Category	Diastolic BP (mmHg)
<120	Normal	<80
120-139	Prehypertension	80-89
140-159	Stage 1 hypertension	90-99
≥160	Stage 2 hypertension	≥100

[a]For individuals not taking antihypertensive medication and not acutely ill. Based on average of two or more readings on two or more occasions.

[b]When systolic and diastolic pressures fall into different categories, use the higher category for classification.

Data from The Seventh Report of the Joint National Committee on Detection, Evaluation, and Treatment of High Blood Pressure, 2003, *Hypertension* 42: 1206-1252.

Table 2.4 Classification of TC, LDL-C, Triglycerides, and HDL-C (mg·dl⁻¹)

TOTAL CHOLESTEROL, LOW-DENSITY LIPOPROTEIN CHOLESTEROL, AND TRIGLYCERIDES

Classification	TC	LDL-C	Triglycerides
Optimal or desirable	<200	<100	<150
Near or above optimal	–	100-129	–
Borderline high	200-239	130-159	150-199
High	≥240	160-189	200-499
Very high	–	≥190	≥500

HIGH-DENSITY LIPOPROTEIN CHOLESTEROL

Classification	HDL-C
Low	<40
Normal	40-59
High	≥60

Data from National Cholesterol Education Program Committee, 2001, "Executive Summary of the Third Report of the National Cholesterol Education Program (NCEP) Expert Panel on Detection, Evaluation, and Treatment of High Blood Cholesterol in Adults (Adult Treatment Panel III)," *Journal of the American Medical Association* 285(19): 2487.

subtract 1 from the total number of positive risk factors. This information is especially helpful in classifying the individual for exercise testing and in designing safe exercise programs.

Disease Risk Classification

On the basis of the results from the coronary risk factor analysis, you should classify individuals as low, moderate, or high risk. According to the American College of Sports Medicine (ACSM 2010), the low CHD risk category comprises individuals who are asymptomatic with no more than one major risk factor (see table 2.2). Individuals having two or more risk factors are classified as moderate CHD risk. The high CHD risk category includes individuals who have one or more signs or symptoms of cardiovascular, pulmonary, or metabolic disease or individuals with known cardiovascular, pulmonary, or metabolic disease (see p. 320).

Lifestyle Evaluation

Planning a well-rounded physical fitness program for an individual requires that you obtain information concerning the client's living habits. The lifestyle assessment provides useful information regarding the individual's risk factor profile. Factors such as smoking, lack of physical activity, and diets high in saturated fats or cholesterol increase the risk of CHD, atherosclerosis, and hypertension. These factors can be used to pinpoint patterns and habits that need modification and to assess the likelihood of the client's adherence to the exercise program. You can obtain a lifestyle profile for your clients by using either the Lifestyle Evaluation form or the Fantastic Lifestyle Checklist provided in appendix A.5, page 326. The Fantastic Lifestyle Checklist is a self-administered tool designed to assess a client's present health-related behaviors.

Informed Consent

Before conducting any physical fitness tests or exercise programs, you should see that each participant signs the informed consent (see appendix A.6, "Informed Consent," p. 330). This form explains the purpose and nature of each physical fitness test, any inherent risks in the testing, and the expected benefits of these tests. The informed consent also assures your clients that test results will remain confidential and that their participation is strictly voluntary. If your client is underage (<18 yr), a parent or guardian must also sign the informed consent. All consent forms should be approved by your institutional review board or legal counsel.

Clinical Tests

For a comprehensive health screening, you will need to evaluate information and data obtained from the physician's medical examination and clinical tests. Clinical tests provide data about your client's blood chemistry, blood pressure, cardiopulmonary function, and aerobic capacity.

Physical Examination

Your prospective exercise program participants should obtain a physical examination and a signed medical clearance from a physician (appendix A.4, "PARmed-X," p. 322), especially if they are

- men ≥45 yr of age or women ≥55 yr of age;
- individuals of any age with two or more major risk factors;
- individuals of any age with one or more signs or symptoms of cardiovascular or pulmonary disease; or
- individuals of any age with known cardiovascular, pulmonary, or metabolic disease.

The physical examination should focus on signs and symptoms of CHD and should include an evaluation of body weight; orthopedic problems; edema; acute illness; pulse rate; cardiac regularity; blood pressure (supine, sitting, and standing); and auscultation of the heart, lungs, and major arteries. The physical examination and medical history may reveal signs or symptoms of CHD particularly if accompanied by shortness of breath, chest pains, leg cramps, or high blood pressure. Clients with these symptoms must obtain a signed medical clearance (p. 322) from their physician prior to exercise testing or exercise participation.

Blood Chemistry Profile

Information obtained from a complete blood analysis is used to assess your client's overall health status and readiness for exercise. Table 2.5 provides normal values for selected blood variables. If any of these values fall outside of the normal range, refer your clients to their physician. Pay special attention to your client's fasting blood glucose and blood lipid values.

Table 2.5 Normal Values for Selected Blood Variables

Variable	Ideal or typical values
Triglycerides	<150 mg·dl⁻¹
Total cholesterol	<200 mg·dl⁻¹
LDL-cholesterol	<100 mg·dl⁻¹
HDL-cholesterol	≥40 mg·dl⁻¹
TC/HDL-cholesterol	<3.5
Blood glucose	60-109 mg·dl⁻¹
Hemoglobin	13.5-17.5 g·dl⁻¹ (men)
	11.5-15.5 g·dl⁻¹ (women)
Hematocrit	40-52% (men)
	36-48% (women)
Potassium	3.5-5.5 meq·dl⁻¹
Blood urea nitrogen	4-24 mg·dl⁻¹
Creatinine	0.3-1.4 mg·dl⁻¹
Iron	40-190 μg·dl⁻¹ (men)
	35-180 μg·dl⁻¹ (women)
Calcium	8.5-10.5 mg·dl⁻¹

The National Cholesterol Education Program (NCEP) (2001) established guidelines for classifying lipoprotein levels and major risk factors that modify low-density lipoprotein cholesterol (LDL-C) treatment goals. For adults aged 20 yr or older, NCEP (2001) recommends that a fasting lipoprotein profile (i.e., total cholesterol, LDL-C, HDL-C, and triglycerides) be obtained every 5 yr. To classify your client's lipoprotein values, use the NCEP (2001) guidelines (see table 2.4). For nonfasting lipoprotein tests, only the total cholesterol (TC) and HDL-C values can be evaluated. If your client's TC is borderline high (200 to 239 mg·dl⁻¹) or high (≥240 mg·dl⁻¹), and the HDL-C level is less than 40 mg·dl⁻¹, a follow-up fasting lipoprotein test will be needed to assess LDL-C. Refer clients to their physicians for an extensive clinical evaluation and dietary therapy if they have high (160 to 189 mg·dl⁻¹) or very high (>190 mg·dl⁻¹) LDL-C values. Treatment goals for lowering LDL-C depend on the number of major risk factors (exclusive of LDL-C) that the client has. To determine your client's risk category, focus on the following risk factors in table 2.2: cigarette smoking, hypertension, low HDL-C, family history of premature CHD, and age (men ≥45 yr; women ≥55 yr). Table 2.6 is NCEP's listing of three risk categories that modify LDL-C treatment goals. The NCEP (2001) dietary therapy guidelines for individuals with high LDL-C are included in table 9.4, page 241.

In addition to TC and lipoproteins, you can evaluate your client's triglyceride value and the ratio of TC to HDL-C. Clients with triglyceride levels of ≥150 mg·dl⁻¹ or TC/HDL-C ratios >5.0 are at higher risk for CHD.

Table 2.6 Three Risk Categories That Modify LDL-C Goals (NCEP 2001)

Risk category	LDL-C goal (mg·dl⁻¹)
CHD and CHD risk equivalents[a]	<100
Multiple (2+) risk factors[b]	<130
0-1 risk factor	<160

[a]CHD risk equivalents include diabetes and atherosclerotic disease (i.e., peripheral arterial disease, abdominal aortic aneurysm, and symptomatic carotid artery disease).

[b]Risk factors include cigarette smoking, hypertension, low high-density lipoprotein cholesterol, family history of premature CHD, and age.

Resting Blood Pressure

Blood pressure (BP) is a measure of the force or pressure exerted by the blood on the arteries. The highest pressure (**systolic blood pressure, SBP**) reflects the pressure in the arteries during systole of the heart when myocardial contraction forces a large volume of blood into the arteries. Following systole, the arteries recoil and the pressure drops during diastole, or the filling phase of the heart. **Diastolic blood pressure (DBP)** is the lowest pressure in the artery during the cardiac cycle. The difference between the systolic and diastolic BPs is known as the **pulse pressure.** The pulse pressure creates a pulse wave that can be palpated at various sites in the body to determine pulse rate and to estimate BP.

Values used for classification of resting BP are presented in table 2.3 (Chobanian et al. 2003). Normal BP (**normotensive**) is defined as values less than 120/80 mmHg. The prehypertension category (systolic BP = 120-139 mmHg; diastolic BP = 80-89 mmHg) is added to identify individuals at high risk of developing hypertension. Hypertension is defined as a resting BP equaling or exceeding 140/90 mmHg on two or more occasions.

Although prehypertension is not considered a disease, prehypertensive individuals are encouraged to modify their lifestyle in order to reduce their risk of developing hypertension by

- losing body weight if overweight;
- adopting a healthy eating plan that includes a diet rich in fruits, vegetables, and low-fat dairy products but reduced in cholesterol, saturated fat, and total fat;
- restricting dietary sodium intake to no more than 2.4 g (100 mmol) per day;
- engaging in aerobic physical activities at least 150 min/wk; and
- limiting alcohol consumption to no more than 1 oz (29.6 ml) per day for men and 0.5 oz (14.8 ml) per day for women.

When lifestyle modifications are ineffective, pharmacological therapy may be required to lower BP. There are numerous drugs available to treat hypertension (see Chobanian et al. 2003), including

- diuretics to rid the body of excess salt and fluids;
- beta-blockers to reduce heart rate and cardiac output;
- sympathetic nerve inhibitors to prevent constriction of arterioles;
- vasodilators to induce relaxation in smooth muscles of arterial walls; and
- angiotensin-converting enzyme inhibitors to disrupt the body's production of angiotensin, which constricts arterioles.

Additional Clinical Tests

For individuals with known or suspected CHD, additional tests may be indicated. These may include a resting 12-lead ECG, angiogram, echocardiogram, and a physician-monitored graded exercise test. A chest X-ray, comprehensive blood chemistry, and complete blood count should also be obtained (ACSM 2010). For clients with known pulmonary disease, ACSM (2010) recommends a chest X-ray, pulmonary function tests, and specialized pulmonary tests (e.g., blood gas analysis).

Graded Exercise Test

Coronary heart disease often is not detectable from the resting ECG, and abnormalities may not appear until the individual engages in relatively strenuous exercise. The client's physician may recommend administration of a graded exercise test as part of the health evaluation to assess functional aerobic capacity of some individuals. Graded exercise tests should be administered only by trained, professionally certified personnel such as exercise scientists, physicians, and nurses.

Use the client's risk classification to determine whether the test should be a maximal or a submaximal exercise test and whether a physician needs to be present during the exercise testing (table 2.7). Also, you need to be familiar with medical conditions that are absolute and relative contraindications to exercise testing in an out-of-hospital setting (see "Absolute and Relative Contraindications to Exercise Testing" on p. 22). Individuals with absolute contraindications should not be given a graded exercise test unless their condition has been sta-

---

Table 2.7   ACSM Guidelines for Medical Examination and Exercise Testing Prior to Participation Based on Risk Classification (ACSM 2010)[a]

	Low risk	Moderate risk	High risk
MEDICAL EXAM AND EXERCISE TEST RECOMMENDED PRIOR TO PARTICIPATION IN:			
Moderate exercise (3-6 METs or 40-60% $\dot{V}O_2$max)	0[b]	0	+[c]
Vigorous exercise (>6 METs or >60% $\dot{V}O_2$max)	0	+	+
PHYSICIAN SUPERVISION RECOMMENDED DURING EXERCISE TEST[d]			
Submaximal test	0	0	+
Maximal test	0	+	+

[a]For definitions of low, moderate, or high risk, see page 24, "Disease Risk Classification."

[b]0 indicates that item is not necessary; however, it should not be viewed as inappropriate.

[c]+ indicates that item is recommended.

[d]For physician supervision—this suggests that a physician be in close proximity and readily available should there be an emergent need.

bilized or medically treated. In cases in which the benefits outweigh the risks, individuals with relative contraindications may perform exercise tests. These tests, however, should use low-level endpoints and be administered with caution (ACSM 2010).

The ACSM (2010) recommends a maximal exercise test for older men (≥45 yr) and women (≥55 yr) before they begin a vigorous (>6 METs [metabolic equivalents] or >60% of functional aerobic capacity) exercise program (see table 2.7). These maximal exercise tests should be administered with physician supervision. For low-risk individuals of any age, submaximal exercise testing can be done without physician supervision. However, the exercise tests should be conducted by exercise specialists, who are preferably ACSM certified and who are well trained and experienced in monitoring exercise tests and handling emergencies (ACSM 2010). The results from these tests provide a basis for prescription of exercise for healthy and coronary-prone individuals, as well as for cardiopulmonary patients.

TESTING PROCEDURES FOR BLOOD PRESSURE, HEART RATE, AND ELECTROCARDIOGRAM

One of your major responsibilities as an exercise scientist is to become proficient at measuring BP, heart rate, and ECGs during rest and exercise. During a graded exercise test, you will be expected to be able to obtain accurate and precise measurements of BP and heart rate while the client is exercising. Because of their importance and complexity, this section is devoted to a thorough discussion of these procedures.

Measuring Blood Pressure

Blood pressure can be measured directly or indirectly. The "gold standard" for assessing BPs is the direct measurement of intra-arterial BP. This method is invasive and requires catheterization. Therefore, in clinical or field settings, BP is typically measured indirectly by auscultation or oscillometry.

For **auscultation**, a stethoscope and a **sphygmomanometer** consisting of a BP cuff (cloth cover and bladder) and either a mercury column or an aneroid manometer are used. Step-by-step instructions for the auscultatory method are presented in "Resting Blood Pressure Measurement" on page 28. **Oscillometry** uses an automated electronic manometer to measure oscillations in pressure (i.e., waveforms) when the cuff is deflated. Systolic and diastolic BPs are calculated with the use of proprietary algorithms provided by each manufacturer.

Blood Pressure Measurement Techniques

Measure resting BP in the supine and exercise (sitting or standing) positions prior to testing. The client should be wearing a short-sleeved or sleeveless garment and should be seated in a quiet room. Take BP measurements rapidly, and completely deflate the cuff for at least 30 sec between consecutive readings. For more accurate results, obtain two or three determinations of pressure from each arm.

It takes a great deal of practice to become proficient at measuring BPs. When you are first learning this method, it is highly recommended that you practice with a trained BP technician, using a dual- or multiple-head stethoscope so that you can listen simultaneously and compare BP readings for the same trial.

Sources of Measurement Error

Sources of error in measuring BP are numerous (Reeves 1995). You need to be aware of the following sources of error and do as much as possible to control them:

- Inaccurate sphygmomanometer
- Improper cuff width or length
- Cuff not centered, too loose, or over clothing
- Arm unsupported or elbow lower than heart level
- Poor auditory acuity of technician
- Improper rate of inflation or deflation of the cuff pressure
- Improper stethoscope placement or pressure
- Expectation bias and inexperience of the technician
- Slow reaction time of the technician
- Parallax error in reading the manometer
- Background noise
- Client holding treadmill handrails or cycle ergometer handlebars

To measure resting BP (seated position), use the following recommended procedures (Reeves 1995):

1. Seat the client in a quiet room for at least 5 min. The client's bare arm should be resting on a table so that the middle of the arm is at the level of the heart.

2. Estimate the client's arm circumference or measure it at the midpoint between the acromion process of the shoulder and the olecranon process of the elbow (see appendix D.4, "Standardized Sites for Circumference Measurements," p. 369, for description of measuring arm circumference) using an anthropometric tape measure. The bladder of the cuff should encircle 80% of an adult's arm and 100% of a child's arm.

3. Palpate the brachial artery pulse on the anteromedial aspect of the arm below the belly of the biceps brachii and 2 to 3 cm (1 in.) above the antecubital fossa. Wrap the deflated cuff firmly around the upper arm so that the midline of the cuff is over the brachial artery pulse. The lower edge of the cuff should be approximately 2.5 cm (1 in.) above the antecubital fossa. If the cuff is too loose, BP will be overestimated. Avoid placing the cuff over clothing; and if the shirtsleeve is rolled up, make certain that it is not occluding the circulation.

4. Position the manometer so that the center of the mercury column or dial is at eye level and the cuff's tubing is not overlapping or obstructed.

5. Locate and palpate the radial pulse (see p. 33 for anatomical description of this site), close the valve of the BP unit completely by screwing it away from you, and rapidly inflate the cuff to 70 mmHg. Then slowly increase the pressure in 10 mmHg increments while palpating the radial pulse, and note when the pulse disappears (estimate of systolic BP). Partially open the valve by unscrewing it toward you to slowly release the pressure at a rate of 2 to 3 mmHg/sec, and note when the pulse reappears (estimate of diastolic BP). Fully open the valve to completely release the pressure in the cuff. The estimate of systolic BP from the palpatory method is then used to determine how much the cuff needs to be inflated for measuring BP by means of the auscultatory technique. In this way, you can avoid over- or underinflating the cuff for clients with low or high BPs, respectively.

6. Position the earpieces of the stethoscope so that they are aligned with the auditory canals (i.e., angled anteriorly).

7. Place the head (bell) of the stethoscope over the brachial pulse (about 1 cm superior and medial to the antecubital fossa). Make certain that the entire head of the stethoscope is contacting the skin. To avoid extraneous noise, do not place any part of the head of the stethoscope underneath the cuff.

8. Close the valve, and quickly and steadily inflate the cuff pressure to about 20 to 30 mmHg above the estimated systolic pressure previously determined by palpation.

9. Partially open the valve to slowly release the pressure at a rate of 2 to 3 mmHg/sec. Note when you hear the first sharp thud caused by the sudden rush of blood as the artery opens. This is known as the first Korotkoff sound and corresponds to the systolic pressure (Phase I).

10. Continue reducing the pressure slowly (no more than 2 mmHg/sec), noting when the metallic tapping sound becomes muffled (Phase IV diastolic pressure) and when the sound disappears (Phase V diastolic pressure). Typically, the Phase V value is used as the index of diastolic pressure. However, both Phase IV and V diastolic pressures should be noted. During rhythmic exercise, the Phase V pressure tends to decrease because of reduction in peripheral resistance. In some cases, it may even drop to zero.

11. After noting the Phase V pressure, continue deflating the cuff for at least 10 mmHg, making certain that no additional sounds are heard. Then rapidly and completely deflate the cuff.

12. Record all three BP values (Phase I, IV, and V) to the nearest 2 mmHg. Wait at least 30 sec and repeat the measurement. Use the average of the two measurements for each of the three values.

The following section addresses questions about measuring BP and provides tips for taking more accurate BP measurements during rest or exercise.

■ *Which type of sphygmomanometer—mercury column or aneroid—provides more valid and reliable measures of resting blood pressure?*

For over a century, the mercury column manometer has been considered the gold standard for indirect measurement of BP. Calibrated, aneroid manometers may yield values similar to those of mercury column manometers (Dorigatti et al. 2007); however, the latter are preferred for a number of reasons. Mercury column manometers are based on gravity, leaving little room for mechanical errors. In contrast, the aneroid manometer is a spring-based device that can fatigue with use and thereby lose its calibration more easily. It can become inaccurate without the technician's awareness. Therefore, aneroid manometers must be calibrated frequently (at least every 6 mo). Often when the aneroid manometer fails the calibration test, it must be returned to the manufacturer for repair. For a complete list of recommended aneroid sphygmomanometers, see www.dableducational.org.

■ *How can I check the accuracy of an aneroid manometer?*

To check the accuracy of an aneroid manometer against a mercury unit, follow the procedure suggested by Reeves (1995):

■ Disconnect the bulbs of both cuffs and reconnect the bulb and dial of the aneroid unit to the cuff of the mercury unit.

■ Loosely roll up the cuff, secure the Velcro strips, and hold the cuff steady while gradually inflating it.

■ Hold the dial of the aneroid manometer close to the mercury column and compare the two readings at several pressures throughout the measurement scale (e.g., throughout 40-220 mmHg). If the aneroid and mercury manometer pressures differ by more than 2 to 3 mmHg, send the aneroid manometer to the manufacturer for adjustment.

■ *What criteria are used to judge the accuracy of devices that measure blood pressure?*

The Association for the Advancement of Medical Instrumentation (AAMI) and the British Hypertension Society (BHS) established separate criteria for judging the accuracy of BP devices. Most validation studies use one or both of these sets of criteria. For either set, measured values from the device are compared to those obtained from a mercury sphygmomanometer. To meet AAMI criteria, the measured average BP (systolic and diastolic) should not differ from the mercury standard by more than 5 mmHg, and the standard deviation should not exceed 8 mmHg. For the BHS criteria (O'Brien et al. 2001), differences in both systolic and diastolic BPs are graded as A, B, C, or D depending on the cumulative percentage of absolute individual difference scores falling within three categories: 5, 10, and 15 mmHg (see table 2.8). To be recommended, a device must achieve at least a B; A and D denote the greatest and least degree of agreement with the mercury standard.

Table 2.8   British Hypertension Society Validation Criteria for Blood Pressure Measuring Devices[a]

	CATEGORY		
Grade[b]	≤5 mmHg	≤10 mmHg	≤15 mmHg
A	60%	85%	95%
B	50%	75%	90%
C	40%	65%	85%
D	Worse than C		

[a]Values are the cumulative percentage of absolute difference scores between the mercury standard and the test device.

[b]All three percentages must be greater than or equal to the values shown for a specific grade to be awarded.

The European Society of Hypertension (ESH) updated the BHS validation criteria (O'Brien et al. 2002). The ESH protocol, also known as the International Protocol, is more complex. Basically, it categorizes mean differences in BP as follows: 0 to 5 mmHg = very accurate, 6 to 10 mmHg = slightly inaccurate, 11 to 15 mmHg = moderately inaccurate, and >15 mmHg = very inaccurate. The number of comparisons cumulatively falling within 5, 10, and 15 mmHg is counted (i.e., the 5 mmHg zone represents all values falling within 0-5 mmHg; the 10 mmHg zone represents all values falling within 0-5 mmHg and 6-10 mmHg; the 15 mmHg zone represents all values falling within 0-5 mmHg, 6-10 mmHg, and 10-15 mmHg). These values are then compared to standards set for each of two phases of the validation process. Devices recommended for clinical use must pass both phases of the validation process. For a detailed description of the International Protocol, see the work of O'Brien and colleagues (2002).

The Dabl Educational Trust has a Web site that provides up-to-date, evidence-based information about BP measurement techniques and devices (www.dableducational.org). Here you will find tables evaluating the validity of various types of BP devices according to AAMI, BHS, and International Protocol criteria.

■ *In the future, will the mercury column manometer be banned? If so, what types of devices will replace it?*

Because of the toxic effects of mercury on the environment, future use of mercury manometers and thermometers in the United States and European countries may be restricted or even banned. Many hospitals and health care facilities in Europe are voluntarily removing mercury manometers and replacing them with aneroid or automated measuring devices. In Sweden and the Netherlands, the use of mercury in hospital settings is already banned (Beevers, Lip, and O'Brien 2001b). Although no health care agencies in the United States presently forbid mercury manometers, some experts predict that the manometers are destined for the museum shelves (Markandu 2000; O'Brien 2003). The American Heart Association (AHA) encourages the continued use of mercury manometers until other devices are better validated (Jones et al. 2001).

In countries banning use of mercury manometers, aneroid and oscillometric devices are being used even though they have not been accepted as being as accurate as mercury (Pickering et al. 2005). The AHA also made the following recommendations for health care and fitness settings that exclusively use aneroid or automated devices (Jones et al. 2001):

- Select only devices that satisfy the validation criteria of the AAMI or similar organizations.
- Schedule regular maintenance and calibration.
- Insist on the use of mercury manometers for calibration.
- Ensure regular training of personnel who measure BP.

Hybrid sphygmomanometers, which combine features of both electronic and auscultatory devices, are now being developed. With the hybrid sphygmomanometer, the mercury column is replaced with an electronic pressure gauge. The technician uses a stethoscope to listen for the Korotkoff sounds. When systolic and diastolic pressures are heard, the technician presses a button next to the deflation knob to freeze the display showing the systolic and diastolic pressures. The pressure is displayed digitally or as a simulated mercury column or aneroid display. The hybrid sphygmomanometer combines some of the best features of mercury and electronic devices and may be a good candidate to replace the mercury sphygmomanometer as the gold standard in clinical settings (Pickering et al. 2005).

■ *How accurate are automated blood pressure devices?*

There are many automated devices available for clinical and home use. These automated devices inflate and deflate a cuff that is placed over the brachial artery (upper arm device), radial artery (wrist device), or digital artery (finger device). The automated electronic manometer assesses oscillations in pressure while the cuff is gradually deflated. The maximum oscillation corresponds to mean arterial pressure; and algorithms, which vary among manufacturers, are used to calculate systolic and diastolic pressures. Unfortunately, most of these devices have not been independently evaluated for accuracy.

In a review of various types of BP devices, only 5 of 23 upper arm models of automated devices for self-measurement of BP passed both the AAMI and BHS validation criteria and received the recommendation of the ESH (O'Brien et al. 2001). The recommended models, all manufactured by Omron Healthcare, Inc., included the HEM-705CP, HEM-713C, HEM-722C, HEM-735C, and HEM-737 Intellisense. Studies indicated that the Omron HEM-907, an automated, oscillometric device, met the AAMI validation criteria (Elliott et al. 2007); also the Omron M7 (model HEM-780-E) and the Omron M6 (model HEM-7001-E), which measure BP at the upper arm, fulfilled the validation criteria of the International Protocol in a population of normal-weight and obese adults with arm circumferences ranging from 32 to 42 cm (Altunkan et al. 2007; El Feghali et al. 2007). For a complete list of recommended, not recommended, and questionable automated upper arm sphygmomanometers, see www.dableducational.org.

Generally, automated upper arm devices are more accurate than automated wrist devices for measuring resting BP. Wrist devices become inaccurate if the arm is not kept at heart level during measurement, and the position of the wrist during measurement may also influence the accuracy of the measurement. O'Brien (2001) reported that none of the four automated wrist models tested in his study passed the EHS validation criteria. However, a number of different wrist devices have recently met International Protocol criteria and are recommended for self-measurement of BP: Citizen CH-656C, Microlife BP W200-1, Omron 637IT, Omron R5-I, and Omron R7 (Altunkan and Altunkan 2006; Altunkan, Oztas, and Altunkan 2006; Cotte et al. 2008; Omboni et al. 2007; Palatini et al. 2008; Topouchian et al. 2006). For a complete list of recommended, questionable, and not recommended automated wrist sphygmomanometers, see www.dableducational.org.

Finger devices generally are not recommended for measuring BP. Although Schutte and colleagues (2004) reported that the Finometer satisfied the criteria of the AAMI and BHS for measuring the resting BP of black women, other studies indicated that this device does not meet the AAMI or BHS validation criteria (see www.dableducational.org). Therefore, finger devices should not be used for clinical measurement of BP.

■ Can automated devices be used to measure blood pressure during exercise?

The validity and accuracy of automated devices for measuring exercise BP have not yet been firmly established (Griffin, Roberts, and Heyward 1997). To date, no criteria have been established to evaluate the accuracy of devices for measuring BP under stress (e.g., exercise). The accuracy of some finger devices (i.e., Finapres and Portapres Model 2) designed for continuous, noninvasive, ambulatory BP monitoring has been assessed during incremental cycle ergometer exercise (Blum et al. 1997; Eckert and Horstkotte 2002; Idema, van den Meiracker, and Imholz 1989). In these studies, the mean differences between the automated (Finapres and Portapres Model 2) and the intra-arterial measures of BP during low-intensity (~100 W) exercise

ranged from 12 to 22 mmHg for systolic pressure and from –5 to –9.8 mmHg for diastolic pressure. During exercise, these automated finger devices systematically underestimated and overestimated systolic and diastolic BPs, respectively, and average differences increased as exercise intensity increased. Therefore, these devices should not be used to measure BP during exercise.

■ How do body position and arm position affect blood pressure measurements?

Posture affects BP; generally, BP increases from lying (supine) to sitting to standing. Usually, resting BP is measured in the sitting position. Regardless of body position, the upper arm must be held or supported horizontally at the level of the heart (right atrium); the midsternal level most closely approximates the level of the right atrium. Raising the arm above heart level underestimates BP, and positioning the arm below heart level tends to overestimate BP. Also, the accuracy of automated wrist devices is greatly affected if the wrist is not held at heart level (Beevers, Lip, and O'Brien 2001a). Generally, the arm should be supported at heart level during the measurement of sitting and standing BP; diastolic BP may increase as much as 10% when the arm is extended and unsupported (Beevers et al. 2001a). Typically, the arm is supported by resting it on a table or by having the technician hold it at the elbow. Even when supine BP is measured, a pillow should be placed under the upper arm to support it at heart level.

■ What is white coat hypertension?

In the condition known as white coat hypertension, individuals who have normal BP outside of the clinical environment become hypertensive when their BP is measured by a health professional. White coat hypertension appears to be more common in women and in the elderly (Chung and Lip 2003). To confirm this condition, BP should be measured outside of the clinical environment via self-measurement at home or via 24 hr ambulatory BP monitoring. Recent studies suggest that white coat hypertension is not benign (Chung and Lip 2003; Gustavsen et al. 2003). A 10 yr follow-up study of 420 patients with stage 1 or 2 hypertension (of whom 18% had white coat hypertension) showed that individuals with white coat hypertension have an increased risk of CVD compared to normotensive individuals (Gustavsen et al. 2003). This finding suggests that one should consider white coat hypertension when evaluating cardiovascular risk factors.

■ *What are miscuffing and cuff hypertension?*

Miscuffing (i.e., undercuffing or overcuffing) is a serious source of measurement error caused by using a BP cuff with a bladder that is not appropriately scaled for the client's arm circumference. Experts recommend using a cuff with a bladder width that is 40% of the measured upper arm circumference and a length that encircles at least 80% of the arm circumference. Undercuffing occurs when the bladder is too small for the arm circumference, leading to the overestimation of BP, known as cuff hypertension. Conversely, overcuffing underestimates BP because the bladder is too large for the arm circumference (Beevers et al. 2001a). To avoid these problems, the correct cuff and bladder size must be selected for each client.

■ *How can I determine the appropriate cuff size for my client?*

To ensure accurate BP readings, you need to select a cuff size appropriate for your client's arm circumference. Generally, four cuff sizes are commercially available: children, standard adult, large adult, and obese (i.e., thigh). To select the proper cuff size, measure your client's arm circumference (see appendix D.4, "Standardized Sites for Circumference Measurements," p. 369, for a description of measuring arm circumference). You should not assume that a child's cuff is appropriate for all children. Comparing National Health and Nutrition Examination (NHANES) data from 1999 through 2004, Prineas and colleagues (2007) reported that average midarm circumference for children and adolescents increased during this time. Approximately 52% of boys and 42% of girls aged 13-17 yr required a standard adult cuff fit. If arm circumference cannot be measured directly, you can estimate it using gender-specific prediction equations (see Ostchega et al. 2004). Table 2.9 presents recommended cuff and bladder sizes for measured or estimated arm circumferences.

■ *How can I measure exercise blood pressure more accurately?*

Measuring BP during exercise is much more difficult than doing so during rest. You should not attempt to measure exercise BP until you have demonstrated competency and have confidence in your ability to measure resting BP. It is particularly difficult to accurately measure BP when the client is running on the treadmill because of extraneous noise and arm movement during running. Sometimes you will not be able to determine diastolic BP during exercise because of the noise and vibration. Novice technicians should first practice taking BPs during cycle ergometer exercise and then try measuring BP during treadmill exercise. See "Tips for Measuring Exercise Blood Pressure" for pointers on improving your BP measurements during exercise.

Measuring Heart Rate

The average resting heart rate for adults is 60 to 80 beats per minute (bpm), with the average resting heart rate of women typically 7 to 10 bpm higher than that of men. Heart rates as low as 28 to 40 bpm have been reported for highly conditioned endurance athletes, whereas poorly trained, sedentary individuals may have heart rates that exceed 100 bpm.

Do not use resting heart rate as a measure of cardiorespiratory fitness. There is wide variability

Table 2.9 Recommended Cuff and Bladder Sizes for Arm Circumferences		
Cuff type	**Arm circumference (cm)**	**Bladder width × length (cm)**
Smaller child	≤17	4 × 13
Larger child	18-25	10 × 18
Standard adult	26-33	12 × 26
Larger adult	34-42	16 × 33
Obese adult (thigh cuff)	43-50	20 × 42

Data compiled from Beevers et al. 2001a and Ostchega et al. 2004.

Tips for Measuring Exercise Blood Pressure

When measuring exercise BP, take extra precautions to ensure accurate readings:

- Instruct the client to refrain from grasping the handlebars or handrails of the exercise apparatus during the BP measurement.
- Position the cuff on the arm so that the tubing protruding from its bladder is superior instead of inferior. This position lessens extraneous noise caused by the tubing contacting the stethoscope during exercise.
- Limit arm movement during the BP measurement; stabilize the client's arm at heart level by placing and holding it firmly between your arm and trunk.
- Inflate the cuff well above the anticipated value or reading obtained during the previous stage of the graded exercise test, keeping in mind that systolic BP increases with exercise intensity.
- Position the manometer so that it is no more than 3 ft (92 cm) away and is at eye level so that you can read the scale easily. Errors will occur if you do not keep your eyes close to the level of the meniscus of the mercury column or perpendicular to the aneroid scale. For mercury column sphygmomanometry, use a model that is mounted on a stand with wheels so that the manometer can be properly positioned during incremental stages of the exercise test. Positioning is particularly important when the client is performing graded treadmill tests that progressively increase the incline of the treadmill.

---

in resting heart rate within the population, and a low resting heart rate is not always indicative of cardiorespiratory fitness level. In some cases, a low resting heart rate indicates a diseased heart. The following general guidelines may be used to classify resting heart rate:

1. <60 bpm = **bradycardia** (slow rate)
2. 60 to 100 bpm = normal rate
3. >100 bpm = **tachycardia** (fast rate)

Before you measure resting heart rate, your client should rest for 5 to 10 min in either a supine or a seated position. It is important that you measure resting heart rate carefully because this value is sometimes used in the calculation of target exercise heart rates for submaximal exercise tests, as well as for exercise prescriptions. You can measure heart rate using auscultation, palpation, heart rate monitors, or ECG recordings.

Auscultation

When measuring resting heart rate by auscultation, place the bell of the stethoscope over the third intercostal space to the left of the sternum. The sounds arising from the heart are counted for 30 or 60 sec. The 30 sec count is multiplied by 2 to convert it to beats per minute.

Palpation

With use of the **palpation** technique for determining heart rate, the pulse is palpated at one of the following sites:

- Brachial artery—on the anteromedial aspect of the arm below the belly of the biceps brachii, approximately 2 to 3 cm (1 in.) above the antecubital fossa
- Carotid artery—in the neck just lateral to the larynx
- Radial artery—on the anterolateral aspect of the wrist directly in line with the base of the thumb
- Temporal artery—along the hairline of the head at the temple

For precautions necessary to be sure your measurement is accurate, refer to "Heart Rate Determination by Palpation."

Heart Rate Monitors and Electrocardiogram Recordings

Heart rate also can be measured using heart rate monitors or an ECG monitoring system. Generally, heart rate monitors are designed to detect either the pulse or the ECG electrical signal from the heart, and provide a digital display of the heart rate. Pulse monitors use infrared sensors attached to the client's fingertip,

---

Heart Rate Determination by Palpation

Follow these procedures when determining heart rate by palpation:

- Use the tips of the middle and index fingers. Do not use your thumb; it has a pulse of its own and may produce an inaccurate count.

- When palpating the carotid site, do not apply heavy pressure to the area. Baroreceptors in the carotid arteries detect this pressure and cause a reflex slowing of the heart rate.

- If you start the stopwatch simultaneously with the pulse beat, count the first beat as zero. If the stopwatch is running, count the first beat as 1. Continue counting either for a set period of time (6, 10, 15, 30, or 60 sec) or for a set number of beats. When the heart rate is counted for less than 1 min, use the following multipliers to convert the count to beats per minute: 6 sec count times 10; 10 sec count times 6; 15 sec, 4; 30 sec, 2. Typically, shorter time intervals (i.e., 6 or 10 sec counts) are used to measure exercise and postexercise heart rates during and immediately following exercise. Because there is a rapid and immediate decline in heart rate when a person stops exercising, the 6 or 10 sec count reflects the individual's actual exercise heart rate more accurately than the longer counts do.

---

earlobe, or wrist (i.e., heart rate watch) to detect pulsations in blood flow during the cardiac cycle. Chest-strap wire and wireless ECG-type monitors tend to be more accurate and reliable than pulse monitors, especially during vigorous exercise. However, the accuracy of wireless chest-strap monitors may be affected by electrical equipment (such as some treadmills, stair climbers, rowing machines, and video screens) generating radio or magnetic interference. Generally, heart rate monitors provide an accurate measure of ECG heart rate during rest and exercise (Vehrs et al. 2002).

Most ECG monitoring systems provide a continuous digital display of the heart rate. This value is usually recorded at the top of the ECG strip recording. If your equipment does not provide a digital readout, you can use a heart rate ruler that converts the distance of two cardiac cycles to beats per minute.

No matter which technique is used to measure heart rate, you should be aware that heart rate fluctuates easily due to temperature, anxiety, exercise, stress, eating, smoking, drinking coffee, time of day, and body position. In a supine position, the resting heart rate is lower than in either a sitting or a standing position.

Twelve-Lead Electrocardiogram

The **electrocardiogram (ECG)** is a composite record of the electrical events in the heart during the cardiac cycle. As the heart depolarizes and repolarizes during contraction, an electrical impulse spreads to the tissues surrounding the heart. Electrodes placed on opposite sides of the heart transmit the electrical potential to an ECG recorder.

In addition to providing baseline data, the resting ECG is used to detect such contraindications to exercise testing as evidence of previous myocardial infarction, ischemic ST-segment changes, conduction defects, and left ventricular hypertrophy. The reading and interpretation of ECGs require a high degree of skill and practice. As an exercise technician you can administer the resting 12-lead ECG, but a qualified physician should interpret the results. This chapter includes only basic information about administering an ECG. You should consult other references for more detailed information concerning the reading and interpretation of ECG abnormalities (Dubin 2000; Dunbar and Saul 2009; Thaler 2010).

Electrocardiogram Basics

A typical normal ECG (figure 2.1) is composed of a **P wave** that represents depolarization of the atria. The **PR interval** indicates the delay in the impulse at the atrioventricular node. Electrical currents generated during ventricular depolarization and contraction produce the **QRS complex.** The **T wave** and **ST segment** correspond to ventricular repolarization.

A lead is a pair of electrodes placed on the body and connected to an ECG recorder. An axis is an imaginary line connecting the two electrodes. A standard 12-lead ECG consists of three limb leads, three augmented unipolar leads, and six chest leads. Each of the 12 ECG leads records a different view of the heart's electrical activity. Thus, the tracings from the various leads differ from one another.

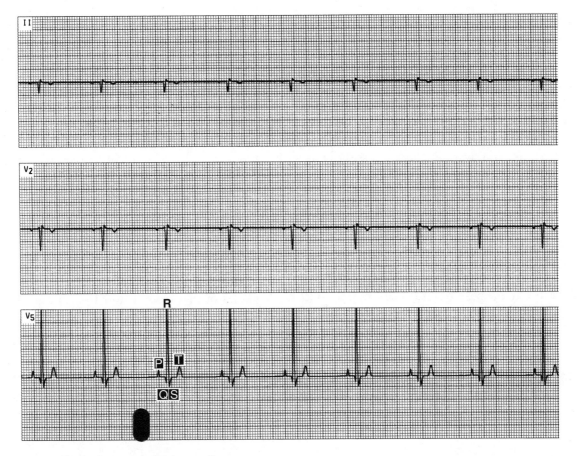

Figure 2.1 Typical normal electrocardiogram.

Resting 12-Lead Electrocardiogram Procedures

To measure the 12 leads, 10 electrodes are used. The electrodes for the three **limb leads** (I, II, and III) are placed on the right arm, left arm, and left leg. A ground electrode is placed on the right leg. This is electronically equivalent to placing the electrodes at the shoulders and the symphysis pubis. Limb lead I measures the voltage differential between the left and right arm electrodes. Limb leads II and III measure the voltage between the left leg and right (lead II) and left (lead III) arms. Figure 2.2 shows

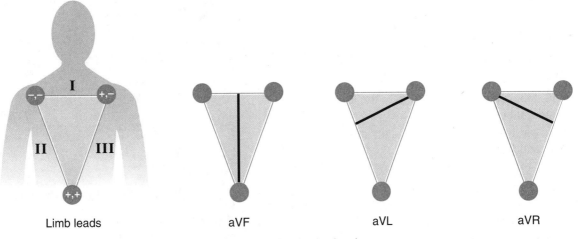

Limb leads   aVF   aVL   aVR

Figure 2.2 Three limb leads and three augmented unipolar leads.

the three limb leads and three augmented unipolar leads.

The three **augmented unipolar leads** are aVF (feet), aVL (left), and aVR (right). The augmented unipolar lead compares the voltage across one of the limb electrodes with the average voltage across the two opposite electrodes. Lead aVL, for example, records the voltage across an electrode placed on the left arm and the average voltage across the other two limb electrodes (see figure 2.2).

The six **chest leads** (V_1 to V_6) measure the voltage across a specific area of the chest, with the average voltage across the other three limb leads. Figure 2.3 illustrates electrode placement for the chest leads, V_1 through V_6.

During the resting ECG, the client should lie quietly in a supine position on a table. The electrode sites should be shaved if hair is present and should be cleaned with alcohol. Remove the superficial layer

of skin at each site by rubbing it with fine-grain emery paper or a gauze pad. Disposable electrodes contain electrode gel and adhesive discs. After applying the electrode, tap it firmly to test for noisy leads. You should always calibrate the ECG recorder prior to use by recording the standard 1 mV deflection per centimeter. Also, to standardize the time base for the ECG, set the paper speed to 25 mm/sec.

The Twelve-Lead Exercise ECG

To avoid poor ECG tracings caused by moving limbs during exercise, the electrode configuration is modified slightly for an exercise 12-lead ECG. The right and left arm electrodes are placed below the right and left clavicles, respectively. The right and left leg electrodes are attached to the right and left sides of the trunk, below the rib cage on the anterior axillary line. The six chest electrodes are positioned as previously described (see figure 2.4).

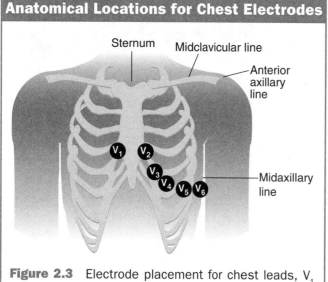

Figure 2.3 Electrode placement for chest leads, V_1 to V_6.

- V_1—fourth intercostal space to the right of the sternal border
- V_2—fourth intercostal space to the left of the sternal border
- V_3—at the midpoint of a straight line between V_2 and V_4
- V_4—fifth intercostal space along the midclavicular line
- V_5—horizontal to V_4 on the anterior axillary line
- V_6—horizontal to V_4 and V_5 on the midaxillary line

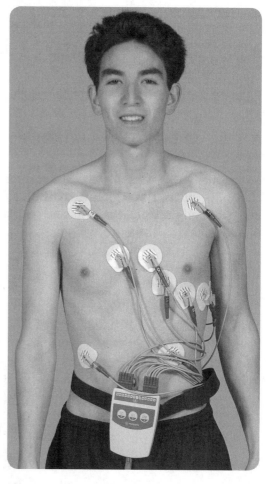

Figure 2.4 Electrode placement for 12-lead exercise electrocardiogram.

Sources for Equipment

Product	Manufacturer's Address
Anaeroid or mercury sphygmomanometer and blood pressure cuffs	W.A. Baum Co. (888) 281-6061 www.wabaum.com
Automated electronic blood pressure devices	Omron Healthcare, Inc. (847) 680-6200 www.omronhealthcare.com
Electrocardiograph	GE Healthcare Bio-Science Corp. (800) 526-3593 www.gehealthcare.com
Heart rate monitors	Creative Health Products (800) 742-4478 www.chponline.com

KEY POINTS

- The purpose of the health evaluation is to detect disease and to assess disease risk.

- Important components of the health evaluation are a medical history, CHD risk factor analysis, physical examination, clinical tests, and medical clearance.

- The lifestyle evaluation includes information about the diet, tobacco and alcohol use, physical activity, and psychological stress levels of the individual.

- All clients are required to sign an informed consent prior to taking any physical fitness tests or participating in an exercise program.

- The resting evaluation of cardiorespiratory function includes heart rate, BP, and a 12-lead ECG that is interpreted by a qualified physician.

- Resting BP can be assessed using auscultation or automated BP devices.

- Heart rate may be taken using auscultation, palpation, heart rate monitors, or ECG recordings.

- The 12-lead ECG includes three limb leads (I, II, III), three augmented unipolar leads (aVF, aVR, aVL), and six chest leads (V_1 through V_6).

- A graded maximal exercise test is the best way to assess functional aerobic capacity.

- Unless contraindications to exercise are observed, a maximal exercise test is recommended for men 45 yr or older and women 55 yr or older before they begin a vigorous exercise program.

KEY TERMS

Learn the definition for each of the following key terms. Definitions of key terms can be found in the glossary on page 411.

augmented unipolar leads	low CHD risk	P wave
auscultation	miscuffing	QRS complex
bradycardia	moderate CHD risk	sphygmomanometer
chest leads	normotensive	ST segment
cuff hypertension	oscillometry	systolic blood pressure (SBP)
diastolic blood pressure (DBP)	overcuffing	tachycardia
electrocardiogram	palpation	T wave
high CHD risk	prehypertension	undercuffing
hypertension	PR interval	white coat hypertension
limb leads	pulse pressure	

REVIEW QUESTIONS

In addition to being able to define each of the key terms, test your knowledge and understanding of the material by answering the following review questions.

1. Identify the purpose of each component of the comprehensive health evaluation.

2. At minimum, a pretest health screening should include four items. Name these.

3. Identify cardiovascular, pulmonary, metabolic, and musculoskeletal diseases or disorders that warrant referral to a physician for medical clearance (name three signs or symptoms for each category).

4. Identify the positive and negative risk factors for CHD. Specify the criteria for each of these risk factors.

5. Identify the cutoff values for classifying resting BPs.

6. Identify the cutoff values for classifying TC, LDL-C, HDL-C, and triglycerides.

7. List the three ACSM risk stratification categories and the criteria for each category.

8. Describe the criteria used to determine whether or not an individual needs a physical examination and medical clearance prior to exercise testing or exercise participation.

9. Name three methods for measuring BP. Which one is considered to be the "gold standard" method?

10. Name three sources of error in measurement of BP.

11. Describe three things you should do to ensure accurate BP readings during exercise.

12. Describe the effects of miscuffing on BP readings.

13. What effect do arm position and body posture have on BP readings?

14. Name three methods for measuring heart rate.

15. Identify the component parts of a typical normal ECG tracing. What does each component represent relative to the cardiac cycle?

16. Describe the anatomical locations for placement of the 10 electrodes used to obtain a 12-lead ECG recording.

17. Identify ACSM's guidelines for medical examinations and exercise testing for low-, moderate-, and high-risk individuals.

18. Name three absolute and three relative contraindications to exercise testing.

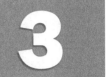

Principles of Assessment, Prescription, and Exercise Program Adherence

KEY QUESTIONS

- What are the essential components of a physical fitness profile?

- What are the purposes of physical fitness tests, and how can I use the results?

- Several physical fitness tests are available; how do I select the best test for my client?

- Are field tests as good as laboratory tests for measuring physical fitness?

- What is the best way to interpret test results for my client?

- What are the essential elements of an exercise prescription?

- Is one type of exercise better than others for improving each component of physical fitness?

- Does high-intensity exercise improve physical fitness faster than low-intensity exercise?

- Is it safe to exercise every day?

- When should I increase the frequency, intensity, and duration in an exercise prescription? Can these elements be increased simultaneously?

- Do older people benefit as much from exercise as younger people?

- How can I get my clients to stick with their exercise programs?

- How can technology be used to promote physical activity?

- Do I need to be professionally certified or licensed in order to work in this field?

Health and fitness professionals need to master the basic principles of physical fitness assessment and exercise prescription. You must know how to use the results of physical fitness tests to plan scientifically sound exercise programs that are individualized to meet your client's needs, interests, and abilities. With your knowledge, leadership, and guidance, your clients can reduce their risk of disease and improve their health and physical fitness levels safely and effectively.

✴ As an exercise specialist, you will have diverse responsibilities, such as

- educating clients about the positive benefits of regular physical activity;

- conducting pretest health evaluations to screen clients for exercise participation (see chapter 2);

- selecting, administering, and interpreting tests designed to assess each component of physical fitness;

- designing individualized exercise programs;

- leading exercise classes;

- analyzing your clients' exercise performance and correcting performance errors;

- educating your clients about the "do's and don'ts" of exercise; and

- motivating your clients to improve their adherence to exercise.

Exercise specialists play many roles: educator, leader, technician, and artist. To be effective in these roles, you must integrate knowledge from many disciplines such as anatomy, physiology, chemistry, nutrition, education, and psychology, as well as refine your exercise testing, prescription, and leadership skills.

This chapter presents principles of exercise testing and prescription, along with information about exercise program adherence, use of technology to promote physical activity, and the importance of professional certification for individuals in the field of exercise science.

PHYSICAL FITNESS TESTING

There are several areas that you must understand in order to plan and administer physical fitness tests. These comprise

- the components of physical fitness to be tested;

- purposes of physical fitness testing;

- testing order and the testing environment;

- test validity, reliability, and objectivity;

- prediction equation evaluation; and

- test administration and interpretation.

Components of Physical Fitness

Physical fitness is the ability to perform occupational, recreational, and daily activities without becoming unduly fatigued. As an exercise specialist, one of your primary responsibilities is to assess each of the following physical fitness components:

1. **Cardiorespiratory endurance. Cardiorespiratory endurance** is the ability of the heart, lungs, and circulatory system to supply oxygen and nutrients efficiently to working muscles. Exercise physiologists measure the **maximum oxygen consumption** ($\dot{V}O_2$max), or the rate of oxygen utilization of the muscles during aerobic exercise, in order to assess cardiorespiratory endurance and functional aerobic capacity. Physical fitness evaluations should include a test of cardiorespiratory function during rest and exercise. Graded exercise tests (GXTs) are used for this purpose. Improved cardiorespiratory endurance is one of the most important benefits of aerobic exercise training programs. Chapters 4 and 5 present detailed information about graded exercise testing and aerobic exercise programs.

2. **Musculoskeletal fitness. Musculoskeletal fitness** refers to the ability of the skeletal and muscular systems to perform work. This requires muscular strength, muscular endurance, and bone strength. **Muscular strength** is the maximal force or tension level that can be produced by a muscle group; **muscular endurance** is the ability of a muscle to maintain submaximal force levels for extended periods; **bone strength** is directly related to the risk of bone fracture and is a function of the mineral content and density of the bone tissue. Resistance training is one of the most effective ways to improve the strength of muscles and bones and to develop muscular endurance. Chapters 6 and 7 provide detailed information about assessing musculoskeletal fitness and designing resistance training programs.

3. **Body weight and body composition. Body weight** refers to the size or mass of the individual. **Body composition** refers to body weight in terms of the absolute and relative amounts of muscle, bone, and fat tissues. Aerobic exercise and resistance training are effective in altering body weight and composition. Chapters 8 and 9 discuss body composition assessment techniques and exercise programs for weight management.

4. **Flexibility. Flexibility** is the ability to move a joint or series of joints fluidly through the complete range of motion. Flexibility is limited by factors such as bony structure of the joint and the size and strength of muscles, ligaments, and other connective tissues. Daily stretching can greatly improve flexibility. Chapters 10 and 11 give more information about assessing flexibility and designing stretching programs.

5. **Balance. Balance** is the ability to keep the body's center of gravity within the base of support when maintaining a static position, performing voluntary movements, or reacting to external disturbances. **Functional balance** refers to the ability to perform daily movement tasks requiring bal-

ance such as picking up an object from the floor, dressing, and turning to look at something behind you. Tai chi and yoga are two examples of activities that can be used to improve balance. Chapter 12 addresses the assessment of balance and design of programs for improving balance.

Purposes of Physical Fitness Testing

As mentioned in chapter 2, it is imperative that you carefully screen your clients for exercise testing, classify their disease risk, identify any contraindications to exercise testing, and obtain their informed consent before conducting any physical fitness tests. You can use laboratory and field tests to assess each component of physical fitness and to develop physical fitness profiles for your clients. Results from these tests enable you to identify strengths and weaknesses and to set realistic and attainable goals for your clients. Data from specific tests (e.g., heart rates from a GXT) will help you make accurate and precise exercise prescriptions for each client. Also, you can use baseline and follow-up data to evaluate the progress of exercise program participants.

Testing Order and the Testing Environment

When you administer a complete battery of physical fitness tests in a single session, use the following test sequence to minimize the effects of previous tests on subsequent test performance:

- Resting blood pressure and heart rate
- Body composition and balance
- Cardiorespiratory endurance
- Muscular fitness
- Flexibility

Often clients are apprehensive about taking physical fitness tests. Test anxiety may affect the validity and reliability of test results. Therefore, you should put your client at ease by establishing good rapport; projecting a sense of relaxed confidence; and creating a testing environment that is friendly, quiet, private, safe, and comfortable. Room temperature should be maintained at 70 to 74° F (21 to 23° C), and the relative humidity should be controlled whenever possible. For pretest health screening and interpretation of the client's test results, the room should have comfortable chairs and a table for completing questionnaires and paperwork, as well as an examination table or bed for the resting evaluation of heart rate, blood pressure, and the 12-lead electrocardiogram. All equipment used for physical testing should be carefully calibrated and prepared before your client arrives for testing. This will ensure valid test data and efficient use of time.

Test Validity, Reliability, and Objectivity

To accurately assess your client's physical fitness status, you must select tests that are valid, reliable, and objective. It is necessary to understand these basic concepts fully in order to evaluate the relative worth of specific physical fitness tests and prediction equations.

Test Validity

With regard to physical fitness testing, test validity is the ability of a test to *measure accurately,* with minimal error, a specific physical fitness component. **Reference** or **criterion methods** are used to obtain *direct* measures of physical fitness components. However, some physical fitness components cannot always be measured directly, requiring the use of *indirect* measures for estimation of the value of the reference measure. For example, exercise physiologists consider the direct measurement of $\dot{V}O_2max$ (i.e., collection and analysis of expired gas samples) during maximal exercise to be the criterion measure of cardiorespiratory fitness. Direct measurement of $\dot{V}O_2max$, however, requires expensive equipment and considerable technical expertise. Therefore in the laboratory setting, $\dot{V}O_2max$ is usually estimated using formulas to convert the amount of work output during a GXT to oxygen consumption (see chapter 4). In field settings, prediction equations are used to estimate $\dot{V}O_2max$ from a combination of physiological, demographic, and performance predictor variables.

One way in which researchers quantify the validity of physical fitness tests is by calculating the relationship between predicted scores (y') and the criterion scores (y) using correlation coefficients ($r_{y,y'}$). This value, $r_{y,y'}$, is known as the **validity coefficient.** The magnitude of the validity coefficient cannot exceed 1.0. The closer the value is to 1.0, the greater the validity of the test. Valid physical fitness field tests and prediction equations typically have validity coefficients in excess of $r_{y,y'} = 0.80$.

Because field tests indirectly estimate a physical fitness component, there will be a difference between the measured (reference) and predicted values for that component. This difference (y – y') is called the **residual score**. The **standard error of estimate (SEE)** is a measure of prediction error and is used to quantify the accuracy of the prediction equation and the validity of the field test. The magnitude of the *SEE* depends on the size of the residual scores and reflects the average degree of deviation of individual data points around the line of best fit or regression line depicting the linear relationship between the measured and the predicted scores. When individual data points fall close to the regression line, the *SEE* is small (see figure 3.1). A valid field test has a high validity coefficient and a small prediction error.

In addition to test validity, test sensitivity and specificity are often reported. **Sensitivity** refers to the probability of correctly identifying individuals who have risk factors for a specific disease or syndrome (e.g., the probability of correctly diagnosing individuals with cardiovascular disease risk factors using body mass index and waist circumference cutoff values). **Specificity** is a measure of the ability to correctly identify individuals with no risk factors. Given that the sensitivity and specificity of tests are typically less than 1.00 (i.e., <100% correct), some individuals will be identified as having risk factors even though they have none (**false positive**), and some will be identified as having no risk factors when they do have some (**false negative**).

Test Reliability

Reliability is the ability of a test to yield *consistent* and *stable* scores across trials and over time. For example, the skinfold test is considered to be reliable because a trained skinfold technician obtains similar skinfold values when taking duplicate measurements on the same person. Researchers quantify reliability by calculating the relationship between trial 1 and trial 2 test scores or day 1 and day 2 test scores. This value, $r_{x1,x2}$, is known as the **reliability coefficient.** The magnitude of the reliability coefficient cannot exceed 1.0. In general, physical fitness tests have high reliability coefficients, typically exceeding $r_{x1,x2} = 0.90$.

It is important to know that test reliability affects test validity. Tests with poor reliability also have poor validity because unreliable tests fail to produce consistent test scores. It is possible, however, for a test to have excellent reliability ($r_{x1,x2} > 0.90$) but poor validity. Even when a test yields stable and precise values across trials or between days, it may not validly measure a specific physical fitness component. For example, researchers reported high test–retest reliability ($r_{x1,x2} = 0.99$) for the sit-and-reach test, but also noted that this test has poor validity ($r_{y,y'} = 0.12$) as a measure of low back flexibility in women (Jackson and Langford 1989).

Test Objectivity

Objectivity is also known as intertester reliability. Objective tests yield similar test scores for a given individual when the same test is administered by different technicians. Objectivity is quantified by calculating the correlation between pairs of test scores measured on the same individuals by two different technicians. This value, $r_{1,2}$, is known as the **objectivity coefficient.** As with validity and reliability coefficients, the magnitude of the objectivity coefficient cannot exceed 1.0. Most physical fitness tests have high objectivity coefficients ($r_{1,2} > 0.90$), especially when technicians are highly trained, practice together, and carefully follow standardized testing procedures.

Prediction Equation Evaluation

Although reference measures obtained in the laboratory setting provide the most valid assessment

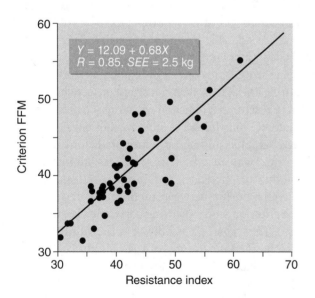

Figure 3.1 Line of best fit and *SEE* (prediction error).

of each physical fitness component, these tests are expensive and time-consuming and require considerable technical expertise. In field and clinical settings, you can obtain estimates of these reference measures by selecting valid field tests and prediction equations that have good predictive accuracy. Table 3.1 provides an overview of the types of tests used in laboratory and field settings to assess each physical fitness component.

To select the most appropriate tests for measuring your client's physical fitness, it is important to be able to evaluate the relative worth of the fitness tests and their prediction equations. To do this, you should ask the following questions:

■ *What reference measure was used to develop the prediction equation?*

As mentioned earlier, the reference or criterion measure of a specific physical fitness component is obtained by directly measuring the component. Reference measures are used as the "gold standard" to validate field tests and to develop prediction equa-

tions that accurately estimate the reference measure. For example, skinfold prediction equations are developed and cross-validated through comparison of the estimated body density, calculated from the skinfold equation, to the reference measure of body density typically obtained from hydrodensitometry (underwater weighing). Similarly, the validity of the sit-and-reach test for measuring low back flexibility was tested by comparing sit-and-reach scores to range of motion values (reference measure) directly measured by X-ray or goniometric methods. Table 3.1 lists reference measures that experts commonly use to assess each physical fitness component. Field tests and prediction equations developed using indirect methods instead of reference methods as a criterion have questionable validity.

■ *How large was the sample used to develop the prediction equation?*

Large randomly selected samples ($N = 100$ to 400 subjects) generally are needed to ensure that the data are representative of the population for

Table 3.1 Direct (Reference) and Indirect (Field) Measures of Physical Fitness Components

Physical fitness component	Reference measure	Laboratory or reference method	Indirect measures or field tests	Group prediction error (*SEE* and *TE*)	Individual prediction error*	Chapter
Cardiorespiratory endurance	Direct measurement of $\dot{V}O_2$max ($ml \cdot kg^{-1} \cdot min^{-1}$)	Maximal GXT	Submaximal GXT, distance run/walk tests, step tests	<5.0 $ml \cdot kg^{-1} \cdot min^{-1}$	± 10 $ml \cdot kg^{-1} \cdot min^{-1}$	4
Body composition	Db ($g \cdot cc^{-1}$), FFM (kg), or %BF	Hydrodensitometry or dual-energy X-ray absorptiometry	Bioimpedance, skinfolds, anthropometry	<0.0080 $g \cdot cc^{-1}$ <3.5 kg FFM (men) <2.8 kg FFM (women) <3.5 %BF	± 6.0 kg ± 5.0 kg ± 7.0%	8
Muscular strength	Maximal force (kg) or torque (Nm)	Isokinetic or 1-RM tests	Submaximal tests (2- to 10-RM value)	<2.0 kg	± 4 kg	6
Bone strength	Bone mineral content and bone density	Dual-energy X-ray absorptiometry	Anthropometric measures of bony width	NR	NR	8
Flexibility	ROM at joint (degrees)	X ray or goniometry	Linear measures of ROM	$<6°$	$\pm 12°$	10
Balance	None	Computerized balance assessment	Timed performance on balance tasks; distance reached	NR	NR	12

Db = total body density; FFM = fat-free mass; %BF = relative body fat; *SEE* = standard error of estimate; *TE* = total error; GXT = graded exercise test; ROM = range of motion; RM = repetition maximum; NR = not reported; Nm = newton-meter.

*95% limits of agreement.

whom the prediction equation was developed. Also, equations based on large samples tend to have more stable regression weights for each predictor variable in the equation.

■ *What is the ratio of sample size to the number of predictor variables in the equation?*

In multiple regression, the correlation between the reference measure of the physical fitness component and the predictors in the equation is represented by the **multiple correlation coefficient (R_{mc})**. The larger the R_{mc} (up to maximum value of 1.00), the stronger the relationship. The size of R_{mc} will be artificially inflated if there are too many predictors in the equation compared to the total number of subjects. Statisticians recommend that there should be a minimum of 20 to 40 subjects per predictor variable. For example, if a skinfold (SKF) prediction equation has three predictors (e.g., triceps SKF, calf SKF, and age), then the minimum sample size needs to be 60 to 120 subjects. Prediction equations that are based on small samples or that have a poor subject-to-predictor ratio are suspect and should not be used.

■ *What were the sizes of the R_{mc} and the standard error of estimate for the prediction equation?*

In general, the R_{mc} for equations predicting physical fitness components exceeds 0.80. This means that at least 64% [$R^2 = 0.80^2 \times 100$] of variance in the reference measure can be accounted for by the predictors in the equation. As you can easily see, the larger the R_{mc}, the greater the amount of shared variance between the reference measure and predictor variables. When you evaluate the relative worth of a prediction equation, it is more important to focus on the size of the prediction error (*SEE*) than on the R_{mc} because the magnitude of R_{mc} is greatly affected by sample size and variability of the data. Keep in mind that *SEE* reflects the degree of deviation of individual data points (participants' scores) around the line of best fit through the entire sample's data points. In multiple regression, the **line of best fit** is the **regression line** that depicts the linear relationship between the reference measure and all of the predictor variables in the equation. Table 3.1 presents standard values for evaluating prediction errors of physical fitness prediction equations.

■ *To whom is the prediction equation applicable?*

To answer this question, you need to pay close attention to the physical characteristics of the sample used to derive the equation. Factors such as age, gender, race, fitness level, and body fatness need to be examined carefully. Prediction equations are either **population specific** or **generalized**. Population-specific equations are intended only for individuals from a specific homogeneous group. For example, separate SKF equations have been developed for prepubescent boys and girls (see table 8.3, p. 204). Population-specific equations are likely to systematically over- or underestimate the physical fitness component if they are applied to individuals who do not belong to that population subgroup. On the other hand, there are generalized prediction equations that can be applied to individuals who differ greatly in physical characteristics. Generalized equations are developed using diverse, heterogeneous samples and account for differences in physical characteristics by including these variables as predictors in the equation. For example, the prediction equation for the Rockport walking test (see chapter 4) is a generalized equation because gender and age are predictors in this equation.

■ *How were the variables measured by the researchers who developed the prediction equation?*

It is important to know not only which variables are included in a prediction equation, but also how each one of these predictors was measured by the researchers developing the equation. Although it is highly recommended that standardized procedures be used for all physical fitness testing, this is not always done. For example, the suprailiac SKF used in the SKF equations developed by Jackson, Pollock, and Ward (1980) is measured above the iliac crest at the anterior axillary line. In contrast, the *Anthropometric Standardization Reference Manual* (Lohman, Roche, and Martorell 1988) recommends that the suprailiac SKF be measured above the iliac crest at the midaxillary line. For most individuals, there will be a difference between SKF thicknesses measured at these two sites. Thus, larger than expected prediction errors may result if physical fitness variables are not measured according to the descriptions provided by the researchers who developed the equation.

■ *Was the prediction equation cross-validated on another sample from the population?*

An equation must be tested on other samples from the population before its validity or predictive accuracy can be determined. For example, the Rockport 1.0-mile walking test was originally developed to assess the cardiorespiratory fitness of women and men ages 20 to 69 yr (Kline et al. 1987). Other researchers cross-validated this equation to establish its predictive accuracy for women 65 yr of age or older (Fenstermaker, Plowman, and Looney 1992). In general, prediction equations that have not been cross-validated on the original study sample or on additional samples in other studies should not be used.

■ *What were the sizes of the validity coefficient ($r_{y,y'}$) and the prediction errors when this equation was applied to the cross-validation sample (i.e., what is the group predictive accuracy of the equation)?*

An equation with good predictive accuracy has a moderately high validity coefficient ($r_{y,y'}$ >0.80) and an acceptable prediction error (see table 3.1, Group prediction error). In cross-validation studies, the accuracy of an equation for estimating the reference values of a group is assessed by analyzing two types of prediction error: the *SEE* and the total error (*TE*). As mentioned, the *SEE* reflects the average deviation of individual data points from the regression line or line of best fit (see figure 3.1). The **total error (*TE*)** is the average degree of deviation of individual data points from the line of identity (see figure 3.2). The **line of identity** has a slope of 1.0 and a y-intercept equal to 0. When an equation closely predicts the actual or measured scores of the cross-validation sample, individual data points fall close to the line

of identity (i.e., *TE* is small). Acceptable values for evaluating group prediction errors (*SEE* and *TE*) are presented in table 3.1.

■ *Was the average predicted score similar to the average reference score for the cross-validation sample?*

The prediction equation should yield similar mean values for the actual (measured or reference) and predicted scores of the cross-validation sample. The **constant error (*CE*)** is the difference between the actual and predicted means. The means are compared using a paired *t*-test and should not differ significantly from each other. A large significant difference indicates a **bias** or systematic difference (i.e., over- or underestimation) between the original validation sample and the cross-validation sample. This difference is caused by technical error or biological variability between the samples.

■ *How good is the prediction equation for estimating reference values of individual clients (i.e., what is the individual predictive accuracy of the equation)?*

Although a prediction equation may accurately estimate the average reference score for a specific group, it may not necessarily give accurate estimates for all individuals composing that group. To evaluate how well a prediction equation works for individuals, researchers use the **Bland and Altman method** (1986), which sets **limits of agreement** around the average difference ($\bar{d}$) between the actual

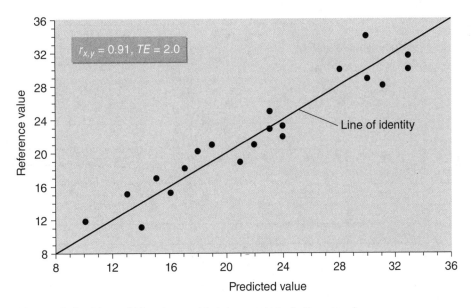

Figure 3.2 Line of identity and total error (prediction error).

and predicted scores for the sample. With this method, difference scores (actual – predicted values) and average scores [(actual + predicted values) / 2] are calculated for each individual in the sample and are plotted on a graph (see figure 3.3). When the difference scores are normally distributed, 95% lie within ±2 standard deviations from the overall mean difference $(\overline{d})$ for the group. In this case, the standard deviation of the difference scores (S_d) is used to set the upper $(+2S_d)$ and lower $(-2S_d)$ limits of agreement. Smaller 95% limits of agreement indicate that the equation has a better individual predictive accuracy. The limits of agreement estimate how well you will be able to predict your client's actual value when using the equation. In the example in figure 3.3, the predictive accuracy of the equation for estimating the actual %BF of individual clients is approximately ±6% BF (note the upper and lower limits of agreement on the y-axis of the graph).

In summary, you should apply all of the following evaluation criteria when selecting field tests and prediction equations that indirectly assess the physical fitness of your clients:

- An acceptable method is used to derive reference measures of the physical fitness component.
- A large sample (N = 100-400) and 20 to 40 subjects per predictor variable are used to develop the equation.

- The sizes of the multiple correlation and validity coefficients exceed 0.80.
- The group prediction errors (SEE and TE) are acceptable (see table 3.1).
- Demographic characteristics (e.g., age, gender, race, fitness status) of the validation and cross-validation samples are described.
- The prediction equation is cross-validated in the original study or on independent samples from other studies.
- The constant error (bias), or difference between the measured and predicted means for the cross-validation sample, is not statistically significant.
- The 95% limits of agreement are acceptable (see table 3.1).

Physical Fitness Tests: Administration and Interpretation

To obtain good test results, it is important to prepare your clients for physical fitness testing by giving them appropriate instructions at least 1 day before the scheduled exercise tests.

Pretest Instructions

Give the client directions to the testing facility and make special arrangements if the facility requires a parking pass. Make sure the client has the following instructions in preparation for the test:

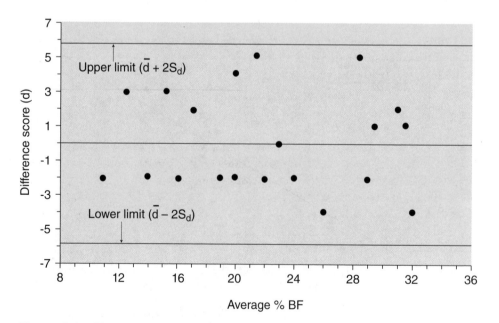

Figure 3.3 Bland-Altman plot with 95% limits of agreement.

- Wear comfortable clothing, socks, and athletic shoes if available.
- Drink plenty of fluids during the 24 hr period before the test.
- Refrain from eating, smoking, and drinking alcohol or caffeine for 3 hr prior to the test.
- Do not engage in strenuous physical activity the day of the test.
- Get adequate sleep (6 to 8 hr) the night before the test.

Test Administration

Later chapters give detailed procedures for administering laboratory and field tests for each physical fitness component. Your technical skills and expertise in administering these tests are directly related to your mastery of standardized testing procedures and the amount of time you spend practicing testing techniques. For example, to become a proficient SKF technician, you probably should practice on at least 50 to 100 people (Jackson and Pollock 1985). You also need a great deal of practice in order to measure exercise blood pressures and heart rates accurately and to coordinate the timing of these measurements during a GXT on the treadmill or cycle ergometer. Remember that you cannot obtain valid test scores if you do not follow the standardized testing procedures.

Test Interpretation

After collecting the test data, you must analyze and interpret the results for your client. Computer software programs are available that display and compare the client's test results to normative data. Some graphs display the individual's physical fitness profile so that you and your client can easily pinpoint strengths, as well as physical fitness components in need of improvement.

To classify your client's physical fitness status, you should compare test scores to established norms. For this purpose, age–gender norms are provided for many of the cardiorespiratory fitness, muscular fitness, body composition, flexibility, and balance tests included in this book. For some tests, percentile rankings are used to classify a client's performance. To illustrate the interpretation of a percentile ranking, let's use the example of a 35 yr old male client whose sit-and-reach score ranks in the 60th percentile. This ranking means that his score is better than 60% of the scores of all males the same age taking this test.

When interpreting results for clients, use lay language, rather than highly technical terms and jargon, to explain their test scores. Whenever possible, try to phrase poor results in positive terms. For example, if a female client's body fat level is classified as obese, do not embarrass and alarm her by saying, "Your underwater weighing test indicates that you are obese and need to lose at least 20 pounds to achieve a healthy body fat level in order to reduce your risk of diseases linked to obesity. You need to decrease your caloric intake and increase your caloric expenditure by dieting and exercising. The sooner you start a weight management program, the better."

Instead, you should use a more positive and less intimidating approach when interpreting this result. The following approach is more appropriate, especially for clients with low self-efficacy or motivation to initiate and adhere to an exercise program: "People with more than 35% body fat are at risk for disease. If you wish, I will evaluate your daily calorie intake and suggest healthy foods you like to eat that are low in fat. Also, we can discuss ways to increase your physical activity level. I think we can find some activities that you will enjoy and have time for, so that you'll burn more calories each day. With these changes, you should be able to lower your body fat to a healthy level in a reasonable amount of time."

BASIC PRINCIPLES FOR EXERCISE PROGRAM DESIGN

A number of basic training principles apply to all types of exercise programs, whether they are designed to improve cardiorespiratory fitness, musculoskeletal fitness, body composition, flexibility, or balance.

- **Specificity-of-training principle.** The **specificity principle** states that the body's physiological and metabolic responses and adaptations to exercise training are specific to the type of exercise and the muscle groups involved. For example, physical activities requiring continuous, dynamic, and rhythmical contractions of large muscle groups are best suited for stimulating improvements in cardiorespiratory endurance; stretching exercises develop range of joint motion and flexibility; and resistance exercises are effective for improving muscular strength and muscular endurance. Furthermore, the gains in muscular fitness are specific to the exercised muscle groups, type and speed of contraction, and training intensity.

■ **Overload training principle.** To promote improvements in physical fitness components, the physiological systems of the body must be taxed using loads that are greater (**overload principle**) than those to which the individual is accustomed. Overload can be achieved through increases in the frequency, intensity, and duration of aerobic exercise. Muscle groups can be effectively overloaded through increases in the number of repetitions, sets, or exercises in programs designed to improve muscular fitness and flexibility.

■ **Principle of progression.** Throughout the training program, you must progressively increase the training volume, or overload, to stimulate further improvements (i.e., **progression principle**). The progression needs to be gradual because "doing too much, too soon" may cause musculoskeletal injuries and is a major reason why some individuals drop out of exercise programs.

■ **Principle of initial values.** Individuals with low initial physical fitness levels will show greater relative (%) gains and a faster rate of improvement in response to exercise training than individuals with average or high fitness levels (**initial values principle**). For example, during the first month of an aerobic exercise program, the $\dot{V}O_2$max of a client with poor cardiorespiratory endurance capacity may improve 12% or more, whereas a highly trained endurance athlete may improve only 1% or less.

■ **Principle of interindividual variability.** Individual responses to a training stimulus are quite variable and depend on a number of factors such as age, initial fitness level, and health status (i.e., **interindividual variability principle**). You therefore must design exercise programs with the specific needs, interests, and abilities of each client in mind and develop personalized exercise prescriptions that take into account individual differences and preferences.

■ **Principle of diminishing returns.** Each person has a genetic ceiling that limits the extent of improvement that is possible due to exercise train-

ing. As individuals approach their genetic ceiling, the rate of improvement in physical fitness slows and eventually levels off (i.e., **diminishing return principle**).

■ **Principle of reversibility.** The positive physiological effects and health benefits of regular physical activity and exercise are reversible. When individuals discontinue their exercise programs (detraining), exercise capacity diminishes quickly; and within a few months most of the training improvements are lost (i.e., **reversibility principle**).

The Art and Science of Exercise Prescription

Traditionally, some exercise specialists have focused on rigidly applying scientific principles of exercise prescription and devoted little or no attention to the *art* of exercise prescription. As an exercise programming artist, you need to be creative, flexible, and able to modify the exercise prescription based on your client's goals, behaviors, and responses to the exercise. Using both a scientific and an artistic approach will enable you to personalize the exercise prescription, increasing the probability of your clients' making long-term commitments to including physical activity and exercise as an indispensable part of their lifestyles.

Basic Elements of the Exercise Prescription

Although prescriptions are individualized for each client, there are basic elements common to all exercise prescriptions. These basic elements include mode, intensity, duration, frequency, and progression.

Mode

As mentioned earlier, the specificity-of-training principle implies that certain types of exercise training are better suited than others to developing specific components of physical fitness. Table 3.2 presents types of training and examples of exercise modes that optimize improvements for each physical fitness component.

To promote changes in body composition and bone strength, many experts recommend using more than one type of exercise training. For body composition changes, you should prescribe a combination of aerobic exercise to reduce body fat

Table 3.2 Types of Training and Exercise Modes for Improving Physical Fitness Components

Physical fitness component	Type of training	Exercise modes
Cardiorespiratory endurance	Aerobic exercise	Walking, jogging, cycling, rowing, stair climbing, simulated cross-country skiing, aerobic dance, step aerobics, and elliptical activity
Muscular strength and muscular endurance	Resistance exercise	Free weights, exercise machines, and exercise bands
Bone strength	Weight-bearing aerobic exercise and resistance exercise	Walking, jogging, aerobic dance, step aerobics, stair climbing, simulated cross-country skiing, free weights, and exercise machines
Body composition	Aerobic exercise and resistance exercise	Same modes as listed for cardiorespiratory endurance and muscular strength
Flexibility	Stretching exercise	Static stretches, PNF stretches, yoga, tai chi, and Pilates
Balance	Balance training	Tai chi, yoga, Pilates, and balance exercises

PNF = proprioceptive neuromuscular facilitation.

and resistance exercise to build muscle and bone. Similarly, weight-bearing, aerobic activities and resistance training are both effective for building bone mass for improved bone health.

Intensity

Exercise intensity dictates the specific physiological and metabolic changes in the body during exercise training. As mentioned previously, the initial exercise intensity in the exercise prescription depends on the client's program goals, age, capabilities, preferences, and fitness level and should stress, but not overtax, the cardiopulmonary and musculoskeletal systems. Later chapters provide detailed information and guidelines on selecting exercise intensities for the development of each physical fitness component, as well as for the progression of exercise intensity.

Duration

Duration and intensity of exercise are inversely related; the higher the intensity, the shorter the duration of the exercise. Exercise duration depends not only on the intensity of exercise but also on the client's health status, initial fitness level, functional capability, and program goals. For improved health benefits, the American College of Sports Medicine (ACSM) and the American Heart Association (Nelson et al. 2007) recommend that every individual accumulate 150 min/wk or more of moderate-intensity aerobic exercise. This amount

of physical activity can be achieved in either one continuous bout (30 min) of exercise on each of 5 days or in multiple bouts of shorter duration throughout the day (e.g., 10 min bouts, three times a day), depending on the client's functional capacity and time constraints.

As the client adapts to the exercise training, the duration of exercise may be slowly increased about every 2 or 3 wk. For older and less fit individuals, ACSM (2010) recommends increasing exercise duration, rather than intensity, in the initial stages of the exercise program. For most clients, the duration of aerobic, resistance, and flexibility exercise workouts should not exceed 60 min. This will lessen the chance of overuse injuries and exercise "burnout."

Frequency

Frequency typically refers to the total number of weekly exercise sessions. Research shows that exercising 3 days a week on alternate days is sufficient to improve various components of physical fitness. However, frequency is related to the duration and intensity of exercise and varies depending on the client's program goals and preferences, time constraints, and functional capacity. Sedentary clients with poor initial fitness levels may exercise more than once a day. When improved health is the primary goal of the exercise program, ACSM and the American Heart Association (AHA) recommend either 3 days/wk of vigorous-intensity exercise or

5 days/wk of moderate-intensity exercise. If you prescribe daily physical activity for an apparently healthy client, it is important to vary the type of exercise (i.e., aerobic, resistance, flexibility, and balance exercises) or exercise mode (e.g., walking, cycling, and weightlifting) to lessen the risk of overuse injuries to the bones, joints, and muscles.

Progression of Exercise

Throughout the exercise program, physiological and metabolic changes enable the individual to perform more work. For continued improvements, the cardiopulmonary and musculoskeletal systems must be progressively overloaded through periodic increases in the frequency, intensity, and duration of the exercise.

When applying the principle of progression to an exercise prescription, you should increase the frequency, intensity, and duration gradually, and you should do so one element at a time. A simultaneous increase in frequency, intensity, and duration, or in any combination of these elements, may overtax the individual's physiological systems, thereby increasing the risk of exercise-related injuries and exercise burnout. Generally, for older and less fit clients, it is better to increase exercise duration, instead of exercise intensity, especially during the initial stage of their exercise prescriptions.

Stages of Progression in the Exercise Program

Most individualized exercise programs include initial conditioning, improvement, and maintenance stages. The **initial conditioning stage** typically lasts 1 to 6 wk and serves as a primer to familiarize the client with exercise training. During this stage, you should prescribe stretching exercises, light calisthenics, and low-intensity aerobic or resistance exercises. Have your clients progress slowly by increasing exercise duration first, followed by small increases in exercise intensity. The initial stage of the exercise program may be skipped for some physically active individuals provided that their initial fitness level is good to excellent and that they are accustomed to the exercise modes prescribed for their programs.

The **improvement stage** of the exercise program typically lasts 4 to 8 mo, and the rate of progression is more rapid than in the initial conditioning stage.

During this stage, the frequency, intensity, and duration are systematically and slowly advanced, one element at a time, until the client's fitness goal is reached.

The **maintenance stage** of the exercise program is designed to preserve the level of fitness achieved by the client at the end of the improvement stage. This stage should continue on a regular, long-term basis. The amount of exercise required to maintain the client's physical fitness level is less than that needed to improve specific fitness components. Thus, the frequency of a specific mode of exercise used to develop any given fitness component can be decreased and that mode replaced with other types of physical activities. By the end of the improvement stage, for example, a client may be jogging 5 days a week. For maintenance, jogging may be reduced to 2 or 3 days a week, and different aerobic activities (e.g., in-line skating and stair climbing) or other types of exercise and sport activities (e.g., weightlifting or tennis) may be substituted the other 3 days. Including a variety of enjoyable physical activities during this stage helps to counteract boredom and to maintain the client's interest level.

EXERCISE PROGRAM ADHERENCE

Exercise professionals face the challenge of convincing individuals to start exercising and getting them to make a lifelong commitment to a physically active lifestyle. Approximately one of every two adults (49%) in the United States does not get the recommended amount of physical activity, and 24% of the adult population report no physical activity at all (CDC 2005). Exercise specialists play an important role in educating the public about why regular physical activity is absolutely essential for good health and how to exercise safely and effectively.

Of those individuals starting an exercise program, almost 50% will drop out within 1 yr. As an exercise specialist, you must help the client to develop a positive attitude toward physical activity and to make a firm commitment to the exercise program. To increase adherence, you need to be aware of factors related to exercise attrition.

Many factors influence regular participation in physical activity and adherence to an exercise program (see table 3.3). Knowing the factors associated

Table 3.3 Factors Related to Physical Activity Participation and Exercise Program Adherence

Category	Positive factors	Negative factors
Demographic and biological	Education Gender[a] Socioeconomic status	Age Race[b] Overweight or obesity
Psychological, cognitive, emotional	Enjoyment of exercise Expected benefits of exercise Perceived health and fitness Self-efficacy Self-motivation	Barriers to exercise Mood disturbance
Behavioral	Activity history during adulthood Healthy dietary habits	Smoking
Social-cultural	Physician influence Support from spouse, family, friends, or peers	Social isolation
Environmental	Access to exercise facilities Satisfaction with exercise facility Exercise equipment at home Enjoyable scenery Observing others exercising Neighborhood safety	Climate or season Urban location
Program	Exercise leadership and supervision Variety of exercise modes and activities	Initial exercise intensity Perceived effort

[a]Males are more likely to be physically active than females.

[b]Whites are more physically active than non-whites.

Data compiled from comprehensive reviews of research studies dealing with this topic (Sallis and Owen 1999; Trost et al. 2002).

with continued participation in physical activity will direct your approach and the steps you take in order to facilitate your clients' adherence to their exercise programs. You should focus on factors that are potentially modifiable such as exercise facilities; program variables (e.g., exercise intensity and perceived exertion); enjoyable scenery during exercise; and support from spouse, family, friends, and peers.

As an exercise specialist, you also need to understand and implement psychological models related to successful behavior change. For an excellent overview of behavior change theories and discussion of strategies you can use to help your clients adopt and maintain a physically active lifestyle, see Napolitano and colleagues 2010. The following are models that may be useful for encouraging exercise and improving adherence to exercise:

- Behavior modification
- Health belief model
- Social cognitive model

- Transtheoretical model of health behavior change (stages of motivational readiness for change)
- Decision-making theory
- Theory of reasoned action and theory of planned behavior
- Self-determination theory

With use of the behavior modification model, clients become actively involved in the change process by setting realistic short- and long-term goals, developing a plan to achieve these goals, and signing a contract that describes each goal and how it may be achieved. Throughout the exercise program, you should provide your client with feedback and revise the plan as needed. You can help your clients adopt physical activity into their lifestyle by implementing behavior counseling strategies such as having clients keep a diary of their physical activity and developing a social support system for a client. Sometimes it can be effective to give rewards like

T-shirts, certificates, emblems, and pins to recognize the attainment of specific goals, such as walking a total of 50 mi (80.5 km) in 1 mo. Help your client set both short-term and long-term goals that are attainable. For this purpose, you can periodically reevaluate your client's fitness levels to assess improvement. You can state goals in performance or physiological terms. An example of a short-term performance goal is to complete a 3 mi (4.8 km) fun run in less than 33 min. A long-term physiological goal might be to increase maximum oxygen uptake ($\dot{V}O_2$max) by 15% in 4 mo. As the exercise specialist, you must help each individual set realistic goals.

The **health belief model** is based on the assumption that individuals will engage in exercise on a regular basis because they perceive the threat of disease and believe that this threat is severe and that they are susceptible to disease. When the benefits outweigh the barriers, individuals will take action and adopt exercise into their lifestyle. Self-efficacy and cues to action are important components of this model (ACSM 2010).

The **social cognitive model**, developed by Bandura (1982), is based on the concepts of self-efficacy and outcome expectation. The likelihood that people will engage in a specific behavior, like exercising regularly, depends on their **self-efficacy** or perception of their ability to perform the task, as well as their confidence about making the behavioral change (Grembowski et al. 1993). To assess self-efficacy, have your clients rate, on a scale of 0% to 100%, their confidence in making the specific behavior change. Individuals with high self-efficacy ratings (70%) believe they have the knowledge and skill to exercise successfully. As a result, they are more likely to succeed in making a long-term behavior change. To increase self-efficacy, you should educate your clients so that they fully understand their beliefs and should help them identify specific barriers to engaging in physical activity. Techniques to improve your client's exercise self-efficacy include performance mastery (e.g., teach your clients scientifically sound and safe exercise principles and techniques and allow them to practice these techniques); modeling (e.g., give clients an opportunity to observe role models who are performing the exercise successfully); positive reinforcement (e.g., compliment clients when they perform activities correctly or improve a specific physical fitness component); and emotional arousal (e.g., educate clients about the health benefits of

physical activity and exercise). Schlicht, Godin, and Camaione (1999) provide more detailed descriptions of how you can incorporate these techniques into your clients' exercise programs.

The **transtheoretical model** describes the process that clients go through when adopting a change in health behavior (e.g., exercising). The following are the basic concepts of this model:

- Clients progress through five stages of change at different rates.
- In this process, clients may move back and forth through the stages of change.
- Clients use different cognitive and behavioral strategies in this process.
- Clients weigh the costs and benefits of the health behavior change.

To effectively apply this model, the exercise specialist needs to be aware of the client's stage of readiness for participating in exercise. The **stages of motivational readiness for change model** is based on the premise that individuals move through a series of stages as they adopt and maintain a new habit (Prochaska and DiClemente 1982). This model has been used to facilitate long-term changes in health behaviors such as smoking, weight management, dietary modification, and stress management (Riebe and Niggs 1998) as well as in physical activity behaviors (Dunn et al. 1999; Marcus et al. 1998). Your clients' abilities to make a long-term commitment to an exercise program or to daily physical activity are based on their motivational readiness for change. The following example illustrates the five stages of motivational readiness in terms of changing exercise behavior:

1. **Precontemplation:** Client does not exercise and does not intend to start exercising.
2. **Contemplation:** Client is not exercising but intends to start.
3. **Preparation:** Client is exercising but is not meeting the recommended amount of physical activity.
4. **Action:** Client has been performing the recommended amount of exercise regularly for less than 6 mo.
5. **Maintenance:** Client has been exercising regularly at the recommended amount for 6 mo or longer.

Individuals are at different stages of readiness for change; therefore, you need to match intervention strategies to the client's stage and tailor your approach to meet the individual's needs, interests, and concerns. Detailed descriptions of how to plan and deliver physical activity intervention strategies specific to the stages of change are available (see ACSM 2010; Marcus and Forsyth 2003; Marcus and Lewis 2003).

The **decision-making theory** proposes that individuals decide whether or not to engage in a behavior by weighing the perceived benefits and costs of that behavior. Clients are more likely to exercise when they perceive that the benefits outweigh the costs (e.g., "I feel better about myself when I exercise even though it takes time from my busy schedule"). Clients in early stages of motivational change (e.g., precontemplation stage) tend to perceive more disadvantages compared to clients in later stages (e.g., action stage) of change (Marcus and Forsyth 2003). To assess your clients' motivational readiness and decisional balance for exercise, you may use a 16-item self-report tool (see Marcus, Rakowski, and Rossi 1992).

The **theory of reasoned action** proposes a way to understand and predict an individual's behavior. According to this theory, intention is the most important determinant of behavior; intention is highly influenced by the individual's attitudes and subjective behavioral norms. For example, believing that exercise results in positive outcomes leads to a favorable attitude about engaging in physical activity and the intention to do so. Subjective behavioral norms, or perceptions about what others think or believe about exercise, also may influence your client's intention (Downs 2006). The **theory of planned behavior** extends the theory of reasoned action by taking into consideration the client's perception of behavioral control (i.e., perceived power and control belief). This theory proposes that individuals intend to perform a specific behavior (e.g., exercising) if they evaluate it positively (e.g., attitude), believe that others think it is important (subjective norms), and perceive the behavior to be under their control (e.g., power). Although these theories provide useful information about the role of intention for adopting exercise behavior, intention alone is insufficient for predicting whether or not your client will engage in physical activity on a regular basis (Napolitano et al. 2010).

In helping your clients adopt and maintain a physically active lifestyle, it is also important to understand their motivation or degree of determination for changing or avoiding this behavior. Motivation is a complex construct; it may be described as falling along a continuum, ranging from no motivation (i.e., amotivation) to intrinsic motivation. The **self-determination theory** describes how the presence or absence of specific psychological needs (i.e., autonomy, competence, and relatedness) affects behavior through a continuum of motivation (Deci and Ryan 2000). According to this theory, four levels of motivation with respect to exercise may be identified (Mears and Kilpatrick 2008):

1. Amotivation: The individual has no intention or desire to engage in exercise.
2. Other-determined motivation: The individual is motivated to exercise by outside factors such as rewards, guilt, fear, or pressure; long-term adherence is unlikely. Possible motives for exercising may be "I exercise to lose weight" or "My partner thinks I should exercise more."
3. Self-determined extrinsic motivation: The individual values exercise, is motivated by extrinsic factors like improved health or gains in fitness, and freely chooses (i.e., autonomously) to exercise without a sense of outside pressure. A possible motive for exercising may be "I exercise because it is an important part of my healthy lifestyle."
4. Intrinsic motivation: The individual engages in exercise for the sheer enjoyment and satisfaction it brings to his or her sense of well-being; enjoying exercise for its own sake leads to adherence. The probable motive for exercising is "I am a physically active person, and I exercise because I like doing it."

The ultimate goal of this approach is to get clients to value physical activity and to think of themselves as exercisers rather than using exercise to attain an external goal like weight loss. Some individuals may never reach the point of exercising for sheer enjoyment of the activity; however, valuing exercise may be enough to get clients to adhere to their exercise regimens (Rodgers and Loitz 2009).

Questionnaires have been developed to assess your client's exercise motivation. The *Behavioral Regulation in Exercise Questionnaire* measures your client's level of motivation on the continuum ranging from amotivation to intrinsic motivation

(Markland and Tobin 2004). The *Exercise Motivation Inventory* identifies and measures specific motives (i.e., guilt, enjoyment, fitness) for engaging in exercise (Markland and Ingledew 1997). You can use results from questionnaires to help your clients understand their level of motivation and to develop ways to improve their exercise motivation. Rodgers and Loitz (2009) offer suggestions and steps you can take to understand and improve your client's motivation to exercise (see "Tips to Enhance Exercise Motivation").

Tips to Enhance Exercise Motivation (Rodgers and Loitz 2009)

Try to understand why the client is there:

- Is the motive an external one? Try to move the client's focus to a value motive.
- Focus on integrating the exercise with the client's sense of self.

Create opportunities to experience competence:

- Put clients in a position where they can easily see and hear you and receive direction from you.
- Celebrate meaningful successes; don't overemphasize trivial accomplishments.
- Use clear, appropriate communication strategies; avoid jargon.
- Be respectful of your client's efforts.

Create opportunities for autonomy:

- Give choices and options.
- Relate the exercises to your client's goals.
- Avoid coercive and controlling encouragement.

Create opportunities for relatedness:

- Introduce the client to other participants.
- Give tips and instructions on the expected behavior, including proper etiquette.
- Communicate understanding of your client's perspective.

Bottom line:

- Pay attention to factors that create opportunities for your clients to feel competent, related, and autonomous.
- Encourage value motives for exercising; downplay external reasons for exercising.

As an exercise specialist, you need to integrate principles from each of these models and implement strategies to improve your clients' exercise program adherence. The ACSM (2006) recommends program modifications and motivational strategies to increase long-term adherence to an exercise program (see "Strategies to Increase Exercise Program Adherence"). The key to increasing exercise program adherence lies in the leadership, education, and motivation that you provide. First, you must be a positive role model. You also must be knowledgeable, able to educate clients about exercise and fitness, and able to provide motivation and encourage social support.

Strategies to Increase Exercise Program Adherence

- Recruiting physician support of the exercise program
- Prescribing moderate-intensity exercise to minimize injury and complications
- Advocating exercising with others
- Offering a variety of exercise and fitness activities that are enjoyable
- Providing positive reinforcement through periodic testing
- Recruiting support of the program from clients' families and friends
- Adding optional recreational games to the conditioning program
- Using progress charts to record exercise achievements
- Establishing a reward system to recognize participant accomplishments
- Providing qualified exercise professionals who are well trained, innovative, and enthusiastic

---

USING TECHNOLOGY TO PROMOTE PHYSICAL ACTIVITY

Technology is a double-edged sword. Computers, for example, contribute to sedentary leisure-time behaviors (e.g., playing sedentary computer games). On the other hand, technology has been used to promote physical activity and change exercise behavior. For years, pedometers, accelerometers, and heart rate monitors have been used as motivational tools. Newer technologies and approaches being used to promote physical activity include global positioning system (GPS), geographic information systems (GIS), interactive video games, and persuasive technology. Also, experts suggest that Internet-based physical activity interventions should be used by clinicians to promote and change exercise behavior (Marcus, Ciccolo, and Sciamanna 2009).

Pedometers

Pedometers count and monitor the number of steps taken throughout the day. Most pedometers provide a fairly accurate count of steps taken during ambulatory activities such as walking, jogging, and running. Estimates of the distance walked and caloric expenditure are less accurate. Some newer devices also provide an estimate of the total time spent during continuous walking at a moderate intensity for durations of 10 min or more. To provide accurate step counts, most pedometers need to be attached to a firm waistband; however, some can be carried in a shirt pocket, a pants pocket, or a bag held close to the body. Studies show that some pedometers provide a valid (bias <3%) and reliable (coefficient of variation <2.1%) measure of steps during constant- and variable-speed walking for both healthy and overweight adults when the pedometer is placed on the waistband (sides and back), in a shirt pocket, or around the neck; however, positioning the pedometer in a pants pocket or in a backpack decreases accuracy (Hasson et al. 2009; Holbrook, Barreira, and Kang 2009).

Studies show that pedometer-based walking increases physical activity (Williams et al. 2008). In a synthesis of studies addressing the use of pedom-

eters to increase physical activity, Bravata and colleagues (2007) reported that on average, pedometer users increase their physical activity by 27% over baseline levels. A key predictor of increased physical activity is setting a step goal (e.g., 10,000 steps per day) for participants. Pedometer-based walking programs are associated with significant decreases in body mass index, body weight, and systolic blood pressure (Bravata et al. 2007; Richardson et al. 2008).

Thresholds for health benefits from walking have been established using pedometers. Accumulating 8000 to 9000 steps per day at a rate of no less than 100 steps·min^{-1} is equivalent to 30 min of moderate physical activity, the health benefit threshold. For weight loss, accumulating 11,000 to 13,000 steps per day is recommended. Using criterion-referenced approaches, youth-specific thresholds for good health are being established. In the future, minimal levels of steps per day may be used to identify health risk thresholds for cardiovascular diseases, obesity, and osteoporosis. Table 3.4 presents classification of physical activity levels for adults and children based on the number of steps taken daily (Tudor-Locke et al. 2005, 2008). Additional information about the validity and accuracy of pedometers is available (Holbrook, Barreira, and Kang 2009; Lamonte, Ainsworth, and Reis 2006; Tudor-Locke et al. 2002, 2006).

Accelerometers

Accelerometers record body acceleration minute to minute, providing detailed information about the frequency, duration, intensity, and patterns of movement. Counts from accelerometers are used to estimate energy expenditure. Recently, accelerometers were used to provide an objective measure of compliance with physical activity recommendations for the U.S. population (Troiano et al. 2008).

Table 3.4   Classification of Pedometer-Based Activity for Adults and Children

Classification[a]	Adults	Girls (6-12 yr)	Boys (6-12 yr)
Sedentary	<5000	<7000	<10,000
Low active	5000-7499	7000-9499	10,000-12,499
Somewhat active	7500-9999	9500-11,999	12,500-14,999
Active	10,000-12,499	12,000-14,499	15,000-17,499
Highly active	≥12,500	≥14,500	≥17,500

[a]These descriptors are used for adults; for children, the following descriptors are used: copper, bronze, silver, gold, and platinum (copper and platinum representing the lowest and highest levels of activity, respectively).

Accelerometer data indicated that less than 5% of adults in the United States engaged in 30 min per day of moderate exercise, 5 to 7 days per week. This is substantially lower than the self-reported value (49%) from national surveys. Also, only 8% of adolescents reached the goal of exercising 60 min per day, 5 to 7 days per week, based on accelerometer data. The relatively higher cost of accelerometers (about $300 per unit) compared to pedometers ($10 to $30 per unit) limits their use in large-scale physical activity interventions. In the future, lower-cost units may be developed and be more widely used in national surveys and community-based interventions. Detailed information about best practices and research recommendations for using accelerometers are available (see Ward et al. 2005).

Heart Rate Monitors

Heart rate monitors are used primarily to assess and monitor exercise intensity. These devices are especially useful for monitoring exercise intensity of individuals in cardiac rehabilitation programs and highly-trained, competitive athletes. Because heart rate is linearly related to oxygen uptake, it can be used to estimate the individual's exercise energy expenditure. However, estimates of energy expenditure from heart rate may be affected by factors such as temperature, humidity, hydration, and emotional stress.

Combined Heart Rate Monitoring and Accelerometry

The prediction of energy expenditure during physical activity is improved by 20% when data from heart rate monitors are used in conjunction with accelerometer measures of physical activity (Strath, Brage, and Ekelund 2005). New devices that simultaneously monitor heart rate and body motion provide valid and reliable measures of physical activity of children, adolescents, and adults in free-living conditions (Barreira et al. 2009; Crouter, Churilla, and Bassett 2008; Zakeri et al. 2008).

Global Positioning System and Geographic Information System

Global positioning system (GPS) uses 24 satellites and ground stations as reference points to calculate geographic locations and accurately track a specific activity. For example, using a portable GPS unit provides information about altitude, distance, time, and average velocity during hiking. A graph depicting the uphill and downhill portions of the terrain is also provided. Global positioning system can be used in conjunction with accelerometers to assess and monitor physical activity (Rodriguez, Brown, and Troped 2005; Schutz and Herren 2000; Troped et al. 2008). As small receivers become more affordable and accessible to the general public (e.g., in laptop computers and mobile telephones), GPS may be more widely used to assess and to promote physical activity.

The geographic information system (GIS) is a computer system that stores information about location and the surrounding environment. With use of GIS, the impact of the environment (i.e., its form and design) on physical activity can be assessed (Zhu 2008). Detailed information about using GIS to assess environmental supports for physical activity is available (Porter et al. 2004).

Interactive Video Games

Although interactive video games like Dance Dance Revolution (DDR), Wii Sports, and Wii Fit were designed to create more engaging game play, studies show that these games increase energy expenditure and may produce positive health benefits (Chamberlain and Gallagher 2008; Graves et al. 2007; Zhu 2008). Many fitness centers, schools, and senior centers are now offering interactive games to promote physical activity of children, adolescents, and older adults. These interactive games are well suited for playing alone or with others, require little training or skill, provide an alternative to exercising in bad weather, and may serve as a transition to actually participating in sport and physical activities (Chamberlain and Gallagher 2008). Warburton and colleagues (2009) reported that interactive video game cycling significantly increased steady-state heart rate and energy expenditure compared to traditional cycling at constant, submaximal workloads; the two forms of cycling (traditional and interactive video game cycling) resulted in similar ratings of perceived exertion.

Dance Dance Revolution is a video game with a floor pad controller that has a grid of arrow panels. Because dancing is a good aerobic activity, DDR has been used to promote physical activity and weight loss in obese children and adults (Epstein et al. 2007; Zhu 2008). On the basis of the popularity of DDR, Zhu (2008) reported that more than 1500 schools in the United States were planning to use DDR in physical education classes by the end of 2010. Sell and colleagues (2008) reported that energy expenditure of participants playing the DDR video game depends on their experience. On average, DDR was classified as a moderate-intensity (47% $\dot{V}O_2$ reserve and 10.5 kcal·min^{-1}) activity. For inexperienced participants, DDR was equivalent to light intensity (18% $\dot{V}O_2$ reserve and 4.8 kcal·min^{-1}).

Wii Sports is a home video game that uses a wireless, handheld remote controller to detect movement in multiple dimensions while mimicking sport activities. The games include tennis, golf, bowling, and boxing. Although playing Wii Sports will not burn as many calories as actually playing the sport, Wii bowling, tennis, golf, and boxing games increased energy expenditure by 2% compared to sedentary computer games (Graves et al. 2007). Also, energy expenditure and heart rate were significantly greater in Wii boxing (3.2 METs), bowling (2.2 METs), and tennis (2.4 METs) compared to values in sedentary (1.4 METs) gaming (Graves, Ridgers, and Stratton 2008)

In 2008, Wii Fit was launched by Nintendo. This interactive video game offers over 40 training activities categorized into four areas: aerobics (e.g., hula hoops and running), strength training (e.g., lunges and leg extensions), yoga, and balance training. This exercise game uses the handheld Wii remote controller and a balance board peripheral for some of the activities (e.g., running in place and yoga poses). In light of the positive response that Wii Sports and Wii Fit have received, many fitness centers, senior centers, hospitals, and physical therapy centers are now incorporating this interactive technology into their exercise and rehabilitation programs (Zhu 2008). Research is needed to assess the usefulness of interactive video game technology for promoting healthy behavior and physical activity of children, youth, and sedentary adults.

Persuasive Technology

Persuasive technology is defined as a computer system, device, or application that is intentionally designed to change a person's attitude or behavior (Fogg 2003). This technology uses tools (e.g., pedometer or balance board), media (e.g., video, audio, or both), and social interaction (e.g., playing with another person) to persuade individuals to adopt the behavior without their actually knowing it. Although the DDR was not developed specifically to promote physical activity, it has changed exercise attitudes and behavior of children and youth using principles of persuasive technology. Dance Dance Revolution uses video, music, and a dance platform to capture interest and engage children in the activity without their being fully aware that they are exercising. The emerging field of persuasive technology has enormous potential for promoting physical activity and healthy behaviors (Fogg and Eckles 2007; Zhu 2008).

EXERCISE SCIENCE AS A PROFESSION

Exercise professionals need to have extensive knowledge and technical skills in order to work safely and effectively. Historically, individuals working in exercise settings, such as health or fitness clubs, were not necessarily required to have specialized education and training in exercise science. However, survey research indicates that a bachelor's degree in exercise science and an ACSM or a National Strength and Conditioning Association (NSCA) certification are strong predictors of a personal trainer's knowledge. Contrary to popular belief, experience was not related to knowledge (Malek et al. 2002). These findings suggest that formal education and certification by professional organizations should be required for personal fitness trainers and exercise science professionals. To promote exercise science as a profession, issues surrounding accreditation, certification, National Boards, and licensure need to be understood and addressed.

Accreditation

Organizations and programs are awarded accreditation by meeting or exceeding standards established by an independent, third-party accrediting agency. In a survey designed to identify worldwide trends in the fitness field, Thompson (2008) reported that the number one trend for 2009 is having more fully accredited educational programs and certification programs for health/fitness and clinical exercise professionals. Exercise science professionals seem to agree that some form of regulation is needed.

Independent, third-party accrediting agencies such as the Commission on Accreditation of

Allied Health Education Programs (CAAHEP) and the National Commission for Certifying Agencies (NCCA) may serve this purpose. The CAAHEP accredits academic programs—graduate programs in exercise physiology, baccalaureate programs in exercise science, and certificate/associate degree programs for personal fitness trainers. Also, the American Society of Exercise Physiologists (ASEP) has developed standards of practice for exercise physiologists as well as accreditation standards for universities and colleges offering academic degrees in exercise science (American Society of Exercise Physiologists 2004; Wattles 2002). The NCCA accredits certification programs; many organizations that provide professional credentialing or licensing exams in the allied health professions are accredited through the NCCA.

Certification

Fitness and exercise science professionals obtain certification(s) by passing examinations developed by professional organizations. These organizations typically offer education and training programs, administer their own examinations (written, practical, or both), and issue certifications to individuals passing the examinations. These certifications are generally issued for a 2 yr period; people maintain certification by taking continuing education courses. Some certification programs are accredited by third-party agencies like the NCCA.

There are more than 75 organizations offering over 250 certifications for exercise science and fitness professionals (Cohen 2004; Pierce and Herman 2004). Given that there is no governing entity to oversee the development of certification examinations and eligibility requirements, inequalities exist among the certifications available to exercise science professionals. Some certification programs are more rigorous than others, having stringent eligibility requirements; others may or may not be accredited by a third-party accrediting agency like the NCCA. To address the inequality among certification programs, the NCCA formally reviews applications for the accreditation of certification programs. In 2004, the International Health, Racquet, and Sportsclub Association (IHRSA) recommended that all health clubs belonging to their organization hire only personal fitness trainers certified by an NCCA-accredited organization or agency. The bottom line is that all exercise science and fitness certifications are not equal. This leads to confusion for the consumer in terms of knowing who is and who is not highly trained and qualified as an exercise professional. It also complicates selecting the most appropriate certification for oneself. Some agencies sponsor certification programs primarily for financial gain while others certify professionals in order to promote exercise science as a profession. Table 3.5 lists some of the organizations that offer certifications accredited by the NCCA.

National Boards

Some professional organizations in the fitness industry believe that there should be alternatives

---

Table 3.5 Selected Organizations Associated With NCCA and NBFE

NCCA affiliates	NBFE affiliates
American Council on Exercise (ACE)	Aerobics and Fitness Association of America (AFAA)
American College of Sports Medicine (ACSM)	American Aerobic Association International/International Sports Medicine Association (AAAI/ISMA)
Cooper Institute for Aerobics Research	International Sports Sciences Association (ISSA)
National Exercise and Sport Trainers Association (NESTA)	National Association for Fitness Certification (NAFC)
National Exercise Trainers Association (NETA)	National Council for Certified Personal Trainers (NCCPT)
National Federation of Professional Trainers (NFPT)	National Exercise and Sports Trainers Association (NESTA)
National Strength and Conditioning Association (NSCA)	National Gym Association (NGA)
International Fitness Professionals Association (IFPA)	National Personal Training Institute
National Council on Strength and Fitness (NCSF)	National Strength Professionals Association (NSPA)
National Academy of Sports Medicine (NASM)	World Instructor Training Schools (WITS)

to accreditation of certification programs by the NCCA or other third-party agencies. One such alternative is the establishment of National Board examinations for fitness professionals. Unlike the multitude of certification examinations developed by individual organizations and agencies, National Boards are standardized tests used to assess the knowledge, skill, and competence of professionals. Most medical and allied health professions utilize National Boards.

In 2003, the National Board of Fitness Examiners (NBFE) was founded as a nonprofit organization with the twin purposes of defining scopes of practice for all fitness professionals and determining standards of practice for various fitness professionals including floor instructors, group exercise instructors, personal fitness trainers, specialists in youth and senior fitness, and medical exercise specialists. The NBFE established national standards of excellence that certifying organizations and colleges or universities may adopt. The written portion of the National Boards for personal fitness trainers is now offered through the NBFE (for additional information, visit www.NBFE.org). The practical portion of this exam is still being developed and validated under the supervision of the National Board of Medical Examiners (NBME). The NBME and the NBFE are engaged in preliminary discussions and planning that will allow certification organizations to assist in the delivery of practical exams for personal trainers.

To be eligible to sit for the National Boards, personal fitness trainers must successfully complete a personal training certification program from an approved NBFE affiliate. Affiliate status is available to qualified groups from the areas of medicine, certification organizations, fitness professionals, health clubs, and higher education. In the future, the NBFE's National Boards may be used by certifying organizations, colleges and universities, and state licensing programs to test the knowledge, skill, and competence of fitness professionals (American Fitness Professionals and Associates 2004). Table 3.5 lists some of the organizations offering personal training certifications that are affiliated with the NBFE.

Licensure

Although many practitioners in the fitness and exercise science fields agree that certification ensures professional competency, other professionals believe that licensure is better suited for protecting consumers and for enhancing the credibility and professionalism of exercise science and fitness professionals (Eickhoff-Shemek and Herbert 2007). Licensure is decided at the state level; therefore, requirements may vary from state to state. Louisiana was the first state in the United States to pass a law requiring licensure of all clinical exercise physiologists (Herbert 1995). Licensure of clinical exercise physiologists also has been considered in Kentucky, Massachusetts, North Carolina, and Utah. In addition, Georgia, Maryland, Massachusetts, New Jersey, Nevada, and Oregon have considered licensure for personal trainers (Eickhoff-Shemek and Herbert 2008b; Herbert 2004).

To promote exercise science and exercise physiology as a profession, ASEP is working with exercise professionals throughout the United States to develop uniform state licensure requirements for exercise physiologists. Licensure would place exercise physiologists and personal trainers on a par with other allied health professionals (e.g., nurses, nutritionists, physical therapists, and occupational therapists) who are required to have licenses to practice. Licensed fitness professionals may be more likely to obtain referrals from health care professionals and to receive reimbursement for services from third parties (e.g., insurance companies). Along with advantages, there are added responsibilities and disadvantages associated with state licensure. Licensure may limit the scope of practice and services that exercise professionals are currently able to provide to the public. For example, Louisiana licensure law requires clinical exercise physiologists to work under the direction of a licensed physician. Also, the costs of licensure, continuing education for licensure, and professional liability insurance may be greater than the cost of certifications. Professionals moving from one state to another may be required obtain another license because each state could require different credentials for licensure (Eickhoff-Shemek and Herbert 2008a, 2008b).

Statutory Certification

Instead of licensure, some states use statutory certification for allied health professionals. Statutory certification regulates what titles professionals can use and the qualifications needed to obtain these titles. Only certified professionals with the required credentials are allowed to use the specific title (e.g., certified nutritionist). Other professionals without the necessary credentials can still practice in the state but must use a different title. This approach could be promoted by the fitness and exercise professions to prevent the use of titles, such as personal trainer or exercise physiologist, by individuals having no formal education or professional certifications.

All of these approaches demonstrate that there is an urgent need to get a handle on certifications for exercise professionals so that we gain control of who is practicing in our field. This will ensure the safety of exercise program participants and enable individuals working in the fitness field to be recognized as exercise science professionals. Until these issues are resolved and a list of accredited certification agencies and organizations is finalized, you should select a professional certification that matches your level of education and career goals. Table 3.6 compares certifications offered by selected professional organizations. For more information about certification programs, visit the Web sites of professional organizations (addresses are listed in appendix A.7, p. 332).

Many advantages are associated with obtaining either state licensure or certification by professional organizations. You will have a better chance of finding

Table 3.6   Comparison of Professional Certifications

Professional organization	Certification	ELIGIBILITY REQUIREMENTS			Scope of practice
		Education	Field	Experience	
ACSM (www.acsm.org)	Certified Personal Trainer (PT)	High school diploma or equivalent	NA	18 yr or older; current adult CPR certification with practical skills component	Lead and demonstrate safe and effective methods of exercise; write exercise recommendations; motivate clients to adopt and maintain healthy behaviors
	Certified Health Fitness Specialist (HFS)	2 or 4 yr associate's or bachelor's degree	Health related	Current CPR certification with practical skills component	Conduct risk stratification and fitness assessments; prescribe exercise programs for apparently healthy clients with or without medically controlled diseases; motivate clients to adopt and maintain healthy behaviors
	Certified Clinical Exercise Specialist (CES)	4 yr bachelor's degree	Allied health	600 hr in clinical exercise program or clinical exercise testing; current certification as Basic Life Support Provider or CPR for Professional Rescuer	Identify risk factors; conduct exercise assessment; deliver training, rehabilitation, and lifestyle management services
	Registered Clinical Exercise Physiologist (RCEP)	Graduate degree	Exercise science, exercise physiology, or kinesiology	Either ACSM CES certification or 600 hr of clinical experience; current certification as Basic Life Support Provider or CPR for Professional Rescuer	Perform exercise testing, exercise prescription, exercise and physical activity counseling, exercise supervision, exercise and health education, and evaluation of exercise and physical activity outcome measures
ACSM/ACS (www.acsm.org)	Cancer Exercise Trainer (CET)	4 yr bachelor's degree **or** No degree	Any field	500 hr training older adults or individuals with chronic conditions **or** 10,000 hr training older adults or individuals with chronic conditions; current certification in adult CPR and AED	Train adults diagnosed with cancer and apparently healthy adults or adults with known stable CV diseases; perform fitness assessments and design and modify exercise programs based on the cancer diagnosis and treatment

Professional organization	Certification	Education	Field	Experience	Scope of practice
ACSM/NCPAD (www.acsm.org)	Certified Inclusive Fitness Trainer (CIFT)	NA	NA	Current ACSM certification or current NCCA-accredited fitness-related certification; current adult CPR and AED with practical skills component	Assess, develop, and implement exercise programs for persons with physical, sensory, or cognitive disability; lead safe, effective, adapted methods of exercise; write adapted exercise recommendations
ACE (www.acefitness.org)	Group Fitness Instructor	NA	NA	18 yr or older; current CPR and AED certification	Teach safe and effective group fitness classes
	Personal Trainer	NA	NA	18 yr or older; current CPR and AED certification	Provide one-on-one or small-group fitness instruction
	Advanced Health & Fitness Specialist	4 yr bachelor's degree or ACE certification*	Exercise science or related field	18 yr or older; current CPR and AED certification; 300 hr of related experience	Design and implement exercise programs for healthy individuals or high-risk individuals, or both
	Lifestyle + Weight Management Consultant	4 yr bachelor's degree or ACE certification*	Exercise science or related field	18 yr or older; current CPR and AED certification	Develop sound, balanced weight management programs incorporating nutrition, exercise, and lifestyle change; identify lifestyle barriers and design plans to overcome them
ASEP (www.asep.org)	Exercise Physiologist Certified (EPC)	4 yr degree with grade of C or better in five of nine core courses	Exercise physiology or exercise science	Current membership in ASEP	Measure, examine, analyze, and instruct to evaluate and improve physical fitness components of both apparently healthy and at-risk individuals as well as persons with known disease
CSEP (www.csep.ca)	Certified Personal Trainer (CSEP CPT)	2 yr college diploma or 2 yr university degree credits in seven core areas	NA	Current CPR and first aid certification	Administer the CPAFLA to healthy populations; develop and implement a tailored physical activity and fitness plan
	Certified Exercise Physiologist (CSEP CEP)	4 yr university degree	Exercise science, physical activity, kinesiology, or human kinetics	300+ hr of fitness-related experience with healthy populations and populations with medical conditions or disability; current CPR at Basic Rescuer Level and first aid certification	Assess, prescribe, and supervise exercise; provide counseling and healthy lifestyle education for apparently healthy individuals, populations with medical conditions or disabilities, or both
NSCA (www.nsca-cc.org)	Certified Strength and Conditioning Specialist (CSCS)	4 yr bachelor's degree or chiropractic medicine degree	Any field	Current CPR and AED certification with practical skills component	Design and implement safe and effective strength and conditioning programs for athletes
	Certified Personal Trainer (CPT)	High school diploma or equivalent	NA	18 yr or older; current CPR and AED certification with practical skills component	Assess, motivate, educate, and train clients about health and fitness; design safe and effective exercise programs

*Currently holding one of the following ACE certifications: Personal Trainer, Lifestyle + Weight Management Consultant, Advanced Health & Fitness Specialist, Group Fitness Instructor, or a NCCA-accredited certification.

ACSM = American College of Sports Medicine; ACE = American Council on Exercise; ACS = American Cancer Society; ASEP = American Society of Exercise Physiologists; CPAFLA = Canadian Physical Activity and Fitness Lifestyle Assessment; CSEP = Canadian Society for Exercise Physiology; NA = not applicable; NCPAD = National Center on Physical Activity and Disability; NSCA = National Strength and Conditioning Association.

a job in the health and fitness fields because many employers are now hiring only professionally certified health and fitness instructors. Certification by reputable professional organizations upgrades the quality of the typical person working in the field and assures employers and their clientele that employees have mastered the knowledge and skills needed to be competent exercise science professionals. Hence, the likelihood of lawsuits resulting from negligence or incompetence may be lessened. Also, certification and licensure help to validate exercise specialists as health professionals who are deserving of the respect afforded to professionals in other allied health professions.

KEY POINTS

- The essential components of physical fitness are cardiorespiratory endurance, musculoskeletal fitness, body composition, flexibility, and balance.

- Valid, reliable, and objective laboratory and field tests have been developed to assess each fitness component.

- Test validity refers to the ability of a physical fitness test to accurately measure a specific fitness component.

- Test reliability is the ability of a test to yield consistent and stable scores across trials and over time.

- Objective tests give similar test scores when different technicians administer the test to the same client.

- All physical fitness prediction equations need to be validated and cross-validated to determine their applicability and suitability for use in the field.

- The line of best fit is a regression line depicting a linear relationship between a reference measure and all of the predictor variables in the regression equation.

- The *SEE* is a type of prediction error that reflects the degree of deviation of individual data points around the line of best fit or regression line.

- The *TE* is a type of prediction error that reflects the degree of deviation of individual data points around the line of identity.

- Sensitivity and specificity are measures of the ability of a test to correctly identify individuals with and without risk factors for diseases.

- Standard evaluation criteria are used to judge the relative worth of newly developed physical fitness tests and prediction equations.

- The Bland and Altman method evaluates how well a prediction equation works for estimating a physical fitness component of an individual within a group.

- To obtain valid and reliable test results, one must follow standardized testing procedures and have technical skills.

- Established norms for most tests are available and are used to classify physical fitness status based on the client's test scores.

- When interpreting test results to clients, one needs to be positive and to use simple, nontechnical terms.

- To design an effective exercise program, it is necessary to understand and apply training principles. These principles include specificity, overload, progression, initial values, interindividual variability, diminishing returns, and reversibility.

- The basic elements of an exercise prescription are mode, intensity, duration, and frequency.

- The exercise prescription should be individualized to meet the needs, interests, and abilities of the client.

- The three stages of an exercise program are initial conditioning, improvement, and maintenance.

- Throughout the improvement stage of an exercise program, the frequency, intensity, and duration of exercise are increased, one at a time.

- Physical activity participation and exercise adherence are related to demographic, biological, psychological, cognitive, emotional, behavioral, social, cultural, and environmental factors.

- When developing strategies for increasing exercise program adherence, it is important to integrate principles and concepts from psychological models and theories related to successful behavior change.

- To promote physical activity participation and adherence, pedometers, accelerometers, heart rate monitors, GPS, and GIS can be used.

■ Persuasive technology uses tools, media, and social interaction to promote physical activity and healthy behaviors.

■ Accreditation, professional certification, and licensure are ways to ensure competency of professionals working in the exercise science field.

KEY TERMS

Learn the definition for each of the following key terms. Definitions of key terms can be found in the glossary on page 411.

accelerometer

balance

behavior modification model

bias

Bland and Altman method

body composition

body weight

bone strength

cardiorespiratory endurance

constant error *(CE)*

criterion method

decision-making theory

diminishing return principle

false negative

false positive

flexibility

functional balance

generalized prediction equations

geographic information system (GIS)

global positioning system (GPS)

health belief model

heart rate monitor

improvement stage

initial conditioning stage

initial values principle

interindividual variability principle

limits of agreement

line of best fit

line of identity

maintenance stage

maximum oxygen consumption

multiple correlation coefficient (R_{mc})

muscular endurance

muscular strength

musculoskeletal fitness

objectivity

objectivity coefficient

overload principle

pedometer

persuasive technology

physical fitness

population-specific equations

progression principle

reference method

regression line

reliability

reliability coefficient

residual score

reversibility principle

self-determination theory

self-efficacy

sensitivity

social cognitive model

specificity

specificity principle

stages of motivational readiness for change model

standard error of estimate *(SEE)*

theory of reasoned action

theory of planned behavior

total error *(TE)*

transtheoretical model

validity

validity coefficient

REVIEW QUESTIONS

In addition to being able to define each of the key terms, test your knowledge and understanding of the material by answering the following review questions.

1. Define physical fitness. Name and define the five components of physical fitness.

2. What is the recommended sequence of testing for administering a complete physical fitness test battery?

3. Identify the reference or criterion method for each of the five components of physical fitness.

4. Which is more important: test validity or test reliability? Explain your choice.

5. Select one physical fitness component and explain how you can determine the relative worth or predictive accuracy of a field test developed to assess this component.

6. Select one physical fitness component and give an example of how each of the seven training principles can be applied to this component.

7. Identify exercise modes suitable to develop each of the five components of fitness.

8. Identify the three elements of an exercise prescription. For older or less fit clients, which of the elements should be increased first during the initial stage of their exercise programs?

9. Name the three stages of an exercise program. On average, how long should each stage last?

10. Identify three positively related and three negatively related factors associated with physical activity participation.

11. Choose one of the psychological models related to successful behavior change and give specific examples of how this model could be applied to a client undertaking a resistance training program to develop muscular fitness.

12. What is persuasive technology and how can it be used to promote physical activity?

13. What are the advantages of becoming a professionally certified exercise scientist?

Assessing Cardiorespiratory Fitness

One of the most important components of physical fitness is cardiorespiratory endurance. Cardiorespiratory endurance is the ability to perform dynamic exercise involving large muscle groups at moderate-to-high intensity for prolonged periods (American College of Sports Medicine [ACSM] 2010). Every physical fitness evaluation should include an assessment of cardiorespiratory function during both rest and exercise.

This chapter presents guidelines for graded exercise testing, as well as maximal and submaximal exercise test protocols and procedures. Although many of the graded exercise test protocols presented in this chapter were developed years ago, these classic protocols are still widely used in research and clinical settings. In addition, each of these protocols meets the ACSM (2010) guidelines for graded exercise tests. The chapter also addresses graded exercise testing for children and older adults and includes a discussion of cardiorespiratory field tests. All of the test protocols included in this chapter are summarized in appendix B.1, "Summary of Graded Exercise Test and Cardiorespiratory Field Test Protocols," on page 334.

DEFINITION OF TERMS

Exercise physiologists consider directly measured **maximum oxygen uptake ($\dot{V}O_2max$)** the most valid measure of functional capacity of the cardiorespiratory system. The $\dot{V}O_2max$, or rate of oxygen uptake during maximal exercise, reflects the capacity of the heart, lungs, and blood to deliver oxygen to the working muscles during dynamic exercise involving large muscle mass. The $\dot{V}O_2max$ is widely accepted as the criterion measure of cardiorespiratory fitness.

Traditionally, a plateau in oxygen consumption despite an increase in workload is the criterion used to determine the attainment of a true $\dot{V}O_2max$ during a maximum exercise tolerance test. Over the last decade, however, evidence suggests that the incidence of a $\dot{V}O_2$ plateau during incremental exercise testing is highly variable, ranging from 16% to 94% (Day et al. 2003; Rossiter, Kowalchuk, and Whipp 2006; Yoon, Kravitz, and Robergs 2007). In fact, these studies established that a "plateau phenomenon" is not a prerequisite for identifying a true $\dot{V}O_2max$ in the majority of individuals (Noakes 2008).

Ramp-type protocols elicit a peak rather than a maximum rate of oxygen consumption. **$\dot{V}O_2$peak** is the highest rate of oxygen consumption measured during the exercise test, regardless of whether or not a $\dot{V}O_2$ plateau is reached. $\dot{V}O_2$ peak may be higher, lower, or equal to $\dot{V}O_2max$. For many individuals who do not reach an actual $\dot{V}O_2$ plateau, the $\dot{V}O_2$peak attained during a maximum-effort, incremental test to the limit of tolerance is a valid index of $\dot{V}O_2max$ (Day et al. 2003; Hawkins et al. 2007; Howley 2007).

Maximal and submaximal $\dot{V}O_2$ are expressed in absolute or relative terms. **Absolute $\dot{V}O_2$** is measured in liters per minute ($L \cdot min^{-1}$) or milliliters per minute ($ml \cdot min^{-1}$) and provides a measure of energy cost for non-weight-bearing activities such as leg or arm cycle ergometry. Absolute $\dot{V}O_2$ is directly related to body size; thus men typically have a larger absolute $\dot{V}O_2max$ than women.

Because absolute $\dot{V}O_2$ depends on body size, $\dot{V}O_2$ is typically expressed relative to body weight, that is, in $ml \cdot kg^{-1} \cdot min^{-1}$. **Relative $\dot{V}O_2max$** is used to classify an individual's cardiorespiratory (CR) fitness level or to compare fitness levels of individuals differing in body size. Relative $\dot{V}O_2$ can also be used to estimate the energy cost of weight-bearing activities such as walking, running, and stair climbing. However, although the relationship between absolute $\dot{V}O_2max$ and body mass is strong ($r = 0.86$), it is not perfect ($r = 1.00$). Therefore, when $\dot{V}O_2max$ is expressed simply as a linear function of body mass, CR fitness levels of heavier (>75.4 kg) and lighter (<67.7 kg) individuals may be under- or overclassified, respectively (Heil 1997). Some experts propose scaling $\dot{V}O_2$ to an exponential

function of body mass (Buresh and Berg 2002; Heil 1997). Heil (1997) suggested using a body mass exponent of 0.67 to compare individuals of similar height, age, and training status and an exponent of 0.75 to compare heterogeneous groups (e.g., older vs. younger or trained vs. sedentary individuals). A current limitation of this exponential approach is that the norms used to classify CR fitness levels were established for relative $\dot{V}O_2max$ values expressed as $ml \cdot min^{-1} \cdot kg^{-1}$ and not as $ml \cdot min^{-1} \cdot kg^{0.67 \text{ or } 0.75}$.

Sometimes $\dot{V}O_2$ is expressed relative to the individual's fat-free mass (see chapter 8), that is, as $ml \cdot kgFFM^{-1} \cdot min^{-1}$. For example, your client's improvement in relative $\dot{V}O_2max$ following a 16 wk aerobic exercise program may reflect both improved capacity of the cardiorespiratory system (increase in absolute $\dot{V}O_2max$) and weight loss (increase in relative $\dot{V}O_2$ expressed as $ml \cdot kg^{-1} \cdot min^{-1}$ due to a decrease in body weight). Thus, expressing $\dot{V}O_2max$ relative to fat-free mass, instead of body weight, provides you with an estimate of cardiorespiratory endurance that is independent of changes in body weight.

The rate of oxygen consumption can also be expressed as a gross $\dot{V}O_2$ or net $\dot{V}O_2$. **Gross $\dot{V}O_2$** is the total rate of oxygen consumption and reflects the caloric costs of both rest and exercise (gross $\dot{V}O_2$ = resting $\dot{V}O_2$ + exercise $\dot{V}O_2$). On the other hand, **net $\dot{V}O_2$** represents the rate of oxygen consumption in excess of the resting $\dot{V}O_2$ and is used to describe the caloric cost of the exercise. Both gross and net $\dot{V}O_2$ can be expressed in either absolute (e.g., $L \cdot min^{-1}$) or relative ($ml \cdot kg^{-1} \cdot min^{-1}$) terms. Unless specified as a net $\dot{V}O_2$, the $\dot{V}O_2$ values reported throughout this book refer to gross $\dot{V}O_2$.

GRADED EXERCISE TESTING: GUIDELINES AND PROCEDURES

Exercise scientists and physicians use exercise tests to evaluate functional cardiorespiratory capacity ($\dot{V}O_2max$) objectively. The $\dot{V}O_2max$, determined from graded maximal or submaximal exercise tests, is used to classify the cardiorespiratory fitness level of your client (see table 4.1). You can use baseline and follow-up data to evaluate the progress of exercise program participants and to set realistic goals for your clients. You can use the heart rate (HR) and oxygen uptake data obtained during the graded exercise test to make accurate, precise exercise prescriptions.

As discussed in chapter 2, before the start of a vigorous (>60% $\dot{V}O_2$max or >6 METs [metabolic equivalents]) exercise program, ACSM (2010) recommends a graded **maximal exercise test** for

- older men (≥45 yr) and women (≥55 yr);
- individuals of any age with moderate risk (two or more coronary heart disease risk factors);
- high-risk individuals with one or more signs or symptoms of cardiovascular and pulmonary disease; and
- high-risk individuals with known cardiovascular, pulmonary, or metabolic disease.

However, you may use **submaximal exercise tests** for low-risk individuals, as well as clients with moderate risk, if they are starting a moderate (40-60% $\dot{V}O_2$max or 3-6 METs) exercise program (ACSM 2010). For medical conditions that are absolute and relative contraindications to exercise testing, see chapter 2, page 22.

General Guidelines for Exercise Testing

You may use a maximal or submaximal **graded exercise test (GXT)** to assess the cardiorespiratory fitness of the individual. The selection of a maximal or submaximal GXT depends on

- your client's age and risk stratification (low risk, moderate risk, or high risk),
- your reasons for administering the test (physical fitness testing or clinical testing), and
- the availability of appropriate equipment and qualified personnel.

In clinical and research settings, $\dot{V}O_2$max is typically measured directly and requires expensive equipment and experienced personnel. Although $\dot{V}O_2$max can be predicted from maximal exercise intensity with a fair degree of accuracy, submaximal tests also provide a reasonable estimate of your client's cardiorespiratory fitness level and are less costly, time-consuming, and risky. Submaximal exercise testing, however, is considered less sensitive as a diagnostic tool for coronary heart disease (CHD).

In either case, the exercise test should be a multistage, graded test. This means that the individual exercises at gradually increasing submaximal workloads. Many commonly used exercise test protocols require that each workload be performed for 3 min. The GXT measures maximum functional capacity ($\dot{V}O_2$max) when the oxygen uptake plateaus and does not increase by more than 150 ml·min^{-1} with a further increase in workload. However, given that

---

Table 4.1 Cardiorespiratory Fitness Classifications: $\dot{V}O_2$max (ml·kg^{-1}·min^{-1})

Age (yr)	Poor	Fair	Good	Excellent	Superior
WOMEN					
20-29	≤35	36-39	40-43	44-49	50+
30-39	≤33	34-36	37-40	41-45	46+
40-49	≤31	32-34	35-38	39-44	45+
50-59	≤28	29-30	31-34	35-39	40+
60-69	≤25	26-28	29-31	32-36	37+
70-79	≤23	24-26	27-29	30-36	37+
MEN					
20-29	≤41	42-45	46-50	51-55	56+
30-39	≤40	41-43	44-47	48-53	54+
40-49	≤37	38-41	42-45	46-52	53+
50-59	≤34	35-37	38-42	43-49	50+
60-69	≤30	31-34	35-38	39-45	46+
70-79	≤27	28-30	31-35	36-41	42+

Data from *Physical Fitness Specialist Manual* (2005). The Cooper Institute for Aerobics Research, Dallas, TX. Used with permission.

many individuals do not attain a $\dot{V}O_2$ plateau, other criteria may be used to indicate the attainment of a true $\dot{V}O_2$max:

- Failure of the HR to increase with increases in exercise intensity
- Venous lactate concentration exceeding 8 mmol·L^{-1}
- **Respiratory exchange ratio (RER)** greater than 1.15
- Rating of perceived exertion greater than 17 using the original Borg scale (6-20)

If the test is terminated before the person reaches a plateau in $\dot{V}O_2$ and an RER greater than 1.15, the GXT is a measure of $\dot{V}O_2$peak rather than $\dot{V}O_2$max. Children, older adults, sedentary individuals, and clients with known disease are more likely than other groups to attain a $\dot{V}O_2$peak rather than a $\dot{V}O_2$max. For CHD screening and classification purposes, bringing a person to at least 85% of the age-predicted maximal HR is desirable, because some electrocardiogram (ECG) abnormalities do not appear until the HR reaches this level of intensity.

Evidence suggests that maximal exercise tests are no more dangerous than submaximal tests provided you carefully follow guidelines for exercise tolerance testing and monitor the physiological responses of the exercise participant continuously. Shephard (1977) predicted one fatality in every 10 to 20 yr for a population of 5 million middle-aged Canadians who undergo maximal exercise testing. For high-risk patients, he estimated one fibrillation per 5000 submaximal exercise tests and one fibrillation per 3000 maximal exercise tests. For clinical testing, the risk of an exercise test being fatal is approximately 0.4 to 0.5 per 10,000 tests (Atterhog, Jonsson, and Samuelsson 1979; Rochmis and Blackburn 1971), and the risk of myocardial infarction is estimated to be four per 10,000 tests (Thompson 1993). The overall risk of exercise testing in a mixed population is six cardiac events (e.g., myocardial infarction, death, and dysrhythmias) per 10,000 tests (ACSM 2010). The risk for apparently healthy individuals (without known disease) is very low, with no complications occurring in 380,000 exercise tests done on young individuals (Levine, Zuckerman, and Cole 1998).

General Procedures for Cardiorespiratory Fitness Testing

At least 1 day before the exercise test, you should give your client pretest instructions (see chapter 3, p. 46). Prior to graded exercise testing, the client should read and sign the informed consent and complete the PAR-Q; see appendix A.1, "Physical Activity Readiness Questionnaire (PAR-Q)," p. 316).

Step-by-step procedures, as recommended by ACSM (2010), for administering a GXT are listed on page 69.

Pretest, exercise, and recovery HRs can be measured using the palpation or auscultation technique (see chapter 2) if a HR monitor or ECG recorder is unavailable. Because of extraneous noise and vibration during exercise, it may be difficult to obtain accurate measurements of BP, especially when your client is running on the treadmill. To become proficient at taking exercise BP, you need to practice as much as possible.

For years, the Borg scales have been used to obtain **ratings of perceived exertion (RPE)** during exercise testing. The original scale (6 to 20) and the revised scale (0 to 10) allow clients to rate their degree of exertion subjectively during exercise and are highly related to exercise HRs and $\dot{V}O_2$. Both RPE scales take into account the linear rise in HR and $\dot{V}O_2$ during exercise. The revised scale also reflects nonlinear changes in blood lactate and ventilation during exercise. Ratings of 6 on the original scale and 0 on the revised scale correspond to no exertion at all; ratings of 10 on the revised scale and 19 on the original scale usually correspond with the maximal level of exercise (Borg 1998). Moderate-intensity exercise is rated between 12 and 14 on the original scale and rated 5 or 6 on the revised scale. Ratings of perceived exertion are useful in determining the endpoints of the GXT, particularly for patients who are taking beta-blockers or other medications that may alter the HR response to exercise. You can teach your clients how to use the RPE scales to monitor relative intensities during aerobic exercise programs.

Alternatively, you may use OMNI scales to obtain your client's RPE for various modes of exercise testing. The OMNI scales can be used to measure RPE for the overall body, the limbs, and the chest. These scales were originally developed for children and adolescents using a picture system to illustrate intensity (0 = extremely easy to 10 = extremely hard) of effort during exercise. Later the scales were modi-

⭐ PROCEDURES FOR ADMINISTERING A GRADED EXERCISE TEST

- Measure the client's resting HR and blood pressure (BP) in the exercise posture (see chapter 2 for these procedures).

- Begin the GXT with a 2 to 3 min warm-up to familiarize clients with the exercise equipment and prepare them for the first stage of the exercise test.

- During the test, monitor HR, BP, and ratings of perceived exertion (RPEs) at regular intervals. Measure HR at least two times during each stage, near the end of the second and third minutes of each stage. A steady-state HR (two HR measurements within ±5 bpm) should be reached for each stage of the test. Do not increase the workload until a steady-state HR is reached.

- Blood pressure should be measured during the last minute of each stage of the test and repeated if a hypotensive or hypertensive response is observed.

- Rating of perceived exertion should be assessed near the end of the last minute of each exercise stage using either the Borg or OMNI scales.

- Throughout the exercise test, continuously monitor the client's physical appearance and symptoms.

- Discontinue the GXT when the test termination criteria are reached, if the client requests stopping the test, or if any of the indications for stopping an exercise test are apparent (see p. 70).

- Have the client cool down by exercising at a low work rate that does not exceed the intensity of the first stage of the exercise test (e.g., walking on the treadmill at 2 mph [53.6 m·min^{-1}] and 0% grade, or cycling on the cycle ergometer at 50 to 60 revolutions per minute [rpm] and zero resistance). Active recovery reduces the risk of hypotension from venous pooling in the extremities.

- During recovery, continue measuring postexercise HR and BP for at least 5 min. If an abnormal response occurs, extend the recovery period. The HR and BP during active recovery should be stable but may be higher than preexercise levels. Continue monitoring the client's physical appearance during recovery.

- If your client has signs of discomfort or if an emergency occurs, use a passive cool-down with the client in a sitting or supine position.

---

fied for use with adults engaging in cycle ergometer, treadmill, stepping, and resistance exercises. As part of the validation testing for the cycling and treadmill scales, the OMNI RPE values were correlated with HR and $\dot{V}O_2$ data. Concurrent validity coefficients ranged from 0.82 to 0.94 for HR and OMNI RPE; likewise, the validity coefficients ranged between 0.88 and 0.95 for $\dot{V}O_2$ and OMNI RPE (Robertson 2004). For resistance exercise, RPE values from the OMNI scale were correlated with weight lifted, yielding validity coefficients ranging from 0.72 to 0.91 (Robertson 2004; Robertson et al. 2005). Appendix B.4 contains sample instructions, procedures, and OMNI pictorial scales for boys, girls, and adults engaging in cycling, treadmill walking/running, stepping, and resistance exercise. Like the Borg scales, the OMNI scales can be used by your clients to monitor intensity of their workouts during aerobic and resistance exercise training. For a detailed discussion of how to use these scales, refer to the work of Robertson (2004). Table 4.2 summarizes the verbal cues corresponding to the numerical values of the OMNI RPE scales.

Table 4.2 Verbal Cues for OMNI RPE Scales

Adults	Children
Extremely easy = 0	Not tired at all = 0
Easy = 2	A little tired = 2
Somewhat easy = 4	Getting more tired = 4
Somewhat hard = 6	Tired = 6
Hard = 8	Really tired = 8
Extremely hard = 10	Very, very tired = 10

Test Termination

In a maximal or submaximal GXT, the exercise usually continues until the client voluntarily terminates the test or a predetermined endpoint is reached. As an exercise technician, however, you must be acutely aware of all indicators for stopping a test. If you notice any of the following signs or symptoms, you should stop the exercise test prior to the client's reaching $\dot{V}O_2max$ (for a maximal GXT) or the predetermined endpoint (for a submaximal GXT).

General Indications for Termination of a Graded Exercise Test in Low-Risk Adults[a]

1. Onset of angina or angina-like symptoms
2. Drop in systolic BP of >10 mmHg from baseline BP despite an increase in workload
3. Excessive rise in BP: systolic pressure >250 mmHg or diastolic pressure >115 mmHg
4. Shortness of breath, wheezing, leg cramps, or claudication
5. Signs of poor perfusion (e.g., ataxia, dizziness, pallor, cyanosis, cold or clammy skin, or nausea)
6. Failure of HR to rise with increased exercise intensity
7. Noticeable change in heart rhythm
8. Client's request to stop
9. Physical or verbal manifestations of severe fatigue
10. Failure of the testing equipment

[a]For definitions of specific terms, refer to the glossary on page 411.

From Gibbons, R.J. et al. 2002. ACC/AHA 2002 Guideline update for exercise testing. A report of the American College of Cardiology/American Heart Association Task Force on Practice Guidelines (Committee on Exercise Testing). www.acc.org/qualityandscience/clinical/guidelines/exercise/exercise_clean.pdf.

MAXIMAL EXERCISE TEST PROTOCOLS

Many maximal exercise test protocols have been devised to assess cardiorespiratory capacity. As the exercise technician, you must be able to select an exercise mode and test protocol that are suitable for your clients given their age, gender, and health and fitness status. Commonly used modes of exercise are treadmill walking or running and stationary cycling. Arm ergometry is useful for persons with paraplegia and clients who have limited use of the lower extremities. Also, combined leg and arm ergometry and total body recumbent stepper exercise tests may be suitable alternatives to treadmill testing for assessing the cardiorespiratory fitness of older persons with balance deficits, gait impairments, and decreased coordination (Billinger, Loudon, and Gajewski 2008; Loudon et al. 1998). Bench stepping is not highly recommended but could be useful in field situations when large groups need to be tested. Whichever mode of exercise you choose, be sure to adhere to the principles explained in "General Principles of Exercise Testing" on page 71.

The exercise test may be continuous or discontinuous. A continuous test is performed with no rest between work increments. **Continuous exercise tests** can vary in the duration of each exercise stage and the magnitude of the increment in exercise intensity between stages. The ACSM (2010) recommends total test duration between 8 and 12 min to increase the probability of individuals reaching $\dot{V}O_2max$. However, Midgley and colleagues (2008) challenged this recommendation based on an extensive review of studies dealing with this topic. They concluded that duration of cycle ergometer tests should be between 7 and 26 min and that treadmill tests should be between 5 and 26 min to yield a valid determination of $\dot{V}O_2max$. This recommendation assumes that an adequate warm-up precedes the shorter-duration tests and that the treadmill grade does not exceed 15% during the protocol. For most continuous exercise test protocols, the exercise intensity is increased gradually (2 to 3 METs for low-risk individuals) throughout the test, and the duration of each stage is usually 2 or 3 min, allowing most individuals to reach a steady-state $\dot{V}O_2$ during each stage. Across the stages of this type of GXT, the workload may increase linearly or nonlinearly. Each increment in workload is dictated by the specific protocol and does not vary among individuals. Although this type of GXT is widely used in research and clinical settings, it may not be optimal for assessing the functional capacity of all individuals, especially those with low-exercise tolerance.

GENERAL PRINCIPLES OF EXERCISE TESTING[a]

1. Typically, you will use either a treadmill or stationary cycle ergometer for graded exercise testing. All equipment should be calibrated before use.

2. Begin the GXT with a 2 to 3 min warm-up to orient the client to the equipment and prepare the client for the first stage of the GXT.

3. The initial exercise intensity should be considerably lower than the anticipated maximal capacity.

4. Exercise intensity should be increased gradually throughout the stages of the test. Work increments may be 2 METs or greater for apparently healthy individuals and as small as 0.5 MET for patients with disease.

5. Closely observe contraindications for testing and indications for stopping the exercise test. When in any doubt about the safety or benefits of testing, do not perform the test at that time.

6. Monitor the HR at least two times, but preferably each minute, during each stage of the GXT. Heart rate measurements should be taken near the end of each minute. If the HR does not reach steady state (two HRs within ±5 or 6 bpm), extend the work stage an additional minute or until the HR stabilizes.

7. Measure BP and RPE once during each stage of the GXT, in the later portion of the stage.

8. Continually monitor client appearance and symptoms.

9. For submaximal GXTs, terminate the test when the client's HR reaches 70% HRR (heart rate reserve) or 85% HRmax (maximal heart rate), unless the protocol specifies a different termination criterion. Also, stop the test immediately if there is an emergency situation, if the client fails to conform to the exercise protocol, or if the client experiences signs of discomfort.

10. The test should include a cool-down period of at least 5 min, or longer if abnormal HR and BP responses are observed. During recovery, HR and BP should be monitored each minute. For active recovery, the workload should be no more than that used during the first stage of the GXT. A passive recovery is used in emergency situations and when clients experience signs of discomfort and cannot perform an active cool-down.

11. Exercise tolerance in METs should be estimated for the treadmill or ergometer protocol used, or directly assessed if oxygen uptake is measured during the GXT.

12. The testing area should be quiet and private. The room temperature should be 21° to 23° C (70° to 72° F) or less and the humidity 60% or less if possible.

[a]Physician supervision is recommended for maximal exercise tests of moderate- or high-risk clients, as well as submaximal exercise tests for high-risk clients.

Today, continuous ramp-type tests are gaining popularity and are widely used because they can be individualized for the client's estimated exercise tolerance. For example, increments in work rate during a ramp protocol are much higher for endurance-trained athletes than for sedentary individuals (e.g., 30 W·min^{-1} vs. 10 W·min^{-1}). Also, each exercise stage for ramp protocols is much shorter (e.g., 20 sec) than that of the traditional continuous GXT protocols (2-3 min). **Ramp protocols** provide continuous and frequent increments in work rate throughout the test so that the $\dot{V}O_2$ increases linearly; they are designed to bring individuals to their limit of exercise tolerance in approximately 10 min.

In a study comparing four ramp protocol durations (5, 8, 12, and 16 min) during incremental cycling exercise, Yoon and colleagues (2007) reported that the optimal protocol duration to elicit $\dot{V}O_2$max of healthy, moderately to highly trained men and women is between 8 and 10 min.

Because of the frequent (e.g., every 10 or 20 sec) increases in work rate with ramp protocols, $\dot{V}O_2$ plateaus are rarely observed. However, as previously mentioned, the $\dot{V}O_2$peak from ramp-type protocols appears to be a valid index of $\dot{V}O_2$max even without a plateau in $\dot{V}O_2$ (Day et al. 2003). This ramp approach potentially improves the prediction of $\dot{V}O_2$max given that $\dot{V}O_2$ increases linearly across work rates. Ramp protocols allow some individuals to reach a higher exercise tolerance compared to traditional GXT protocols. However, there are disadvantages. To design an individualized ramp protocol, the maximum work rate for each client must be predetermined or accurately estimated from training records or questionnaires so that you can select a work rate that allows the individual to reach his or her peak exercise tolerance in approximately 10 min. Also, ramp protocols increase work rate frequently (e.g., 25-30 stages in a 10 min test), requiring more expensive electromagnetically braked cycle ergometers and programmable treadmills that make rapid and smooth transitions between the stages of the exercise test. Lastly, inexperienced technicians may have difficulty measuring exercise BP during each minute of the ramp protocol.

For **discontinuous exercise tests**, the client rests 5 to 10 min between workloads. The workload is progressively increased until the client reaches maximum exercise tolerance (exhaustion). Typically, each stage of the discontinuous protocol lasts 5 or 6 min, allowing $\dot{V}O_2$ to reach a steady state. On average, discontinuous tests take five times longer to administer than do continuous tests. Similar $\dot{V}O_2$max values are attained using discontinuous and continuous (increasing workload every 2-3 min) protocols (Maksud and Coutts 1971); therefore, continuous tests are preferable in most research and clinical settings.

McArdle, Katch, and Pechar (1973) compared the $\dot{V}O_2$max scores as measured by six commonly used continuous and discontinuous treadmill and cycle ergometer tests. They noted that the $\dot{V}O_2$max scores for the cycle ergometer tests were approximately 6% to 11% lower than for the treadmill tests. Many subjects identified local discomfort and fatigue in the thigh muscles as the major factors limiting further work on both the continuous and discontinuous cycle ergometer tests. For the treadmill tests, subjects indicated windedness and general fatigue as the limiting factors and complained of localized fatigue and discomfort in the calf muscles and lower back.

Treadmill Maximal Exercise Tests

For treadmill maximal exercise tests, the exercise is performed on a motor-driven treadmill with variable speed and incline (see figure 4.1). Speed varies up to 25 mph (40 km·hr⁻¹), and incline is measured

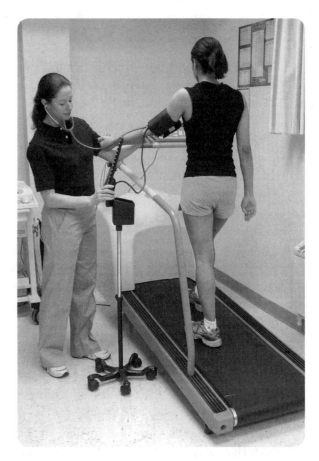

Figure 4.1 Treadmill.

in units of elevation per 100 horizontal units and is expressed as a percentage. The workload on the treadmill is raised through increases in the speed or incline or both. Workload is usually expressed in miles per hour and percent grade.

It is difficult and expensive to measure the oxygen consumption during exercise. Therefore, ACSM (2010) has developed equations (table 4.3) to estimate the metabolic cost of exercise ($\dot{V}O_2$). These equations provide a valid estimate of $\dot{V}O_2$ for steady-state exercise only. When used to estimate the maximum rate of energy expenditure ($\dot{V}O_2$max), the measured $\dot{V}O_2$ will be less than the estimated $\dot{V}O_2$ if steady state is not reached. Also, because maximal exercise involves both aerobic and anaerobic components, the $\dot{V}O_2$max will be overestimated since the contribution of the anaerobic component is not known.

Before using any of the ACSM metabolic equations to estimate $\dot{V}O_2$, make certain that all units of measure match those in the equation (see "Converting Units of Measure").

Table 4.3 Metabolic Equations for Estimating Gross $\dot{V}O_2$ (ACSM 2010)

Exercise mode gross $\dot{V}O_2$ (ml·kg^{-1}·min^{-1})	Resting $\dot{V}O_2$ (ml·kg^{-1}·min^{-1})	Comments
Walking $\dot{V}O_2 = S^a \times 0.1 + S \times G^b \times 1.8$	+3.5	1. For speeds of 50-100 m·min^{-1} (1.9-3.7 mph) 2. 0.1 ml·kg^{-1}·m^{-1} = O_2 cost of walking horizontally 3. 1.8 ml·kg^{-1}·m^{-1} = O_2 cost of walking on incline (% grade of treadmill)
Running $\dot{V}O_2 = S^a \times 0.2 + S \times G^b \times 0.9$	+3.5	1. For speeds >134 m·min^{-1} (>5.0 mph) 2. If truly jogging (not walking), this equation can also be used for speeds of 80-134 m·min^{-1} (3-5 mph) 3. 0.2 ml·kg^{-1}·m^{-1} = O_2 cost of running horizontally 4. 0.9 ml·kg^{-1}·m^{-1} = O_2 cost of running on incline (% grade of treadmill)
Leg ergometry $\dot{V}O_2 = W^c / M^d \times 1.8 + 3.5$	+3.5	1. For work rates between 50 and 200 W (300-1200 kgm·min^{-1}) 2. kgm·min^{-1} = kg × m·rev^{-1} × rev·min^{-1} 3. Monark and Bodyguard = 6 m·rev^{-1}; Tunturi = 3 m·rev^{-1} 4. 1.8 ml·kg^{-1}·min^{-1} = O_2 cost of cycling against external load (resistance) 5. 3.5 ml·kg^{-1}·min^{-1} = O_2 cost of cycling with zero load
Arm ergometry $\dot{V}O_2 = W^c / M^d \times 3.0 + none$	+3.5	1. For work rates between 25 and 125 W (150-750 kgm·min^{-1}) 2. kgm·min^{-1} = kg × m·rev^{-1} × rev·min^{-1} 3. 3.0 ml·kg^{-1}·min^{-1} = O_2 cost of cycling against external load (resistance) 4. None = due to small mass of arm musculature, no special term for unloaded (zero load) cycling needed
Stepping $\dot{V}O_2 = F^e \times 0.2 + F \times ht^f \times 1.8 \times 1.33$	+3.5	1. Appropriate for stepping rates between 12 and 30 steps·min^{-1} and step heights between 0.04 m (1.6 in.) and 0.40 m (15.7 in.) 2. 0.2 ml·kg^{-1}·m^{-1} = O_2 cost of moving horizontally 3. 1.8 ml·kg^{-1}·m^{-1} = O_2 cost of stepping up (bench height) 4. 1.33 includes positive component of stepping up (1.0) + negative component of stepping down (0.33)

[a]S = speed of treadmill in m·min^{-1}; 1 mph = 26.8 m·min^{-1}.

[b]G = grade (% incline) of treadmill in decimal form (e.g., 10% = 0.10).

[c]W = work rate in kgm·min^{-1}; 1 Watt = 6 kgm·min^{-1}.

[d]M = body mass in kilograms; 1 kg = 2.2 lb.

[e]F = frequency of stepping in steps per minute.

[f]ht = bench height in meters; 1 in. = 0.0254 m.

CONVERTING UNITS OF MEASURE

- Convert body mass (M) in pounds to kilograms (1 kg = 2.2 lb). For example, 170 lb / 2.2 = 77.3 kg.

- Convert treadmill speed (S) in miles per hour to meters per minute (1 mph = 26.8 m·min^{-1}). For example, 5.0 mph × 26.8 = 134.0 m·min^{-1}.

- Convert treadmill grade (G) from percent to decimal form by dividing by 100. For example, 12% / 100 = 0.12.

- Convert METs to ml·kg^{-1}·min^{-1} by multiplying (1 MET = 3.5 ml·kg^{-1}·min^{-1}). For example, 6 METs × 3.5 = 21.0 ml·kg^{-1}·min^{-1}.

- Convert kgm·min^{-1} to watts (W) (1 W = 6 kgm·min^{-1}) by dividing. For example, 900 kgm·min^{-1} / 6 = 150 W.

- Convert step height in inches to meters (1 in. = 0.0254 m) by multiplying. For example, 8 in. × 0.0254 = 0.2032 m.

The ACSM metabolic equations in table 4.3 are useful in clinical settings for estimating the total rate of energy expenditure (gross $\dot{V}O_2$) during steady-state treadmill walking or running. The total energy expenditure, in ml·kg^{-1}·min^{-1}, is a function of three components: *speed, grade,* and *resting energy expenditures.* For treadmill walking, the oxygen cost of raising one's body mass against gravity (vertical work) is approximately 1.8 ml·kg^{-1}·m^{-1}, and 0.1 ml·kg^{-1}·m^{-1} of oxygen is needed to move the body horizontally. For treadmill running, the oxygen cost for vertical work is one-half that for treadmill walking (0.9 ml·kg^{-1}·m^{-1}), whereas the energy expenditure for running on the treadmill (0.2 ml·kg^{-1}·m^{-1}) is twice that for walking. See "ACSM Walking Equation" for an example of how to take these three factors into account when figuring $\dot{V}O_2$.

The $\dot{V}O_2$ estimated from the ACSM walking equation (see table 4.3) is reasonably accurate for walking speeds between 50 and 100 m·min^{-1} (1.9 to 3.7 mph). However, since the equation is more accurate for walking up a grade than on the level, $\dot{V}O_2$ may be underestimated as much as 15% to 20% during walking on the level (ACSM 2010). For the ACSM running or jogging equations, the $\dot{V}O_2$ estimates are relatively accurate for speeds exceeding 134 m·min^{-1} (5 mph) and speeds as low as 80 m·min^{-1} (3 mph) provided that the client is jogging and not walking (ACSM 2010).

Figure 4.2 illustrates commonly used treadmill exercise test protocols. These protocols conform to the general guidelines for maximal exercise testing. Some of the protocols are designed for a specific population, such as well-conditioned athletes or high-risk cardiac patients. The exercise intensity for each stage of the various treadmill test protocols can be expressed in METs. The MET estimations for each stage of some commonly used treadmill protocols are listed in table 4.4.

Population-specific and generalized equations have been developed to estimate $\dot{V}O_2$max from exercise time for some treadmill protocols (see table 4.5). It is important for exercise technicians to keep in mind that the initial workload in some of the protocols designed for highly trained athletes is too intense (exceeding 2 to 3.5 METs) for the average individual. The Balke and Bruce protocols are well suited for low-risk individuals, and the Bruce protocol is easily adapted for high-risk individuals using an initial workload of 1.7 mph at 0% to 5% grade.

Balke Treadmill Protocol

To administer the Balke and Ware (1959) exercise test protocol (see figure 4.2), set the treadmill speed at 3.4 mph (91.1 m·min^{-1}) and the initial grade of the treadmill at 0% during the first minute of exercise. Maintain a constant speed on the treadmill throughout the entire exercise test. At the start of

---

ACSM WALKING EQUATION

To calculate the gross $\dot{V}O_2$ for a 70 kg (154 lb) subject who is walking on the treadmill at a speed of 3.5 mph and a grade of 10%, follow these steps:

$\dot{V}O_2$ = speed + (grade × speed)
    + resting $\dot{V}O_2$ (ml·kg^{-1}·min^{-1})

= [speed (m·min^{-1}) × 0.1] + [grade (decimal)
    × speed (m·min^{-1}) × 1.8] + 3.5

1. Convert the speed in mph to m·min^{-1}; 1 mph = 26.8 m·min^{-1}.

    3.5 mph × 26.8 = 93.8 m·min^{-1}

2. Calculate the speed component (S).

    S = speed (m·min^{-1}) × 0.1

      = 93.8 m·min^{-1} × 0.1

      = 9.38 ml·kg^{-1}·min^{-1}

3. Calculate the grade × speed component (G × S). Convert % grade into a decimal by dividing by 100.

    G × S = grade (decimal) × speed × 1.8

        = 0.10 × (93.8 m·min^{-1}) × 1.8

        = 16.88 ml·kg^{-1}·min^{-1}

4. Calculate the total gross $\dot{V}O_2$ in ml·kg^{-1}·min^{-1} by adding the speed, grade × speed, and resting $\dot{V}O_2$ (R).

    $\dot{V}O_2$ = S + (S × G) + R

      = (9.38 + 16.88 + 3.5) ml·kg^{-1}·min^{-1}

      = 29.76 ml·kg^{-1}·min^{-1}

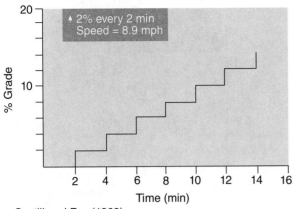

Costill and Fox (1969)
For: highly trained
Warm-up: 10-min walk or run
Initial workload: 8.9 mph, 0%, 2 min

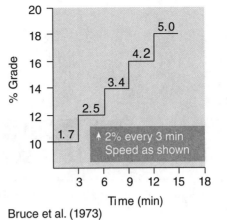

Bruce et al. (1973)
For: normal and high risk
Initial workload: 1.7 mph, 10%, 3 min = normal
1.7 mph, 0-5%, 3 min = high risk

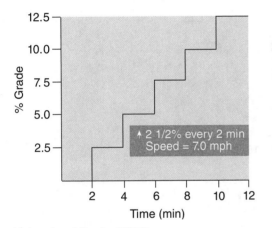

Maksud and Coutts (1971)
For: highly trained
Warm-up: 10-min walking, 3.5 mph, 0%
Initial workload: 7 mph, 0%, 2 min

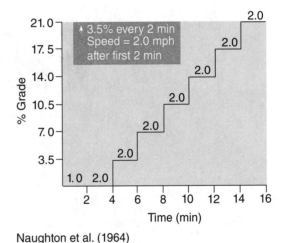

Naughton et al. (1964)
For: cardiac and high risk
Initial workload: 1.0 mph, 0%, 2 min

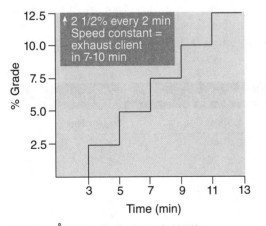

Modified Åstrand (Pollock et al. 1978)
For: highly trained
Warm-up: 5-min walk or jog
Initial workload: 5-8 mph, 0%, 3 min

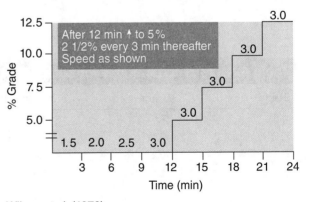

Wilson et al. (1978)
For: cardiac and high risk
Initial workload: 1.5 mph, 0%, 3 min

(continued)

Figure 4.2 Treadmill exercise test protocols.

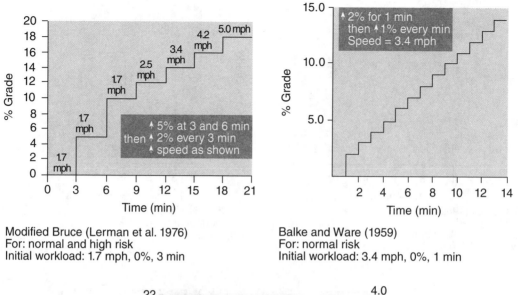

Modified Bruce (Lerman et al. 1976)
For: normal and high risk
Initial workload: 1.7 mph, 0%, 3 min

Balke and Ware (1959)
For: normal risk
Initial workload: 3.4 mph, 0%, 1 min

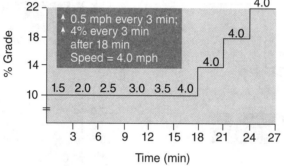

Kattus (1968)
For: cardiac and high risk
Initial workload: 1.5 mph, 10%, 3 min

Figure 4.2 *(continued)*

the second minute of exercise, increase the grade to 2%. Thereafter, at the beginning of every additional minute of exercise, increase the grade by only 1%.

Use the prediction equation for the Balke protocol in table 4.5 to estimate your client's $\dot{V}O_2$max from exercise time. Alternatively, you can use a nomogram (see figure 4.3) developed for the

Table 4.4	MET Estimations for Each Stage of Commonly Used Treadmill Protocols			
Stage[a]	Bruce	Modified Bruce[b]	Balke	Naughton
1	4.6	2.3	3.6	1.8
2	7.0	3.5	4.5	3.5
3	10.2	4.6	5.0	4.5
4	12.1	7.0	5.5	5.4
5	14.9	10.2	5.9	6.4
6	17.0	12.1	6.4	7.4
7	19.3	14.9	6.9	8.3

[a]Percent grade and speed for each stage are illustrated in figure 4.2.

[b]Stage 1 = 0% grade, 1.7 mph; Stage 2 = 5% grade, 1.7 mph.

Table 4.5 Population-Specific and Generalized Equations for Treadmill Protocols

Protocol	Population	Reference	Equation
Balke	Active and sedentary men	Pollock et al. (1976)	$\dot{V}O_2max = 1.444(time) + 14.99$ $r = 0.92$, $SEE = 2.50$ $(ml \cdot kg^{-1} \cdot min^{-1})$
	Active and sedentary women[a]	Pollock et al. (1982)	$\dot{V}O_2max = 1.38(time) + 5.22$ $r = 0.94$, $SEE = 2.20$ $(ml \cdot kg^{-1} \cdot min^{-1})$
Bruce[b]	Active and sedentary men	Foster et al. (1984)	$\dot{V}O_2max = 14.76 - 1.379(time) + 0.451(time^2) - 0.012(time^3)$ $r = 0.98$, $SEE = 3.35$ $(ml \cdot kg^{-1} \cdot min^{-1})$
	Active and sedentary women	Pollock et al. (1982)	$\dot{V}O_2max = 4.38(time) - 3.90$ $r = 0.91$, $SEE = 2.7$ $(ml \cdot kg^{-1} \cdot min^{-1})$
	Cardiac patients and elderly persons[c]	McConnell and Clark (1987)	$\dot{V}O_2max = 2.282(time) + 8.545$ $r = 0.82$, $SEE = 4.9$ $(ml \cdot kg^{-1} \cdot min^{-1})$
Naughton	Male cardiac patients	Foster et al. (1983)	$\dot{V}O_2max = 1.61(time) + 3.60$ $r = 0.97$, $SEE = 2.60$ $(ml \cdot kg^{-1} \cdot min^{-1})$

[a]For women, the Balke protocol was modified: speed 3.0 mph; initial workload 0% grade for 3 min, increasing 2.5% every 3 min thereafter.

[b]For use with the standard Bruce protocol, cannot be used with modified Bruce protocol.

[c]This equation is used only for treadmill walking while holding the handrails.

SEE = standard error of estimate.

Balke treadmill protocol to calculate the $\dot{V}O_2max$ of your client. To use this nomogram, locate the time corresponding to the last complete minute of exercise during the protocol along the vertical axis labeled "Balke time," and draw a horizontal line from the time axis to the oxygen uptake axis. Be certain to plot the exercise time of women and men in the appropriate column when using this nomogram.

Bruce Treadmill Protocol

The Bruce, Kusumi, and Hosmer (1973) exercise test is a multistaged treadmill protocol (see figure 4.2). The protocol increases the workload by changing both the treadmill speed and percent grade. During the first stage (minutes 1 to 3) of the test, the normal individual walks at a 1.7 mph pace at 10% grade. At the start of the second stage (minutes 4 to 6), increase the grade by 2% and the speed to 2.5 mph (67 m·min^{-1}). In each subsequent stage of the test, increase the grade 2% and the speed by either 0.8 or 0.9 mph (21.4 or 24.1 m·min^{-1}) until the client is exhausted. Prediction equations for this protocol have been developed to estimate the $\dot{V}O_2max$ of active and sedentary women and men, cardiac patients, and people who are elderly (see table 4.5). As an alternative, you may use the nomogram (see

figure 4.4) developed for the Bruce protocol. Plot the client's exercise time for this protocol along the vertical axis labeled "Bruce time," and draw a horizontal line from the time axis to the oxygen uptake. Again, be certain to use the appropriate column for men and women.

Modified Bruce Protocol

The modified Bruce protocol (see figure 4.2) is more suitable than the Bruce protocol for high-risk and elderly individuals. However, with the exception of the first two stages, this protocol is similar to the standard Bruce protocol. Stage 1 starts at 0% grade and a 1.7 mph walking pace. For stage 2, the % grade is increased to 5%. McInnis and Balady (1994) compared physiological responses to the standard and modified Bruce protocols in patients with CHD and reported similar HR and BP responses at matched exercise stages despite the additional 6 min of low-intensity exercise performed using the modified Bruce protocol.

Note that the prediction equations for the Bruce protocol (see table 4.5) can be used for only the standard, not the modified, Bruce protocol. To estimate $\dot{V}O_2$ for the modified Bruce protocol, use the ACSM metabolic equation for walking (see table 4.3).

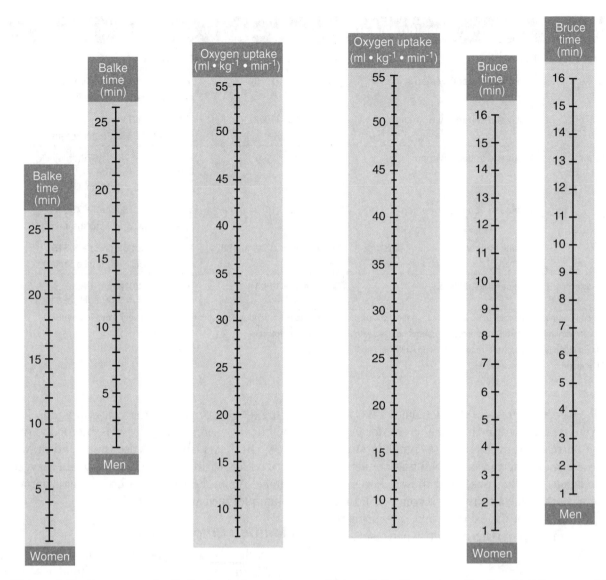

Figure 4.3 Nomogram for Balke graded exercise test.

Reprinted, by permission, from N. Ng, 1995, *METCALC* (Champaign, IL: Human Kinetics), 30.

Figure 4.4 Nomogram for standard Bruce graded exercise test.

Reprinted, by permission, from N. Ng. 1995, *METCALC* (Champaign, IL: Human Kinetics), 32.

Treadmill Ramp Protocols

Kaminsky and Whaley (1998) developed a standardized ramp protocol (i.e., BSU/Bruce ramp protocol) for assessing the functional cardiorespiratory capacity of symptomatic, sedentary, and apparently healthy individuals. For this protocol, the treadmill speed increases gradually (in 0.1-0.4 mph, or 2.68-10.72 m·min⁻¹, increments) every minute. The minimum speed is 1.0 mph (26.8 m·min⁻¹); the maximum speed is 5.8 mph (155 m·min⁻¹). The treadmill grade also increases gradually (by 0-5%) every minute. The minimum grade is 0%; the maximum grade is 20%. Every 3 min during this ramp protocol, the

work rates (i.e., speed and grade) equal those of the traditional Bruce protocol (see table 4.6). For example, during the sixth minute of exercise, the treadmill speed (2.5 mph, or 53.6 m·min⁻¹) and grade (12%) are the same, allowing comparisons between the two types of protocols. The ramp approach has the advantage of avoiding large, unequal increments in workload. Also, it results in uniform increases in hemodynamic and physiological responses to incremental exercise and more accurately estimates exercise capacity and ventilatory threshold.

Porszasz and colleagues (2003) devised a ramp protocol that increases work rate linearly so that

Table 4.6 Comparison of Work Rates for the Standard Bruce Protocol and the Bruce Ramp Protocol

Minute[a]	SPEED IN MPH[b]		GRADE (%)	
	SB	BR	SB	BR
1	1.7	1.0	10	0
2	1.7	1.3	10	5
3	*1.7*	*1.7*	*10*	*10*
4	2.5	2.1	12	10
5	2.5	2.3	12	11
6	*2.5*	*2.5*	*12*	*12*
7	3.4	2.8	14	12
8	3.4	3.1	14	13
9	*3.4*	*3.4*	*14*	*14*
10	4.2	3.8	16	14
11	4.2	4.1	16	15
12	*4.2*	*4.2*	*16*	*16*
13	5.0	4.5	18	16
14	5.0	4.8	18	17
15	*5.0*	*5.0*	*18*	*18*
16	5.5	5.3	20	18
17	5.5	5.6	20	19
18	5.5	5.8	20	20

SB = standard Bruce protocol; BR = Bruce ramp protocol.

[a]Boldfaced italics identify the times during the two protocols when the work rates are equivalent.

[b]To convert mph to m·min⁻¹, multiply by 26.8.

the individual walking on a treadmill reaches exhaustion in approximately 10 min. To linearly increase work rate over time, it is necessary to couple linear increases in walking speed with curvilinear increases in treadmill grade. Because this protocol starts with slow walking (i.e., 0.5-1.0 mph, or 13.4-26.8 m·min⁻¹), it is suitable for individuals with low-exercise tolerance as well as for sedentary individuals with a range of exercise tolerances. As with all types of ramp protocols, this protocol is individualized. The peak work rate, a comfortable range of walking speeds, and the increments in treadmill incline or grade are determined for each client.

This protocol compares favorably to cycle ergometer ramp protocols that increment work rate linearly so that maximum exercise tolerance is reached in ~10 min. The slope of the relationship between $\dot{V}O_2$ and work rate, however, is consistently steeper on the treadmill than on the cycle ergometer

(Porszasz et al. 2003). This steeper slope reflects additional use of the limbs (i.e., swinging the arms and legs) and frictional force as treadmill speed increases. For each individual, the time course for the grade increments needed to elicit a linear increase in work rate can be calculated with a prediction equation based on the client's body weight, desired initial and final walking speeds, initial grade, and estimated peak work rate (see Porszasz et al. 2003). These individual variables, along with the prediction equation for increasing grade, can be programmed into the computer of a contemporary treadmill. Thus, each individualized ramp protocol is controlled by the computer so that the frequent increases in speed and grade are smooth and rapid.

Cycle Ergometer Maximal Exercise Tests

The cycle ergometer is a widely used instrument for assessing cardiorespiratory fitness. On a friction-type cycle ergometer (see figure 4.5), resistance is applied against the flywheel using a belt and weighted pendulums. The hand wheel adjusts the workload by tightening or loosening the brake belt. The workload on the cycle ergometer is raised through increases in the resistance on the flywheel. The power output is usually expressed in kilogram-meters per minute (kgm·min⁻¹) or watts (1 W = 6 kgm·min⁻¹) and is easily measured using the equation:

$$\text{power} = \text{force} \times \text{distance} / \text{time}$$

where force equals the resistance or tension setting on the ergometer (kilograms) and distance is the distance traveled by the flywheel rim for each revolution of the pedal times number of revolutions per minute. On the Monark and Bodyguard cycle ergometers, the flywheel travels 6 m per pedal revolution. Therefore, if a resistance of 2 kg is applied and the pedaling rate is 60 rpm, then

$$\text{power} = 2 \text{ kg} \times 6 \text{ m} \times 60 \text{ rpm} = 720 \text{ kgm·min}^{-1},$$
$$\text{or } 120 \text{ W.}$$

To calculate the distance traveled by the flywheel of cycle ergometers with varying-sized flywheels, measure the circumference (in meters) of the resistance track on the flywheel and multiply the circumference by the number of flywheel revolutions during one complete revolution (360°) of the pedal (Gledhill and Jamnik 1995).

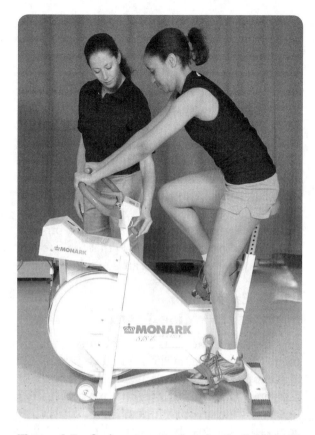

Figure 4.5 Cycle ergometer (mechanically braked).

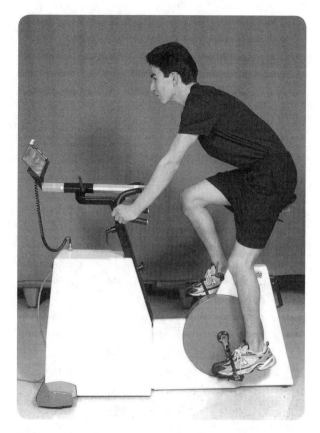

Figure 4.6 Cycle ergometer (electrically braked).

When you are standardizing the work performed on a friction-type cycle ergometer, the client should maintain a constant pedaling rate. Some cycle ergometers have a speedometer that displays the individual's pedaling rate. Check this dial frequently to make certain that your client is maintaining a constant pedaling frequency throughout the test. If a speedometer is not available, use a metronome to establish your client's pedaling cadence. Controlling the pedaling rate on an electrically braked cycle ergometer (figure 4.6) is unnecessary. An electromagnetic braking force adjusts the resistance for slower or faster pedaling rates, thereby keeping the power output constant. This type of cycle ergometer, however, is difficult to calibrate.

Most cycle ergometer test protocols for untrained cyclists use a pedaling rate of 50 or 60 rpm, and power outputs are increased by 150 to 300 kgm·min^{-1} (25 to 50 W) in each stage of the test. However, you can use higher pedaling rates (≥80 rpm) for trained cyclists. A pedaling rate of 60 rpm produces the highest $\dot{V}O_2$max when compared with rates of 50, 70, or 80 rpm (Hermansen and Saltin

1969). Figure 4.7 illustrates some widely used discontinuous and continuous maximal exercise test protocols for the cycle ergometer. Guidelines for use of cycle ergometers are presented in "Testing With Cycle Ergometers" on page 81.

To calculate the energy expenditure for cycle ergometer exercise, use the ACSM equations provided in table 4.3. The total energy expenditure or gross $\dot{V}O_2$, in ml·kg^{-1}·min^{-1}, is a function of the oxygen cost of pedaling against resistance (power output in watts), the oxygen cost of unloaded cycling (approximately 3.5 ml·kg^{-1}·min^{-1} at 50 to 60 rpm with zero resistance), and the resting oxygen consumption. The cost of cycling against an external load or resistance is approximately 1.8 ml·kg^{-1}·m^{-1}. For a sample calculation, see "ACSM Leg Ergometry Equation" on page 82.

Keep in mind that the leg and arm ergometry equations are accurate in estimating $\dot{V}O_2$ only if the client attains a steady state during the maximal GXT. If, for example, the client is able to complete only 1 min of exercise during the last stage of the maximal test protocol, the power output from the previous stage (in which the client reached steady

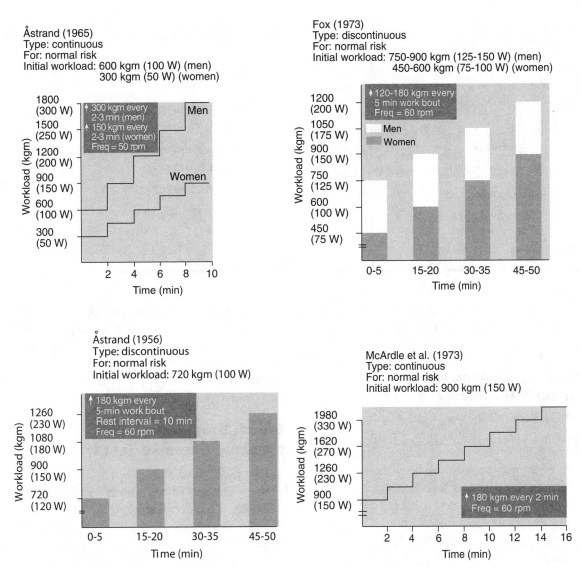

Figure 4.7 Cycle ergometer exercise test protocols.

TESTING WITH CYCLE ERGOMETERS

The following guidelines are suggested for the use of cycle ergometers:

1. Calibrate the cycle ergometer often by hanging known weights from the belt of the flywheel and reading the dial on the hand wheel.

2. Always release the tension on the belt between tests.

3. Establish pedaling frequency before setting the workload.

4. Check the load setting frequently during the test because it may change as the belt warms up.

5. Set the metronome so that one revolution is completed for every two beats (e.g., set the metronome at 120 for a test requiring a pedaling frequency of 60 rpm).

6. Adjust the height of the seat so the knee is slightly flexed (about 5°) at maximal leg extension with the ball of the foot on the pedal.

7. Have the client assume an upright, seated posture with hands properly positioned on the handlebars.

ACSM LEG ERGOMETRY EQUATION

To calculate the energy expenditure of a 62 kg (136 lb) woman cycling at a work rate or power output of 360 kgm·min^{-1}, follow these steps:

1. Calculate the energy cost of cycling at the specified power output.

$\dot{V}O_2$ = work rate[a] (W) / body mass (M) × 1.8

= 360 kgm·min^{-1}/ 62 kg × 1.8

= 10.45 ml·kg^{-1}·min^{-1}

2. Add the estimated cost of cycling at zero load (i.e., 3.5 ml·kg^{-1}·min^{-1}).

$\dot{V}O_2$ = 10.45 ml·kg^{-1}·min^{-1} + 3.5 ml·kg^{-1}·min^{-1}

= 13.95 ml·kg^{-1}·min^{-1}

3. Add the estimated resting energy expenditure (3.5 ml·kg^{-1}·min^{-1}).

$\dot{V}O_2$ = 13.95 ml·kg^{-1}·min^{-1} + 3.5 ml·kg^{-1}·min^{-1}

= 17.45 ml·kg^{-1}·min^{-1}

[a]Work rate is in kgm·min^{-1}.

---

state) should be used to estimate $\dot{V}O_2$max rather than the power output corresponding to the last stage.

Åstrand Cycle Ergometer Maximal Test Protocol

For the Åstrand (1965) continuous test protocol (see figure 4.7), the initial power output is 300 kgm·min^{-1} (50 W) for women and 600 kgm·min^{-1} (100 W) for men. Because the pedaling rate is 50 rpm, the resistance is 1 kg for women (1 kg × 6 m × 50 rpm = 300 kgm·min^{-1}) and 2 kg for men (2 kg × 6 m × 50 rpm = 600 kgm·min^{-1}). Have your client exercise at this initial workload for 2 min. Then increase the power output every 2 to 3 min in increments of 150 kgm·min^{-1} (25 W) and 300 kgm·min^{-1} (50 W) for women and men, respectively. Continue the test until the client is exhausted or can no longer maintain the pedaling rate of 50 rpm. Use the ACSM metabolic equation for leg ergometry to estimate $\dot{V}O_2$ from your client's power output during the last steady-state stage of the GXT.

Fox Cycle Ergometer Maximal Test Protocol

The Fox (1973) protocol is a discontinuous test consisting of a series of 5 min exercise bouts with 10 min rest intervals. The starting workload is between 750 (125 W) and 900 kgm·min^{-1} (150 W) for men and 450 (75 W) and 600 kgm·min^{-1} (100 W) for women. The progressive increments in work depend on the client's HR response and usually are between 120 and 180 kgm·min^{-1} (20 and 30 W). The client exercises until exhausted or until no longer able to pedal for at least 3 min at a power output that is 60 to 90 kgm·min^{-1} (10 to 15 W) higher than the previous workload. You can use the metabolic equations to convert the power output from the last steady-state stage of this protocol to $\dot{V}O_2$max.

Bench Stepping Maximal Exercise Tests

The least desirable mode of exercise for maximum exercise testing is bench stepping. During bench stepping, the individual is performing both positive (up phase) and negative (down phase) work. Approximately one-quarter to one-third less energy is expended during negative work (Morehouse 1972). This factor, coupled with adjusting the step height and stepping rate for differences in body weight, makes standardization of the work extremely difficult.

General Procedures

Most step test protocols increase the intensity of the work by gradually increasing the height of the bench or stepping rate. The work (W) performed can be calculated using the equation W = F × D, where F is body weight in kilograms and D is bench height times number of steps per minute. For example, a 50 kg (110 lb) woman stepping at a rate of 22 steps·min^{-1} on a 30 cm (0.30 m) bench is performing 330 kgm·min^{-1} of work (50 kg × 0.30 m × 22 steps·min^{-1}).

The following equations can be used to adjust the step height and stepping rate for differences in body weight to achieve a given work rate (Morehouse 1972):

$$\text{step height (cm)} = \text{work (kgcm·min}^{-1}) / \text{body weight (kg)} \times \text{stepping rate}$$

$$\text{stepping rate (steps·min}^{-1}) = \text{work (kgcm·min}^{-1}) / \text{body weight (kg)} \times \text{step height (cm)}$$

For example, if you devise a graded step test protocol that requires a client weighing 60 kg (132 lb) to exercise at a work rate of 300 kgm·min^{-1}, and the stepping rate is set at 18 steps·min^{-1}, you need to determine the step height that corresponds to the work rate:

$$\text{step height} = 300 \text{ kgm·min}^{-1} / 60 \text{ kg} \times 18 \text{ steps·min}^{-1}$$

$$= 0.28 \text{ m, or } 28 \text{ cm}$$

Alternatively, you may choose to keep the step height constant and vary the stepping cadence for each stage of the GXT. For example, if the step height is set at 30 cm (0.30 m), and the protocol requires that a client weighing 60 kg (132 lb) exercise at a work rate of 450 kgm·min^{-1}, you need to calculate the corresponding stepping rate for this client:

$$\text{stepping rate} = 450 \text{ kgm·min}^{-1} / 60 \text{ kg} \times 0.30 \text{ m}$$

$$= 25 \text{ steps·min}^{-1}$$

You can calculate the energy expenditure in METs using the ACSM metabolic equation for stepping exercise (see table 4.3). The total gross $\dot{V}O_2$ is a function of step frequency, step height, and the resting energy expenditure. The oxygen cost of the horizontal movement is approximately 0.2 ml·kg^{-1}·m^{-1} for each four-count stepping cycle. The oxygen demand for stepping up is 1.8 ml·kg^{-1}·m^{-1}; approximately one-third more must be added (i.e., constant of 1.33 in equation) to account for the oxygen cost of stepping down. For an example of such calculations, see "ACSM Stepping Equation."

Nagle, Balke, and Naughton Maximal Step Test Protocol

Nagle, Balke, and Naughton (1965) devised a graded step test for assessing work capacity. Have your client step at a rate of 30 steps·min^{-1} on an automatically adjustable bench (2 to 50 cm). Set the initial bench height at 2 cm and increase the height 2 cm every minute of exercise. Use a metronome to establish the stepping cadence (four beats per stepping cycle). To establish a cadence of 30 steps·min^{-1}, set the metronome at 120 (30 × 4). Terminate the test when the subject is fatigued or can no longer maintain the stepping cadence. Use the ACSM metabolic equation for stepping exercise to calculate

---

ACSM STEPPING EQUATION

To calculate the energy expenditure for bench stepping using a 16 in. (about 40 cm) step height at a cadence of 24 steps·min^{-1}, use the following procedure:

$$\dot{V}O_2 \text{ in ml·kg}^{-1}\text{·min}^{-1} = [\text{frequency (F) in steps·min}^{-1} \times 0.2] + (\text{step height in m/step} \times \text{F in steps·min}^{-1} \times 1.33 \times 1.8) + \text{resting } \dot{V}O_2$$

1. Calculate the $\dot{V}O_2$ for the stepping frequency (F).

$$\dot{V}O_2 = \text{stepping frequency (F)} \times 0.20$$

$$= 24 \text{ steps·min}^{-1} \times 0.20$$

$$= 4.8 \text{ ml·kg}^{-1}\text{·min}^{-1}$$

2. Convert the bench height to meters (1 in. = 2.54 cm or 0.0254 m).

$$\text{ht} = 16 \text{ in.} \times 0.0254 \text{ m}$$

$$= 0.4064 \text{ m}$$

3. Calculate the $\dot{V}O_2$ for the vertical work performed during stepping.

$$\dot{V}O_2 = \text{bench ht} \times \text{stepping rate} \times 1.33 \times 1.8$$

$$= 0.4064 \text{ m} \times 24 \text{ steps·min}^{-1} \times 1.33 \times 1.8$$

$$= 23.35 \text{ ml·kg}^{-1}\text{·min}^{-1}$$

4. Add resting $\dot{V}O_2$ to the calculated $\dot{V}O_2$ from steps 1 and 3.

$$\dot{V}O_2 = 4.8 \text{ ml·kg}^{-1}\text{·min}^{-1} + 23.35 \text{ ml·kg}^{-1}\text{·min}^{-1} + 3.5 \text{ ml·kg}^{-1}\text{·min}^{-1}$$

$$= 31.65 \text{ ml·kg}^{-1}\text{·min}^{-1}$$

the energy expenditure ($\dot{V}O_2$max) corresponding to the step height and stepping cadence during the last work stage of this protocol.

Recumbent Stepper Maximal Exercise Test

Billinger and colleagues (2008) developed a maximum exercise test using a total body recumbent stepper (NuStep TRS 4000). This device has 10 settings ranging from 50 to 290 watts (W). The protocol begins with a 2 min warm-up at load setting 1 (50 W). Immediately following the warm-up, the initial workload is set to 4 (75 W), and the resistance is increased progressively until the participant reaches test termination criteria. A constant cadence (115 steps·min^{-1}) is used throughout the exercise protocol. Compared to treadmill testing (Bruce protocol), the recumbent stepper test elicited a lower HRmax (181 vs. 188 bpm) and $\dot{V}O_2$ (3.13 vs. 3.67 L·min^{-1}) on average. These differences are expected given the seated posture during the recumbent stepper exercise test. The correlation coefficients for $\dot{V}O_2$max ($r = 0.92$) and HRmax ($r = 0.96$) indicated a strong relationship between the Bruce protocol and the recumbent stepper protocol.

This test modality may be especially useful for assessing the cardiorespiratory fitness of individuals with neuromuscular disorders that impair gait, coordination, and balance. Seated steppers are now widely used as a training modality in rehabilitation, fitness centers, and retirement communities.

SUBMAXIMAL EXERCISE TEST PROTOCOLS

It is desirable to directly determine the functional cardiorespiratory capacity of the individual for classifying the aerobic fitness level and prescribing an aerobic exercise program. However, this is not always practical to do. The actual measurement of $\dot{V}O_2$max requires expensive laboratory equipment, a considerable amount of time to administer, and a high level of motivation on the part of the client.

Alternatively, you can use submaximal exercise tests to predict or estimate the $\dot{V}O_2$max of the individual. Many of these tests are similar to the maximal exercise tests described previously but differ in that they are terminated at some predetermined

HR intensity. You will monitor the HR, BP, and RPE during the submaximal exercise test. The treadmill, cycle ergometer, and bench stepping exercises are commonly used for submaximal exercise testing.

Assumptions of Submaximal Exercise Tests

Submaximal exercise tests assume that a *steady-state HR* is achieved and is consistent for each exercise work rate. Steady-state HR usually is achieved in 3 to 4 min at a constant, submaximal work rate. Also, it is assumed that a *linear relationship exists between $\dot{V}O_2$ and HR* within the range of 110 to 150 bpm. The HR and work rate from two submaximal work outputs can be plotted (i.e., HR–$\dot{V}O_2$ relationship) and extrapolated to HRmax to estimate $\dot{V}O_2$max from submaximal data (see figure 4.10, p. 89). Although the linear relationship between HR and $\dot{V}O_2$ holds for light-to-moderate workloads, the relationship between oxygen uptake and work rate becomes curvilinear at heavier workloads. If your clients are taking medications that alter HR, you should not use submaximal HR data to estimate their $\dot{V}O_2$max.

Another assumption of submaximal testing is that the *mechanical efficiency during cycling or treadmill exercise is constant for all individuals.* However, a client with poor mechanical efficiency while cycling has a higher submaximal HR at a given workload, and the actual $\dot{V}O_2$max is underestimated due to this inefficiency. As a result, $\dot{V}O_2$max predicted by submaximal exercise tests tends to be overestimated for highly trained individuals and underestimated for untrained, sedentary individuals.

Submaximal tests also assume that the *HRmax for clients of a given age is similar.* The HRmax, however, has been shown to vary as much as ±11 bpm, even after controlling for variability due to age and training status (Londeree and Moeschberger 1984). Also, for submaximal tests, the HRmax is estimated from age. The equation HRmax = 220 – age is widely used. The HRmax of approximately 5% to 7% of men and women is more than 15 bpm less than their age-predicted HRmax. On the other hand, 9% to 13% have HRmax values that exceed their age-predicted HRmax by more than 15 bpm (Whaley et al. 1992). Because of interindividual variability in HRmax and the potential inaccuracy with use of age-predicted HRmax, there may be considerable error (±10% to 15%) in estimating your client's $\dot{V}O_2$max, especially when submaximal data are extrapolated to an age-predicted HRmax.

In addition, Tanaka, Monahan, and Seals (2001) noted that the traditional age-predicted HRmax equation (220 – age) overestimates the measured HRmax of younger individuals and increasingly underestimates the actual HRmax of individuals older than 40 yr. Using data from a meta-analysis of 351 studies that included over 18,000 healthy, nonsmoking adults and from a controlled laboratory-based study of 514 healthy adults (18-81 yr), the authors reported that age singly accounts for 80% of the variance in HRmax, independent of gender and physical activity status. They derived the following equation to predict HRmax from age: HRmax = 208 – (0.7 × age). HRmax estimates from this equation differ from those of the traditional equation, particularly in older (>40 yr) adults. For example, the age-predicted HRmax for a 60 yr old client is 166 bpm for the revised equation (208 – 0.7 × 60 = 166 bpm) and 160 bpm for the traditional equation (220 – 60 = 160 bpm).

Gellish and colleagues (2007) used longitudinal modeling to track the relationship between HRmax and age as individuals age. Their data yielded a linear prediction equation [HRmax = 207 – (0.7 × age)] that is similar to the equation derived by Tanaka and colleagues (2001). The confidence interval for predicting HRmax of adults 30 to 75 yr was ±5 to 8 bpm. Using a nonlinear model produced a tighter confidence interval of only ±2 to 5 bpm; however, this quadratic equation, HRmax = 192 – 0.007 × age^2, is not as practical to use.

Because of interindividual variability in HRmax and the potential inaccuracy of age-predicted HRmax equations, the actual HRmax should be measured directly (by ECG or HR monitor) whenever possible. An accurate HRmax is particularly important in situations in which

- the exercise test is terminated at a predetermined percentage of either HRmax (%HRmax method) or heart rate reserve [HRR = %(HRmax – HRrest) + HRrest],
- the client's $\dot{V}O_2$max is estimated from submaximal exercise test data that are extrapolated to an age-predicted HRmax, or
- HRmax is used to determine target exercise HRs for aerobic exercise prescriptions (see chapter 5).

Treadmill Submaximal Exercise Tests

Treadmill submaximal tests provide an estimate of functional cardiorespiratory capacity ($\dot{V}O_2$max) and assume a linear increase in HR with successive increments in workload. Compared to clients with low cardiorespiratory fitness levels, the well-conditioned individual presumably is able to perform a greater quantity of work at a given submaximal HR.

You can use treadmill maximal test protocols (figure 4.2) to identify the slope of the individual's HR response to exercise. The $\dot{V}O_2$max can be predicted from either one (single-stage model) or two (multistage model) submaximal HRs. The accuracy of the single-stage model is similar to that of the multistage model.

Multistage Model

To estimate $\dot{V}O_2$max with the multistage model, use the HR and workload data from two or more submaximal stages of the treadmill test. Be sure your client reaches steady-state HRs between 115 and 150 bpm (Golding 2000). Determine the slope (*b*) by calculating the ratio of the difference between the two submaximal (SM) workloads (expressed as $\dot{V}O_2$) and the corresponding change in submaximal HRs:

$$b = (SM_2 - SM_1) / (HR_2 - HR_1)$$

Calculate the $\dot{V}O_2$ for each workload using the ACSM metabolic equation (table 4.3), and use the following equation to predict $\dot{V}O_2$max:

$$\dot{V}O_2max = SM_2 + b(HR_{max} - HR_2)$$

If the actual maximal HR is not known, estimate it using one of age-predicted HRmax equations previously mentioned. See "Multistage Model for Estimating $\dot{V}O_2$max" on page 86 for an example that illustrates how $\dot{V}O_2$max is estimated from submaximal treadmill test data for a 38 yr old male. In this example, the Bruce protocol was administered to the client. Please note that this model may be used for any multistage GXT tests.

Single-Stage Model

To estimate $\dot{V}O_2$max with the single-stage model, use one submaximal HR and one workload. The steady-state submaximal HR during a single-stage GXT should reach 130 to 150 bpm. "Formulas for Men and Women" shows formulas that have been developed (Shephard 1972).

Multistage Model for Estimating $\dot{V}O_2$max

Submaximal Data From Bruce Protocol

Stage 2[a]	Stage 1[a]
$\dot{V}O_2{}^b$ = 24.5 ml·kg^{-1}·min^{-1} (SM$_2$)	16.1 ml·kg^{-1}·min^{-1} (SM$_1$)
HR = 145 bpm (HR$_2$)	130 bpm (HR$_1$)

Maximal HR: 220 – age = 182 bpm

$$\text{Slope } (b) = (SM_2 - SM_1) / (HR_2 - HR_1)$$
$$b = (24.5 - 16.1) / (145 - 130)$$
$$b = 8.4 / 15$$
$$b = 0.56$$

$\dot{V}O_2$max: = SM$_2$ + b(HR$_{max}$ – HR$_2$)

$$= 24.5 + 0.56(182 - 145)$$
$$= 24.5 + 20.72$$
$$\dot{V}O_2\text{max} = 45.22 \text{ ml·kg}^{-1}\text{·min}^{-1}$$

---

[a]Stages 1 and 2 refer to the last two stages of the GXT completed by the client, and not the first and second stage of the test protocol. For example, if the client completes three stages of the submaximal exercise test protocol, data from stage 2 and stage 3 are used to estimate $\dot{V}O_2$.

[b]$\dot{V}O_2$ is calculated using ACSM metabolic equations (see table 4.3). $\dot{V}O_2$ can be expressed in L·min^{-1}, ml·kg^{-1}·min^{-1}, or METs.

Single-Stage Model for Estimating $\dot{V}O_2$max

Submaximal Data From Balke Protocol: Stage 3

$$\dot{V}O_2 = 5.0 \text{ METs } (SM_{\dot{V}O_2})$$
$$HR = 148 \text{ bpm } (HR_{SM})$$

Maximal HR: 220 – age = 175 bpm

$$\dot{V}O_2\text{max: } = SM_{\dot{V}O_2} \times [(HR_{max} - 72) / (HR_{SM} - 72)]$$
$$= 5 \times [(175 - 72) / (148 - 72)]$$
$$= 5 \times (103 / 76)$$
$$= 6.8 \text{ METs}$$

Formulas for Men and Women

Men

$$\dot{V}O_2\text{max} = SM_{\dot{V}O_2} \times [(HR_{max} - 61) / (HR_{SM} - 61)]$$

Women

$$\dot{V}O_2\text{max} = SM_{\dot{V}O_2} \times [(HR_{max} - 72) / (HR_{SM} - 72)]$$

$SM_{\dot{V}O_2}$ is calculated using the ACSM metabolic equations (see table 4.3). Estimate HR_{max} (if not known) using one of the age-predicted HRmax formulas; HR_{SM} is the submaximal HR.

"Single-Stage Model for Estimating $\dot{V}O_2$max" provides an example to illustrate how this model is used to predict $\dot{V}O_2$max from submaximal tread-mill data for a 45 yr old female. In this example, the Balke protocol was administered. Please note that this model may be used for any GXT protocol.

Single-Stage Treadmill Walking Test

Ebbeling and colleagues (1991) developed a single-stage treadmill walking test suitable for estimating $\dot{V}O_2$max of low-risk, healthy adults 20 to 59 yr. For this protocol, walking speed is individualized and ranges from 2.0 to 4.5 mph (53.6 to 120.6 m·min^{-1}) depending on your client's age, gender, and fitness level. Establish a walking pace during a 4 min warm-up at 0% grade. The warm-up work bout should produce a HR within 50% to 70% of the individual's age-predicted HRmax. The test consists of brisk walking at the selected pace for an additional 4 min at 5% grade. Record the steady-state HR at this workload, and use it in the following equation to estimate $\dot{V}O_2$max:

$$\dot{V}O_2\text{max} = 15.1 + 21.8(\text{speed in mph})$$
$$\text{(ml·kg}^{-1}\text{·min}^{-1}) \quad - 0.327(\text{HR in bpm})$$
$$- 0.263(\text{speed} \times \text{age in years})$$
$$+ 0.00504(\text{HR} \times \text{age})$$
$$+ 5.48(\text{gender: female} = 0; \text{male} = 1)$$

Single-Stage Treadmill Jogging Test

You can estimate the $\dot{V}O_2$max of younger adults (18 to 28 yr) using a single-stage treadmill jogging test

(George et al. 1993). For this test, select a comfortable jogging pace ranging from 4.3 to 7.5 mph (115.2 to 201 m·min^{-1}), but not more than 6.5 mph (174.2 m·min^{-1}) for women and 7.5 mph (201 m·min^{-1}) for men. Have the client jog at a constant speed for about 3 min. The steady-state exercise HR should not exceed 180 bpm. Estimate $\dot{V}O_2$max using the following equation:

$$\dot{V}O_2max = 54.07 - 0.1938(\text{body weight in kg})$$
$$(ml·kg^{-1}·min^{-1}) \quad + 4.47(\text{speed in mph})$$
$$- 0.1453(\text{HR in bpm})$$
$$+ 7.062(\text{gender: female = 0; male = 1})$$

Cycle Ergometer Submaximal Exercise Tests

Cycle ergometer multistage submaximal tests can be used to predict $\dot{V}O_2$max. These tests are either continuous or discontinuous and are based on the assumption that HR and oxygen uptake are linear functions of work rate. The HR response to submaximal workloads is used to predict $\dot{V}O_2$max.

Åstrand-Ryhming Cycle Ergometer Submaximal Exercise Test Protocol

The Åstrand-Ryhming protocol (1954) is a single-stage test that uses a nomogram to predict $\dot{V}O_2$max from HR response to one 6 min submaximal workload. A power output is selected that produces a HR between 125 and 170 bpm. The initial workload is usually 450 to 600 kgm·min^{-1} (75 to 100 W) for trained, physically active women and 600 to 900 kgm·min^{-1} (100 to 150 W) for trained, physically active men. An initial workload of 300 kgm·min^{-1} (50 W) may be used for unconditioned or older individuals.

During the test, measure the HR every minute and record the average HR during the fifth and sixth minutes. If the difference between these two HRs exceeds 5 or 6 bpm, extend the work bout until a steady-state HR is achieved. If the HR is less than 130 bpm at the end of the exercise bout, increase the workload by 300 kgm·min^{-1} (50 W) and have the client exercise an additional 6 min.

To estimate $\dot{V}O_2$max for this protocol, use the modified Åstrand-Ryhming nomogram (see figure 4.8). This nomogram estimates $\dot{V}O_2$max (in L·min^{-1}) from submaximal treadmill, cycle ergometer, and step test data. For each test mode, the submaximal HR is plotted with either oxygen cost for treadmill

exercise ($\dot{V}O_2$ in L·min^{-1}), power output (kgm·min^{-1}) for cycle ergometer exercise, or body weight (kg) for stepping exercise. For the cycle ergometer test, plot the client's power output (kgm·min^{-1}) and the steady-state exercise HR in the corresponding columns of the Åstrand-Ryhming nomogram (see figure 4.8). Connect these points with a ruler and read the estimated $\dot{V}O_2$max at the point where the line intersects the $\dot{V}O_2$max column.

The correlation between measured $\dot{V}O_2$max and the $\dot{V}O_2$max estimated from this nomogram is $r = 0.74$. The prediction error is ±10% and ±15%,

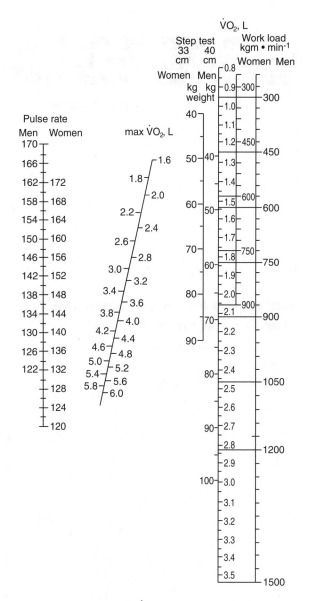

Figure 4.8 Modified Åstrand-Ryhming nomogram.

From "Aerobic Capacity in Men and Women with Special Reference to Age" by I. Åstrand, 1960. *Acta Physiologica Scandinavica* 49 (Suppl. 169), p. 51. Copyright 1960 by *Acta Physiologica Scandinavica*. Reprinted by permission.

respectively, for well-trained and untrained individuals (Åstrand and Rodahl 1977). A cross-validation study of this protocol and nomogram yielded a validity coefficient of 0.82 and a prediction error of 5.1 ml·kg^{-1}·min^{-1} for estimating the $\dot{V}O_2$max of adults 18 to 44 yr (Swain et al. 2004).

For clients younger or older than 25 yr, you must use the following age-correction factors to adjust the $\dot{V}O_2$max predicted from the nomogram for the effect of age. For example, if the estimated $\dot{V}O_2$max from the nomogram is 3.2 L·min^{-1} for a 45 yr old client, the adjusted $\dot{V}O_2$max is 2.5 L·min^{-1} (3.2 × 0.78 = 2.5 L·min^{-1}).

Age-Correction Factors for Åstrand-Ryhming Nomogram

Age	Correction factor
15	1.10
25	1.00
35	0.87
40	0.83
45	0.78
50	0.75
55	0.71
60	0.68
65	0.65

YMCA Cycle Ergometer Submaximal Exercise Test Protocol

The YMCA protocol (Golding 2000) is a cycle ergometer submaximal test for women and men. This protocol uses three or four consecutive 3 min workloads on the cycle ergometer designed to raise the HR to between 110 bpm and 85% of the age-predicted HRmax for at least two consecutive workloads. The pedal rate is 50 rpm, and the initial workload is 150 kgm·min^{-1} (25 W). Using a friction-type cycle ergometer, set the resistance to 0.5 kg (0.5 kg × 50 rpm × 6 m = 150 kgm·min^{-1}). To achieve this work rate using a plate-loaded cycle ergometer, use one weight plate (1.0 kg) and reduce the pedaling frequency to 25 rpm (1.0 kg × 25 rpm × 6 m = 150 kgm·min^{-1}). Use the HR during the last minute of the initial workload to determine subsequent workloads (see figure 4.9). If the HR is less than 86 bpm, set the second workload at 600 kgm·min^{-1}. If HR is 86 to 100, the workload is 450 kgm·min^{-1} for the second stage of the protocol. If the HR at the end of the first workload exceeds 100 bpm, set the second workload at 300 kgm·min^{-1}.

Set the third and fourth workloads accordingly (see figure 4.9). Measure the HR during the last 30 sec of minutes 2 and 3 at each workload. If these HRs differ by more than 5 or 6 bpm, extend the workload an additional minute until the HR stabilizes. If the client's steady-state HR reaches or exceeds 85% of the age-predicted HRmax during the third workload, terminate the test.

Calculate the energy expenditure ($\dot{V}O_2$) for the last two workloads using the ACSM metabolic equations (see table 4.3). To estimate $\dot{V}O_2$max from these data, use the equations for the multistage model to calculate the slope of the line depicting the HR response to the last two workloads. Alternatively, you can graph these data to estimate $\dot{V}O_2$max (see figure 4.10). To do this, plot the $\dot{V}O_2$ for each workload and corresponding HRs. Connect these two data points with

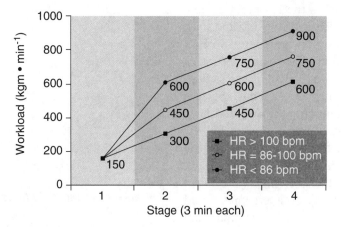

Figure 4.9 YMCA cycle ergometer protocol.

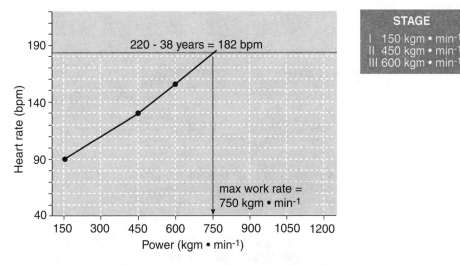

STAGE		HR
I	150 kgm • min⁻¹	91
II	450 kgm • min⁻¹	130
III	600 kgm • min⁻¹	155

Figure 4.10 Plotting heart rate versus submaximal work rates to estimate maximal work capacity and $\dot{V}O_2$max.

a straight edge, extending the line so that it intersects the predicted maximal HR line. To extrapolate $\dot{V}O_2$max, drop a perpendicular line from the point of intersection to the *x*-axis of the graph. If this is done carefully, the graphing method and multistage method will yield similar estimates of $\dot{V}O_2$max.

Swain Cycle Ergometer Submaximal Exercise Test Protocol

Swain and colleagues (2004) devised a submaximal cycle ergometry protocol for estimating $\dot{V}O_2$ max based on the relationship between heart rate reserve (HRR) and $\dot{V}O_2$ reserve ($\dot{V}O_2$R) rather than on the HR–$\dot{V}O_2$ relationship. This protocol gradually approaches a target HR of 65% to 75% HRR in 1 min stages. This target HR zone is equivalent to 65% to 75% $\dot{V}O_2$R. When the client reaches her target HR, she continues to exercise at that workload for an additional 5 min. The initial work rate and increments in work rate differ depending on the client's body mass and activity level (see figure 4.11). The predictive validity of this test was good (*r* = 0.89; *SEE* = 4.0 ml·kg⁻¹·min⁻¹) for estimating the $\dot{V}O_2$max of adults ages 18 to 44 yr. However, more cross-validation studies are needed to determine this test's applicability to older or high-risk clients.

Figure 4.11 illustrates the Swain test protocols for active and inactive clients who weigh <90 kg or ≥90 kg (198 lb). To select the appropriate protocol and to calculate your client's estimated $\dot{V}O_2$max, follow the preliminary procedures and general instructions for all clients shown on page 91 (Swain et al. 2004).

Fox Single-Stage Cycle Ergometer Test Protocol

You can modify the maximal exercise test protocol (see figure 4.7) designed by Fox (1973) to predict $\dot{V}O_2$max (ml·min⁻¹). Have your client perform a single workload (i.e., 900 kgm·min⁻¹ or 150 W) for 5 min. The standard error of estimate for this test is ±246 ml·min⁻¹, and the standard error of prediction is ±7.8%. The correlation between actual and predicted $\dot{V}O_2$max is *r* = 0.76. To estimate $\dot{V}O_2$max, measure the HR at the end of the fifth minute of exercise (HR₅) and use the following equation:

$$\dot{V}O_2max \ (ml·min^{-1}) = 6300 - 19.26(HR_5)$$

Bench Stepping Submaximal Exercise Tests

Although there are many step tests available to evaluate cardiorespiratory fitness, few provide equations for predicting $\dot{V}O_2$max. Only step test protocols with prediction equations are included in this section.

Åstrand-Ryhming Step Test Protocol

As mentioned previously, you can use the Åstrand-Ryhming nomogram (see figure 4.8, p. 87) to predict $\dot{V}O_2$max from postexercise HR and body weight during bench stepping. For this protocol, the client steps at a rate of 22.5 steps·min⁻¹ for 5 min. The bench height is 33 cm (13 in.) for women and 40 cm (15.75 in.) for men. Measure the postexercise HR by counting the number of beats between 15 and

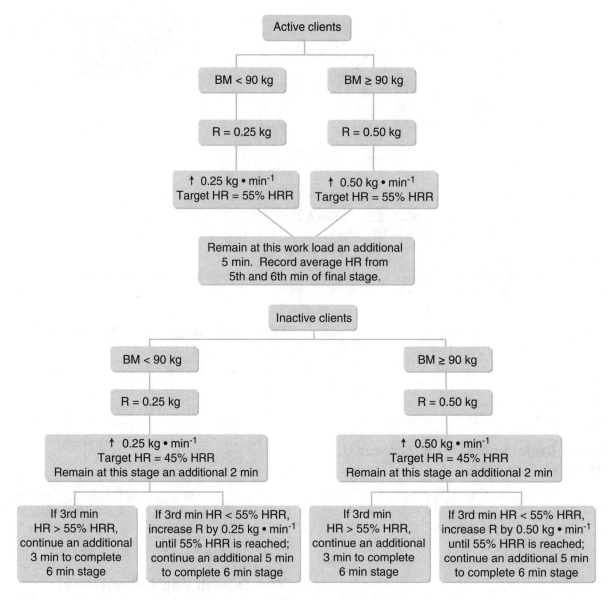

Figure 4.11 Swain cycle ergometer protocol for active clients and inactive clients.

30 sec immediately after exercise (convert this 15 sec count to beats per minute by multiplying by 4). Correct the predicted $\dot{V}O_2$max from the nomogram if your client is older or younger than 25 yr (using the age-correction factors).

Queens College Step Test Protocol

In a step test to predict $\dot{V}O_2$max devised by McArdle and colleagues (1972), the client steps at a rate of 22 steps·min^{-1} (females) or 24 steps·min^{-1} (males) for 3 min. The bench height is 16.25 in. (41.3 cm). Have your client remain standing after the exercise. Wait 5 sec and then take a 15 sec HR count. Convert the count to beats per minute by multiplying by 4. If

you are administering this test simultaneously to more than one client, you should teach your clients how to measure their own pulse rates (see p. 93). To estimate $\dot{V}O_2$max in ml·kg^{-1}·min^{-1}, use the equations listed in table 4.7. The standard error of prediction for these equations is ±16%.

Additional Modes for Submaximal Exercise Testing

If you are working in the context of a health or fitness club, you may have access to stair climbers and rowing ergometers. You can use some of these exercise machines for submaximal exercise testing of your clients.

Stair Climbing Submaximal Test Protocols

In light of the popularity of and continued interest in step aerobic training, you may choose to use a simulated stair climbing machine to estimate the aerobic fitness of some clients. The StairMaster 4000 PT and 6000 PT are two step ergometers commonly used in health and fitness settings. The StairMaster 4000 PT has step pedals that go up and down, whereas the 6000 PT model has a revolving staircase. Howley, Colacino, and Swensen (1992) reported that the HR response to increasing submaximal workloads (4.7 and 10 METs) on the StairMaster 4000 PT step ergometer was linear. Also, compared to values with treadmill exercise, the HRs measured during stepping were systematically higher (7 to 11 bpm) at each submaximal intensity. However, the MET values read from the step ergometer were about 20% higher than the measured MET values. To obtain more accurate MET values for each submaximal intensity, use the following equation:

$$\text{actual METs} = 0.556 + 0.745(\text{StairMaster 4000 PT MET value})$$

The StairMaster 4000 PT test protocol, developed by the manufacturer, provides a relatively more accurate estimate of $\dot{V}O_2$max for young women (20-25 yr) who use this device for aerobic training (r = 0.57; *SEE* = 5.3 ml·kg^{-1}·min^{-1}; *CE* = 1.0 ml·kg^{-1}·min^{-1}) as compared to estimates for their untrained counterparts (r = 0.00; *SEE* = 6.7 ml·kg^{-1}·min^{-1}; *CE* = 6.9 ml·kg^{-1}·min^{-1}) (Roy et al. 2004). This finding illustrates that the exercise testing mode should match the exercise training mode (i.e., application of the specificity principle).

To estimate $\dot{V}O_2$max, measure the steady-state HR and calculate the corrected MET value for each of two submaximal exercise intensities (e.g., 4 and 7 METs). Each stage of the test should last 3 to 6 min in order to produce steady state. Then use either the multistage model formulas (see p. 85) or the graphing method (see figure 4.10) to predict $\dot{V}O_2$max.

Table 4.7	Prediction Equations for Cardiorespiratory Field Tests	
Field test	Equation[a]	Source
	DISTANCE RUN/WALK	
1.0 mi steady-state jog	$\dot{V}O_2max = 100.5 - 0.1636(BW, kg) - 1.438(time, min) - 0.1928(HR, bpm)$ $+ 8.344(gender)^{[b]}$	George et al. (1993)
1.0 mi run/walk (8-17 yr)	$\dot{V}O_2max = 108.94 - 8.41(time, min) + 0.34(time, min)^2 + 0.21(age \times gender)^{[b]}$ $- 0.84(BMI)^{[c]}$	Cureton et al. (1995)
1.5 mi run/walk	$\dot{V}O_2max = 88.02 - 0.1656(BW, kg) - 2.76(time, min) + 3.716(gender)^{[b]}$	George et al. (1993)
1.5 mi run/walk	$\dot{V}O_2max = 100.16 + 7.30(gender)^{[b]} - 0.164(BW, kg) - 1.273(time, min)$ $- 0.1563(HR, bpm)$	Larsen et al. (2002)
12 min run	$\dot{V}O_2max = 0.0268(distance, m) - 11.3$	Cooper (1968)
15 min run	$\dot{V}O_2max = 0.0178(distance, m) + 9.6$	Balke (1963)
1.0 mi walk	$\dot{V}O_2max = 132.853 - 0.0769(BW, lb) - 0.3877(age, years) + 6.315(gender)^{[b]}$ $- 3.2649(time, min) - 0.1565(HR, bpm)$	Kline et al. (1987)
	STEP TESTS	
Åstrand	Men: $\dot{V}O_2max$ (L·min^{-1}) $= 3.744 [(BW + 5) / (HR - 62)]$ Women: $\dot{V}O_2max$ (L·min^{-1}) $= 3.750 [(BW - 3) / (HR - 65)]$	Marley and Linnerud (1976)
Queens College	Men: $\dot{V}O_2max = 111.33 - (0.42 HR, bpm)$ Women: $\dot{V}O_2max = 65.81 - (0.1847 HR, bpm)$	McArdle et al. (1972)

[a]All equations estimate $\dot{V}O_2max$ in ml·kg^{-1}·min^{-1} unless otherwise specified.

[b]For gender, substitute 1 for males and 0 for females.

[c]BMI = body mass index or body weight (body weight [BW] in kg)/ht^2 (in meters).

HR = heart rate; m = meters.

During the test, clients may hold the handrail lightly for balance but should not support their body weight. If they support their body weight, $\dot{V}O_2max$ will be overestimated (Howley et al. 1992). Also, compared to the value with treadmill testing, your client's estimated $\dot{V}O_2max$ may be lower because stair climbing produces systematically higher HRs at any given submaximal exercise intensity.

Rowing Ergometer Submaximal Test Protocols

Submaximal exercise protocols have been developed for the Concept II rowing ergometer and can be used to estimate your client's $\dot{V}O_2max$. The Hagerman (1993) protocol is designed for noncompetitive or unskilled rowers. Before beginning the test, set the fan blades in the fully closed position and select the small axle sprocket. For this test, select a submaximal exercise intensity (the HR should not exceed 170 bpm) that the client can sustain for 5 to 10 min. Measure the exercise HR at

the end of each minute. Continue the rowing exercise until the client achieves a steady-state HR. Use the Hagerman (1993) nomogram (see figure 4.12) to estimate $\dot{V}O_2max$ from the submaximal power output (watts) and the steady-state HR during the last minute of exercise.

FIELD TESTS FOR ASSESSING AEROBIC FITNESS

The maximal and submaximal exercise tests using the treadmill or cycle ergometer are not well suited for measuring the cardiorespiratory fitness of large groups in a field situation. Thus, a number of performance tests such as distance runs have been devised to predict $\dot{V}O_2max$ (see table 4.7). These tests are practical, inexpensive, less time-consuming than the treadmill or cycle ergometer tests, easy to administer to large groups, and suitable for personal training settings; they can be used to

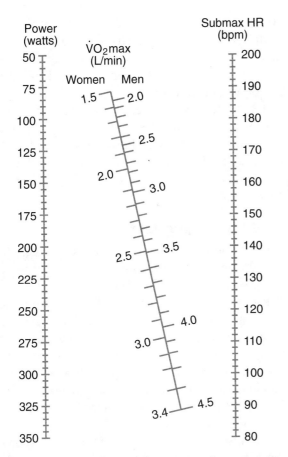

Figure 4.12 Concept II nomogram for estimating $\dot{V}O_2max$ in noncompetitive and unskilled male and female rowers.

From *Concept II Rowing Ergometer Nomogram for Prediction of Maximal Oxygen Consumption* by Dr. Fritz Hagerman, Ohio University, Athens, OH. The nomogram is not appropriate for use with non-Concept II ergometers and is designed to be used by noncompetitive or unskilled rowers participating in aerobic conditioning programs. Adapted by permission of Concept II, INC., RR1, Box 110, Morrisville, VT. (800) 245-5676.

classify the cardiorespiratory fitness level of healthy men (≤45 yr) and women (≤55 yr). You cannot use field tests to detect CHD because HR, ECG, and BP are usually not monitored during the performance. Most field tests used to assess cardiorespiratory endurance involve walking, running, swimming, cycling, or bench stepping; they require that clients be able to accurately measure their postexercise HR. Pollock, Broida, and Kendrick (1972) found that with practice, men could learn to measure their own pulse rates accurately. The correlation between manual and electronic measurements of pulse rate ranged between $r = 0.91$ and 0.94. Similar results ($r = 0.95$) were reported for college women for pulse rates measured manually and electronically (Witten 1973). Prior to administering field tests that require

HOW TO MEASURE YOUR PULSE RATE

1. Use your middle and index fingers to locate the radial pulse on the outside of your wrist just below the base of your thumb. Do not use your thumb to feel the pulse because it has a pulse of its own and may produce an inaccurate count.

2. If you cannot feel the radial pulse, try locating the carotid pulse by placing your fingers lightly on the front of your neck, just to the side of your voice box. Do not apply heavy pressure because this will cause your HR to slow down.

3. Use a stopwatch or the second hand of your wristwatch and count the number of pulse beats for a 6, 10, or 15 sec period.

4. Convert the pulse count to beats per minute using the following multipliers: 6 sec count times 10; 10 sec count times 6; and 15 sec count times 4.

5. Remember this value and record it on your scorecard.

the measurement of HR, you should teach your clients how to measure their pulse rates using the palpation technique described in "How to Measure Your Pulse Rate."

Distance Run Tests

The most commonly used distance runs involve distances of 1.0 or 1.5 mi (1600 or 2400 m) to evaluate aerobic fitness. Distance run tests are based on the assumption that the more fit individual will be able to run a given distance in less time or to run a greater distance in a given period of time. Using factor analysis, Disch, Frankiewicz, and Jackson (1975) noted that runs greater than 1.0 mi tended to load exclusively on the endurance factor rather than the speed factor.

You should be aware that the relationship between distance runs and $\dot{V}O_2max$ has not been firmly established. Although performance on a distance run can be accurately measured, it may not be an accurate index of $\dot{V}O_2max$ or a substitute for the direct measurement of $\dot{V}O_2max$. Endurance running performance may be influenced by other factors such as motivation, percent fat (Cureton et al. 1978; Katch et al. 1973), running efficiency (pacing ability), and lactate threshold (Costill and Fox 1969; Costill, Thomason, and Roberts 1973).

The correlations between distance run tests and $\dot{V}O_2$max tend to vary considerably ($r = 0.27$ to 0.90) depending on the subjects, sample size, and testing procedures (George et al. 1993; Rikli, Petray, and Baumgartner 1992; Zwiren et al. 1991). Generally, the longer the run, the higher the correlation with $\dot{V}O_2$max. On the basis of this observation, it is recommended that you select a test with a distance of at least 1.0 mi (1600 m) or a duration of at least 9 min.

The most widely used distance run tests are the 9 and 12 min runs and the 1.0 and 1.5 mi runs. Some physical fitness test batteries for children and adolescents recommend using either the 9 min or 1.0 mi run test.

9 or 12 Min Run Tests

To administer the 9 or 12 min run test, use a 400 m track or flat course with measured distances so that the number of laps completed can be easily counted and multiplied by the course distance. Place markers to divide the course into quarters or eighths of a mile so that you can quickly determine the exact distance covered in 9 or 12 min. Instruct your clients to run as far as possible. Walking is allowed, but the objective of these tests is to cover as much distance as possible in either 9 or 12 min. At the end of the test, calculate the total distance covered in meters and use the appropriate equation in table 4.7 to estimate the client's $\dot{V}O_2$max.

1.5-Mile Run/Walk Test

The 1.5 mi run/walk test is conducted on a 400 m track or flat measured area. To measure the course, use an odometer or measuring wheel. For the 1.5 mi run, instruct your clients to cover the specified distance in the fastest possible time. Walking is allowed, but the objective is to cover the distance in the shortest possible time while maintaining a steady exercise pace. Call out the elapsed time (in minutes and seconds) as the client crosses the finish line. You can use a HR monitor to ensure that your client maintains a steady exercise pace during this test. Instruct your clients to keep their target HR between 60% and 90% HRmax. The exercise HR at the end of the test, along with gender, body mass, and elapsed exercise time, can be substituted into the Larsen equation (see table 4.7) to estimate the $\dot{V}O_2$max of young (18-29 yr) adults (Larsen et al.

2002). Cross-validation of this equation yielded a high validity coefficient ($r = 0.89$) and small prediction errors ($SEE = 2.5$ ml·kg^{-1}·min^{-1}; $TE = 2.68$ ml·kg^{-1}·min^{-1}) for a sample of young military personnel (Taylor et al. 2002).

To use the $\dot{V}O_2$max prediction equations for the 1.5 mi run/walk test (see table 4.7), convert the seconds to minutes by dividing the seconds by 60. For example, if a client's time for the test is 12:30, the exercise time is converted to 12.5 min (30 / 60 sec = 0.5 min).

1.0-Mile Jogging Test

One limitation of distance run tests is that individuals are encouraged to run as fast as possible and give a maximal effort, thereby increasing the risk of cardiovascular and orthopedic injuries. The potential risk is even greater for untrained individuals who do not run or jog regularly and have difficulty selecting a proper jogging pace. To address this problem, George and colleagues (1993) developed a submaximal 1 mi track jogging test for 18 to 29 yr old women and men that requires only moderate steady-state exertion.

For this test, instruct your clients to select a comfortable, moderate jogging pace and to measure their postexercise HR immediately following the test. The elapsed time for 1 mi should be at least 8 min for males and 9 min for females, and the postexercise HR (15 sec count × 4) should not exceed 180 bpm. To help establish a suitable pace, precede the timed 1 mi test with a 2 to 3 min warm-up. Use either an indoor or outdoor track for this test. Record the time required to jog 1 mi in minutes, and have your clients measure their postexercise HRs using the palpation technique (radial or carotid sites). Estimate the client's $\dot{V}O_2$max using the prediction equation for the 1.0 mi steady-state jog test (see table 4.7).

Walking Test

The Rockport Walking Institute (1986) has developed a walking test to assess cardiorespiratory fitness for men and women ages 20 to 69 yr. Because this test requires only fast walking, it is useful for testing older or sedentary individuals (Fenstermaker, Plowman, and Looney 1992). The test was developed and validated for a large, heterogeneous sample of 86 women and 83 men (Kline et al. 1987). The cross-validation analysis resulted in a high validity coefficient and small standard error of estimate (*SEE*), indicating that the 1.0 mi walking test yields a valid submaximal assessment of estimated $\dot{V}O_2$max. Other researchers have substantiated the predictive accuracy of this equation for women 65 yr of age and older (Fenstermaker et al. 1992).

To administer this test, instruct your clients to walk 1.0 mi as quickly as possible and to take their HR immediately at the end of the test by counting the pulse for 15 sec. It is important that clients know how to take their pulse accurately. The walking course should be a measured mile that is flat and uninterrupted, preferably a 400 m track. Clients should warm up for 5 to 10 min before the test and wear good walking shoes and loose-fitting clothes.

To estimate your client's $\dot{V}O_2$max, use the generalized equation for the 1.0 mi walking test (see table 4.7). Alternatively, you can use the Rockport relative fitness charts (appendix B.2, p. 336) to classify your client's cardiorespiratory fitness level. Locate the walking time and corresponding postexercise HR (bpm) on the appropriate chart for the individual's age and gender. These charts are based on body weights of 125 lb for women and 170 lb for men. If the client weighs substantially more than this, the cardiorespiratory fitness level will be overestimated.

⎯ Step Tests

The major advantage of using step tests to assess cardiorespiratory fitness is that they can be administered to large groups in a field situation without requiring expensive equipment or highly trained personnel. Most of these step tests use postexercise and recovery HRs to evaluate aerobic fitness, but they do not provide an estimate of the individual's $\dot{V}O_2$max. Step test protocols and scoring procedures are described in appendix B.3, "Step Test Protocols," page 338.

The validity of step tests is highly dependent on the accurate measurement of pulse rate. Step tests that use recovery HR tend to possess lower validity than those using the time required for the HR to reach a specified level during performance of a standardized workload (Baumgartner and Jackson 1975). The correlation coefficients between step test performance and $\dot{V}O_2$max range between $r = 0.32$ and 0.77 (Cureton and Sterling 1964; deVries and Klafs 1965; McArdle et al. 1972).

Additional Field Tests

In addition to running, walking, and step tests, cycling and swimming tests have been devised for use in field situations (Cooper 1977). The 12 min cycling test, using a bike with no more than three speeds, is conducted on a hard, flat surface when the wind velocity is less than 10 mph (268 m·min^{-1}). These conditions limit the effect of outside influences on the rider's performance. Five- and 10-speed bikes are not employed unless use of the lower gears can be restricted. Use an odometer to measure the distance traveled in 12 min. In the 12 min swimming test, the client may use any stroke and rest as needed. Norms for the 12 min cycling test and 12 min swimming test are available (Cooper 1977).

Of these two tests, the swimming test is the less preferred because the outcome is highly skill dependent. For example, a skilled swimmer with an average cardiorespiratory fitness level will probably be able to swim farther in 12 min than a poorly skilled swimmer with an above-average cardiorespiratory fitness level. In fact, Conley and colleagues (1991, 1992) reported that the 12 min swim has low validity ($r = 0.34$ to 0.42) as a cardiorespiratory field test for male and female recreational swimmers. Whenever possible, select an alternative field test and avoid using the 12 min swim test.

EXERCISE TESTING FOR CHILDREN AND OLDER ADULTS

You may need to modify the generic guidelines for exercise testing (see "General Principles of Exercise Testing," p. 71) of low-risk adults when you are assessing cardiorespiratory fitness of children and older adults. You must take into account growth, maturation, and aging when selecting exercise testing modes and protocols for these groups.

Assessing Cardiorespiratory Fitness of Children

In the laboratory setting, you can assess the cardiorespiratory fitness of children using either the treadmill or cycle ergometer. Treadmill testing is usually preferable, especially for younger children, because their shortened attention span may not allow them to maintain a constant pedaling rate during a cycle ergometer test. Also, children younger than 8 yr or shorter than 50 in. (127 cm) may not be tall enough to use a standard cycle ergometer. To accommodate children, modify the seat height, pedal crank length, and handlebar position.

For treadmill testing, you may choose to use the modified Balke protocol (see table 4.8) because the speed is constant and the means of increasing intensity is to change the grade. The ACSM (2010) recommends using either the modified Balke protocol or the modified Bruce protocol (i.e., 2 min instead of 3 min stages). Age and gender endurance time norms for children (4-18 yr) for the modified Bruce protocol are available elsewhere (Wessel, Strasburger, and Mitchell 2001). For cycle ergometer testing, you can use the McMaster protocol (see table 4.8). For this protocol, the pedaling frequency is 50 rpm, and increments in work rate are based on the child's height.

Field tests, such as the 1.0 mi (1600 m) run/walk, are widely used to assess the cardiorespiratory fitness of children 5 to 17 yr of age. These tests are part of the Physical Best Program (American Alliance for Health, Physical Education, Recreation and Dance 1988), Fitnessgram (Cooper Institute for Aerobics Research 1994), and the President's Challenge Test (President's Council on Physical Fitness and Sports 1997), as well as national physical fitness surveys of children and youth (Ross and Pate 1987). To estimate $\dot{V}O_2$peak of 8 to 17 yr olds for the 1.0 mi run/walk test, you can use a generalized prediction equation (see table 4.7) (Cureton et al. 1995). For younger children (5 to 7 yr), the 0.5 mi run/walk test is recommended (Rikli, Petray, and Baumgartner 1992). Criterion-referenced standards for the 1.0 mi test are available elsewhere (American Alliance for Health, Physical Education, Recreation and Dance 1988; Cooper Institute for Aerobics Research 1994).

In Canada and Europe, the multistage 20 m shuttle run test, developed by Leger and colleagues (1988), is a popular alternative to distance running/walking field tests to estimate the aerobic fitness of children (8-19 yr) in educational settings. This test has been cross-validated using other samples of European and Canadian children (Anderson 1992; vanMechelen, Holbil, and Kemper 1986).

For this test, children run back and forth continuously on a 20 m (indoor or outdoor) course. The running speed is set using a sound signal emitted from a prerecorded tape. The starting pace is 8.5 km·hr[-1], and the speed is increased 0.5 km·hr[-1] each minute until they can no longer maintain the pace. The maximal aerobic speed at this stage is used, in combination with age, in the following equation to estimate $\dot{V}O_2$max:

$$\dot{V}O_2\text{max} = 31.025 + 3.238(\text{speed, km·hr}^{-1})$$
$$(\text{ml·kg}^{-1}\text{·min}^{-1}) \quad - 3.248(\text{age, yr})$$
$$+ 0.1536(\text{age} \times \text{speed})$$

Table 4.8 Graded Exercise Test Protocols for Children (Skinner 1993)

MODIFIED BALKE TREADMILL PROTOCOL

Activity classification	Speed (mph)	Initial grade (%)	Increment (%)	Duration (min)
Poorly fit	3.0	6	2	2
Sedentary	3.25	6	2	2
Active	5.0	0	2.5	2
Athletes	5.25	0	2.5	2

MCMASTER CYCLE ERGOMETER PROTOCOL

Height (cm)	Initial work rate: kgm·min⁻¹ (watts)	Increments: kgm·min⁻¹ (watts)	Duration (min)
<120	75 (12.5)	75 (12.5)	2
120-139.9	75 (12.5)	150 (25)	2
140-159.9	150 (25)	150 (25)	2
≥160	150 (25)	300 (50) for boys 150 (25) for girls	2

Assessing Cardiorespiratory Fitness of Older Adults

To assess the cardiorespiratory fitness of elderly clients, you can use modified treadmill and cycle ergometer protocols. The following modifications for standard GXT protocols are recommended:

- Extend the warm-up to more than 3 min.
- Set an initial exercise intensity of 2 to 3 METs; work increments should be 0.5 to 1.0 MET (e.g., Naughton treadmill protocol; see table 4.4, p. 76).
- Adjust (reduce) the treadmill speed to the walking ability of your client when needed.
- Extend the duration of each work stage (at least 3 min), allowing enough time for the client to attain steady state.
- Select a protocol likely to produce a total test time of 8 to 12 min.

Select treadmill protocols that increase grade, instead of speed, especially for older clients with poor ambulation. You can modify the standard Balke protocol (see figure 4.2) by having the client walk at 0% grade and 3.0 (4.8 km·hr⁻¹) mph or slower initially and by increasing the duration of each stage to at least 3 min. If elderly clients are more comfortable holding on to the handrails during a treadmill test, you can use the standard Bruce protocol and the McConnell and Clark (1987) prediction equation to estimate their $\dot{V}O_2$max (see table 4.5). Alternatively, you could use cycle ergometer GXTs for older individuals with poor balance, poor neuromuscular coordination, or impaired vision. You can also use field tests to estimate the cardiorespiratory fitness of your older (60-94 yr) clients. The Senior Fitness Test Battery (Rikli and Jones 2001) includes two measures of aerobic endurance: the 6 min walking test and the 2 min step test.

6 Min Walking Test

Purpose: Assess aerobic endurance.

Application: Measure ability to perform activities of daily living such as walking, stair climbing, shopping, and sightseeing.

Equipment: You will need a 5 × 20 yd (4.6 × 18.3 m) rectangular walking area, a measuring tape, a stopwatch, four cones, masking tape, index cards, and chairs.

Test procedures: Use masking tape or chalk to mark 5 yd (4.6 m) lines on a flat, rectangular course. Place cones on the inside corners of the rectangle. Instruct participants to walk (not jog) as fast as possible around the course for 6 min. Partners can keep track of the total number of laps and distance covered by marking the index card each time a lap is completed. Administer one trial; measure total distance to the nearest 5 yd. Test two or more people at a time for motivation.

Scoring: Calculate the total distance covered in 6 min. Each mark on the index card represents 50 yd (45.6 m). Use table 4.9 to determine a client's percentile ranking.

Safety tips: Place chairs around the outside of the walking course in case a client needs to sit and rest during the test. Select a well-lit, level walking area with a nonslip surface. Discontinue the test if the client shows signs of overexertion. Have the client cool down by stepping in place for 1 min.

Validity and reliability: The 6 min walking distance was positively related ($r = 0.78$) to submaximal treadmill walking time (Bruce protocol, time to reach 85% HRmax). This walking test detects the expected performance declines across age groups and discriminates between individuals with high and low physical activity levels and functional ability test scores. The test–retest reliability was $r = 0.94$.

2 Min Step Test

Purpose: Alternative test of aerobic endurance when time, space, or weather prohibits administering the 6 min walking test.

Application: Measure ability to perform activities of daily living such as walking, stair climbing, shopping, and sightseeing.

Equipment: You will need a stopwatch, a tape measure, masking tape, and a tally counter to count steps.

Test procedures: Determine the minimum knee-stepping height of the client by identifying the midpoint between the kneecap (midpatellar level) and iliac crest. Mark this point on the anterior aspect of the client's thigh and on a nearby wall or chair. These marks are used to monitor knee height during the test. Ask the client to step in place for 2 min, lifting the right knee as high as the target level marked on the wall. Use the tally counter to count the number of times the right knee reaches the target level.

Table 4.9 6 Min Walking Test Norms for Older Adults[a]

Percentile rank	60-64 YR		65-69 YR		70-74 YR		75-79 YR		80-84 YR		85-89 YR		90-94 YR	
	F	M	F	M	F	M	F	M	F	M	F	M	F	M
95	741	825	734	800	709	779	696	762	654	721	638	710	564	646
90	711	792	697	763	673	743	655	716	612	678	591	659	518	592
85	690	770	673	738	650	718	628	686	584	649	560	625	488	557
80	674	751	653	718	630	698	605	661	560	625	534	596	463	527
75	659	736	636	700	614	680	585	639	540	604	512	572	441	502
70	647	722	621	685	599	665	568	621	523	586	493	551	423	480
65	636	710	607	671	586	652	553	604	508	571	476	532	406	461
60	624	697	593	657	572	638	538	586	491	554	458	512	388	440
55	614	686	581	644	561	625	524	571	477	540	443	495	373	422
50	603	674	568	631	548	612	509	555	462	524	426	477	357	403
45	592	662	555	618	535	599	494	539	447	508	409	459	341	384
40	582	651	543	605	524	586	480	524	433	494	394	442	326	366
35	570	638	529	591	510	572	465	506	416	477	376	422	308	345
30	559	626	515	577	497	559	450	489	401	462	359	403	291	326
25	547	612	500	562	482	544	433	471	384	444	340	382	273	304
20	532	597	483	544	466	526	413	449	364	423	318	358	251	279
15	516	578	463	524	446	506	390	424	340	399	292	329	226	249
10	495	556	439	499	423	481	363	394	312	370	261	295	196	214
5	465	523	402	462	387	445	322	348	270	327	214	244	150	160

F = females; M = males.

[a]Values represent distance in yards; to convert yards to meters, multiply by 0.91.

Adapted, by permission, from R. Rikli and C. Jones, 2001, *Senior fitness test manual* (Champaign, IL: Human Kinetics), 125.

Table 4.10 2 Min Step Test Norms for Older Adults[a]

Percentile rank	60-64 YR		65-69 YR		70-74 YR		75-79 YR		80-84 YR		85-89 YR		90-94 YR	
	F	M	F	M	F	M	F	M	F	M	F	M	F	M
95	130	135	133	139	125	133	123	135	113	126	106	114	92	112
90	122	128	123	130	116	124	115	126	104	118	98	106	85	102
85	116	123	117	125	110	119	109	119	99	112	93	100	80	96
80	111	119	112	120	105	114	104	114	94	107	88	95	76	91
75	107	115	107	116	101	110	100	109	90	103	85	91	72	86
70	103	112	104	113	97	107	96	105	87	99	81	87	69	83
65	100	109	100	110	94	104	93	102	84	96	79	84	66	79
60	97	106	96	107	90	101	90	98	81	93	76	81	63	76
55	94	104	93	104	87	98	87	95	78	90	73	78	61	72
50	91	101	90	101	84	95	84	91	75	87	70	75	58	69
45	88	98	87	98	81	92	81	87	72	84	67	72	55	66
40	85	96	84	95	78	89	78	84	69	81	64	69	53	62
35	82	93	80	92	74	86	75	80	66	78	61	66	50	59
30	79	90	76	89	71	83	72	77	63	75	59	63	47	55
25	75	87	73	86	68	80	68	73	60	71	55	59	44	52
20	71	83	68	82	63	76	64	68	56	67	52	55	40	47
15	66	79	63	77	58	71	59	63	51	62	47	50	36	42
10	60	74	57	72	52	66	53	56	46	56	42	44	31	36
5	52	67	47	67	43	67	45	47	37	48	39	36	24	26

F = females; M = males.

[a]Values represent number of times right knee reaches target level.

Adapted, by permission, from R. Rikli and C. Jones, 2001, *Senior fitness test manual* (Champaign, IL: Human Kinetics), 126.

If the proper knee height cannot be maintained, ask the client to slow down or stop until he can execute proper form; keep the stopwatch running. Administer one trial.

Scoring: Count the number of times the right knee reaches the target level in 2 min. Use table 4.10 to determine your client's percentile ranking.

Safety tips: Clients with poor balance should stand close to a wall, doorway, or chair for support in case they lose their balance during the test. Spot each client carefully. Have the client cool down after the test by walking slowly for 1 min. Discontinue the test if your client shows signs of overexertion.

Validity and reliability: The 2 min step test scores were moderately correlated ($r = 0.73-0.74$) with Rockport 1 mi walking scores and treadmill walking (Bruce protocol, time to reach 85% HRmax) in older adults. This step test detected expected performance declines across age groups and discriminated between exercisers and nonexercisers. The test–retest reliability was $r = 0.90$.

Sources for Equipment

Product	Supplier's contact information	
Cycle ergometer (Lode, electronically braked)	AEI Technologies, Inc. (800) 793-7751 www.aeitechnologies.com	
Cycle ergometer (Monark)	Claflin Medical Equipment Co. (800) 338-2372 www.claflinequip.com	
Cycle ergometer (Bodyguard, Tunturi, Schwinn)	U.S. Fitness Products (888) 761-1638 www.usafitness.com	
Elliptical trainers	Life Fitness (800) 351-3737 www.lifefitness.com	Precor (800) 786-8404 www.precor.com
Nordic ski machine	Nordic Track (888) 308-9616 www.nordictrack.com	
Recumbent stepper	NuStep, Inc. (800) 322-4434 www.nustep.com	
Rowing ergometer	Concept 2, Inc. (800) 245-5676 www.concept2.com	
Stair climbing machines	Nautilus, Inc. (800) 628-8458 www.nautilus.com	
Treadmill (Quinton)	Cardiac Science (800) 426-0337 www.cardiacscience.com	

- The best way to assess cardiorespiratory capacity (cardiorespiratory fitness) is through a GXT in which the functional $\dot{V}O_2$max is measured.

- Unless contraindications to exercise are observed, you should administer a maximal exercise test to moderate-risk men ($\geq$45 yr) and women ($\geq$55 yr) before they begin a vigorous exercise program.

- Before, during, and after a maximal or submaximal exercise test, closely monitor the HR, BP, and RPE.

- Treadmill, cycle ergometer, and bench stepping are the most commonly used modes of exercise for exercise testing.

- The choice of exercise mode and exercise test protocol depends on the age, gender, purpose of the test, and the health and fitness status of the individual.

- Submaximal exercise tests are used to estimate the functional cardiorespiratory capacity by predicting the $\dot{V}O_2$max of the individual. Failure to meet the assumptions underlying submaximal exercise tests produces a ±10% to 20% error in the prediction of $\dot{V}O_2$max from submaximal HR data.

- Field tests are the least desirable way of assessing aerobic fitness and should not be used for diagnostic purposes. However, field tests are useful for assessing the cardiorespiratory fitness of large groups.

- Commonly used field tests include distance runs, walking tests, and step tests.

- Distance runs should last at least 9 min to assess aerobic function. Distance runs usually range between 1 and 2 mi (1600 and 3200 m) or 9 and 12 min.

- The validity of step tests for assessing cardiorespiratory fitness is highly dependent on the accurate measurement of HR and is usually somewhat lower than the validity of distance run tests.

- For children and older adults, select a treadmill protocol that increases grade rather than speed.

- The 6 min walking test or 2 min step test can be used to assess cardiorespiratory fitness of older adults in field settings.

Learn the definition for each of the following key terms. Definitions of key terms can be found in the glossary on page 411.

absolute $\dot{V}O_2$

cardiorespiratory endurance

continuous exercise test

discontinuous exercise test

graded exercise test (GXT)

gross $\dot{V}O_2$

maximal exercise test

maximum oxygen uptake ($\dot{V}O_2$max)

net $\dot{V}O_2$

ramp protocols

rating of perceived exertion (RPE)

relative $\dot{V}O_2$max

respiratory exchange ratio (RER)

submaximal exercise test

$\dot{V}O_2$max

$\dot{V}O_2$peak

REVIEW QUESTIONS

In addition to being able to define each of the key terms listed, test your knowledge and understanding of the material by answering the following review questions.

1. What is the most valid and direct measure of functional cardiorespiratory capacity?

2. What is the difference between absolute and relative $\dot{V}O_2$?

3. What is the difference between gross and net $\dot{V}O_2$?

4. What is the difference between $\dot{V}O_2$max and $\dot{V}O_2$peak?

5. What factors should you consider when choosing a maximal or submaximal exercise test protocol for your client?

6. Identify the ACSM criteria for attainment of $\dot{V}O_2$max during a GXT.

7. During a GXT, what three variables are monitored at regular intervals?

8. List three reasons for stopping a GXT.

9. What is active recovery, and why is it recommended for graded exercise testing?

10. What is the difference between continuous, discontinuous, and ramp exercise testing protocols?

11. Calculate the gross $\dot{V}O_2$ for a 60 kg woman running on a treadmill at a speed of 6.0 mph and a grade of 10%.

12. Calculate the gross $\dot{V}O_2$ for an 80 kg man cycling on Monark cycle ergometer at a pedaling frequency of 70 rpm and a resistance of 3.5 kg.

13. Calculate the energy expenditure for bench stepping using an 8 in. step and a cadence of 30 steps·min^{-1}.

14. Name three types of field tests for estimating aerobic capacity.

15. Which type of testing, treadmill or cycle ergometer, should be used for assessing the cardiorespiratory fitness of children?

16. How should standard GXT protocols be modified for testing of older adults?

Designing Cardiorespiratory Exercise Programs

- What are the basic components of an aerobic exercise prescription?
- How is the aerobic exercise prescription individualized to meet each client's goals and interests?
- What methods are used to prescribe and monitor exercise intensity?
- Which exercise modes are best suited for an aerobic exercise prescription?
- How often does a client need to exercise to improve and maintain aerobic fitness?
- How long does a client need to exercise to improve aerobic fitness?
- Is discontinuous aerobic training as effective as continuous training?
- How effective are multimodal, cross-training programs?
- What are the physiological benefits of aerobic exercise training?

Once you have assessed an individual's cardiorespiratory fitness status, you are responsible for planning an aerobic exercise program to develop and maintain the cardiorespiratory endurance of that program participant—a program designed to meet the individual's needs and interests, taking into account age, gender, physical fitness level, and exercise habits. Appendix A.5, "Lifestyle Evaluation," page 326, provides forms that will help you determine your clients' exercise patterns and preferences.

In designing the exercise prescription, keep in mind that some people engage in aerobic exercise to improve their health status or reduce their disease risk, while others are primarily interested in enhancing their physical fitness (VO_2max) levels. Given that the quantity of exercise needed to promote health is less than that needed to develop and maintain higher levels of physical fitness, you must adjust the exercise prescription according to your client's primary goal.

This chapter provides guidelines for writing individualized exercise prescriptions that promote health status as well as develop and maintain cardiorespiratory fitness. The chapter compares various training methods and aerobic exercise modes, and presents examples of individualized exercise programs.

THE EXERCISE PRESCRIPTION

It is important to consider your client's goals and purposes for engaging in an exercise program. The primary goal for exercising may affect the mode, intensity, frequency, duration, and progression of the exercise prescription. For example, the quantity of physical activity needed to achieve health benefits or reduce one's risk of illness and death is less than the amount of activity typically prescribed when the client's goal is to make substantial improvements in cardiorespiratory fitness. When the primary goal for the exercise prescription is improved health, refer to "Guidelines for Exercise Prescription for Improved Health."

On the other hand, when the primary goal for the exercise prescription is to improve cardiorespiratory fitness, refer to "ACSM and AHA Guidelines for Exercise Prescription for Improved Health and Cardiorespiratory Fitness" on page 105.

Elements of a Cardiorespiratory Exercise Workout

Each exercise workout of the aerobic exercise prescription and program should include the following phases:

- Warm-up (5-10 min)
- Endurance conditioning (20-60 min)
- Cool-down (5-10 min)
- Stretching (≥10 min)

The purpose of the warm-up is to increase blood flow to the working cardiac and skeletal muscles, increase body temperature, decrease the chance of muscle and joint injury, and lessen the chance of abnormal cardiac rhythms. During the warm-up, the tempo of the exercise is gradually increased to prepare the body for a higher intensity of exercise performed during the conditioning phase. The warm-up starts with 5 to 10 min of low-intensity (<40% VO_2reserve [VO_2R]) to moderate-intensity

(40%-60% $\dot{V}O_2 R$) aerobic activity (e.g., brisk walking for clients who jog or slow jogging for clients who run during their endurance conditioning phase).

During the endurance conditioning phase of the workout, the aerobic exercise is performed according to the exercise prescription following the **FITT principle** (i.e., F = frequency; I = intensity; T = time, duration; and T = type, mode of activity). This phase usually lasts 20 to 60 min, depending on the exercise intensity. Exercise bouts of 10 min are acceptable as long as your client accumulates at least 20 to 60 min that day. The conditioning phase is followed immediately by the cool-down phase.

A cool-down phase immediately after endurance exercise is needed to reduce the risk of cardiovascular complications caused by stopping exercise suddenly. During cool-down, the individual continues exercising (e.g., walking, jogging, or cycling) at a low intensity for about 5 to 10 min. This light activity allows the heart rate (HR) and blood pressure (BP) to return to near baseline levels, prevents the pooling of blood in the extremities, and reduces the possibility of dizziness and fainting. The continued pumping action of the muscles increases the venous return and speeds up the recovery process.

The stretching phase usually lasts at least 10 min and is performed after the warm-up or cool-down phase. Usually static stretching exercises for the legs, lower back, abdomen, hips, groin, and shoulders are included (for specific exercises, see appendix F.1, "Selected Flexibility Exercises," p. 390). Stretching exercises after the cool-down phase may help to reduce the chance of muscle cramps or muscle soreness.

GUIDELINES FOR EXERCISE PRESCRIPTION FOR IMPROVED HEALTH

The following guidelines are from the U.S. Department of Health and Human Services (2008).

1. Mode: Select endurance-type physical activities.

2. Intensity: Prescribe at least moderate-intensity physical activities (3 to 6 METs [metabolic equivalents]).

3. Frequency and duration: Schedule at least 150 to 300 min per week (e.g., 30 min, 5 days per week or 60 min, 3 days per week). Duration varies according to the type and intensity of activity (see "Examples of Moderate-Intensity and Vigorous-Intensity Aerobic Activities," chapter 1, p. 6).

ACSM AND AHA GUIDELINES FOR EXERCISE PRESCRIPTION FOR IMPROVED HEALTH AND CARDIORESPIRATORY FITNESS

These are the American College of Sports Medicine (ACSM 2010) guidelines:

1. Mode: Select rhythmical aerobic activities that can be maintained continuously and that involve large muscle groups and require little skill to perform (see "Classification of Aerobic Exercise Modalities," p. 106).

2. Intensity: Prescribe moderate-intensity (3.0 to 6.0 METs or 40% to <60% $\dot{V}O_2R$) or vigorous-intensity (>6.0 METs or ≥60% $\dot{V}O_2R$) or a combination of moderate- and vigorous-intensity exercise. Intensity varies depending on client's cardiorespiratory fitness classification.

3. Frequency: Schedule moderate-intensity exercise at least 5 days/wk; vigorous-intensity exercise at least 3 days/wk; or a combination of moderate- and vigorous-intensity exercise 3 to 5 days/wk.

4. Duration: Schedule 20 to 60 min of continuous or intermittent activity, depending on the exercise intensity. Intermittent exercise bouts of at least 10 min may be accumulated throughout the day to reach the target duration of 20 to 60 min.

5. Rate of progression: Adjust the exercise prescription for each client in accordance with the conditioning effect, participant characteristics, new exercise test results, or performance during the exercise sessions. The rate of progression depends on the individual's age, functional capacity, health status, and goals. For apparently healthy adults, the aerobic exercise prescription consists of three stages: initial conditioning, improvement, and maintenance.

Modes of Exercise

If the primary goal of the exercise program is to develop and maintain cardiorespiratory fitness, prescribe aerobic activities using large muscle groups in a continuous, rhythmical fashion. In the initial and improvement stages of the exercise program, it is important to closely monitor the exercise intensity. Therefore, you should select modes of exercise that allow the individual to maintain a constant exercise intensity and are not highly dependent on the participant's skill. **Type A activities** require minimal skill or physical fitness to perform. Activities such as walking, cycling, and aqua-aerobics are best suited for this purpose. **Type B activities** are vigorous-intensity exercises that require minimal skill but average physical fitness. Jogging, step aerobics, and spinning are examples of type B activities. You may prescribe type B activities in the initial and improvement stages for individuals who exercise regularly. **Type C activities** include endurance activities that require both skill and average physical fitness levels. Swimming, skating, and cross-country skiing should be prescribed only for individuals who have acquired these skills or who possess adequate physical fitness levels to learn these skills. **Type D activities** are recreational sports that may improve physical fitness and should be performed in addition to the person's regular aerobic exercise program. Examples of type D activities are racket sports, hiking, soccer, basketball, and downhill skiing. You should consider using type C and D activities to add variety in the later stages (maintenance stage) of your client's exercise program.

In addition to walking, jogging, and cycling, there are other exercise modalities that provide a sufficient cardiorespiratory demand for improving aerobic fitness. Exercise modalities such as bench step aerobics, machine-based stair climbing, elliptical training, and rowing offer your exercise program participants a variety of options for their exercise prescription. Many individuals prefer to cross-train to add variety and enjoyment to their aerobic workouts. But are these exercise modes just as effective as traditional type A and B activities (walking, jogging, and cycling)? The answer to this

Classification of Aerobic Exercise Modalities[a]

This list contains examples of moderate amounts of physical activity. More vigorous activities, such as stair walking and running, require less time (15 minutes). On the other hand, less vigorous activities, like washing and waxing the car, require more time (45 to 60 minutes).

Type A activities	Type B activities	Type C activities	Type D activities
■ Cycling (indoors)	■ Jogging and running	■ Aerobic dancing	■ Basketball
■ Walking	■ Rowing[b]	■ Bench step aerobics	■ Downhill skiing
■ Aqua-aerobics	■ Stair climbing[b]	■ In-line skating	■ Handball
■ Slow dancing	■ Simulated climbing[b]	■ Nordic skiing (outdoors)	■ Racket sports
	■ Nordic skiing[b]	■ Rope skiing	■ Hiking
	■ Elliptical training[b]	■ Swimming	
	■ Spinning		
	■ Fast dancing		

[a]Type A activities require minimal skill and physical fitness; type B activities require average physical fitness but minimal skill; type C activities require both skill and average physical fitness levels; type D activities are recreational sports and should be prescribed only in addition to a regular, aerobic exercise program.

[b]Machine-based activities.

question is not simple and depends on the method (%$\dot{V}O_2$max or perceived exertion) used to equate different exercise modalities.

During exercise at a prescribed percentage of $\dot{V}O_2$max, Thomas and colleagues (1995) noted that six different aerobic exercise modes (treadmill jogging, Nordic skiing, shuffle skiing, stepping, cycling, and rowing) produced relatively similar cardiovascular responses (see figure 5.1), but that cycling resulted in a significantly higher perceived exertion (RPE) compared to the other modes. Likewise, other researchers have reported that the relationship between HR and $\dot{V}O_2$ at constant, submaximal intensities was similar for treadmill jogging, in-line skating (Wallick et al. 1995), and aerobic dancing with arms used extensively above the head or kept below the shoulders (Berry et al. 1992). In contrast, Parker and colleagues (1989) reported that the average steady-state HR during 20 min of aerobic dancing was significantly higher than that for treadmill jogging when the subjects exercised at the same relative intensity (60% $\dot{V}O_2$ max). Likewise, Howley, Colacino, and Swensen (1992) noted that HR response during electronic stepping ergometer exercise was systematically higher than that with treadmill exercise at the same submaximal $\dot{V}O_2$. Also, supporting the body weight during step

ergometer exercise significantly reduced the HR and oxygen consumption compared to lightly holding on to the handrails for balance.

When exercise modes are equated using subjective ratings of perceived exertion (RPEs), research suggests that treadmill jogging may be superior to other aerobic exercise modes in terms of total oxygen consumption and rate of energy expenditure (Kravitz, Robergs, and Heyward 1996; Kravitz et al. 1997b; Zeni, Hoffman, and Clifford 1996). Subjects exercising on seven different modalities at a somewhat hard (RPE = 13 or 14) intensity for 15 to 20 min experienced a greater total oxygen consumption for treadmill jogging compared to stepping, rowing, Nordic skiing, cycling, shuffle skiing, and aerobic riding (Kravtiz et al. 1997b; Thomas et al. 1995). Also, the rate of energy expenditure during treadmill exercise was 20% to 40% greater than during stationary cycling (Kravitz et al. 1997b; Zeni et al. 1996) and 57% greater than during aerobic riding (Kravitz et al. 1996, Kravitz et al. 1997b). In addition, steady-state exercise HRs were higher (see figure 5.2) for treadmill jogging compared to cycling and aerobic riding (Kravitz, Robergs, and Heyward 1996; Kravitz et al. 1997b; Zeni et al. 1996).

When selecting aerobic exercise modes for your client's exercise prescription, you should consider

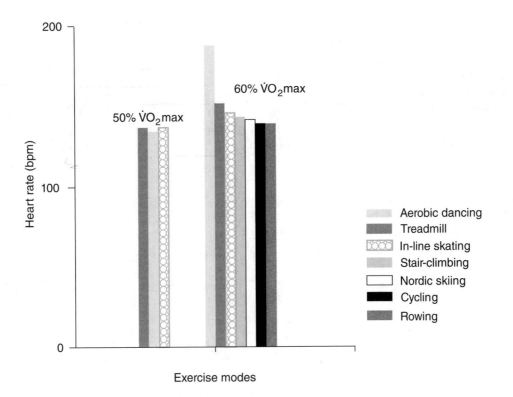

Figure 5.1 Comparison of steady-state heart rate response at submaximal exercise intensities for various aerobic exercise modes.

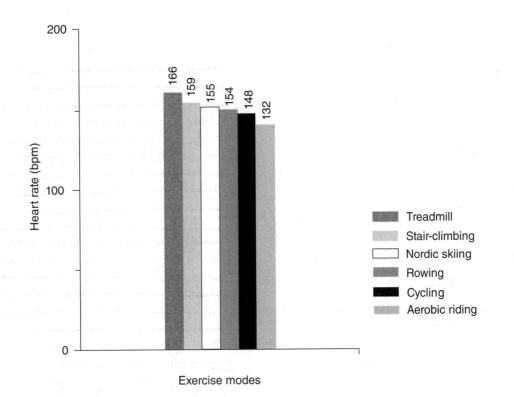

Figure 5.2 Comparison of steady-state heart rate response at somewhat hard intensity (rating of perceived exertion = 13 or 14) for various aerobic exercise modes.

how easily the exercise intensity can be graded and adjusted in order to overload the cardiorespiratory system throughout the improvement stage. For aerobic dance and bench step aerobic exercise, work rates can be progressively increased by means of quicker cadences, different bench heights (Olson et al. 1991), and upper body exercise using light (1 to 4 lb [0.45 to 1.8 kg]) handheld weights (Kravitz et al. 1997a). The intensity of in-line skating can be effectively graded by increasing the skating velocity (Wallick et al. 1995). The intensity of rowing, stair climbing, and simulated whole-body climbing exercise can be incremented progressively using a variety of exercise machines (Brahler and Blank 1995; Howley et al. 1992).

Prescribe rope-skipping activities with caution; the exercise intensity for skipping 60 to 80 skips·min^{-1} is approximately 9 METs. This value exceeds the maximum MET capacity of most sedentary individuals. Also, the exercise intensity is not easily graded because doubling the rate of skipping increases the energy requirement by only 2 to 3 METs. Town, Sol, and Sinning (1980) reported an average energy expenditure of 11.7 to 12.5 METs for skipping at rates of 125, 135, and 145 skips·min^{-1}. They concluded that rope skipping is a strenuous exercise that may not serve well as a form of graded aerobic exercise.

When selecting exercise modes for your older clients, you need to consider their functional aerobic capacity, musculoskeletal problems, and neuromuscular coordination (impaired vision or balance). Select activities that are enjoyable and convenient. For many older adults, walking is an excellent mode. Stationary cycling and aquatic exercise can be used for individuals with impaired vision or balance. Research suggests that tai chi increases balance, muscular strength, and flexibility as well as cardiorespiratory fitness ($\dot{V}O_2$peak) of older adults (Chewning, Yu, and Johnson 2000; Lan et al. 1998).

Intensity of Exercise

Traditionally, exercise intensity has been expressed as a straight percentage of either the individual's maximal aerobic capacity ($\dot{V}O_2$max), peak oxygen consumption ($\dot{V}O_2$peak), or heart rate reserve (HRR). However, research has suggested that the %$\dot{V}O_2$max is not equivalent (1:1 ratio) to the %HRR for cycling and treadmill exercise (Swain and Leutholtz 1997; Swain et al. 1998). Therefore, ACSM changed its

recommendation regarding the method used to calculate exercise intensity for aerobic exercise prescriptions. Instead of expressing relative intensity as a straight percentage of $\dot{V}O_2$max (%$\dot{V}O_2$max), ACSM recommends using the **percent $\dot{V}O_2$max reserve (%$\dot{V}O_2$R)**. The $\dot{V}O_2$R is the difference between the $\dot{V}O_2$max and resting oxygen consumption ($\dot{V}O_2$rest). With this modification, percent values for the %$\dot{V}O_2$R and %HRR methods for prescribing exercise intensity are approximately equal, thereby improving the accuracy of calculating a target $\dot{V}O_2$, particularly for clients who are engaging in low-intensity aerobic exercise (Swain 1999).

Regardless of the method used, intensity and duration of exercise are indirectly related. In other words, the higher the exercise intensity, the shorter the duration of exercise required and vice versa. Before prescribing the exercise intensity for aerobic exercise, carefully evaluate the individual's initial cardiorespiratory fitness classification, goals for the program, exercise preferences, and injury risks. Your client can improve cardiorespiratory fitness with either lower-intensity, longer-duration exercise or higher-intensity, shorter-duration exercise. For most individuals, low-to-moderate intensities of longer duration are recommended; higher-intensity exercise increases the risk of orthopedic injury and discourages continued participation in the exercise program.

Part of the art of exercise prescription is being able to select an exercise intensity that is adequate to stress the cardiovascular system without overtaxing it. According to ACSM (2010), the initial exercise intensity for apparently healthy adults is 40% to 85% $\dot{V}O_2$R, depending on their initial physical fitness classification (i.e., fair to excellent cardiorespiratory fitness level). Lower-intensity exercise (30%-45% $\dot{V}O_2$R) may be sufficient to provide important health benefits for sedentary clients or older individuals with poor initial cardiorespiratory fitness levels. For most individuals, intensities of 55% to 80% $\dot{V}O_2$R are sufficient to improve cardiorespiratory fitness. As a general rule, the more fit the individual, the higher the exercise intensity needs to be to produce further improvement in cardiorespiratory fitness. Exercise intensity can be prescribed using the $\dot{V}O_2$ reserve, HR, or RPE method.

$\dot{V}O_2$Reserve (MET) Method

First, measure the client's functional aerobic capacity ($\dot{V}O_2$max or $\dot{V}O_2$peak) using a graded exercise test (see chapter 4). Express the client's $\dot{V}O_2$max in relative terms, that is, ml·kg^{-1}·min^{-1} or METs (metabolic equivalents). Given that 1 MET approximately equals 3.5 ml·kg^{-1}·min^{-1}, a $\dot{V}O_2$max of 35 ml·kg^{-1}·min^{-1}, for example, would be equivalent to 10 METs (35 / 3.5 = 10 METs).

Next determine the **$\dot{V}O_2$reserve ($\dot{V}O_2$R)**. As mentioned previously, the $\dot{V}O_2$R is the difference between $\dot{V}O_2$max and $\dot{V}O_2$rest ($\dot{V}O_2$R = $\dot{V}O_2$max – $\dot{V}O_2$rest). The percent of $\dot{V}O_2$R depends on the initial cardiorespiratory fitness level of the client. To calculate the target $\dot{V}O_2$ (in METs) based on the $\dot{V}O_2$R, use the following equation:

$$target\ \dot{V}O_2 = [relative\ exercise\ intensity\ (\%) \times \dot{V}O_2R] + \dot{V}O_2rest$$

For example, the target $\dot{V}O_2$ corresponding to 50% $\dot{V}O_2$R for a client with a $\dot{V}O_2$max of 10 METs is calculated as follows:

$$target\ \dot{V}O_2 = [0.50 \times (10 - 1\ MET)] + 1\ MET$$
$$= (0.50 \times 9\ METs) + 1\ MET$$
$$= 4.5 + 1.0\ METs,\ or\ 5.5\ METs$$

The exercise intensity (METs) for walking, jogging, running, cycling, and bench-stepping activities is directly related to the speed of movement, power output, or mass lifted. Use the ACSM equations (table 4.3, p. 73) to calculate the speed or work rates corresponding to a specific MET intensity for the exercise prescription. For example, to estimate how fast a woman should jog on a level course to be exercising at an intensity of 8 METs, follow these steps:

1. Convert the METs to ml·kg^{-1}·min^{-1}.

$$\dot{V}O_2 = 8\ METs \times 3.5\ ml·kg^{-1}·min^{-1}$$
$$= 28\ ml·kg^{-1}·min^{-1}$$

2. Substitute known values into the ACSM running equation and solve for speed.

$$28\ ml·kg^{-1}·min^{-1} = [speed\ (m·min^{-1}) \times 0.2] + 3.5\ ml·kg^{-1}·min^{-1}$$
$$28.0\ ml·kg^{-1}·min^{-1} - 3.5 = speed\ (m·min^{-1}) \times 0.2$$
$$122.5\ m·min^{-1} = speed$$

3. Convert speed to mph.

$$1\ mph = 26.8\ m·min^{-1}$$
$$122.5\ m·min^{-1} / 26.8\ m·min^{-1} = 4.57\ mph$$

4. Convert mph to minute per mile pace.

$$pace = 60\ min/hr / mph$$
$$= 60\ min/hr / 4.57\ mph$$
$$= 13.1\ min·mi^{-1}\ (or\ 8.1\ min·km^{-1})$$

Average MET values for selected conditioning exercises, sports, and recreational activities are presented in appendix E.4, "Gross Energy Expenditure for Conditioning Exercises, Sports, and Recreational Activities," page 382. When estimating MET values for children and adolescents, use the compendium of energy expenditures (MET values) developed for youth (see Ridley, Ainsworth, and Olds 2008). Prescribing exercise intensity using only MET values has certain limitations. The caloric costs (i.e., average MET values) of conditioning exercises are only estimates of energy expenditure. The caloric costs of activities, particularly type C activities, vary greatly with the individual's skill level. Although these MET estimates provide a starting point for prescribing exercise intensity, environmental factors such as heat, humidity, altitude, and pollution may alter the HR and RPE responses to exercise. Therefore, you should use the HR or RPE method along with the MET method to ensure that the exercise intensity does not exceed safe limits.

Heart Rate Methods

There are three ways to prescribe exercise intensity for your clients using HR data. Each of these approaches is based on the assumption that HR is a linear function of exercise intensity (i.e., the higher the exercise intensity, the higher the HR).

Heart Rate Versus MET Graphing Method

When a submaximal or maximal graded exercise test (GXT) is administered, the client's steady-state HR response to each stage of the exercise test can be plotted (see figure 5.3). The HRmax is the HR observed at the highest exercise intensity during a maximal GXT. For submaximal GXTs, you can estimate your client's HRmax using one of the age-predicted HRmax formulas (e.g., 220 – age). From this graph, you can obtain HRs corresponding to given percentages of the estimated functional capacity or $\dot{V}O_2$max. In our example, the functional capacity of the individual is 7.4 METs, and the HRmax is 195 bpm. The HRs corresponding to

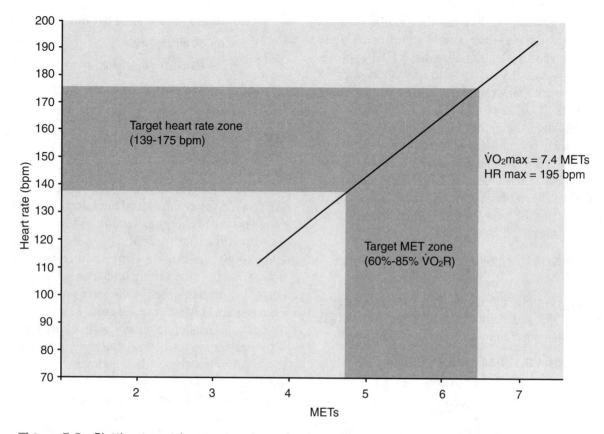

Figure 5.3 Plotting target heart rate zone using graded exercise test data (heart rate vs. METs). HRmax = maximal heart rate; $\dot{V}O_2R$ = oxygen reserve.

exercise intensities of 4.8 and 6.4 METs (60% to 85% $\dot{V}O_2R$) are 139 and 175 bpm, respectively. During exercise workouts, the individual should measure the HR using a HR monitor or palpation to verify that the appropriate exercise intensity is reached.

It is important to note that the HR response to graded exercise is dependent to some extent on the mode of exercise testing. For example, compared to treadmill testing, exercising on an electronic step ergometer elicits higher HRs, and stationary cycling typically results in somewhat lower HRs at the same relative exercise intensities. When using this method to obtain HRs for an exercise prescription, be sure to match the exercise testing and training modes by selecting a testing mode that elicits HR responses that are similar to those obtained for the training mode (see figure 5.1). For example, if your client chooses in-line skating as a training mode, you should administer a treadmill GXT, given that the relationship between HR and $\dot{V}O_2$ at submaximal exercise intensities is similar for these two exercise modes (Berry et al. 1992).

Heart Rate Reserve Method

When HR data from a GXT are not available, you can use the **Karvonen**, or **percent heart rate reserve (%HRR), method** to determine target HRs for your client's exercise prescription. The **heart rate reserve (HRR)** method takes into account the resting HR and maximal HR. The HRR is the difference between the maximal HR and resting HR. A percentage of HRR is added to the client's resting HR to determine the target exercise HR:

target HR = [% exercise intensity × (HRmax – HRrest)] + HRrest

As previously mentioned, the percent values for the HRR method closely approximate the percent values for the $\dot{V}O_2R$ method (Swain and Leutholtz 1997; Lounana et al. 2007). The ACSM (2010) recommends using 40% to 85% HRR. For example, if

maximal HR = 178 bpm,

resting HR = 68 bpm, and

exercise intensity = 60% HRR, then

$$\text{target exercise HR} = 0.60(178 - 68) + 68$$
$$\text{or } 134 \text{ bpm.}$$

Percentage of Maximal Heart Rate Method

You also can use a straight percentage of maximal HR (**percent heart rate maximum, %HRmax**) to estimate exercise intensity and determine target exercise HR. This method is based on the fact that the %HRmax is related to %$\dot{V}O_2$R and %HRR. In table 5.1, we can see that 67% and 94% HRmax correspond to exercise intensities of 45% and 85% $\dot{V}O_2$R or HRR. The ACSM (2010) recommends prescribing target HRs between 64% and 94% HRmax depending on the fitness level of your client.

With use of this technique, the actual maximal HR must be known or must be predicted either from the HR response to submaximal workloads or from the HRmax prediction equations such as 220 – age or 206.9 – (0.67 × age). For example, if the age-predicted maximal HR is 180 bpm and the exercise intensity is set at 70% HRmax, the target exercise HR is equal to 126 bpm.

$$\text{\%HRmax} \times \text{HRmax} = \text{target HR}$$
$$0.70 \times 180 \text{ bpm} = 126 \text{ bpm}$$

Compared to the Karvonen (%HRR) method, the %HRmax method tends to give a lower value when the same relative intensity is used. If in our example the client's resting HR is 80 bpm, the target HR using the Karvonen method is 150 bpm [0.70 × (180 – 80) + 80 bpm] compared to 126 bpm for the %HRmax method.

The ACSM (2010) recommends using the %HRmax method to prescribe exercise intensity for your older clients. The %HRmax provides a more accurate estimate of %$\dot{V}O_2$peak of older adults than the %HRR method; using the %HRR method results in a higher than expected percentage of $\dot{V}O_2$max (Kohrt et al. 1998). However, you should measure, not predict (220 – age), the client's HRmax, for two reasons. Older individuals (>65 yr of age) have large variability in HRmax, and they are more likely to be taking medications that affect peak HR.

Limitations of Heart Rate Methods

Exclusive use of HR to develop intensity recommendations for your client's exercise prescription may lead to large errors in estimating relative exercise intensities (%$\dot{V}O_2$R) for some individuals. This is especially true when HRmax is predicted from age (220 – age) instead of being directly measured. In about 30% of the population, an age-predicted prescription of 60% HRR may be as low as 70% or as high as 80% of the actual HRmax (Dishman 1994). Measured HRmax varies with exercise mode. Therefore, your client's perceived effort may differ among exercise modes even during exercise at the same submaximal HR. Also, medications, emotional states, and environmental factors (e.g., temperature, humidity, and air pollution) can affect your client's exercise training HRs. You should consider using RPEs to adjust the exercise intensity in such situations.

Ratings of Perceived Exertion Method

In light of the limitations associated with using HR for setting exercise intensity, consider using a combination of HR and RPE in developing prescriptions for your clients. You can use RPEs to prescribe and monitor exercise intensity (Birk and Birk 1987). The RPE scales (see table 4.2, p. 69, and appendix B.4, p. 341) are valid and reliable tools for assessing the level of physical exertion during continuous aerobic exercise (Birk and Birk 1987; Borg and Linderholm 1967; Dunbar et al. 1992; Robertson 2004).

Table 5.1   Comparison of Methods for Prescribing Exercise Intensity for Healthy Adults

CR fitness classification	%HRR or %$\dot{V}O_2$R	%HRmax	RPE
Poor	30-45	57-67	Light-moderate
Fair	40-55	64-74	Light-moderate
Average	55-70	74-84	Moderate-hard
Good	65-80	80-91	Moderate-hard
Excellent	70-85	84-94	Somewhat hard-hard

HRR = heart rate reserve; RPE = rating of perceived exertion.

During the GXT, the client rates the intensity of each stage of the test using a RPE scale. You can use the intensities (METs) corresponding to somewhat hard (6 on OMNI scale or 12 on Borg RPE scale) to hard (8 on OMNI scale or 16 on Borg RPE scale) to set the minimum and maximum training intensities for the exercise prescription. Compared to the %HRR method, RPEs between 12 and 16 closely approximate 40% and 84% HRR, respectively (Pollock et al. 1998). With practice an individual can learn to associate RPE with a specific target exercise HR, especially at higher exercise intensities (Smutok, Skrinar, and Pandolf 1980). Thus, the RPE can be used instead of HR, or in combination with HR, to monitor training intensity and to adjust the exercise prescription for conditioning effects.

One advantage of RPE as a method of monitoring exercise intensity is that your clients do not need to stop exercising in order to check their HRs. For an extensive review of research pertaining to the use of perceived exertion for prescribing exercise intensity, see the studies of Dishman (1994) and Robertson (2004).

Monitoring Exercise Intensity

Throughout the aerobic exercise program, carefully monitor exercise intensity in order to ensure your client's safety and to confirm that your client is exercising at or near the prescribed intensity. The HR and RPE methods can be used for this purpose. Teach your clients how to monitor exercise intensity using HR palpation techniques (see chapter 2), HR monitors, and the RPE scales (see table 4.2, p. 69).

Some clients may prefer using a talk test to monitor their exertion. The **talk test** is a measure of the client's ability to converse comfortably while exercising and is based on the relationship between exercise intensity and pulmonary ventilation. **Pulmonary ventilation**, or the movement of air into and out of the lungs, increases linearly with exercise intensity ($\dot{V}O_2$) up to a point. At the breaking point, known as the **ventilatory threshold**, pulmonary ventilation increases exponentially relative to the exercise intensity and rate of oxygen consumed. At the ventilatory threshold, it becomes difficult to speak during exercise. Studies of college-age students (Persinger et al. 2004), clinically stable cardiac patients (Voelker et al. 2002), and athletes (Recalde et al. 2002) showed that individuals who pass the talk test are exercising at intensities that are within the accepted guidelines for the exercise prescription. Those failing the talk test are exercising at intensities that exceed the prescribed level. The talk test provides a fairly precise and consistent method for monitoring exercise during stationary cycling and treadmill exercise (Persinger et al. 2004).

Frequency of Exercise

The frequency of the exercise sessions depends on your client's caloric goals, health and fitness level, preferences, and time constraints. For health benefits, individuals should exercise at a moderate intensity on at least 5 days per week. Individuals with fair to excellent cardiorespiratory fitness levels should exercise at a moderate to vigorous intensity a minimum of three to five times per week to produce significant changes in aerobic endurance (ACSM 2010). Individuals with poor cardiorespiratory fitness levels should exercise at light to moderate intensities a minimum of 5 days a week. Multiple daily exercise bouts of at least 10 min duration each may be prescribed for sedentary clients having poor aerobic fitness.

In terms of improving $\dot{V}O_2$max, the sequence of exercise sessions seems to be less important than the total work (volume) performed during the training. Similar improvements were noted for individuals who trained every other day (M-W-F) and three consecutive days (M-T-W) (Moffatt, Stamford, and Neill 1977). The ACSM (2010) recommends exercising on alternate days during the initial stages of training to lessen the chance of bone or joint injury. Also, older adults who can tolerate vigorous exercise should work out at least 3 days/wk with a day of rest between each exercise session (ACSM 2010).

Duration of Exercise

As an exercise specialist, you must prescribe an appropriate combination of exercise intensity and duration so that the individual adequately stresses the cardiorespiratory system without overexertion. As mentioned earlier, the intensity and duration of exercise are inversely related (the lower the exercise intensity, the longer the duration of the exercise). The ACSM (2010) recommends 20 to 60 min of continuous or intermittent activity. Apparently healthy individuals usually can sustain exercise intensities of 60% to 85% $\dot{V}O_2R$ for 20 to 30 min. To improve functional capacity ($\dot{V}O_2$max), exercise of moderate intensity and duration (20-30 min) is recommended for most adults (ACSM 2010). During the improvement stage, duration can be increased every 2 to 3 wk until participants can exercise continuously for 30 min at a moderate to vigorous intensity (ACSM 2010). Poorly conditioned and older individuals may be able to exercise continuously at a low intensity (<40% $\dot{V}O_2R$) for only 5 to 10 min. They may need to perform multiple sessions (e.g., two to three 10 min exercise bouts) in a given day to accumulate 20 to 30 min of aerobic exercise.

An alternative way of estimating the duration of exercise is to use the caloric cost of the exercise. To achieve health benefits, ACSM (2010) recommends target **caloric thresholds** of 150 to 400 kcal·day^{-1}, and a minimal weekly caloric threshold of 1000 kcal from physical activity or exercise.

During the initial stage of the exercise program, however, weekly exercise caloric expenditure may be considerably lower (200 to 600 kcal·wk^{-1}). Throughout the improvement stage, the goal is to increase your client's caloric expenditure from 1000 to 2000 kcal·wk^{-1} by gradually increasing the frequency, intensity, and duration of the exercise. For example, in order for a 60 kg (132 lb) woman who is exercising at an intensity of 7 METs, five times per week, to reach a weekly net caloric threshold of 1500 kcal·wk^{-1}, she needs to expend 300 kcal per exercise session (1500 kcal / 5 = 300 kcal). You can estimate the net caloric cost of her exercise (kcal·min^{-1}) using the following formula:

$$\text{net caloric cost (kcal·min}^{-1}) = \text{METs} \times 3.5 \times \text{body mass in kg} / 200$$

To calculate the net caloric expenditure from her activity, subtract the resting oxygen consumption (1 MET) from the gross $\dot{V}O_2$ ($\dot{V}O_2$ cost of exercise + $\dot{V}O_2$rest) and substitute this value (7 − 1 = 6 METs) into the equation:

$$\text{net caloric cost} = 6 \text{ METs} \times 3.5 \times 60 \text{ kg} / 200$$
$$= 6.3 \text{ kcal·min}^{-1}$$

Therefore, she needs to exercise approximately 48 min (300 kcal/6.3 kcal·min^{-1}), five times per week, in order to achieve her weekly caloric expenditure goal of 1500 kcal.

Rate of Progression

Physiological changes associated with aerobic endurance training (see "Physiological Changes Induced by Cardiorespiratory Endurance Training," p. 114) enable the individual to increase the total work performed. The greatest conditioning effects occur during the first 6 to 8 wk of the exercise program. Aerobic endurance may improve as much as 3% per week during the first month, 2% per week for the second month, and 1% per week or less thereafter. For continued improvements, the cardiorespiratory system must be overloaded through adjustments in the intensity and duration of the exercise to the new level of fitness. The degree and rate of improvement depend on the age, health status, and initial fitness level of the participant. For the average person, aerobic training programs generally produce a 5% to 20% increase in $\dot{V}O_2$max (Pollock 1973). Sedentary, inactive persons may improve as much as 40% in aerobic fitness, while elite athletes may improve only 5% because they begin at a level much closer to their genetic limits. We do not expect older individuals entering the exercise program to improve as quickly as younger individuals even when the initial fitness levels are the same.

Stages of Progression

As discussed in chapter 3, the three stages of progression for cardiorespiratory exercise programs are the initial conditioning, improvement, and maintenance stages (ACSM 2010).

Initial Conditioning

The initial conditioning stage may last 1 to 6 wk, depending on your client's rate of adaptation to the exercise program. In this stage, each exercise session should include a warm-up, moderate-intensity (3-6 METs) aerobic activity, low-intensity muscular fitness exercises, and a cool-down that emphasizes stretching exercises (ACSM 2006). Clients starting a moderate-intensity aerobic conditioning program should exercise a minimum of 3 to 5 days/wk. The duration of the aerobic exercise should be at least 20 min and progress to 30 min. After clients are able to sustain aerobic activity at 55% to 60% HRR for 30 min, they progress to the improvement stage.

Improvement

The improvement stage usually lasts 4 to 8 mo. During this stage, the rate of progression is more rapid. Intensity, duration, and frequency of exercise should always be increased independently. Either

Physiological Changes Induced by Cardiorespiratory Endurance Training

Cardiorespiratory System

Increases

- Heart size and volume
- Blood volume and total hemoglobin
- Stroke volume—rest and exercise
- Cardiac output—maximum
- $\dot{V}O_2max$
- Oxygen extraction from blood
- Lung volumes

Decreases

- Resting heart rate
- Submaximal exercise heart rate
- Blood pressure (if high)

Musculoskeletal System

Increases

- Mitochondria—number and size
- Myoglobin stores
- Triglyceride stores
- Oxidative phosphorylation

Other Systems

Increases

- Strength of connective tissues
- Heat acclimatization
- High-density lipoprotein cholesterol

Decreases

- Body weight (if overweight)
- Body fat
- Total cholesterol
- Low-density lipoprotein cholesterol

duration or frequency should be increased before intensity is increased. Increase the duration no more than 20% per week until your clients are able to sustain moderate-to-vigorous exercise for 20 to 30 min. Frequency should progress from 3 to 5 days/wk. Once the desired duration and frequency are reached, the exercise intensity may be increased by no more than 5% HRR every sixth exercise session (ACSM 2010).

Rate of progression during this stage depends on a number of factors. Cardiac patients, older adults, and less fit individuals may need more time for the body to adapt to a higher conditioning intensity. In such cases, the exercise duration should be at least 20 to 30 min before the exercise intensity increases (ACSM 2010).

Maintenance

After achieving the desired level of cardiorespiratory fitness, an individual enters the maintenance stage

of the exercise program. This stage continues on a regular, long-term basis if the individual has made a lifetime commitment to exercise.

The goal of this stage is to maintain the cardiorespiratory fitness level and the weekly exercise caloric expenditure achieved during the improvement stage. Have your client accomplish this goal by engaging in aerobic activities 3 to 5 days/wk at the intensity and duration that were reached at the end of the improvement stage. Reducing the training frequency from 5 to 3 days/wk does not adversely affect $\dot{V}O_2max$ as long as the training intensity remains the same. However, clients should participate in other activities an additional 2 or 3 days/wk. To this end, a variety of enjoyable activities from the type C and D classifications may be selected to counteract boredom and to maintain the interest level of the participant. For example, an individual who was running 5 days/wk at the end of the improvement stage may choose to run only 3 days/wk and substitute in-line skating and racquetball on the other 2 days.

AEROBIC TRAINING METHODS AND MODES

Either continuous or discontinuous training methods can improve cardiovascular endurance. **Continuous training** involves one continuous aerobic exercise bout performed at low-to-moderate intensities without rest intervals. Discontinuous training consists of several intermittent low- to high-intensity exercise bouts interspersed with rest periods. Both training methods produce significant improvements in $\dot{V}O_2$max (Morris et al. 2002). Recent research suggests that when the volume of exercise is controlled, high-intensity endurance interval training (90-95% HRmax; 95% $\dot{V}O_2$R) improves $\dot{V}O_2$max more than continuous, moderate-intensity (70% HRmax; 50% $\dot{V}O_2$R) aerobic exercise training in healthy adults (Gormley et al. 2008; Helgerud et al. 2007). However, one concern about high-intensity intermittent training is the possibility of exercise burnout. Pollock and colleagues (1977) reported that the dropout rate of adults in a high-intensity interval (discontinuous) training program was twice that of those in a continuous jogging program. Thus, for the typical client, high-intensity interval training may be better suited for stimulating short-term (e.g., 4 wk) improvements in cardiorespiratory fitness and for adding variety to the exercise program. Future research needs to address the long-term health benefits of interval training and its effects on exercise adherence for the general population.

Continuous Training

All of the exercise modes listed as type A or B activities (see p. 106) are suitable for continuous training. One advantage of continuous training is that the prescribed exercise intensity (e.g., 75% HRR) is maintained fairly consistently throughout the duration of the steady-paced exercise. Generally, continuous exercise at low-to-moderate intensities is safer, more comfortable, and better suited for individuals initiating an aerobic exercise program.

Walking, Jogging, and Cycling

The most popular modes of continuous training are walking, jogging or running, and cycling. Exercise programs using walking, jogging, and cycling provide similar cardiovascular benefits (Pollock, Cureton, and Greninger 1969; Pollock et al. 1971, 1975; Wilmore et al. 1980). Improvements in $\dot{V}O_2$max are comparable for most commonly used exercise modes. Pollock and colleagues (1975) compared running, walking, and cycling exercise programs of middle-aged men who trained at 85% to 90% HRmax. All three groups showed significant improvements in $\dot{V}O_2$max. These results indicate that improvement in $\dot{V}O_2$max is independent of the mode of training when frequency, intensity, and duration of exercise are held constant and are prescribed in accordance with sound, scientific principles.

Aerobic Dance

Since the early 1970s, aerobic dance has continued to be a popular mode of exercise for improving and maintaining cardiorespiratory fitness. A number of excellent books provide detailed information about aerobic dance methods and techniques (Kuntzelman 1979; Wilmoth 1986). A typical aerobic dance workout consists of 8 to 10 min of stretching, calisthenics, and low-intensity exercise. This is followed by 15 to 45 min of either high- or low-impact aerobic dancing at the target training intensity. Handheld weights (1 to 4 lb [0.45 kg to 1.8 kg]) can be used to increase exercise intensity. Heart rates should be monitored at least six times during the exercise to ensure that the HR stays within the target zone. The 10 min cool-down period usually includes more stretching and calisthenic-type exercises.

Several studies conducted to assess the cardiorespiratory effect of aerobic dance training have documented average increases in $\dot{V}O_2$max of 10% or greater (Blessing et al. 1987; Milburn and Butts 1983; Parker et al. 1989; Williford et al. 1988). Milburn and Butts (1983) reported that aerobic dance was as effective as jogging for improving cardiorespiratory endurance when performed at similar intensity, frequency, and duration. The subjects trained 30 min, 4 days/wk for 7 wk, at 83% to 84% HRmax.

Bench Step Aerobics

Health and fitness clubs throughout the United States are promoting bench step training as an effective high-intensity, low-impact aerobic exercise mode. Step training uses whole-body movements on steps or benches, ranging in height from 4 to 12 in. (10.2 to 30.5 cm). Choreographed movement routines are performed to music. A typical bench step aerobic workout consists of 5 to 10 min of warm-up and 20 to 30 min of step training. This is followed by a short (3 to 5 min) cool-down.

Exercise training intensity can be graded through use of variations in stepping cadence or bench height. To reduce the risk of injury during stepping on and off the bench, bench heights of 6 to 8 in. (15.2-20.3 cm) and stepping cadences ranging from 118 to 128 steps·min^{-1} are recommended. In terms of energy expenditure, increasing bench height is more effective than increasing cadence. In a study comparing the energy expenditure of bench stepping at two different cadences (125 vs. 130 steps·min^{-1}) and bench heights (6 vs. 8 in., or 15.2 vs. 20.3 cm), there was no significant difference in energy expenditure (kcal·min^{-1}) between the two different cadences. Increasing bench height from 6 to 8 in. (15.2 to 20.3 cm), however, increased energy expenditure by 1.04 kcal·min^{-1} (Grier et al. 2002). Thus, it is more effective to alter the intensity of a typical aerobic stepping routine by increasing the step height than by increasing the stepping cadence.

Studies confirm that continuous step training at bench heights ranging from 6 to 12 in. (15.2 to 30.5 cm) provides an adequate training stimulus that meets ACSM (2010) guidelines for intensity and duration (Olson et al. 1991; Petersen et al. 1993; Woodby-Brown, Berg, and Latin 1993). Following 8 to 12 wk of step aerobic training, $\dot{V}O_2$max improves as much as 8% to 16% (Kravitz et al. 1993; Kravitz et al. 1997a; Velasquez and Wilmore 1992). In a study comparing bench step exercise with and without hand weights, use of 2 to 4 lb (0.9 kg to 1.8 kg) hand weights did not result in a greater improvement in $\dot{V}O_2$max than step training without hand weights (Kravitz et al. 1997a).

Step Ergometry and Stair Climbing

Step ergometry (machine-based stair climbing) is a popular exercise mode in health and fitness clubs. Research shows a linear HR response to graded submaximal exercise performed on stair climbing ergometers. However, the MET levels displayed on the StairMaster 4000 PT overestimate the actual MET intensity of the exercise (Howley et al. 1992).

When prescribing exercise intensity using this type of stair climber, be certain to adjust the machine's estimates for each MET level using the following equation:

actual METs = 0.556 + 0.745(StairMaster MET setting)

Although machine-based stair climbing provides a training stimulus that meets guidelines for exercise intensity, there are relatively few studies comparing the effectiveness of stair climbing training to other aerobic training modes (Howley et al. 1992; Thomas et al. 1995).

Elliptical Training

Elliptical training machines have become popular in the fitness industry. Elliptical trainers are designed for either upper body or combined upper and lower body exercise. The lower body motion during exercise on an elliptical trainer is a cross between the actions performed with machine-based stair climbing and upright stationary cycling. With elliptical trainers, the feet move in an egg-shaped or elliptical pattern, and the feet stay in contact with the footpads of the device throughout the exercise. Unlike running or jogging, this form of exercise may provide a high-intensity workout with low-impact forces comparable to those for walking (Porcari, Foster, and Schneider 2000). Although there is no research documenting the long-term effects of this type of training on cardiovascular fitness, preliminary data suggest that this exercise modality meets ACSM (2010) guidelines for developing and maintaining cardiorespiratory fitness (Kravitz et al. 1998; Porcari et al. 2000). Kravitz and colleagues (1998) reported that the average energy expenditure during forward–backward exercise with no resistance and against resistance for 5 min (125 strides·min^{-1}) was, respectively, 8.1 and 10.7 kcal·min^{-1}. Exercise intensities ranged between 72.5% and 83.5% HRmax (age predicted). Compared to treadmill exercise, upper body elliptical training at self-selected intensities produced similar $\dot{V}O_2$, HR, and RPE responses (Crommett et al. 1999; Porcari et al. 2000). Although there was no difference in $\dot{V}O_2$ between combined upper and lower body elliptical training and treadmill exercise, upper and lower body elliptical training produced a significantly higher HR and RPE (Crommett et al. 1999).

Aerobic Riding

Aerobic riding involves both upper and lower body muscle groups. For this reason, some manufacturers claim that this mode of exercise will automatically burn more calories than lower body–only exercise modes such as jogging, cycling, and stair climbing. One study, however, noted that the energy expenditure during 10 min of steady-state exercise at a somewhat hard intensity (RPE = 13) on an aerobic rider was significantly lower than the caloric expenditure for treadmill jogging, stationary cycling, and Nordic skiing (Kravitz et al. 1997b). Subjects reported that they felt a similar workout intensity, in terms of RPE, during aerobic riding. Aerobic riding appears to challenge the muscular system (subjects complained of muscular discomfort) more than the cardiovascular system. In fact, the relative submaximal $\dot{V}O_2$ (47% $\dot{V}O_2$max) for aerobic riding was significantly less than that for treadmill jogging (74% $\dot{V}O_2$max), Nordic skiing (68% $\dot{V}O_2$max), or stationary cycling (64% $\dot{V}O_2$max). Thus, aerobic riding may not be suitable for aerobic exercise prescriptions, particularly for individuals with above-average cardiorespiratory fitness.

Water-Based Exercise

Water-based exercise, such as water aerobics or walking in waist-deep water, has been promoted as an effective way to increase the cardiorespiratory fitness of young, middle-aged, and older adults. This exercise is especially popular among individuals who are older, overweight, or afflicted with orthopedic disabilities. A typical water-based exercise session includes the following phases:

- Warm-up—20 min of stretching before entering the pool, followed by walking slowly in the water
- Endurance phase—30 min of continuous walking and dancing in the water
- Resistance phase—10 min of resistance exercises performed underwater with dumbbells, barbell-like devices, and leg pads
- Cool-down—10 min of relaxation and floor exercises outside of the pool

In older women (60-75 yr) participating in water-based exercise training 3 days/wk for 12 wk, $\dot{V}O_2$peak increased by 12% while total cholesterol and low-density lipoprotein cholesterol decreased by 11% and 17%, respectively. Also, muscle strength and arm and leg power increased significantly in response to exercising the limbs against the resistance of water (Takeshima et al. 2002).

Innovative Aerobic Exercise Modes

New and innovative modes of aerobic exercise are introduced every year by the fitness industry in order to stimulate and maintain exercise participation of clients. Many of these new programs combine traditional exercise modes (e.g., stationary cycling, stepping, tai chi, and martial arts) with music. Fitness centers throughout the country now offer group exercise classes using programs such as BodyCombat, RPM, BodyPump, BodyStep, and Tae Bo. BodyCombat is an aerobic workout that combines movements from karate, boxing, taekwondo, and tai chi with fast-paced music. RPM is an indoor cycling workout to music that includes warm-up, pace, hill, mixed terrain, interval, free spin, mountain climb, and stretch segments. BodyPump is a conditioning class that adds strength training with weights to aerobic workouts choreographed to music. Tae Bo is an aerobic exercise routine that combines music with elements of taekwondo and kick boxing to promote aerobic fitness.

Rixon and colleagues (2006) compared exercise HRs and estimates of energy expenditure for Body-Combat (73% HRmax; 9.7 kcal·min⁻¹), RPM (74.3% HRmax; 9.9 kcal·min⁻¹), BodyStep (72.4% HRmax; 9.6 kcal·min⁻¹), and BodyPump (60.2% HRmax; 8.0 kcal·min⁻¹) routines. With the exception of BodyPump, the intensity and duration of these exercise routines appear to be sufficient to meet physical activity recommendations for improving health and for weight management. Training studies are needed to determine the health benefits and effects of these exercise programs on aerobic fitness.

Discontinuous Training

As mentioned previously, discontinuous training involves a series of low- to high-intensity exercise bouts interspersed with rest or relief periods. All of the exercise modes listed as type A and type B activities (see p. 106) are suitable for discontinuous training. Because of the intermittent nature of this form of training, the exercise intensity and total amount of work performed can be greater than with continuous training, making discontinuous training a versatile method that is widely used by athletes, as well as individuals with low cardiorespiratory fitness. In fact, ACSM (2010) recommends the use of discontinuous (intermittent) training for symptomatic individuals who are able to tolerate only low-intensity exercise for short periods of time (3 to 5 min). Interval training, treading, spinning, and circuit resistance training are examples of intermittent or discontinuous training.

Interval Training

Interval training involves a repeated series of exercise work bouts interspersed with rest or relief periods. This method is popular among athletes because it allows the athlete to exercise at higher relative intensities during the work interval than are possible with longer-duration, continuous training. Interval training programs also can be designed to improve speed and anaerobic endurance, as well as aerobic endurance, simply by means of modifications in the exercise intensity and length of the work and relief intervals.

Each work interval consists of running at a pace such that a distance of 1100 yd (1005 m) is covered in 3 to 4 min. The work interval is followed by a rest–relief interval of 1.5 to 2 min. This sequence is repeated three times. During the rest–relief interval, the individual usually walks or jogs while recovering from the work bout. For aerobic interval training, the ratio of work to rest-relief is usually 1:1 or 1:0.5. Each work interval is 3 to 5 min and is repeated three to seven times. The exercise intensity usually ranges between 70% and 85% $\dot{V}O_2$max. Apply the overload principle by increasing the exercise intensity or length of the work interval, decreasing the length of the rest–relief interval, or increasing the number of work intervals per exercise session. For a discussion of interval training and sample programs, including programs for

AN INTERVAL TRAINING PRESCRIPTION TO DEVELOP AEROBIC ENDURANCE

Sets: One

Repetitions: Three

Distance: 1100 yd (1105 m)

Time: 3 to 4 min

Rest–relief interval: 1.5 to 2 min

developing speed and anaerobic endurance, refer to the work of Janssen (2001).

Treading and Spinning

Treading and spinning are two examples of interval training that have gained popularity in fitness clubs because of the variety and enjoyment they offer. Treading and spinning are group classes that involve walking, jogging, and running at various speeds and grades on a treadmill (treading) or stationary cycling at various cadences and resistances (spinning). A typical treading or spinning workout consists of 1:1 or 1.5:1 work–recovery intervals or stages that are repeated for a specified duration. For example, a 30 min treading class may consist of six stages. Each stage lasts 5 min (i.e., 3 min work interval and 2 min recovery interval). One can advance the intensity of the work interval by increasing the treadmill speed or grade. During the recovery interval, both the speed and grade of the treadmill are decreased (e.g., 2.5 mph [4 km·hr^{-1}] and 0% grade). Instructors individualize and adapt the workouts for their clients by adjusting the duration of the work–recovery intervals and varying the speed and grade.

In one study, researchers designed 30 min treading workouts for walkers and runners (Nichols, Sherman, and Abbott 2000). They reported that the average intensity of the walking protocol was 40% to 49% $\dot{V}O_2$max for male and female walkers, respectively. For the running protocol, the average intensity of the work intervals was 76% to 80% $\dot{V}O_2$max for male and female runners, respectively. The researchers suggested that these average intensities, as well as the duration of the workout (30 min), are sufficient to meet ACSM standards for an aerobic exercise prescription. More research is needed to determine the long-term training effects of treading and spinning on cardiorespiratory fitness.

Circuit Resistance Training

Use of circuit resistance training for the development of aerobic fitness, as well as muscular strength and tone, has received much attention. An example of a circuit resistance training program is presented in chapter 7, page 163 (see figure 7.1). Circuit resistance training usually consists of several circuits of resistance training with a minimal amount of rest between the exercise stations (15 to 20 sec). Alternatively, instead of rest, you can have your clients perform 1 to 3 min of aerobic exercise between each station. The aerobic stations may include activities such as stationary cycling, jogging in place, rope skipping, stair climbing, bench stepping, and rowing. This modification of the circuit is known as **super circuit resistance training**.

Gettman and Pollock (1981) reviewed the research dealing with the physiological benefits of circuit resistance training. Because it produces only a 5% increase in aerobic capacity as compared to a 15% to 25% increase with other forms of aerobic training, the authors concluded that circuit resistance training should not be used to develop aerobic fitness. Rather, it may be used during the maintenance stage of an aerobic exercise program.

PERSONALIZED EXERCISE PROGRAMS

The aerobic exercise prescription should be individualized to meet each client's training goals and interests. To do this, you need to consider your client's age, gender, physical fitness level, and exercise preferences. This section presents a sample case study and examples of individualized exercise prescriptions to illustrate how the exercise prescription may be personalized for each client.

Case Study

Like any preventive or therapeutic intervention, exercise should be prescribed carefully. You must be able to evaluate your client's medical history, medical condition, physical fitness status, lifestyle characteristics, and interests before designing the exercise program. In addition, to test your ability to extract, analyze, and evaluate all pertinent information needed to design a safe exercise program for your client, many professional certification examinations require that you be able to analyze a case study. For these reasons this section includes a sample case study (see p. 122).

A case study is a written narrative that summarizes client information that you will need to develop an accurate and safe individualized exercise prescription (Porter 1988). Important elements to focus on when reading and analyzing a case study are listed in "Essential Elements of a Case Study" (see p. 120). First, identify the client's coronary heart disease (CHD) risk factors by focusing on information provided about family history of CHD, blood lipid profile (total cholesterol, high- and low-density lipoprotein cholesterol [HDL-C and LDL-C]), blood glucose levels, resting BP, physical activity, body fat level, and smoking. Become familiar with ideal or typical values for various blood chemistry tests so that you will be able to recognize normal or abnormal test results. Remember that each of the following factors places individuals at greater risk for CHD:

- Triglycerides $\geq$150 mg·dl^{-1}
- Total cholesterol $\geq$200 mg·dl^{-1}
- LDL-cholesterol $\geq$130 mg·dl^{-1}
- HDL-cholesterol <40 mg·dl^{-1}
- Total cholesterol/HDL ratio >5.0
- Blood glucose $\geq$110 mg·dl^{-1}
- Systolic BP $\geq$140 or diastolic BP $\geq$90 mmHg

Use the demographic data (age and gender) and CHD risk factors to determine the client's CHD risk classification (low, moderate, or high risk). The CHD risk classification dictates how closely the client's exercise program needs to be monitored.

Pay close attention to information about the client's medical history and physical examination results. These may reveal signs or symptoms of CHD, particularly if shortness of breath, chest pains, or leg cramps are reported or if high BP is detected. It is also important to note the types of medication the client is using. Drugs such as digitalis, beta-blockers, diuretics, vasodilators, bronchodilators, and insulin may alter the body's physiological responses during exercise and could affect the HR and BP responses reported for the GXT. Keep in mind that exercise programs need to be modified for individuals with musculoskeletal disorders such as arthritis, low back pain, osteoporosis, and chondromalacia. Next, be certain to key in on information regarding the client's lifestyle. Factors such as smoking, lack of physical activity, or diets high in saturated fats or cholesterol increase the risk of CHD, atherosclerosis, and hypertension. You often can target these factors for modification; they also help you assess the likelihood of the client's adherence to the exercise program (see table 3.3, p. 51).

Examine the BP, HR, and RPE data for the GXT used to assess the client's functional aerobic capacity and cardiorespiratory fitness level. You need to be acutely aware of the normal and abnormal physiological responses to graded exercise. After assessing the client's CHD risk and cardiorespiratory fitness level, you can design an aerobic exercise program using a personalized exercise prescription of intensity, frequency, duration, mode, and progression. To write the exercise prescription, use the results from the GXT (HR, RPE, functional MET capacity).

The sample case study on page 122 is provided to test your ability to evaluate risk factors and GXT results and to prescribe an accurate and safe aerobic exercise program for this individual. See the results of the analysis in appendix B.5, "Analysis of Sample Case Study in Chapter 5," page 344.

Sample Cycling Program

The sample cycling program on page 124 shows a personalized cycling program for a 27 yr old female who was given a maximal GXT on a stationary cycle ergometer. Her measured $\dot{V}O_2$max is 7.4 METs. The exercise intensity is based on a percentage of her $\dot{V}O_2$reserve (%$\dot{V}O_2$R), and the target exercise HRs corresponding to 60% (4.8 METs) and 80% $\dot{V}O_2$R (6.1 METs) are 139 bpm and 168 bpm, respectively (see figure 5.3). Thus, the training exercise HR should fall within this HR range. During the initial stage of the exercise program, the woman will cycle at a work rate corresponding to 60% $\dot{V}O_2$R (4.8 METs) for 2 wk.

Essential Elements of a Case Study

Demographic Factors

- Age
- Gender
- Ethnicity
- Occupation
- Height
- Body weight
- Family history of coronary heart disease

Medical History

Present symptoms

- Dyspnea or shortness of breath
- Angina or chest pain
- Leg cramps or claudication
- Musculoskeletal problems or limitations
- Medications

Past history

- Diseases
- Injuries
- Surgeries
- Lab tests

Lifestyle Assessment

- Alcohol and caffeine intake
- Smoking
- Nutritional intake, eating patterns
- Physical activity patterns and interests
- Sleeping habits
- Occupational stress level
- Mental status, family lifestyle

Physical Examination

- Blood pressure
- Heart and lung sounds
- Orthopedic problems or limitations

Laboratory Tests (Ideal or Typical Values)

- Triglycerides (<150 mg·dl^{-1})
- Total cholesterol (<200 mg·dl^{-1})
- LDL-cholesterol (<100 mg·dl^{-1})
- HDL-cholesterol (>40 mg·dl^{-1})
- Total cholesterol/HDL-cholesterol (<3.5)
- Blood glucose (60-110 mg·dl^{-1})
- Hemoglobin: 13.5-17.5 g·dl^{-1} (men)
  11.5-15.5 g·dl^{-1} (women)
- Hematocrit: 40-52% (men)
  36-48% (women)
- Potassium (3.5-5.5 meq·dl^{-1})
- Blood urea nitrogen (4-24 mg·dl^{-1})
- Creatinine (0.3-1.4 mg·dl^{-1})
- Iron: 40-190 mg·dl^{-1} (men)
  35-180 mg·dl^{-1} (women)
- Calcium (8.5-10.5 mg·dl^{-1})

Physical Fitness Evaluation

- Cardiorespiratory fitness (HR, BP, $\dot{V}O_2$max)
- Body composition (% body fat)
- Musculoskeletal fitness (muscle and bone strength)
- Flexibility
- Balance

During weeks 1 and 2, the exercise duration is increased by 5 min/wk (from 40 to 45 min). During the third week, relative exercise intensity rather than duration is increased by 5% (from 60% $\dot{V}O_2R$ to 65% $\dot{V}O_2R$). The work rate corresponding to an exercise intensity is calculated using the ACSM formulas for leg ergometry (see table 4.3, p. 73). For example, the work rate corresponding to 60% $\dot{V}O_2R$ (4.8 METs or 16.8 ml·kg^{-1}·min^{-1}) is calculated as follows:

$$\dot{V}O_2 \text{ (ml·kg}^{-1}\text{·min}^{-1}) = W / M \times 1.8 + 3.5 + 3.5$$

where W = work rate in kgm·min^{-1}
and M = body mass in kg.

$$16.8 = W / 70 \text{ kg} \times 1.8 + 7.0$$

$$16.8 - 7.0 = W / 70 \text{ kg} \times 1.8$$

$$9.8 \times 70 \text{ kg} / 1.8 = 381 \text{ kgm·min}^{-1}$$

To calculate the resistance setting corresponding to 381 kgm·min^{-1} for a cycling cadence of 50 rpm, divide the work rate by the total distance the flywheel travels: 381 / 50 rpm × 6 = 1.27 kg, or 1.3 kg.

To calculate the net energy cost (kcal·min^{-1}) of cycling, subtract the resting $\dot{V}O_2$ (1 MET) from the gross $\dot{V}O_2$ for each intensity. Convert this net MET value to kcal·min^{-1} using the following formula:

$$\text{kcal·min}^{-1} = \text{METs} \times 3.5 \times \text{body mass (kg)} / 200$$

(e.g., 4.8 − 1.0 = 3.8 METs; 3.8 × 3.5 × 70 kg / 200

= 4.7 kcal·min^{-1})

In the initial stages of the program, the weekly net energy expenditure is between 752 and 1040 kcal. In the improvement stage, the exercise intensity, duration, and frequency are progressively increased, and the weekly net caloric expenditure ranges between 1040 and 1874 kcal. Only one variable—intensity, duration, or frequency—should be increased at a time. The variable that is increased during each stage of the progression for this exercise program is indicated by boldface. During the improvement stage, this client's net caloric expenditure due to exercise meets the caloric threshold (>1000 kcal per week from physical activity) recommended by ACSM (2010). In the maintenance phase, tennis and aerobic dancing are added to give variety and to supplement the cycling program. The ACSM (2010) guidelines were followed to calculate each component of this exercise prescription.

Sample Jogging Program

The sample jogging program on page 125 is designed for a 29 yr old male who has an excellent cardiorespiratory fitness level. Since a GXT could not be administered, the $\dot{V}O_2$max was predicted from performance on the 12 min distance run test. The maximal HR was predicted using the formula 220 − age. Because this client is accustomed to jogging and his cardiorespiratory fitness level is classified as excellent, he is exempted from the initial stage and enters the improvement stage of the program immediately. During this time (20 wk), the exercise intensity is increased from 70% to 85% of the estimated $\dot{V}O_2R$. The speed corresponding to each MET intensity is calculated using the ACSM formulas for running on a level course (see table 4.3, p. 73). The intensity, duration, and frequency of the exercise sessions provide a weekly net caloric expenditure between 1010 and 2170 kcal. During the first 4 wk of the program, this client's net rate of energy expenditure due to exercise is 10.2 kcal·min^{-1} (8.3 METs × 3.5 × 70 kg / 200 = 10.2 kcal·min^{-1}); thus, he will expend approximately 1010 kcal, jogging 33 min at an 11:06 min per mile pace three times per week (33 min × 10.2 kcal·min^{-1} × 3). To figure the distance covered, the exercise duration is divided by the running pace: 33 min / 11.1 min·mi^{-1} = 3 mi. During the improvement stage, the frequency of exercise sessions gradually progresses from 3 to 5 days/wk. During the maintenance stage, the running is reduced to 3 days/wk, and handball and basketball are added to the aerobic exercise program. The ACSM (2010) guidelines were followed to calculate each component of this exercise prescription.

Sample Multimodal Exercise Program

Some clients may prefer to engage in a variety of exercise modes (**cross training**) to develop their cardiorespiratory fitness (see "Sample Multimodal Exercise Program" on p. 126). In these cases, it is difficult to systematically prescribe increments in exercise intensity using METs or target HRs. Although MET equivalents for various activities are available (see appendix E.4, p. 382), typically a range of values is given, making it difficult for you to accurately prescribe work rates corresponding to specific intensity recommendations in an exercise prescription. Also, the HR response to a given MET level is highly dependent on the exercise mode.

A 28 yr old female police officer (5 ft 5 in. or 165.1 cm; 140 lb or 63.6 kg; 28% body fat) has enrolled in the adult fitness program. Her job demands a fairly high level of physical fitness—a level she was able to achieve 6 yr ago when she passed the physical fitness test battery used by the police department. Before becoming a police officer, she jogged 20 min, usually three times a week. Since starting her job, she has had little or no time for exercise and has gained 15 lb (6.8 kg). She works 8 hr a day, is divorced, and takes care of two children, ages 7 and 9. At least three times a week, she and the children dine out, usually at fast food restaurants like Burger King and Taco Bell. She reports that her job, along with the sole responsibility for raising her two children, is quite stressful. Occasionally she experiences headaches and a tightness in the back of her neck. Usually in the evening she has one glass of wine to relax.

Her medical history reveals that she smoked one pack of cigarettes a day for 4 yr while she was in college. She quit smoking 3 yr ago. Over the past 2 yr she has tried some quick weight loss diets, with little success. She was hospitalized on two occasions to give birth to her children. She reports that her father died of heart disease when he was 52 and that her older brother has high blood pressure. Recently she had her blood chemistry analyzed because she was feeling light-headed and dizzy after eating. In an attempt to lose weight, she eats only one large meal a day, at dinnertime. Results of the blood analysis were total cholesterol = 220 mg·dl^{-1}; triglycerides = 98 mg·dl^{-1}; glucose = 82 mg·dl^{-1}; high-density lipoprotein cholesterol = 37 mg·dl^{-1}; and total cholesterol/high-density lipoprotein cholesterol ratio = 5.9.

The exercise evaluation yielded the following data:

- Mode, protocol: Treadmill, modified Bruce
- Resting data: HR = 75 bpm; BP = 140/82 mmHg
- Endpoint: Stage 4 (2.5 mph [4 km·hr^{-1}], 12% grade). Test terminated because of fatigue.

Stage	METs	Duration (min)	HR (bpm)	BP (mmHg)	RPE
1	2.3	3	126	145/78	8
2	3.5	3	142	160/78	11
3	4.6	3	165	172/80	14
4	7.0	3	190	189/82	18

Analysis

1. Evaluate the client's CHD risk profile. Be certain to address each of the positive and negative risk factors.
2. Describe any special problems or limitations that need to be considered in designing an exercise program for this client.
3. Were the HR, BP, and RPE responses to the GXT normal? Explain.
4. What is the client's functional aerobic capacity in METs? Categorize her cardiorespiratory fitness level (see table 4.1, p. 67).
5. Plot the HR versus METs on graph paper.
6. From the graph, determine the client's target HR zone for the aerobic exercise program. What HRs and RPEs correspond to 60%, 70%, and 75% of the client's $\dot{V}O_2R$?
7. The client expressed an interest in walking outside on a level track to develop aerobic fitness. Calculate her walking speed for each of the following training intensities: 60%, 70%, and 75% $\dot{V}O_2R$. Use the ACSM equations presented in table 4.3, page 73.
8. In addition to starting an aerobic exercise program, what suggestions do you have for this client for modifying her lifestyle?

See appendix B.5, page 344, for answers to these questions.

The degree of muscle mass involved in the activity, as well as whether the body weight is supported during exercise, can affect the HR response to a prescribed exercise intensity. For example, whole-body exercise modes, such as Nordic skiing and aerobic dancing, involve both upper and lower body musculature. These produce higher submaximal HRs than lower body exercise modes (e.g., cycling and jogging). Also, at any given exercise intensity, the HR response during weight-bearing exercise such as jogging is greater than that for non-weight-bearing exercise (e.g., cycling).

Therefore, you should use RPEs to progressively increase exercise intensity throughout the improvement stage of a multimodal aerobic exercise program (see table 4.2, p. 69). To use the RPE safely and effectively, you will need to teach your clients to focus on and learn to monitor important exertional cues such as breathing effort (rate and depth of breathing) and muscular sensations (e.g., pain, warmth, and fatigue). Guidelines for developing multimodal exercise prescriptions are presented on this page.

For **multimodal exercise programs**, you should set exercise frequency and weekly net caloric expenditure goals for each client (see "Sample Multimodal Exercise Program"). Provide your clients with estimates of net energy expenditure ($kcal \cdot min^{-1}$) for each of the aerobic activities they select for their exercise prescriptions. The exercise duration to achieve a specified weekly net caloric expenditure goal will vary depending on the activity mode chosen for each exercise session. Any combination of type A, B, or C activities can be used, provided that the client is able to maintain the prescribed RPE intensity for at least 20 min.

Flexibility is the key to successful multimodal exercise prescriptions. Clients should be free not only to select exercise modes of interest but also to decide on various combinations of frequency and duration as long as they meet the caloric thresholds specified in their exercise prescriptions for each week.

The primary advantages of multimodal exercise programs over single-mode (e.g., jogging or cycling) programs for many of your clients are

- greater likelihood of engaging in a safe and effective exercise program,
- overall greater enjoyment of physical activity and exercise,
- better understanding of how their bodies respond to exercise,
- more direct involvement and sense of control in developing and monitoring their exercise programs, and
- increased likelihood of incorporating physical activity and exercise into their lifestyles.

GUIDELINES FOR MULTIMODAL EXERCISE PRESCRIPTIONS

- Modes: Select at least three per week from type A and B activities.
- Frequency: Three to seven sessions a week. Engage in either type A, B, or C activities at least three times per week.
- Intensity: Rating of perceived exertion between 5 and 9 on 10 point OMNI scale.
- Duration: At least 15 min, preferably 20 to 30 min. Duration depends on energy cost ($kcal \cdot min^{-1}$) of exercise mode.
- Caloric expenditure: 1000 to 2000 kcal/wk. Group C and D activities can be used to reach the weekly caloric expenditure goal but cannot be counted as one of the required aerobic activities.

Sample Cycling Program

Client data

Age	27 yr
Gender	Female
Body weight	70 kg (154 lb)
Resting heart rate	67 bpm
Maximal heart rate	195 bpm (measured)
$\dot{V}O_2max$	26 ml·kg^{-1}·min^{-1} (measured) 7.4 METs
Graded exercise test	Cycle ergometer
Initial cardiorespiratory fitness level	Poor

Exercise prescription

Mode	Stationary cycling
Intensity	60-80% $\dot{V}O_2R$ 16.8-21.4 ml·kg^{-1}·min^{-1} 4.8-6.1 METs
Exercise heart rates (from figure 5.3)	139 bpm minimum 168 bpm maximum
RPE	5-8 (OMNI scale)
Duration	40-60 min
Frequency	4-5 days/wk

Cycling Program[a]

Phase (weeks)	Intensity %$\dot{V}O_2R$	METs	HR (bpm)	RPE	Power output (W)	Resistance (kg)	Pedal rate (rpm)	Net kcal·min^{-1}	Time (min)	Frequency	Weekly net expenditure (kcal)
Initial											
1	60	4.8	139	5	63	1.3	50	4.7	40	4	752
2	60	4.8	139	5	63	1.3	50	4.7	**45**	4	846
3	**65**	5.2	150	5-6	73	1.5	50	5.2	45	4	936
4	65	5.2	150	5-6	73	1.5	50	5.2	**50**	4	1040
Improvement											
5-8	65-**70**	5.2-5.5	150-155	5-6	73-80	1.5-1.6	50	5.2-5.5	50	4	1040-1103
9-12	65-70	5.2-5.5	150-155	5-6	73-80	1.5-1.6	50	5.2-5.5	**55**	4	1144-1210
13-16	70-**75**	5.5-5.8	152-162	6-7	80-86	1.6-1.7	50	5.5-5.9	55	4	1210-1298
17-20	75	5.8	162	7	86	1.7	50	5.9	**60**	4	1416
21-24	75	5.8	162	7	86	1.7	50	5.9	60	**5**	1770
25-28	**80**	6.1	168	8	93	1.9	50	6.2	60	5	1874
Maintenance											
24+											
Cycling	80	6.1	168	8	93	1.9	50	6.2	60	3	1116
Low-impact aerobics	65% HRR	5.0	150	6-7				4.9	60	1	294
Tennis		7.0		7-8				7.4	60	1	440

[a]Values in boldface indicate training variables that were increased during each stage of the exercise progression.

Sample Jogging Program

Client data

Age	29 yr
Gender	Male
Body weight	70 kg (154 lb)
Resting heart rate	50 bpm
Maximal heart rate	191 bpm (age predicted)
$\dot{V}O_2max$	45 ml·kg^{-1}·min^{-1} (predicted) 12.9 METs
Graded exercise test	None
Initial cardiorespiratory fitness level	Excellent

Exercise prescription

Mode	Jogging and running
Intensity	70-85% $\dot{V}O_2R$ 32.5-38.8 ml·kg^{-1}·min^{-1} 9.3-11.1 METs
Exercise heart rates	149 bpm minimum (70% HRR) 170 bpm maximum (85% HRR)
RPE	6-9 (OMNI scale)
Duration	33-35 min
Frequency	3-5 days/wk

Jogging Program[a]

Phase (weeks)	Intensity %$\dot{V}O_2R$	METs	HR (bpm)	RPE	Pace: mph (min·mi^{-1})	Distance (miles)	Net kcal·min^{-1}	Time (min)	Frequency	Weekly net expenditure (kcal)
Improvement										
1-4	70	9.3	149	6	5.4 (11:06)	3.0	10.2	33	3	1010
5-8	70-**80**	9.3-10.5	149-163	6-7	5.4-6.2 (9:40)	3.0-3.4	10.2-11.6	33	3	1010-1148
9-12	70-80	9.3-10.5	149-163	6-7	5.4-6.2 (9:40)	3.0-3.4	10.2-11.6	33	**4**	1347-1531
13-16	80-**85**	10.5-11.1	163-170	7-9	6.2-6.6 (9:05)	3.4-3.6	11.6-12.4	33	4	1531-1637
17-20	80-85	10.5-11.1	163-170	7-9	6.2-6.6 (9:05)	3.4-3.8	11.6-12.4	33-**35**	**5**	1914-2170
Maintenance										
21+										
Jogging	85	11.2	170	7-9	6.6 (9:05)	3.8	12.4	35	3	1302
Handball	60	8.0		6-7			9.2	60	1	552
Basketball	60	8.0		6-7			9.2	60	1	552

[a]Values in boldface indicate training variables that are increased during each stage of the exercise progression.

Sample Multimodal Exercise Program

Client data

Age	44 yr
Sex	Female
Weight	68 kg (150 lb)
Resting heart rate	70 bpm
Maximum heart rate	170 bpm
$\dot{V}O_2max$ (measured)	30 ml·kg^{-1}·min^{-1}
	8.6 METs
Graded exercise test	Treadmill maximal GXT (Bruce protocol)
Initial cardiorespiratory fitness	Fair

Exercise prescription

Modes and estimates of gross caloric expenditure (METs) and net caloric expenditure (kcal·min^{-1})[a]	Stationary cycling (100 W): 5.5 METs; 5.4 kcal·min^{-1} Step aerobics (6-8 in. step): 8.5 METs; 8.9 kcal·min^{-1} Rowing (100 W): 7.0 METs; 7.1 kcal·min^{-1} Swimming (moderate effort): 7.0 METs; 7.1 kcal·min^{-1} Stair climbing (machine): 9.0 METs; 9.5 kcal·min^{-1} Hiking: 6.0 METs; 5.9 kcal·min^{-1} Resistance training (free weights, machines): 3.0 METs; 2.4 kcal·min^{-1}
Intensity	RPE: 5-9 (OMNI scale)
Duration	20 to 60 min
Frequency	3 to 5 days/wk
Weekly caloric expenditure	500 to 1250 kcal·wk^{-1}

Multimodal Exercise Program

Phase (week)	Intensity (RPE)	Minimal duration (min)	Minimal frequency	Average kcal per workout	Weekly caloric goal
Initial					
1-2	5	20	3	133	500
3-4	5	25	3	200	600
Improvement					
5-8	6	25	3	200	700
9-12	6	30	3	233	800
13-16	6-7	30	4	225	900
17-20	7-8	30	4	250	1000
21-24	8-9	30	5	250	1250
Maintenance					
24+	8-9	30	5	250	1250

Examples

Week 1	Activity	Net kcal·min^{-1} estimates	Time (min)	Frequency	Kcal per workout (net)	Activity type[b]
Monday	Stationary cycling	5.4	20	1	108	A
Wednesday	Step aerobics	8.9	20	1	178	C
Friday	Stair climbing	9.5	30	1	285	B
	Totals*:		70	3	571	3
	Goals:		60	3	500	3
Week 21						
Monday	Swimming	7.1	35	1	248	C
Tuesday	Rowing	7.1	35	1	248	B
Wednesday	Stair climbing	9.5	30	1	285	B
Friday	Resistance training	2.4	40	1	96	D
Sunday	Hiking	5.9	60	1	354	D
	Totals*:		200	5	1231	4
	Goals:		150	5	1250	4

[a]Gross MET levels for activities from Ainsworth and colleagues (2000); net energy expenditure in kcal·min^{-1} = net MET level $\times$ 3.5 $\times$ BM (kg) / 200.

[b]Check all type A and B activities

*Compare weekly totals to weekly goals.

KEY POINTS

- Always personalize cardiorespiratory exercise programs to meet the needs, interests, and abilities of each participant.

- The exercise prescription includes mode, frequency, intensity, duration, and progression of exercise.

- Aerobic endurance activities involving large muscle groups are well suited for developing cardiorespiratory fitness. Type A and B activities such as walking, jogging, and cycling allow the individual to maintain steady-state exercise intensities and are not highly dependent on skill.

- Exercise intensity can be prescribed using the HR, $\dot{V}O_2R$, or RPE methods, or a combination of these methods.

- For the average healthy person, the cardiorespiratory exercise program should be at an intensity of 60% to 85% $\dot{V}O_2$max, a duration of 20 to 60 min, and a frequency of 3 to 5 days/wk.

- The cardiorespiratory exercise program includes three stages of progression: initial conditioning, improvement, and maintenance.

- Each exercise session includes warm-up, aerobic conditioning exercise, and cool-down.

- Continuous and discontinuous training methods are equally effective for improving cardiorespiratory fitness.

- Multimodal exercise prescriptions use a variety of type A, B, and C aerobic activities to improve cardiorespiratory endurance.

KEY TERMS

Learn the definition for each of the following key terms. Definitions of key terms can be found in the glossary on page 411.

caloric threshold

continuous training

cross training

discontinuous training

FITT principle

heart rate reserve (HRR)

improvement stage

initial conditioning stage

interval training

Karvonen method

maintenance stage

multimodal exercise program

percent heart rate maximum (%HRmax)

percent heart rate reserve (%HRR) method

percent $\dot{V}O_2$max reserve (%$\dot{V}O_2$R)

pulmonary ventilation

spinning

super circuit resistance training

talk test

treading

type A, B, C, and D aerobic activities

ventilatory threshold

$\dot{V}O_2$reserve ($\dot{V}O_2$R)

REVIEW QUESTIONS

In addition to being able to define each of the key terms, test your knowledge and understanding of the material by answering the following review questions.

1. Name the four components of any aerobic exercise prescription.

2. What are the guidelines for an exercise prescription for improved health?

3. What are the guidelines for an exercise prescription for cardiorespiratory fitness?

4. Identify the three parts of an aerobic exercise workout and state the purpose of each part.

5. To classify an aerobic exercise mode as either a type A, B, C, or D activity, what criteria are used?

6. Give three examples each for type A, B, C, and D aerobic activities.

7. Describe three methods used to prescribe intensity for an aerobic exercise prescription.

8. Using the $\dot{V}O_2$reserve method, calculate the target $\dot{V}O_2$ for a client whose $\dot{V}O_2$max is 12 METs and relative exercise intensity is 70% $\dot{V}O_2$R.

9. Which method of prescribing intensity (%HRR or %HRmax) corresponds 1:1 with the %$\dot{V}O_2$R method?

10. What are the limitations of using HR methods to monitor intensity of aerobic exercise?

11. Describe how RPEs can be used to prescribe and monitor the intensity of aerobic exercise.

12. Describe how your clients can use the talk test to monitor exercise intensity during their aerobic exercise workouts.

13. What target caloric thresholds are recommended by ACSM for aerobic exercise workouts and weekly caloric expenditure from physical activity and exercise?

14. What is the recommended frequency of activity and exercise for improved health benefits? For improved cardiorespiratory fitness?

15. Name the three stages of a cardiorespiratory exercise program. For the average individual, what is the typical length (in weeks) of each stage?

16. What is the difference between continuous and discontinuous aerobic exercise training? Give examples of continuous and discontinuous training methods.

17. What are the essential elements of a client case study?

Assessing Muscular Fitness

KEY QUESTIONS

- How are strength and muscular endurance assessed?
- How does the type of muscle contraction (concentric, eccentric, or isokinetic) affect force production?
- What test protocols can be used to assess a client's muscular fitness?
- What are the advantages and limitations of using free weights and exercise machines to assess muscular strength?
- What are sources of measurement error for muscular fitness tests, and how are they controlled?
- What are the recommended procedures for administering 1-RM strength tests?
- Is it safe to give 1-RM strength tests to children and older adults?
- What tests can be used to assess the functional strength of older adults?

Muscular strength and endurance are two important components of muscular fitness. Minimal levels of muscular fitness are needed to perform activities of daily living, to maintain functional independence as one ages, and to partake in active leisure-time pursuits without undue stress or fatigue. Adequate levels of muscular fitness lessen the chance of developing low back problems, osteoporotic fractures, and musculoskeletal injuries.

This chapter describes a variety of laboratory and field tests for assessing all forms of muscular strength and endurance. In addition, the chapter compares types of exercise machines, addresses factors affecting muscular fitness tests, discusses sources of measurement error, and provides guidelines for testing muscular fitness of children and older adults.

DEFINITION OF TERMS

Muscular strength is defined as the ability of a muscle group to develop maximal contractile force against a resistance in a single contraction. The force generated by a muscle or muscle group, however, is highly dependent on the velocity of movement. Maximal force is produced when the limb is not rotating (i.e., zero velocity). As the speed of joint rotation increases, the muscular force decreases. Thus, *strength for dynamic movements* is defined as the maximal force generated in a single contraction at a specified velocity (Knuttgen and Kraemer 1987). Muscular endurance is the ability of a muscle group to exert submaximal force for extended periods.

Both strength and muscular endurance can be assessed for static and dynamic muscular contractions. If the resistance is immovable, the muscle contraction is **static** or isometric ("iso," same; "metric," length), and there is no visible movement of the joint. **Dynamic contractions,** in which there is visible joint movement, are either concentric, eccentric, or isokinetic (see figure 6.1, *a* and *b*).

If the resistance is less than the force produced by the muscle group, the contraction is **concentric,**

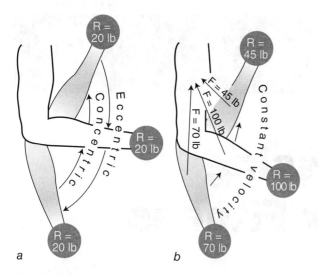

Figure 6.1 Types of muscle contraction.

allowing the muscle to shorten as it exerts tension to move the bony lever. The muscle is also capable of exerting tension while lengthening. This is known as eccentric contraction and typically occurs when the muscles produce a braking force to decelerate rapidly moving body segments or to resist gravity (e.g., slowly lowering a barbell). Both concentric and eccentric contractions are sometimes called isotonic ("iso," same; "tonic," tension). The term "isotonic contraction" is a misnomer because the tension produced by the muscle group fluctuates greatly even though the resistance is constant throughout the range of motion (ROM). This fluctuation in muscular force is due to the change in muscle length

and angle of pull as the bony lever is moved, creating a strength curve that is unique for each muscle group. For example, the strength of the knee flexors is maximal at 160° to 170° (see figure 6.2).

In regular (concentric and eccentric) dynamic exercise, because of the change in mechanical and physiological advantage as the limb is moved, the muscle group is not contracting maximally throughout the ROM. Thus, the greatest resistance that can be used during regular, dynamic exercise is equal to the maximum weight that can be moved at the *weakest* point in the ROM.

Isokinetic contraction (see figure 6.1*b*) is a maximal contraction of a muscle group at a constant velocity throughout the entire range of joint motion ("iso," same; "kinetic," motion). The velocity of contraction is controlled mechanically so that the limb rotates at a set velocity (e.g., 120°·sec⁻¹). Electromechanical devices vary the resistance to match the muscular force produced at each point in the ROM. Thus, isokinetic exercise machines allow the muscle group to encounter variable but maximal resistances during the movement.

STRENGTH AND MUSCULAR ENDURANCE ASSESSMENT

Measures of static or dynamic strength and endurance are used to establish baseline values before training, monitor progress during training, and assess the overall effectiveness of resistance training

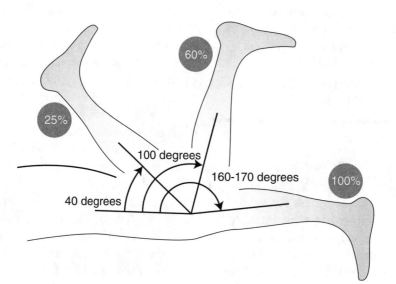

Figure 6.2 Strength variations in relation to knee joint angle.

and exercise rehabilitation programs. Static strength and muscular endurance are measured using dynamometers, cable tensiometers, strain gauges, and load cells. Free weights (barbells and dumbbells), as well as constant-resistance, variable-resistance, and isokinetic exercise machines, are used to assess dynamic strength and endurance (see table 6.1). The testing procedures vary depending on the type of test (i.e., strength or endurance) and equipment.

Isometric Muscle Testing Using Spring-Loaded Dynamometers

Isometric strength is measured as the maximum force exerted in a single contraction against an immovable resistance (i.e., maximum voluntary isometric contraction, or MVIC). For many years, spring-loaded dynamometers have been used to measure static strength and endurance of the grip squeezing muscles and leg and back muscles (see figure 6.3). The handgrip dynamometer has an adjustable handle to fit the size of the hand and measures forces between 0 and 100 kg in 1 kg increments (0 and 220 lb in 2.2 lb increments). The back and leg dynamometer consists of a scale that measures forces ranging from 0 to 2500 lb in 10 lb increments (0 to 1134 kg in 4.5 kg increments). As force is applied to the dynamometer, the spring is compressed and moves the indicator needle a corresponding amount.

Grip Strength Testing Procedures

Before using the handgrip dynamometer, adjust the handgrip size to a position that is comfortable for the individual. Alternatively, you can measure the hand width with a caliper and use this value to set the optimum grip size (Montoye and Faulkner 1964). The individual stands erect, with the arm

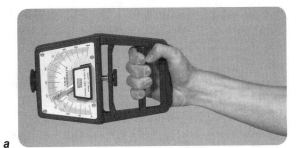

a

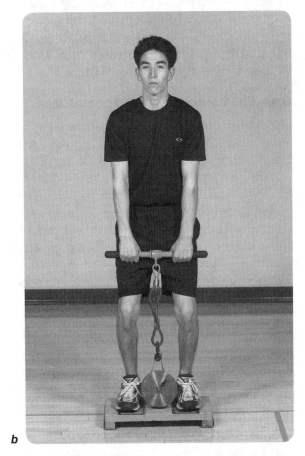

b

Figure 6.3 Spring-loaded dynamometers for measuring static strength and endurance: *(a)* handgrip dynamometer and *(b)* back and leg dynamometer.

Table 6.1	**Strength Training Modes**	
Testing mode	**Equipment**	**Measure***
Static	Isometric dynamometers, cable tensiometers, strain gauges, load cells, and handheld dynamometers	MVIC (kg or N)

Dynamic
  Constant resistance
  Variable resistance
	
	Free weights (barbells and dumbbells) and exercise machines
	Exercise machines
		
		1-RM (lb or kg)
		NA

Isokinetic and omnikinetic	Isokinetic and omnikinetic dynamometers	Peak torque (Nm or ft-lb)

*MVIC = maximal voluntary isometric contraction; NA = not applicable; N = newton; Nm = newton-meter; ft-lb = foot-pound.

and forearm positioned as follows (Fess 1992): shoulder adducted and neutrally rotated, elbow flexed at 90°, forearm in the neutral position, and wrist in slight extension (0° to 30°). For some test protocols, however, the client must keep the arm straight and slightly abducted for measurement of the grip strength of each hand (Canadian Society for Exercise Physiology [CSEP] 2003). The individual squeezes the dynamometer as hard as possible using one brief maximal contraction and no extraneous body movement. Administer three trials for each hand, allowing a 1 min rest between trials, and use the best score as the client's static strength.

Grip Endurance Testing Procedures

Once the grip size is adjusted, instruct the client to squeeze the handle as hard as possible and to continue squeezing for 1 min. Record the initial force and the final force exerted at the end of 1 min. The greater the endurance, the lower the rate and degree of decline in force. The relative endurance score is the final force divided by the initial force times 100.

Alternatively, you can assess static grip endurance by having your client exert a submaximal force, which is a given percentage of the individual's **maximum voluntary isometric contraction (MVIC)** strength (e.g., 50% MVIC). The relative endurance score is the amount of time that this force level is maintained. During the test, the client must watch the dial of the dynamometer and adjust the amount of force exerted as necessary in order to maintain the appropriate submaximal force level.

Leg Strength Testing Procedures

Using the back and leg dynamometer, the individual stands on the platform with trunk erect and the knees flexed to an angle of 130° to 140°. The client holds the hand bar using a pronated grip and positions it across the thighs by adjusting the length of the chain (see figure 6.3b). If a belt is available, attach it to each end of the hand bar after positioning the belt around the client's hips. The belt helps to stabilize the bar and to reduce the stress placed on the hands during the leg lift. Without using the back, the client slowly exerts as much force as possible while extending the knees. The maximum indicator needle remains at the peak force achieved. Administer two or three trials with a 1 min rest interval. Divide the maximum score (in pounds) by 2.2 to convert it to kilograms.

Back Strength Testing Procedures

Using the back and leg dynamometer, the individual stands on the platform with the knees fully extended and the head and trunk erect. The client grasps the hand bar using a pronated grip with the right hand and a supinated grip with the left. Position the hand bar across the client's thighs. Without leaning backward, the client pulls the hand bar straight upward using the back muscles and is instructed to roll the shoulders backward during the pull. Clients should be reminded before lifting to flex the trunk minimally and to keep the head and trunk erect during the test. Administer two trials with a 1 min rest between the trials. Divide the maximum score (in pounds) by 2.2 to convert it to kilograms.

Static Strength Norms for Spring-Loaded Dynamometers

Table 6.2 provides age–gender norms for evaluating the static grip strength of the right and left hands combined. Grip strength norms for each hand are presented in table 6.3. You can also use norms developed for men and women to assess your client's static strength for each dynamometric test item (see table 6.3). Calculate your client's total strength score by adding the right grip, left grip, leg strength, and back strength scores. Before doing this, convert the leg and back strength scores (measured in pounds) to kilograms. To calculate the relative strength score, divide the total strength score by body mass (expressed in kilograms).

Isometric Muscle Testing Using Cable Tensiometers and Strain Gauges

You can use cable tensiometry and strain gauges to assess the static strength of various muscle groups throughout the body. For cable tensiometry, standardized testing procedures have been described in detail and should be followed closely to ensure the validity and reliability of the test results (see Clarke 1966). The instrumentation includes a tensiometer, steel cables, testing table, wall hooks, straps, and goniometer. Attach one end of the cable to the wall or table hooks and, using a strap, attach the other end to the body part to be tested. Always position the cable at a right angle to the pulling bony lever. Use a goniometer to measure the appropriate joint angle. Place the tensiometer on a taut cable. As the

Table 6.2   Age–Gender Norms for Combined Isometric Grip Strength

	GRIP STRENGTH (kg)*											
	15-19 YR		20-29 YR		30-39 YR		40-49 YR		50-59 YR		60-69 YR	
Rating	M	F	M	F	M	F	M	F	M	F	M	F
Excellent	≥108	≥68	≥115	≥70	≥115	≥71	≥108	≥69	≥101	≥61	≥100	≥54
Very good	98-107	60-67	104-114	63-69	104-114	63-70	97-107	61-68	92-100	54-60	91-99	48-53
Good	90-97	53-59	95-103	60-62	95-103	58-62	88-96	54-60	84-91	49-53	84-90	45-47
Fair	79-89	48-52	84-94	52-59	84-94	51-57	80-87	49-53	76-83	45-48	73-83	41-44
Needs improvement	≤78	≤47	≤83	≤51	≤83	≤50	≤79	≤48	≤75	≤44	≤72	≤40

*Combined right- and left-hand grip strength scores.

M = males; F = females.

Source: The Canadian Physical Activity, Fitness & Lifestyle Approach: CSEP-Health & Fitness Program's Health-Related Appraisal and Counselling Strategy, 3rd Edition © 2003. Reprinted with permission of the Canadian Society for Exercise Physiology.

Table 6.3   Static Strength Norms

Classification	Left grip (kg)	Right grip (kg)	Back strength (kg)	Leg strength (kg)	Total strength (kg)	Relative strength*
MEN						
Excellent	>68	>70	>209	>241	>587	>7.50
Good	56-67	62-69	177-208	214-240	508-586	7.10-7.49
Average	43-55	48-61	126-176	160-213	375-507	5.21-7.09
Below average	39-42	41-47	91-125	137-159	307-374	4.81-5.20
Poor	<39	<41	<91	<137	<307	<4.81
WOMEN						
Excellent	>37	>41	>111	>136	>324	>5.50
Good	34-36	38-40	98-110	114-135	282-323	4.80-5.49
Average	22-33	25-37	52-97	66-113	164-281	2.90-4.79
Below average	18-21	22-24	39-51	49-65	117-163	2.10-2.89
Poor	<18	<22	<39	<49	<117	<2.10

*Relative strength is determined by dividing total strength by body mass (kg).

For persons over age 50, reduce scores by 10% to adjust for muscle tissue loss due to aging.

Data from Corbin and colleagues (1978).

individual exerts force on the cable, the riser of the tensiometer is depressed and a maximum indicator needle registers the static strength score. Tensiometers measure forces ranging between 0 and 400 lb (0 to ~181.4 kg). However, the larger tensiometers are less accurate in the lower range; therefore, you should use a small tensiometer, which measures forces between 0 and 100 lb (0 to 45.4 kg), to obtain greater accuracy in the lower range.

Cable tensiometry tests can be used to assess strength impairment at specific joint angles and to monitor progress during rehabilitation. As with all forms of static strength testing, you should be aware that strength is specific to the joint angle and muscle group being tested. Therefore, test at least three to four muscle groups to provide an adequate estimation of static strength.

Test batteries and norms have been developed for males and females 9 yr old through college age (Clarke 1975; Clarke and Monroe 1970). The test battery for males of all ages includes the same three strength tests: shoulder extension, knee extension, and ankle plantar flexion. For elementary and junior high school girls, the test battery includes shoulder extension, hip extension, and trunk flexion. The three test items in the battery developed for senior high school and college women are shoulder flexion, hip flexion, and ankle plantar flexion.

Maximum voluntary isometric contraction testing using strain gauge systems requires the joint being tested to be in gravity neutral position and the strain gauge and strap to be perpendicular to the line of force. Detailed testing procedures and age–gender norms for 11 muscle groups are available (see Meldrum et al. 2003, 2007).

Isometric Muscle Testing Using Digital Handheld Dynamometry

You can use handheld dynamometers that provide a digital display of force production to assess the isometric strength of 11 muscle groups (see figure 6.4, *a* and *b*). This handheld dynamometer digitally displays force measurements up to a maximum of 440 newtons (100 lb in 0.1 lb increments). For this

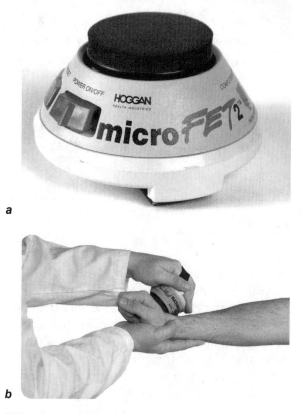

a

b

Figure 6.4 *(a)* Handheld dynamometer for measuring isometric strength and *(b)* the hand being tested.

Courtesy of Hoggan Industries.

type of testing, you place the dynamometer on the limb and hold it stationary while the client exerts maximum force against it. Administer two trials and use either the average or best score for each muscle group. Appendix C.1 describes standardized test protocols for 11 muscle groups. Performance norms for adults (20-79 yr) and children (4-16 yr) are available (see Andrews, Thomas, and Bohannon 1996; Beenakker et al. 2001; Bohannon 1997; van den Beld et al. 2006).

Dynamic Muscle Testing Using Constant-Resistance and Variable-Resistance Modes

Although either a **constant-resistance** or a **variable-resistance exercise** mode can be used to assess dynamic (concentric and eccentric) muscle strength and endurance, you will be better served if you use either free weights or constant-resistance exercise machines.

A major disadvantage of free weights, dumbbells, and constant-resistance exercise machines, however, is that they measure dynamic strength only at the weakest point in the ROM. The reason is that the resistance cannot be varied to account for fluctuations in muscular force caused by the changing mechanical (angle of pull of muscle) and physiological (length of muscle) advantage of the musculoskeletal system during the movement.

In an attempt to overcome this deficiency, equipment manufacturers have designed variable-resistance machines that vary the resistance during the ROM. Variable-resistance machines have a moving connection (i.e., lever, cam, or pulley) between the resistance and the point of force application. As the weight is lifted, the mechanical advantage of the machine decreases. Therefore, more force must be applied to continue moving the resistance. The variable-resistance mode of exercise attempts to match the force capability of the musculoskeletal system throughout the ROM. However, many variable-resistance exercise machines fail to match the strength curves of different muscle groups. Also, with variable-resistance machines it is difficult to assess the client's maximal force or strength because the resistance is modified by the levers, pulleys, and cams, causing the movement velocity to vary. Variable-resistance exercise machines, therefore, have limited usefulness for maximal testing. Still, these types of machines are well suited for resistance training.

Although free weights and constant-resistance exercise machines are generally recommended for muscular fitness testing, there are advantages and limitations to each of these modalities. Compared to exercise machines, free weights require more neuromuscular coordination in order to stabilize body parts and maintain balance during lifting of the barbell or dumbbell. While exercise machines may reduce the need for spotting during the test, these machines limit the individual's range of joint motion and plane of movement. Also, some exercise machines have relatively large weight plate increments so that you must attach smaller weights to the weight stack in order to measure your client's strength accurately.

Lastly, some machines cannot accommodate individuals with short limbs; you may need to use child-sized machines to standardize their starting positions for testing. Clients with long limbs or large body and limb circumferences (e.g., some bodybuilders or obese clients) also may have difficulty using standard exercise machines. Body size and weight increments are less of a problem with free weights.

To overcome some of these limitations, **free-motion machines** that provide constant- and variable-resistance in multiple planes have been developed. These machines have adjustable seats, lever arms, and cable pulleys that can be set to exercise muscle groups in multiple planes. Also, these machines can accommodate smaller or larger individuals, are easy to get in and out of, and have smaller weight increments (5 lb or 2.3 kg) than do older standard machines (typically 10 lb or 4.5 kg). When using free-motion exercise machines for muscular fitness testing, take care to adjust the plane of movement and the seat so that you simulate the starting and ending body positions that were used to develop test norms for older constant-resistance machines. If you use free-motion machines to monitor the progress of your clients, make certain that you use the same settings (i.e., seat and plane-of-movement adjustments) for each test session.

Dynamic Strength Tests

Dynamic strength is usually measured as the **one-repetition maximum (1-RM)**, which is the maximum weight that can be lifted for one complete repetition of the movement. The 1-RM strength value is obtained through trial and error.

Although 1-RM strength tests can be safely administered to individuals of all ages, you should take precautions to decrease the risk of injury when clients attempt to lift maximal loads. Be certain that your client warms up before attempting the lift and starts with a weight that is below the individual's expected 1-RM. When you administer these tests, you should spot your clients and closely monitor their lifting technique and breathing.

The American College of Sports Medicine (ACSM 2010) recommends the bench press and leg press (upper plate of constant-resistance exercise machine) for assessing strength of the upper and lower body, respectively. To determine **relative strength,** divide the 1-RM values by the client's body mass. Norms for men and women are provided in tables 6.4 and 6.5.

Another test of dynamic strength includes six test items: bench press, arm curl, latissimus pull, leg press, leg extension, and leg curl. For each exercise, express and evaluate the 1-RM as a percentage of body mass. For example, if a 120 lb (54.5 kg)

STEPS FOR 1-RM MAXIMUM TESTING

The following basic steps are recommended for 1-RM testing.

1. Have your client warm up by completing 5 to 10 repetitions of the exercise at 40% to 60% of the estimated 1-RM.

2. During a 1 min rest, have the client stretch the muscle group. This is followed by three to five repetitions of the exercise at 60% to 80% of the estimated 1-RM.

3. Increase the weight conservatively, and have the client attempt the 1-RM lift. If the lift is successful, the client should rest 3 to 5 min before attempting the next weight increment. Follow this procedure until the client fails to complete the lift. The 1-RM typically is achieved within three to five trials.

4. Record the 1-RM value as the maximum weight lifted for the last successful trial.

Table 6.4   Age–Gender Norms for 1-RM Bench Press (1-RM/BM)

Percentile rankings* for men	AGE				
	20-29	30-39	40-49	50-59	60+
90	1.48	1.24	1.10	0.97	0.89
80	1.32	1.12	1.00	0.90	0.82
70	1.22	1.04	0.93	0.84	0.77
60	1.14	0.98	0.88	0.79	0.72
50	1.06	0.93	0.84	0.75	0.68
40	0.99	0.88	0.80	0.71	0.66
30	0.93	0.83	0.76	0.68	0.63
20	0.88	0.78	0.72	0.63	0.57
10	0.80	0.71	0.65	0.57	0.53

Percentile rankings* for women	AGE				
	20-29	30-39	40-49	50-59	60-69	70+
90	0.54	0.49	0.46	0.40	0.41	0.44
80	0.49	0.45	0.40	0.37	0.38	0.39
70	0.42	0.42	0.38	0.35	0.36	0.33
60	0.41	0.41	0.37	0.33	0.32	0.31
50	0.40	0.38	0.34	0.31	0.30	0.27
40	0.37	0.37	0.32	0.28	0.29	0.25
30	0.35	0.34	0.30	0.26	0.28	0.24
20	0.33	0.32	0.27	0.23	0.26	0.21
10	0.30	0.27	0.23	0.19	0.25	0.20

*Descriptors for percentile rankings: 90 = well above average; 70 = above average; 30 = below average; 10 = well below average.

Data for women provided by the Women's Exercise Research Center, The George Washington University Medical Center, Washington, D.C., 1998.

Data for men provided by The Cooper Institute for Aerobics Research, *The Physical Fitness Specialist Manual,* The Cooper Institute, Dallas, TX, 2005.

woman bench presses 60 lb (27.2 kg), her strength-to-body mass ratio is 0.50 (60 divided by 120), and she scores 3 points for that exercise. Follow this procedure for each exercise; then add the total points to determine the overall strength and fitness category of the individual. Strength-to-body mass ratios with corresponding point values for college-age men and women are presented in table 6.6.

Dynamic Muscle Endurance Tests

You can assess your client's dynamic muscle endurance by having the individual perform as many repetitions as possible using a weight that is a set percentage of the body weight or maximum strength (1-RM). Pollock, Wilmore, and Fox (1978) recommend using a weight that is 70% of the 1-RM value for each exercise. Although norms for this test have not been established, these authors suggest, on the basis of their testing and research findings, that the

average individual should be able to complete 12 to 15 repetitions.

The YMCA (Golding 2000) and ACSM (2010) recommend using a bench press test to assess dynamic muscular endurance of the upper body. For this absolute endurance test, use a flat bench and barbell. The client performs as many repetitions as possible at a set cadence of 30 repetitions per minute. Use a metronome to establish the exercise cadence. Male clients lift an 80 lb (36.4 kg) barbell, whereas female clients use a 35 lb (15.9 kg) barbell. Terminate the test when the client is unable to maintain the exercise cadence. Table 6.7 presents norms for this test.

Alternatively, you can use a test battery consisting of seven items to assess dynamic muscular endurance. Select the weight to be lifted using a set percentage of the individual's body mass. The client lifts this weight up to a maximum of 15 repetitions.

Table 6.5 Age–Gender Norms for 1-RM Leg Press (1-RM/BM)

Percentile rankings* for men	AGE				
	20-29	30-39	40-49	50-59	60+
90	2.27	2.07	1.92	1.80	1.73
80	2.13	1.93	1.82	1.71	1.62
70	2.05	1.85	1.74	1.64	1.56
60	1.97	1.77	1.68	1.58	1.49
50	1.91	1.71	1.62	1.52	1.43
40	1.83	1.65	1.57	1.46	1.38
30	1.74	1.59	1.51	1.39	1.30
20	1.63	1.52	1.44	1.32	1.25
10	1.51	1.43	1.35	1.22	1.16

Percentile rankings* for women	AGE					
	20-29	30-39	40-49	50-59	60-69	70+
90	2.05	1.73	1.63	1.51	1.40	1.27
80	1.66	1.50	1.46	1.30	1.25	1.12
70	1.42	1.47	1.35	1.24	1.18	1.10
60	1.36	1.32	1.26	1.18	1.15	0.95
50	1.32	1.26	1.19	1.09	1.08	0.89
40	1.25	1.21	1.12	1.03	1.04	0.83
30	1.23	1.16	1.03	0.95	0.98	0.82
20	1.13	1.09	0.94	0.86	0.94	0.79
10	1.02	0.94	0.76	0.75	0.84	0.75

*Descriptors for percentile rankings: 70 = above average; 50 = average; 30 = below average; 10 = well below average.

Data for women provided by the Women's Exercise Research Center, The George Washington University Medical Center, Washington, D.C., 1998.

Data for men provided by The Cooper Institute for Aerobics Research, *The Physical Fitness Specialist Manual,* The Cooper Institute, Dallas, TX, 2005.

Table 6.8 provides percentages for each test item, as well as the scoring system and norms for college-age men and women.

Dynamic Muscle Testing Using Isokinetic and Omnikinetic Exercise Modes

Isokinetic dynamometers provide an accurate and reliable assessment of strength, endurance, and power of muscle groups (see figure 6.5). The speed of limb movement is kept at a constant preselected velocity. Any increase in muscular force produces an increased resistance rather than increased acceleration of the limb. Thus, fluctuations in muscular force throughout the ROM are matched by an equal counterforce or **accommodating resistance.**

Isokinetic dynamometers measure muscular torque production at speeds of 0° to 300°·sec^{-1}.

From the recorded output, you can evaluate peak torque, total work, and power. Some less expensive isokinetic dynamometers lack this recording capability but are suitable for training and rehabilitation exercise.

Omnikinetic exercise dynamometers provide maximum overload at every joint angle throughout the ROM at whatever speed the individual is capable of generating. This testing system provides an accommodating resistance that adjusts to both the force and velocity output of the individual and is not limited to a preset velocity of limb movement. Thus, at any one setting, the individual maximally overloads both the force and velocity production capabilities of the contractile elements. The stronger the individual, the faster the speed of limb movement at any given setting. Also, increasing limb velocity results in increased resistance.

Table 6.6 Strength-to-Body Mass Ratios for Selected 1-RM Tests

Bench press	Arm curl	Lat pull-down	Leg press	Leg extension	Leg curl	Points
			MEN			
1.50	0.70	1.20	3.00	0.80	0.70	10
1.40	0.65	1.15	2.80	0.75	0.65	9
1.30	0.60	1.10	2.60	0.70	0.60	8
1.20	0.55	1.05	2.40	0.65	0.55	7
1.10	0.50	1.00	2.20	0.60	0.50	6
1.00	0.45	0.95	2.00	0.55	0.45	5
0.90	0.40	0.90	1.80	0.50	0.40	4
0.80	0.35	0.85	1.60	0.45	0.35	3
0.70	0.30	0.80	1.40	0.40	0.30	2
0.60	0.25	0.75	1.20	0.35	0.25	1
			WOMEN			
0.90	0.50	0.85	2.70	0.70	0.60	10
0.85	0.45	0.80	2.50	0.65	0.55	9
0.80	0.42	0.75	2.30	0.60	0.52	8
0.70	0.38	0.73	2.10	0.55	0.50	7
0.65	0.35	0.70	2.00	0.52	0.45	6
0.60	0.32	0.65	1.80	0.50	0.40	5
0.55	0.28	0.63	1.60	0.45	0.35	4
0.50	0.25	0.60	1.40	0.40	0.30	3
0.45	0.21	0.55	1.20	0.35	0.25	2
0.35	0.18	0.50	1.00	0.30	0.20	1

Total points	Strength fitness category[a]
48-60	Excellent
37-47	Good
25-36	Average
13-24	Fair
0-12	Poor

[a]Based on data compiled by author for 250 college-age men and women.

Table 6.7 Muscular Endurance Norms for Bench Press[a]

Percentile	AGE GROUP (YR)					
	18-25	26-35	36-45	46-55	56-65	>65
Men						
95	49	48	41	33	28	22
75	34	30	26	21	17	12
50	26	22	20	13	10	8
25	17	16	12	8	4	3
5	5	4	2	1	0	0
Women						
95	49	46	41	33	29	22
75	30	29	26	20	17	12
50	21	21	17	12	9	6
25	13	13	10	6	4	2
5	2	2	1	0	0	0

[a]Score is number of repetitions completed in 1 min using 80 lb barbell for men and 35 lb barbell for women.

Data from YMCA of the USA, 2002, *YMCA fitness testing and assessment manual*, 4th ed. (Champaign, IL: Human Kinetics).

Table 6.8 Dynamic Muscular Endurance Test Battery

Exercise	% BODY MASS TO BE LIFTED		Repetitions (max = 15)
	Men	Women	
Arm curl	0.33	0.25	_____
Bench press	0.66	0.50	_____
Lat pull-down	0.66	0.50	_____
Triceps extension	0.33	0.33	_____
Leg extension	0.50	0.50	_____
Leg curl	0.33	0.33	_____
Bent-knee sit-up			_____
			Total repetitions (max = 105) = _____

Total repetitions	Fitness category[a]
91-105	Excellent
77-90	Very good
63-76	Good
49-62	Fair
35-48	Poor
<35	Very poor

[a]Based on data compiled by author for 250 college-age men and women.

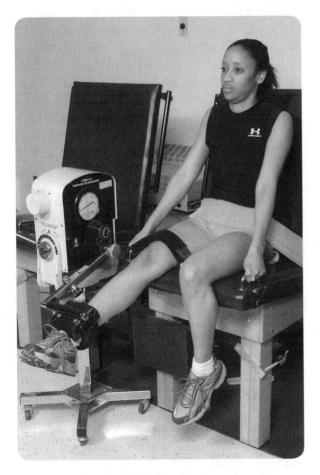

Figure 6.5 Cybex II isokinetic dynamometer.

Even as the muscle fatigues, the individual receives optimal overload with each repetition because the limb speed and resistance decrease. Theoretically, movement at slower speeds will allow recruitment of motor units that were not contributing to the total force production in earlier repetitions performed at faster speeds. Thus, self-accommodating, variable-resistance–variable-velocity exercise devices assess the isokinetic strength and endurance of both fast-twitch and slow-twitch motor units in the muscle group.

Table 6.9 summarizes isokinetic and omnikinetic test protocols for assessing strength, endurance, and power. For detailed descriptions of isokinetic test protocols and test norms, see Perrin 1993. Appendix C.2, "Average Strength, Endurance, and Power Values for Isokinetic (Omni-Tron) Tests" (p. 349), provides omnikinetic performance norms for young and middle-aged men and women, as well as male and female weight trainers.

Calisthenic-Type Strength and Muscular Endurance Tests

In certain field situations, you may not have access to dynamometers, free weights, or exercise machines to assess muscular fitness. As an alternative, you may use calisthenic-type strength and

Table 6.9   Isokinetic and Omnikinetic Test Protocols

Isokinetic tests	Speed setting	Protocol	Measure*
Strength	30° or 60°·sec⁻¹	Two submax practice trials followed by three maximal trials	Peak torque (ft-lb or Nm)
Endurance	120° to 180°·sec⁻¹	One maximal trial	Number of repetitions until torque reaches 50% of initial torque value
Power	120° to 300°·sec⁻¹	Two submax practice trials followed by three maximal trials	Peak torque (ft-lb or Nm)
Omnikinetic tests	Resistance setting	Protocol	Measure*
Strength	10	Three submax trials at resistance setting 2, followed by five maximal trials	Peak torque (ft-lb)
Endurance	3	Three practice trials at resistance setting 2, followed by 20 maximal repetitions	Total work output (ft-lb)
Power	6	Three submax trials followed by one maximal trial	Peak torque or total work (ft-lb)

*ft-lb = foot-pound; Nm = newton-meter; 1 ft-lb = 0.138 Nm.

endurance tests to assess your client's strength and muscular endurance.

Dynamic Strength Tests

You can measure dynamic strength using calisthenic-type exercises by determining the maximum weight, in excess of body mass, that an individual can lift for one repetition of the movement. Because strength is related to the size and body mass of the individual, Johnson and Nelson (1986) recommend using relative strength scores. For each test, attach weight plates (2 1/2, 5, 10, and 25 lb or 1, 2.3, 4.5, and 11.4 kg) to the individual. The relative strength score is the amount of additional weight divided by the body mass. For example, if a 150 lb (68.2 kg) man successfully performs one pull-up with a 30 lb (13.6 kg) weight attached to the waist belt, his relative strength score is 0.20 (30 lb/150 lb). Test protocols and performance norms for the pull-up, dip strength, sit-up, and bench squat are described elsewhere (Johnson and Nelson 1986).

Dynamic Endurance Tests

You can assess dynamic muscular endurance by measuring the maximum number of repetitions of various calisthenic exercises. Pull-up, push-up, and trunk curl (partial curl-up) tests are widely used for this purpose.

Pull-Up Tests

Pull-up tests may be used to measure the dynamic endurance of the arm and shoulder girdle muscles for individuals who are able to lift their body weight. For clients who are unable to perform even one pull-up, you can use modified pull-up and flexed-arm hang tests. Baumgartner (1978) developed a modified pull-up that uses an incline board (at a 30° angle to the floor) with a pull-up bar at the top. A modified scooter board slides along garage door tracks attached to the incline board (Baumgartner et al. 1984). While lying prone on the scooter board, the client pulls up until the chin is over the pull-up bar. Detailed testing procedures, equipment designs, and performance norms for children, adolescents, and college-age women and men are available (see Baumgartner 1978; Baumgartner et al. 1984).

The flexed-arm hang test is scored as the amount of time the client maintains the flexed-arm hanging position (i.e., supporting the body weight with the chin over the pull-up bar). Traditionally, a pronated grip on the pull-up bar is used (i.e., overgrip); however, variations of the flexed-arm hang test include using a supinated grip (i.e., undergrip). Although the flexed-arm hang tests isometric endurance of the arm and shoulder girdle musculature, it has been used for more than three decades as a measure of upper body strength. One study of college women showed that flexed-arm hang time relates more to relative strength (1-RM/body mass) than to absolute strength (1-RM) or to dynamic muscle endurance (measured as repetitions to failure at 70% 1-RM) (Clemons et al. 2004).

Push-Up Tests

The ACSM (2010) and CSEP (2003) recommend using a push-up test to assess endurance of the upper body musculature. To start, clients lie prone on the mat with their legs together and hands pointing forward under the shoulders. Clients push up from the mat by fully extending the elbows and by using either the toes (for males) or the knees (for females) as the pivot point. The upper body should be kept in a straight line and the head should be kept up. The client returns to the down position, touching the chin to the mat. The stomach and thighs should not touch the mat. Clients perform as many consecutive repetitions (no rest between repetitions) as possible; there is no time limit. Repetitions not meeting the stated criteria should not be counted. Terminate the test when the client strains forcibly or is unable to maintain proper push-up technique over two consecutive repetitions, and record the total number of correctly executed repetitions. Table 6.10 provides age–gender norms for the push-up test.

Trunk Curl Tests

Abdominal muscle endurance tests (e.g., trunk curls, partial curl-ups, and sit-ups) are commonly included in health-related fitness test batteries to identify clients at risk for low back pain or injury due to weak abdominal muscles. However, the validity of these tests as measures of abdominal strength or endurance and as predictors of low back pain is questionable. Most trunk curl tests are poorly related to abdominal strength ($r_{x,y} = -0.21$ to 0.36) and only moderately related to abdominal endurance ($r_{x,y} = 0.46$ to 0.50) (Knudson 2001; Knudson and Johnston 1995). Also, Jackson and colleagues (1998) found no relationship between sit-up test scores and incidence of low back pain. Keep these findings in mind when interpreting the results of these tests.

Trunk curl tests differ in duration (60-120 sec), cadence (20-25 reps·min^{-1}), and difficulty. The ACSM (2010) and CSEP (2003) recommend using a timed (1 min) curl-up test with a cadence of 25 reps·min^{-1} to assess the endurance of the abdominal muscles. For this test, the client lies supine on a mat with the knees flexed to 90°, the legs hip-width apart, and the arms fully extended at the sides with the middle finger of both hands touching a piece of masking tape (the zero mark). Place a second piece of masking tape 10 cm (4 in.) beyond the zero mark,

Table 6.10 Age–Gender Norms for Push-Up Test

	AGE (YR)					
	15-19	20-29	30-39	40-49	50-59	60-69
Men						
Excellent	≥39	≥36	≥30	≥25	≥21	≥18
Very good	29-38	29-35	22-29	17-24	13-20	11-17
Good	23-28	22-28	17-21	13-16	10-12	8-10
Fair	18-22	17-21	12-16	10-12	7-9	5-7
Needs improvement	≤17	≤16	≤11	≤9	≤6	≤4
Women						
Excellent	≥33	≥30	≥27	≥24	≥21	≥17
Very good	25-32	21-29	20-26	15-23	11-20	12-16
Good	18-24	15-20	13-19	11-14	7-10	5-11
Fair	12-17	10-14	8-12	5-10	2-6	2-4
Needs improvement	≤11	≤9	≤7	≤4	≤1	≤1

Source: The Canadian Physical Activity, Fitness & Lifestyle Approach: CSEP-Health & Fitness Program's Health-Related Appraisal and Counselling Strategy, 3rd Edition © 2003. Reprinted with permission of the Canadian Society for Exercise Physiology.

and set the metronome to 50 bpm (25 curl-ups per min). Shoes should be worn for this test. Instruct clients to slowly lift their shoulder blades off the mat in time with the metronome. Clients should flex their trunks (curl up) until their fingertips touch the 10 cm mark or their trunk makes a 30° angle with the mat. During the curl-up, the palms of the hands and the heels of the feet must remain in contact with the mat. On the return, the shoulder blades and head must contact the mat, and the fingertips of both hands must touch the zero mark. Score the curl-up test as the total number of consecutive repetitions up to a maximum of 25 in 1 min. Table 6.11 provides age–gender norms for the partial curl-up test.

Other trunk curl tests use a bench (0.46 m or 18 in. high) to protect the lower back by isolating the abdominal muscles. For these tests, the lower legs rest on the top of the bench and the backs of the thighs contact the bench. Instruct your clients to cross their arms so that each hand holds the opposite elbow. During each curl, their forearms must touch the thighs (concentric phase) and their shoulder blades must touch the floor (eccentric phase). The score is the number of correct repetitions completed in 60, 90, or 120 sec. Use a longer duration (90 or 120 sec) for very fit clients and athletes; use 60 sec for individuals of low or average fitness (Knudson and Johnston 1998).

SOURCES OF MEASUREMENT ERROR IN MUSCULAR FITNESS TESTING

The validity and reliability of strength and muscular endurance measures are affected by client factors, equipment, technician skill, and environmental factors. You must control each of these factors to ensure the accuracy and precision of muscular fitness scores.

Client Factors

Before measuring your client's strength or muscular endurance, familiarize the individual with the equipment and testing procedures. Clients with limited or no prior weightlifting experience need time to practice each lift to control for the effects of learning on performance. You should give even experienced weightlifters time to practice so that you can correct any improper lifting techniques prior to testing.

Muscular fitness tests require clients to give a maximal effort. Therefore, clients should get adequate sleep before performing these tests, and you should restrict the use of drugs and medications that may adversely affect their performance.

Table 6.11 Age–Gender Norms for Partial Curl-Up Test

	AGE (YR)					
	15-19	20-29	30-39	40-49	50-59	60-69
Men						
Excellent	25	25	25	25	25	25
Very good	23-24	21-24	18-24	18-24	17-24	16-24
Good	21-22	16-20	15-17	13-17	11-16	11-15
Fair	16-20	11-15	11-14	6-12	8-10	6-10
Needs improvement	≤15	≤10	≤10	≤5	≤7	≤5
Women						
Excellent	25	25	25	25	25	25
Very good	22-24	18-24	19-24	19-24	19-24	17-24
Good	17-21	14-17	10-18	11-18	10-18	8-16
Fair	12-16	5-13	6-9	4-10	6-9	3-7
Needs improvement	≤11	≤4	≤5	≤3	≤5	≤2

Source: The Canadian Physical Activity, Fitness & Lifestyle Approach: CSEP-Health & Fitness Program's Health-Related Appraisal and Counselling Strategy, 3rd Edition © 2003. Reprinted with permission of the Canadian Society for Exercise Physiology.

It is also important that you motivate your clients during testing by encouraging them to do their best and giving them positive feedback after each trial. Adequate rest between trials is necessary in order for clients to obtain scores that truly represent their maximal effort.

Equipment

The design of testing equipment may also affect your client's test scores. Most of the dynamic strength and muscular endurance protocols and norms presented in this chapter were developed using constant-resistance exercise machines. Therefore you should not use free weights or variable-resistance machines when administering these tests. It is also important to calibrate the equipment and make sure that it is in proper working condition prior to testing. Inspection and maintenance of equipment will increase accuracy and decrease risk of accidents. When selecting exercise machines, make sure that the equipment can be properly adjusted to accommodate varying limb lengths and body sizes. Use equipment specifically designed for smaller individuals when testing children and smaller adults.

Technician Skill

All strength testing should be done by qualified, trained technicians who are knowledgeable about proper lifting and spotting techniques and familiar with standardized testing procedures. Explain and demonstrate the proper lifting technique and then correct any performance errors you see as the client practices. During the test, clients may inadvertently "cheat" by moving extraneous body parts to help lift the weight. Carefully observe the client during the test, focusing on the grip used and the starting position. The type of grip (pronated vs. supinated) has a substantial effect on performance. For example, using a narrow grip instead of a wide grip during a lat pull-down exercise increases the amount of weight that can be lifted. Likewise, the client will be able to produce more force during an arm curl using a supinated grip compared to a pronated grip. The client's starting position may also affect strength scores. During the bench press, for example, eccentric movement (i.e., lowering the weight) prior to the concentric phase of the lift will increase maximal muscular force due to the stretch reflex and the tendency for the client to "bounce" the weight off the chest. To obtain accurate assessments of your client's strength, it is important to standardize starting positions and to follow all testing procedures carefully.

Environmental Factors

Factors such as room temperature and humidity may affect test scores. The room temperature should be 70° to 74° F (21° to 23° C) to maximize subject comfort during testing. Ideally, you want a quiet, clean environment with limited distractions (not an overcrowded weight room, for example). When assessing improvements due to training, remember to pretest and posttest your client at the same time of day to control for diurnal variations in strength.

ADDITIONAL CONSIDERATIONS FOR MUSCULAR FITNESS TESTING

This section addresses a number of additional factors and questions regarding the testing and evaluation of your client's muscular fitness.

■ *How can I estimate my client's 1-RM?*

Although 1-RM tests can be safely administered to clients of all ages, sometimes it is preferable to estimate the 1-RM. One-repetition maximum testing can be time-consuming, especially for a large group of clients. Some clients may take 15 min to complete a 1-RM test (multiple attempts and rests). Also, the 1-RM may be underestimated for clients with little or no exercise experience because they are unaccustomed to or may be apprehensive about lifting heavy loads. In these cases, it may be more suitable and practical to estimate 1-RM.

You can estimate the 1-RM of your clients from submaximal muscle endurance tests. Research demonstrates a strong relationship between muscle endurance (measured as the number of repetitions to fatigue) and the percentage of 1-RM lifted (Brzycki 1993). Muscular strength (1-RM) therefore can be predicted from muscular endurance tests with a fair degree of accuracy (Ball and Rose 1991; Braith et al. 1993; Invergo, Ball, and Looney 1991; Kuramoto and Payne 1995; Mayhew et al. 1992). The most frequently used prediction equations are based on the number of repetitions to fatigue in one set. For example, the Brzycki (1993) equation can be used to estimate 1-RM of men. This equation can be used for any combination of submaximal weights and repetitions to fatigue providing that the repetitions to fatigue do not exceed 10.

$$1\text{-RM} = \text{weight lifted (lb)} / [1.0278 - (\text{reps to fatigue} \times 0.0278)]$$

For example, if your client completes seven repetitions to fatigue during a bench press exercise using a 100 lb barbell, the estimated 1-RM is calculated as follows:

$$1\text{-RM} = 100 \text{ lb} / [1.0278 - (7 \text{ reps} \times 0.0278)]$$

$$= 120 \text{ lb } (54.5 \text{ kg})$$

Brzycki (2000) also suggested using a prediction equation based on the number of repetitions to fatigue obtained in *two* submaximal sets to estimate 1-RM. Any two submaximal sets can be used as long as the number of reps to fatigue does not exceed 10. For example, you can determine your client's 5-RM value, or the maximum weight that can be lifted for five reps (e.g., 120 lb for five reps), and the 10-RM value (e.g., 80 lb for 10 reps) and use them in the following equation:

$$\text{predicted 1-RM} = [(SM_1 - SM_2) / (REP_2 - REP_1)] \times (REP_1 - 1) + SM_1$$

$$= [(120 - 80) / (10 - 5)] \times (5 - 1) + 120$$

$$= 152 \text{ lb}$$

In this equation, SM_1 and REP_1 represent the heavier submaximal weight (120 lb) and the respective number of repetitions (five reps) completed, and SM_2 and REP_2 correspond to the lighter submaximal weight (80 lb) and the respective number of repetitions (10 reps) performed.

Alternatively, you can use the average number of repetitions corresponding to various percentages of 1-RM (see table 6.12). This technique and the Brzycki (1993) equation yield similar 1-RM estimates for lifts between 2-RM and 10-RM. To estimate the 1-RM from 2-RM to 10-RM values, divide the weight lifted by the respective %1-RM, expressed as a decimal (%1-RM/100). For example, a client lifting 100 lb (45.4 kg) for eight repetitions would have an estimated 1-RM of 125 lb (56.7 kg):

$$1\text{-RM} = 100 \text{ lb} / 0.80 \text{ or } 125 \text{ lb } (56.7 \text{ kg})$$

Table 6.12 Average Number of Repetitions and %1-RM Values

Repetitions	%1-RM[a]
1	100
2	95
3	93
4	90
5	87
6	85
7	83
8	80
9	77
10	75

[a]These values may vary slightly for different muscle groups and ages.

Data from Baechle, Earle, and Wathen 2000.

Also, gender-specific prediction equations can be used to estimate upper body strength (i.e., the 1-RM bench press) from the YMCA bench press test (see table 6.7) in younger clients (22-36 yr) (Kim, Mayhew, and Peterson 2002):

For Men

$$\text{predicted 1-RM (kg)} = (1.55 \times \text{YMCA test repetitions}) + 37.9$$

$$r = 0.87 \text{ and } SEE = 8.0 \text{ kg.}$$

For Women

$$\text{predicted 1-RM (kg)} = (0.31 \times \text{YMCA test repetitions}) + 19.2$$

$$r = 0.87 \text{ and } SEE = 3.2 \text{ kg.}$$

For example, if a 25 yr old female's YMCA bench press test score is 30 reps, her estimated 1-RM bench press strength is calculated as follows:

$$\text{predicted 1-RM (kg)} = (0.31 \times 30 \text{ reps}) + 19.2$$

$$= 28.5 \text{ kg } (62.8 \text{ lb})$$

■ *How is muscle balance assessed?*

Muscle strength is important for joint stability; however, a strength imbalance between opposing muscle groups (e.g., quadriceps femoris and hamstrings) may compromise joint stability and increase the risk of musculoskeletal injury. For this reason, experts recommend maintaining a balance in strength between agonist and antagonistic muscle groups.

Muscle balance ratios differ among muscle groups and are affected by the force-velocity of muscle groups at specific joints. To control limb velocity during muscle balance testing, you will do best to use isokinetic dynamometers. In field settings, however, you may obtain a crude index of muscle balance by comparing 1-RM values of muscle groups. Based on isokinetic tests of peak torque production at slow speeds (30° to 60°·sec^{-1}), the following muscle balance ratios are recommended for agonist and antagonistic muscle groups:

Muscle groups	Muscle balance ratio
Hip extensors and flexors	1:1
Elbow extensors and flexors	1:1
Trunk extensors and flexors	1:1
Ankle inverters and everters	1:1
Shoulder flexors and extensors	2:3
Knee extensors and flexors	3:2
Shoulder internal and external rotators	3:2
Ankle plantar flexors and dorsiflexors	3:1

Muscle balance between other pairs of muscle groups is also important. The difference in strength between contralateral (right vs. left sides) muscle groups should be no more than 10% to 15%, and the strength-to-body mass (BM) ratio of the upper body (bench press 1-RM/BM) should be at least 40% to 60% of the lower body relative strength (leg press 1-RM/BM). If you detect imbalances, prescribe additional exercises for the weaker muscle groups.

■ Can strength or muscular endurance be assessed by a single test?

Strength and endurance are specific to the muscle group, the type of muscular contraction (static or dynamic), the speed of muscular contraction (slow or fast), and the joint angle being tested (static contraction). There is no single test to evaluate total body muscle strength or endurance. Minimally, the strength test battery should include a measure of abdominal, lower extremity, and upper extrem-

ity strength. In addition, if the individual trains dynamically, select a dynamic, not static, test to assess strength or endurance levels before and after training.

You should also use caution in selecting test items to measure muscle strength. The maximum number of sit-ups, pull-ups, or push-ups that an individual can perform measures muscular endurance, yet maximum-repetition tests have been included in some strength test batteries. This may lead to misinterpretation of the test results.

■ Should absolute or relative measures be used to classify a client's muscle strength?

There is a direct relationship between body size and muscle strength. Generally, larger individuals have more muscle mass, and therefore greater strength, than smaller individuals with less muscle mass.

Because strength directly relates to the body mass and lean body mass of the individual, you should express the test results in relative terms (e.g., 1-RM/BM). This is especially true in comparing your client's score to group norms and in comparing groups or individuals differing in body size and composition (e.g., men vs. women or older vs. younger adults).

Use relative strength scores for assessing individual improvement from training. As a result of resistance training, some individuals may gain body weight while others may lose weight, especially if they are using resistance training as part of a program for weight gain or loss. If you compare the client's relative strength scores (from pre- and posttest training), you will be able to evaluate the change in strength that is independent of a change in body weight.

■ How can the influence of strength on muscular endurance be controlled?

Performance on some endurance tests (e.g., pull-ups and push-ups) is highly dependent on the strength of the individual. It is recommended that you use relative endurance tests that are proportional to the body mass or maximum strength of the individual to assess muscle endurance. You cannot use a pull-up test to assess muscular endurance if the individual is not strong enough to lift the body weight for one repetition of that exercise. Therefore, select a modified or submaximal (percentage of body weight) endurance test.

■ *Are there comprehensive norms that can be used to classify muscular fitness levels of diverse population subgroups?*

Strength norms for women (20 to 82 yr) were developed for the bench press (1-RM), leg press (1-RM), static grip strength, and push-up tests (Brown and Miller 1998). These norms are based on data obtained from 304 independent-living women attending wellness classes at a university medical center. However, there is a lack of up-to-date endurance norms for men and strength and endurance norms for older men. New norms need to be established for this population in particular.

MUSCULAR FITNESS TESTING OF OLDER ADULTS

It is important to accurately assess the muscular fitness of older individuals. Adequate strength in the upper and lower body lessens risk of falls and injuries associated with falling, reduces age-related loss of bone mineral, maintains lean body tissue, improves glucose utilization, and prevents obesity. Moderate-to-high levels of muscular strength enable older adults to maintain their functional independence and to perform activities of daily living as well as fitness and recreational activities. The following sections address tests that you can use to assess the muscular strength and physical performance of older clients.

Strength Testing of Older Adults

Experts agree that it is safe to administer 1-RM tests to older adults if proper procedures (see "Steps for 1-RM Maximum Testing," p. 135) are followed (Shaw, McCully, and Posner 1995). The risk of injury is low, with only 2.4% of older adults (55-80 yr) experiencing an injury during 1-RM assessment (Salem, Wang, and Sigward 2002; Shaw et al. 1995). Salem and colleagues (2002) suggested that at least one pretesting session (i.e., a practice 1-RM test session) is necessary to establish stable baseline 1-RM values for older adults.

Alternatively, you can estimate the 1-RM of older clients from submaximal muscular endurance tests. Kuramoto and Payne (1995) developed prediction equations to estimate 1-RM from a submaximal endurance test in middle-aged and older women. For this endurance protocol, the client completes as

many repetitions as possible using a weight equivalent to 45% of her body mass. To estimate 1-RM, use the following equations:

Middle-Aged Women (40-50 yr)

1-RM = (1.06 × weight lifted in kg) + (0.58 × reps) − (0.20 × age) − 3.41

$r = 0.94$ and *SEE* = 1.85 kg.

Older Women (60-70 yr)

1-RM = (0.92 × weight lifted in kg) + (0.79 × reps) − 3.73

$r = 0.90$ and *SEE* = 2.04 kg.

Knutzen, Brilla, and Caine (1999) tested the validity of selected 1-RM prediction equations for older women (mean age = 69 yr) and men (mean age = 73 yr). On average, these prediction equations underestimated the actual 1-RM for 11 different constant-resistance machine exercises. For exercises such as the biceps curl, the lateral row, the bench press, and ankle plantar and dorsiflexion, the predicted values were on average 0.5 to 3.0 kg less than the actual 1-RM values. However, larger differences (as much as a 10 kg underestimation) were noted for the triceps press-down; the supine leg press; and the hip flexion, extension, abduction, and adduction exercises. The Brzycki (1993) equation gave a closer estimate of actual 1-RMs for hip exercises (extension, flexion, adduction, and abduction) compared to the other equations evaluated; the Wathen (1994a) equation, 1-RM = 100 × weight lifted / [48.8 + 53.8$^{-0.075 \text{(reps)}}$], most closely estimates 1-RM for all upper body exercises, the leg press, and dorsiflexion exercises. The authors concluded that the actual and predicted 1-RM are close enough to warrant using these prediction equations to determine resistance training intensities (i.e., %1-RMs) for older adults. In addition, given that the predicted 1-RM values were consistently less than the actual 1-RM values, the resistance training intensity will not likely exceed the prescribed value.

Functional Fitness Testing of Older Adults

Functional fitness is the ability to perform everyday activities safely and independently without undue fatigue (Rikli and Jones 2001). Functional fitness is multidimensional, requiring aerobic endurance, flexibility, balance, agility, and muscular strength. Older individuals with moderate-to-high functional fitness have the ability to perform normal **activities of daily living (ADL)** such as getting out of a chair or car, climbing stairs, shopping, dressing, and bathing; and these individuals are able to stay strong, active, and independent as they age.

The Senior Fitness Test (Rikli and Jones 2001) assesses the physical capacity and functional fitness of older adults (60-94 yr). This test battery includes two measures of muscular strength: (a) an arm (biceps) curl for upper body strength (figure 6.6) and (b) a 30 sec chair stand for lower body strength (figure 6.7). The ACSM (2010) recommends using these two test items to safely assess the muscular fitness of most older adults.

Arm Curl Test

Purpose: Assess upper body strength.

Application: Measure ability to perform ADL such as lifting and carrying groceries, grandchildren, and pets.

Equipment: You will need a folding or straight-back chair, a stopwatch, and a 5 lb (2.27 kg) dumbbell for women or an 8 lb (3.63 kg) dumbbell for men.

Test procedures: The client sits in the chair with his back straight and his feet flat on the floor. He holds the dumbbell in his dominant hand using a neutral (handshake) grip and lets his arm hang down at his side (see figure 6.6). For each repetition, the client curls the weight by fully flexing the elbow while supinating the forearm and returns the weight to the starting position by fully extending the elbow and pronating the forearm. Instruct your client to keep his upper arm in contact with his trunk during the test. Have your client perform as many repetitions as possible in 30 sec. Administer one trial.

Scoring: Count the number of repetitions executed in 30 sec. If the forearm is more than halfway up when the time expires, count the move as a complete repetition. Use table 6.13 to determine your client's percentile ranking.

Safety tips: Before testing, demonstrate the exercise for your client. Have your client perform one or two repetitions of the exercise without a dumbbell to check body position and lifting technique. Stop the test if the client complains of pain.

Validity and reliability: Arm curl test scores were moderately related ($r_{x,y}$ = 0.84 for men and 0.79 for women) to combined 1-RM values for the chest, upper back, and biceps (criterion-related validity). Average arm curl test scores of physically active older adults were significantly greater than those

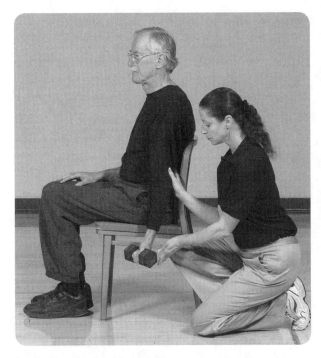
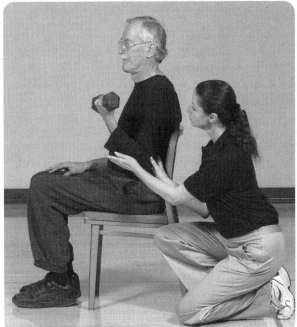

Figure 6.6 Arm curl test for older adults.

Table 6.13   Arm Curl Test Norms for Older Adults*

	60-64 YR		65-69 YR		70-74 YR		75-79 YR		80-84 YR		85-89 YR		90-94 YR	
Percentile rank	F	M	F	M	F	M	F	M	F	M	F	M	F	M
95	24	27	22	27	22	26	21	24	20	23	18	21	17	18
90	22	25	21	25	20	24	20	22	18	22	17	19	16	16
85	21	24	20	24	19	23	19	21	17	20	16	18	15	16
80	20	23	19	23	18	22	18	20	16	20	15	17	14	15
75	19	22	18	21	17	21	17	19	16	19	15	17	13	14
70	18	21	17	21	17	20	16	19	15	18	14	16	13	14
65	18	21	17	20	16	19	16	18	15	18	14	15	12	13
60	17	20	16	20	16	19	15	17	14	17	13	15	12	13
55	17	20	16	19	15	18	15	17	14	17	13	14	11	12
50	16	19	15	18	14	17	14	16	13	16	12	14	11	12
45	16	18	15	18	14	17	13	16	12	15	12	13	10	12
40	15	18	14	17	13	16	13	15	12	15	11	13	10	11
35	14	17	14	16	13	15	12	14	11	14	11	12	9	11
30	14	17	13	16	12	15	12	14	11	14	10	11	9	10
25	13	16	12	15	12	14	11	13	10	13	10	11	8	10
20	12	15	12	14	11	13	10	12	10	12	9	10	8	9
15	11	14	11	13	10	12	9	11	9	12	8	9	7	8
10	10	13	10	12	9	11	8	10	8	10	7	8	6	8
5	9	11	8	10	8	9	7	9	6	9	6	7	5	6

F = females; M = males.

*Values represent number of repetitions in 30 sec.

Adapted, by permission, from R. Rikli and C. Jones, 2001, *Senior fitness test manual* (Champaign, IL: Human Kinetics), 127.

of sedentary older adults (construct validity). Test–retest reliability was *r* = 0.81.

30 Sec Chair Stand Test

Purpose: Assess lower body strength.

Application: Measure ability to perform ADL such as climbing stairs; getting out of a chair, bathtub, or car; and walking.

Equipment: You will need a folding or straight-back chair (seat height = 17 in. or 43 cm) and a stopwatch.

Test procedures: Place the chair against a wall to prevent slipping. Instruct your client to sit erect in the chair with his feet flat on the floor and his arms crossed at the wrists and held against his chest (see figure 6.7). For each repetition, the client rises to a full stand and then returns to the fully seated starting position. Have your client perform as many rep-

etitions as possible in 30 sec. Administer one trial.

Scoring: Count the number of repetitions executed in 30 sec. If the client is more than halfway up when the time expires, count the move as a full stand. Use table 6.14 to determine your client's percentile ranking.

Safety tips: Brace the chair against a wall, watch for balance problems, and stop the test if the client complains of pain. Before testing, demonstrate the movement slowly to show proper form. Have your client perform one or two repetitions to check body position (fully standing and fully seated) for the test.

Validity and reliability: Scores for the chair stand test were moderately related to the 1-RM leg press (criterion-related validity) in older men ($r_{x,y}$ = 0.78) and women ($r_{x,y}$ = 0.71). Average scores were lower for older adults (80+ yr) than for relatively younger

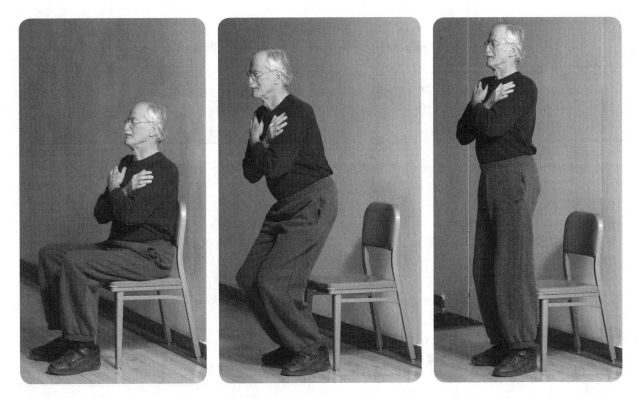

Figure 6.7 30 sec chair stand test for older adults.

Table 6.14   30 Sec Chair Stand Test Norms for Older Adults*

Percentile rank	60-64 YR		65-69 YR		70-74 YR		75-79 YR		80-84 YR		85-89 YR		90-94 YR	
	F	M	F	M	F	M	F	M	F	M	F	M	F	M
95	21	23	19	23	19	21	19	21	18	19	17	19	16	16
90	20	22	18	21	18	20	17	20	17	17	15	17	15	15
85	19	21	17	20	17	19	16	18	16	16	14	16	13	14
80	18	20	16	19	16	18	16	18	15	16	14	15	12	13
75	17	19	16	18	15	17	15	17	14	15	13	14	11	12
70	17	19	15	18	15	17	14	16	13	14	12	13	11	12
65	16	18	15	17	14	16	14	16	13	14	12	13	10	11
60	16	17	14	16	14	16	13	15	12	13	11	12	9	11
55	15	17	14	16	13	15	13	15	12	13	11	12	9	10
50	15	16	14	15	13	14	12	14	11	12	10	11	8	10
45	14	16	13	15	12	14	12	13	11	12	10	11	7	9
40	14	15	13	14	12	13	12	13	10	11	9	10	7	9
35	13	15	12	13	11	13	11	12	10	11	9	9	6	8
30	12	14	12	13	11	12	11	12	9	10	8	9	5	8
25	12	14	11	12	10	11	10	11	9	10	8	8	4	7
20	11	13	11	11	10	11	9	10	8	9	7	7	4	7

(continued)

Table 6.14 *(continued)*

Percentile rank	60-64 YR		65-69 YR		70-74 YR		75-79 YR		80-84 YR		85-89 YR		90-94 YR	
	F	M	F	M	F	M	F	M	F	M	F	M	F	M
15	10	12	10	11	9	10	9	10	7	8	6	6	3	6
10	9	11	9	9	8	9	8	8	6	7	5	5	1	5
5	8	9	8	8	7	8	6	7	4	6	4	4	0	3

F = females; M = males.

*Values represent number of repetitions.

Adapted, by permission, from R. Rikli and C. Jones, 2001, *Senior fitness test manual* (Champaign, IL: Human Kinetics), 128.

adults (60-69 yr) and higher for physically active older adults compared to sedentary older adults (construct validity). Test–retest reliability was *r* = 0.86 and *r* = 0.92 for older men and women, respectively.

MUSCULAR FITNESS TESTING OF CHILDREN

In the past, experts questioned whether or not it was safe to use 1-RM tests to evaluate children. A major concern was the risk of growth plate fractures when the children attempted to lift heavy weights. Experts now agree that it is safe to administer 1-RM tests to children (6-12 yr) if appropriate procedures are followed (Faigenbaum, Milliken, and Westcott 2003).

Results from 1-RM tests may be used to establish baselines for evaluating the progress of children in resistance training programs. You can also use these values to plan a personalized resistance training program for each child, to identify muscle imbalances, and to provide motivation. One shortcoming of 1-RM testing is that it must be closely supervised (one on one) to ensure safety, which limits its usefulness in physical education classes and youth sport programs. Also, child-sized exercise machines must be used; the safety of 1-RM testing using other modes (e.g., dumbbells or barbells) has not been adequately established.

1-RM Testing Guidelines for Children

The following steps are recommended for 1-RM testing of children (Faigenbaum, Milliken, and Westcott 2003):

1. Have a certified, experienced exercise professional administer and closely supervise (one on one) all tests.

2. Before testing, familiarize the children with proper lifting techniques (i.e., proper breathing and controlled movements), allow them to practice these techniques, and answer any questions they may have.

3. Have the child warm up by performing 10 min of low-to-moderate intensity aerobic exercise and stretching.

4. Use dynamic, constant-resistance exercise machines designed specifically for children or individuals with small body frames.

5. Before the 1-RM lift, instruct the child to perform six repetitions with a relatively light load followed by three repetitions with a heavier load. Then gradually increase the weight and have the child attempt the 1-RM lift. Allow at least 2 min of rest between the series of single repetitions with increasing loads. Follow this procedure until the child fails to complete the full ROM of the exercise for at least two attempts. The 1-RM is typically achieved within 7 to 11 trials.

6. Record the 1-RM as the maximum weight lifted for the last successful trial.

7. After testing, have the child stretch the exercised muscle groups for 5 min.

Sources for Equipment

Product	Supplier's contact information
Aquatic exercise equipment	Hydro-Fit, Inc. (800) 346-7295 www.hydrofit.com
Body Masters (constant and variable resistance)	Body Masters Sports Industries, Inc. (800) 325-8964 www.body-masters.com
Cable tensiometer (static)	Pacific Scientific Co., Inc. (815) 226-3100 www.pacsci.com
CAM II (variable resistance)	Keiser Corp. (800) 888-7009 www.keiser.com
Cybex II, Orthotron (isokinetic)	Cybex International (888) 462-9239 www.ecybex.com
Exercise and stability balls	Ball Dynamics International, LLC (800) 752-2255 www.fitball.com
Free-motion machines (constant and variable resistance)	FreeMotion Fitness (877) 363-8449 www.freemotionfitness.com
Free weights (constant resistance)	York Barbell Co. (800) 358-9675 www.yorkbarbell.com
Handgrip dynamometer (static)	Creative Health Products (800) 742-4478 www.chponline.com
Handheld dynamometer (static)	Hoggan Health Industries (800) 678-7888 www.hogganhealth.com
Leg/back dynamometer (static)	Best Priced Products (800) 824-2939 www.best-priced-products.com
Nautilus (variable resistance)	Nautilus, Inc. (800) 864-1270 www.nautilus.com

(continued)

Sources for Equipment *(continued)*

Product	Supplier's contact information
Resistance bands and tubing	Creative Health Products (800) 742-4478 www.chponline.com
Total Gym machines (variable resistance)	Total Gym/EFI (800) 541-4900 www.totalgym.com
Universal gym machines (constant and variable resistance)	Universal Gym Equipment (800) 843-3906 www.universalgymequipment.com

KEY POINTS

- Strength is the ability of a muscle group to exert maximal contractile force against a resistance in a single contraction.

- Muscular endurance is the ability of a muscle group to exert submaximal force for an extended duration.

- Both strength and muscular endurance are specific to the muscle group and to the type of muscle contraction—static, concentric, eccentric, or isokinetic.

- The greatest resistance that can be used during dynamic, concentric muscular contraction with a constant-resistance exercise mode is equal to the maximum weight that can be moved at the weakest point in the ROM.

- Dynamometers, cable tensiometers, strain gauges, and load cells are used to measure static strength and endurance.

- Constant-resistance modes of exercise (free weights and exercise machines) are used to assess dynamic (i.e., concentric and eccentric) strength and endurance.

- The accommodating-resistance mode of exercise is used to assess isokinetic and omnikinetic strength, endurance, and power.

- Free-motion machines allow muscle groups to be exercised in multiple planes.

- Calisthenic-type exercise tests provide a crude index of strength and endurance but can be used when other equipment is not available.

- Strength should be expressed relative to the body mass or lean body mass of the individual.

- Muscular endurance tests should take into account the body mass or maximal strength of the individual.

- Test batteries should include a minimum of three to four items that measure upper body, lower body, and abdominal strength or endurance.

- It is important to follow standardized testing procedures and to control for extraneous variables (e.g., motivation level, time of testing, isolation of body parts, and joint angles) when assessing strength and muscular endurance.

- It is safe to give 1-RM strength tests to children and older adults if appropriate testing procedures are followed.

- Although strength can be predicted from submaximal endurance tests, 1-RM assessments are preferable.

- Use the arm curl test and the 30 sec chair stand test to assess the functional strength of older clients.

KEY TERMS

Learn the definition of each of the following key terms. Definitions of terms can be found in the glossary on page 411.

accommodating-resistance exercise

activities of daily living (ADL)

concentric contraction

constant-resistance exercise

dynamic contraction

eccentric contraction

free-motion machines

functional fitness

isokinetic contraction

isometric contraction

isotonic contraction

maximum voluntary isometric contraction (MVIC)

muscular endurance

muscular strength

omnikinetic exercise

one-repetition maximum (1-RM)

relative strength

static contraction

variable-resistance exercise

REVIEW QUESTIONS

In addition to being able to define each of the key terms, test your knowledge and understanding of the material by answering the following review questions.

1. During dynamic movement, why does muscle force production fluctuate throughout the ROM?

2. Name two methods for assessing static strength and muscular endurance.

3. How do constant-resistance, variable-resistance, accommodating-resistance, and free-motion exercise machines differ?

4. Why are strength test scores typically expressed relative to the client's body mass?

5. Describe the recommended procedures for administering 1-RM strength tests.

6. Identify three sources of measurement error for muscular fitness testing. What can you do to control for these potential errors?

7. Is it safe to give 1-RM tests to children and older adults?

8. Describe two tests that can be used to assess the functional strength of older adults.

9. Why is it important to assess muscle balance?

10. In terms of the specificity principle, explain why a single test cannot be used to adequately assess your client's overall strength. Minimally, what muscle groups should be tested to evaluate overall strength?

11. Identify the test items recommended by ACSM for assessing your client's upper and lower body strength.

12. For certain clients, you may choose not to administer 1-RM strength tests. Describe how you could obtain an estimate of their strength instead.

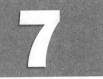
Designing Resistance Training Programs

- How do training principles specifically apply to the design of resistance training programs?
- How are resistance training programs modified to optimize the development of strength, muscular endurance, muscle power, or muscle size?
- What factors do I need to consider when designing individualized exercise prescriptions?
- Is resistance training recommended for children, adolescents, and older adults?
- What methods can be used to design advanced resistance training programs?
- What are the outcomes and health benefits derived from resistance training?
- What is the cause of delayed-onset muscle soreness, and can it be prevented?

Muscular strength and endurance are important to the overall health and physical fitness of your clients, enabling them to engage in physically active leisure-time pursuits, to perform activities of daily living more easily, and to maintain functional independence later in life. Resistance training is a systematic program of exercise for development of the muscular system. Although the primary outcome of resistance training is improved strength and muscular endurance, a number of health benefits are also derived from this form of exercise. Resis-

tance exercise builds bone mass, thereby counteracting the loss of bone mineral (osteoporosis) and risk of falls as one ages. This form of training also lowers blood pressure in hypertensive individuals, reduces body fat levels, and may prevent the development of low back syndrome.

While resistance training has long been widely used by bodybuilders, powerlifters, and competitive athletes to develop strength and muscle size, participation in weightlifting by individuals of all ages and levels of athletic interest has increased dramatically over the past 30 yr. The popularity and widespread appeal of weightlifting exercise for general muscle conditioning challenge exercise specialists and personal trainers to develop resistance training programs that can meet the diverse needs of their clients.

This chapter shows you how to apply basic training principles (see chapter 3) to the design of resistance training programs for novice, intermediate, and advanced weightlifters. The chapter also presents guidelines for developing muscle strength, muscle endurance, muscle size, and muscle power. The chapter addresses various models of periodization, functional training exercise progressions, and guidelines for youth resistance training.

TYPES OF RESISTANCE TRAINING

Muscular fitness can be improved using various types of resistance training—isometric (static), dynamic (concentric and eccentric), and isokinetic.

Although there are general guidelines for designing isometric, dynamic, and isokinetic resistance training programs, each exercise prescription should be individualized to meet the specific needs and goals of your client.

Isometric Training

In 1953, Hettinger and Muller reported that people produce significant gains in isometric strength (5% per week) by holding one 6 sec contraction at two-thirds of maximum intensity, 5 days/wk. This type of training became popular in the late 1950s and early 1960s because the exercises could be performed anywhere and at any time with little or no equipment. A major disadvantage is that strength gains are specific to the joint angle used during training. Thus, to increase strength throughout the range of motion, the exercise needs to be performed at a number of different joint angles (e.g., 30°, 60°, 90°, 120°, and 180° of knee flexion).

Isometric exercise is widely used in rehabilitation programs to counteract strength loss and muscle atrophy, especially in cases in which the limb is temporarily immobilized. This type of training, however, is contraindicated for coronary-prone and hypertensive individuals because the static contraction may produce large increases in intrathoracic pressure. This reduces the venous return to the heart, increases the work of the heart, and causes a substantial rise in blood pressure.

After further research, Hettinger and Muller modified their original exercise prescription. Table 7.1 presents the general guidelines for designing training programs for isometric strength and endurance development. For descriptions and illustrations of isometric exercises for various muscle groups, see appendix C.3, "Isometric Exercises," page 351.

Dynamic Resistance Training

Dynamic resistance training is suitable for developing muscular fitness of men and women of all ages,

as well as children. This type of resistance training involves concentric and eccentric contractions of the muscle group performed against a constant or variable resistance. Typically free weights (barbells and dumbbells) and constant- or variable-resistance machines are used for resistance training.

Several important concepts used to prescribe dynamic resistance training programs are intensity, repetitions, sets, training volume, and order of exercises (Fleck and Kraemer 1997). Intensity is expressed either as a percentage of the individual's 1-repetition maximum (%1-RM) or as the **repetition maximum (RM)**, which is the maximum weight that the person can lift for a given number of repetitions of an exercise (e.g., 8-RM equals the maximum weight that the person can lift for eight repetitions). For the number of repetitions (i.e., 1- to 10-RM) corresponding to various percentages of 1-RM (i.e., 75% to 100% 1-RM), see table 6.12, page 144. The %1-RM values and average number of repetitions for intensities less than 75% 1-RM are as follows:

60% 1-RM = 15- to 20-RM

65% 1-RM = 14-RM

70% 1-RM = 12-RM

Intensity is inversely related to repetitions. In other words, individuals are able to perform more **repetitions** using lighter resistance or weights and fewer repetitions using heavier resistance. A **set** consists of a given number of consecutive repetitions of the exercise. **Training volume** is the total amount of weight lifted during the workout and is calculated by summing the products of the weight lifted, repetitions, and sets for each exercise.

The optimal training stimulus for developing muscular strength or endurance is controversial. Some research supports the conventional prescription of **high–intensity–low-repetition** resistance exercise for strength development and **low–intensity–high-repetition** exercise for muscular endurance (Kraemer et al. 2002; Kraemer and Ratamess

Table 7.1 Guidelines for Designing Isometric Training Programs

Type	Intensity	Duration	Repetitions	Frequency (days/week)	Length of program
Isometric strength	100% MVC*	5 sec per contraction	5-10	5	4 wk or more
Isometric endurance	60% MVC or less	Until fatigued	1 per session	5	4 wk or more

*Maximal voluntary contraction.

2004). To develop muscle strength and muscle mass, the American College of Sports Medicine (ACSM 2010) recommends selecting a resistance that allows the individual to complete 8 to 12 repetitions per set. To improve muscular endurance, a lower resistance (≤50% 1-RM) and higher number of repetitions (15-25 reps) are recommended (ACSM 2010). Table 7.2 summarizes the ACSM (2010) guidelines for the resistance training of healthy populations.

Although this training stimulus may be sufficient for beginner and novice lifters, experts recommend that resistance training programs be tailored to the specific goals of intermediate and advanced lifters (Kraemer et al. 2002; Kraemer and Ratamess 2004). You can design programs to optimize the development of muscle strength, size (hypertrophy), endurance, or power by varying the intensity, repetitions, sets, and frequency of training. Tables 7.3 through 7.5 present guidelines for designing programs for novice, intermediate, and advanced weightlifters. For descriptions of dynamic resistance training exercises, see appendix C.4, "Dynamic Resistance Training Exercises," page 355.

Intensity

As previously mentioned, the %1-RM and RM are widely used to estimate intensity for resistance training programs. The ACSM (2010), however, has stated that the %1-RM does not accurately estimate intensity because the number of repetitions performed at a given %1-RM varies among muscle groups and individuals. Still, many experts endorse the %1-RM to prescribe intensity (Kraemer et al. 2002).

The mean optimal intensity for developing strength ranges between 60% and 100% 1-RM. At these intensities, most individuals are able to perform 1 to 12 repetitions (1-RM to 12-RM). The client's experience with resistance training dictates the optimal intensity for developing strength. Generally, you should prescribe intensities of 60% to 70% 1-RM for novice lifters, 70% to 85% 1-RM for intermediate lifters, and 80% to 100% 1-RM for advanced lifters (Kraemer et al. 2002; Kraemer and Ratamess 2004). Meta-analyses support these recommendations. Rhea and colleagues (2003a) reported that the optimal intensity for strength

Table 7.2 ACSM Guidelines for Resistance Training of Healthy Populations

Goal	Intensity[a]	Repetitions	Sets[b]	Frequency	Number of exercises[c]
Muscle strength and muscle mass	60-80% 1-RM	8-12	2-4	2-3 nonconsecutive days/wk	8-10

[a]To point of momentary muscular fatigue or failure.

[b]Allow 2-3 min rest between sets.

[c]Perform a different exercise for a specific muscle group every two to three sessions.

ACSM 2010

Table 7.3 Guidelines for Resistance Training Programs for Novice Lifters

Goal	Intensity	Volume	Velocity	Frequency	Rest interval
Strength	60-70% 1-RM	1-3 sets of 8-12 reps	Slow to moderate	2-3 days/wk	2-3 min MJ; 1-2 min SJ
Hypertrophy	70-85% 1-RM	1-3 sets of 8-12 reps	Slow to moderate	2-3 days/wk	1-2 min
Endurance	50-70% 1-RM	1-3 sets of 10-15 reps	Slow	2-3 days/wk	<1 min
Power	85-100% 1-RM for force; 30-60% 1-RM for upper body and 0-60% 1-RM for lower body exercises for velocity	1-3 sets of 3-6 reps	Moderate	2-3 days/wk	2-3 min for core exercises (MJ); 1-2 min for SJ

MJ = multijoint exercise; SJ = single-joint exercise.

Kraemer et al. 2002; Ratamess et al. 2009

Table 7.4 Guidelines for Resistance Training Programs for Intermediate Lifters

Goal	Intensity	Volume	Velocity	Frequency	Rest interval
Strength	70-80% 1-RM	1-3 sets of 6-12 reps	Moderate	3 days/wk for whole-body workouts; 4 days/wk for split workouts	2-3 min MJ; 1-2 min SJ
Hypertrophy	70-85% 1-RM	1-3 sets of 8-12 reps	Slow to moderate	3-4 days/wk	1-2 min
Endurance	50-70% 1-RM	1-3 sets of 10-15 reps	Slow to moderate	3-4 days/wk	<1 min
Power	85-100% 1-RM for force; 30-60% 1-RM for upper body and 0-60% 1-RM for lower body exercises for velocity	1-3 sets of 3-6 reps	Moderate	2-4 days/wk	2-3 min for core exercises (MJ); 1-2 min for SJ

MJ = multijoint exercise; SJ = single-joint exercise.

Kraemer et al. 2002; Ratamess et al. 2009

Table 7.5 Guidelines for Resistance Training Programs for Advanced Lifters

Goal	Intensity	Volume	Velocity	Frequency	Rest interval
Strength	80-100% 1-RM, periodized	Multiple sets of 1-12 reps, periodized	Slow to fast	4-6 days/wk	2-3 min MJ; 1-2 min SJ
Hypertrophy	70-100% 1-RM	3-6 sets of 1-12 reps[a], periodized	Slow to moderate	4-6 days/wk	2-3 min MJ; 1-2 min SJ
Endurance	30-80% 1-RM	Multiple sets of 10-25 reps, periodized	Slow for 10-15 reps; moderate to fast for 15-25 reps	4-6 days/wk	<1 min for 10-15 reps; 1-2 min for 15-25 reps
Power	85-100% 1-RM for force; 30-60% 1-RM for velocity	3-6 sets of 1-6 reps, periodized	Fast	4-6 days/wk	2-3 min MJ; 1-2 min SJ

MJ = multijoint exercise; SJ = single-joint exercise.

[a]Greater emphasis on 6RM to 12RM.

For power, emphasize MJ exercises. For strength, hypertrophy, and endurance, use both MJ and SJ exercises; perform MJ before SJ exercises. Exercise larger muscle groups before smaller muscle groups.

Kraemer et al. 2002; Ratamess et al. 2009

gains in untrained (<1 yr of resistance training) and trained (>1 yr) lifters differs (60% 1-RM and 80% 1-RM, respectively). For competitive athletes (college and professional), the optimal training intensity is 85% 1-RM (Peterson, Rhea, and Alvar 2004). Keep in mind that these intensities are averages. Throughout the strength training program, intensity needs to be varied for continued improvement.

To develop muscular endurance, prescribe an intensity of ≤50% 1-RM (ACSM 2010). Although low-to-moderate intensity best suits muscle endurance and toning, it also brings some strength gains. The degree and rate of strength gain, however, will be less than that experienced with a program designed to optimize strength development (specificity principle).

Sets

The optimal number of sets for improving muscular strength is controversial and depends on your client's goal; one or two sets for children and older adults and two to four sets for novice and intermediate lifters are recommended (Kraemer et al. 2002). A major advantage of single-set programs is that they require much less time for a training session than do multiple-set programs (20 vs. 50 min), potentially increasing your client's compliance. Some studies suggest that single sets (one set per exercise) are just as effective as multiple sets (two or three sets per exercise) for increasing the strength of untrained and recreational lifters during the first 3 to 4 mo of resistance training (Feigenbaum and Pollock 1999; Hass et al. 2000).

However, the results from a meta-analysis of 140 strength training studies do not support prescribing single-set programs to develop the strength of untrained and trained recreational lifters (Rhea et al. 2003a). Traditionally, a set refers to the number of consecutive repetitions performed for a specific exercise; however, Rhea and colleagues (2003a) noted that the total number of sets performed for a specific muscle group is a better indicator of training stress than sets per exercise. Using this definition of sets, they reported that an average of four sets during each training session optimizes strength development in untrained and trained lifters. For single-set programs, the authors suggest prescribing multiple exercises for a specific muscle group in order to reach the goal of four sets. The ACSM (2010) stated that each set should be performed to the point of volitional fatigue for each exercise (see table 7.2).

Multiple sets using periodization are recommended for serious athletes, powerlifters, and bodybuilders engaging in advanced strength training and hypertrophy programs (Kraemer et al. 2002). To optimize the strength gains of collegiate and professional athletes, an average of eight sets per muscle group is recommended (Peterson et al. 2004).

Frequency

Muscular fitness may improve from exercising just 1 day/wk, especially in clients with below-average muscular fitness. Recent research, however, suggests that the optimal frequency of strength training for untrained individuals is 3 days/wk. For healthy populations, the ACSM (2010) recommends 2 or 3 nonconsecutive days per week. For advanced lifters, four to six training sessions per week and split routines are recommended (Kraemer et al. 2002). To optimize the strength gains of trained recreational lifters and competitive athletes, each muscle group should be exercised twice a week (Rhea et al. 2003a; Peterson et al. 2004). Advanced lifters and competitive athletes who train 4 to 6 days/wk can accomplish this goal by using split routines (see p. 161, "Variations for Frequency"). You should pre-

scribe 48 hr of rest between workouts to allow the muscles to recuperate and to prevent injury from overtraining.

Volume

Training volume is the sum of the repetitions performed during each training session multiplied by the resistance used (Kraemer et al. 2002). Throughout the resistance training program, volume and intensity must be systematically increased (progression principle) to avoid plateaus and to ensure continued strength improvements. You can alter training volume by changing the number of exercises performed for each session, the number of repetitions performed for each set, or the number of sets performed for each exercise. Several models of periodized training can be used to systematically vary volume and intensity (see p. 161, "Periodization").

Order of Exercises

A well-rounded resistance training program should include at least one exercise for each of the major muscle groups in the body. In this way, **muscle balance**—that is, the ratio of strength between opposing muscle groups (agonists vs. antagonists), contralateral muscle groups (right vs. left side), and upper and lower body muscle groups can be maintained. Order the exercises so that your client first executes multijoint exercises—such as the seated leg press, bench press, and lat pull-down—that involve larger muscles (e.g., gluteus maximus, pectoralis major, and latissimus dorsi) and more muscle groups. Then have your client progress to single-joint exercises for smaller muscle groups (see table 7.6). To avoid muscle fatigue in novice weightlifters, arrange the exercises so that successive exercises do not involve the same muscle group. This allows time for the muscle to recover.

Dynamic Resistance Training Methods

You can use a variety of methods to design dynamic resistance training programs. The majority of these methods are best suited for advanced programs. Each uses a different approach for prescribing sets, order of exercises, or frequency of workouts.

Variations for Sets

You can use either a single set or multiple sets of exercise. For multiple sets, you may choose to have

Table 7.6 Example of Exercise Order for a Basic Resistance Training Program

Body Segment	Type of exercise*	Joint actions	Exercise
1. Hips and thighs	Multijoint	Hip extension and knee extension	Seated leg press
2. Chest	Multijoint	Shoulder horizontal flexion and elbow extension	Flat bench press
3. Upper back and mid back	Multijoint	Shoulder extension/adduction and elbow flexion	Lat pull-down
4. Legs	Single joint	Knee extension	Leg extension
5. Shoulders and upper arms	Multijoint	Shoulder abduction and elbow flexion	Upright row
6. Lower back	Multijoint	Trunk extension and hip extension	Back extension
7. Upper arms	Single joint	Elbow extension	Triceps push-down
8. Leg	Single joint	Knee flexion	Leg curl
9. Upper arms	Single joint	Elbow flexion	Arm curl
10. Calves	Single joint	Ankle plantar flexion	Toe raise
11. Forearms	Single joint	Wrist flexion and extension	Wrist curl
12. Abdomen	Single joint	Trunk flexion	Curl-up

*Multijoint exercises involving larger muscle groups are followed by single-joint exercises for smaller muscle groups.

your client consecutively perform a designated number of sets (usually three or more) at a constant intensity (e.g., 10-RM) for each exercise. Alternatively, you may have your client perform one set of three different exercises for the same muscle group. For example, instead of three consecutive sets of barbell curls for the elbow flexors, you may prescribe one set of incline dumbbell curls, one set of hammer curls, and one set of barbell curls. This adds variety to the program and changes the training stimulus because different muscles or parts of a muscle are used to perform each of these exercises.

A client performing multiple sets of a given exercise may choose to lift the same weight for each set or to vary the intensity of each set by lifting progressively heavier (light-to-heavy sets) or lighter (heavy-to-light sets) weights. **Pyramiding** is a light-to-heavy system in which the client performs as many as six sets of each exercise. In the first set, the client lifts a relatively lighter weight for 10 to 12 repetitions (10- to 12-RM). In subsequent sets the individual lifts progressively heavier weights (i.e., 8-RM, 6-RM, and 4-RM). Because this involves such a large volume of work, you should prescribe the pyramid system for experienced weightlifters only. Bodybuilders commonly use this system to develop muscle size.

Variations for Order and Number of Exercises

Exercise scientists generally recommend ordering the exercises so that large muscle groups are exercised at the beginning of the workout with progression to smaller muscle groups later in the workout. To maximize the overload of muscle groups, however, some clients may choose to pre-exhaust muscle groups by reversing this order. To do this, the individual fatigues smaller muscles by using single-joint exercises prior to performing multijoint exercises.

When you prescribe two or more exercises for a specific muscle group, instruct the average individual to alternate muscle groups so that the muscle can rest and recover between exercises. For example, your client should not perform leg press and leg extension exercises consecutively because the quadriceps femoris is used in both of these exercises. Instead, intersperse one or more exercises using different muscle groups between these two exercises.

In contrast, many advanced weightlifters prefer to do **compound sets** or **tri-sets** in order to completely fatigue a targeted muscle group. To use this training system, the client performs two (compound sets) or three (tri-sets) exercises consecutively for the same muscle group, with little or no rest between the exercises. Many bodybuilders also use a training system called **supersetting.** For supersets, the client exercises agonistic and antagonistic muscle groups consecutively without resting. For example, to superset the quadriceps femoris and hamstrings, follow a leg extension set immediately with a leg curl set.

Variations for Frequency

Traditionally for advanced resistance training programs, exercise scientists have recommended resistance training 3 days/wk on alternate days (e.g., M-W-F) to allow the muscles time to recover. For individuals who want to resistance train 4 to 6 days/wk, prescribe a split routine. With a **split routine,** you are targeting different muscle groups on consecutive days, thereby allowing at least 1 day of recovery for each muscle group. For example, a bodybuilder may exercise the chest and shoulders on Monday and Thursday, the hips and legs on Tuesday and Friday, and the back and arms on Wednesday and Saturday.

Periodization

Periodization systematically varies the intensity and volume of resistance training. The goal of periodization is twofold: (1) to maximize the response of the neuromuscular system (i.e., gains in strength, endurance, power, and hypertrophy) by systematically changing the training or exercise stimulus and (2) to minimize overtraining and injury by planning rest and recovery. The training stimulus may be varied by manipulations in one or more of the following program elements:

- Training volume (number of sets, repetitions, or exercises)
- Training intensity (amount of resistance)
- Type of contraction (concentric, eccentric, or isometric)
- Training frequency

Given the number of program variables, there are numerous possibilities for designing periodized programs. Researchers have identified combinations that optimize the training stimulus for developing strength and muscular endurance (Rhea et al. 2002, 2003b).

The recommended amounts of rest between sets and exercises depend on exercise intensity; a lower intensity requires shorter rests and a higher intensity, longer rests (see "Exercise Intensity and Recommended Rest Periods"). In strength or power training, rests should last at least 3 to 5 min to allow resynthesis of adenosine triphosphate (ATP) and creatine phosphate (CP) and to prevent excessive accumulation of muscle and blood lactate (Kraemer 2003).

Three common periodization models are linear periodization (LP), reverse linear periodization (RLP), and undulating periodization (UP). All periodized training programs are divided into periods, or cycles; however, the duration and the training stimulus differ depending on the model used.

Classic Linear Periodization Model

The classic **linear periodization (LP)** model is divided into three types of cycles. The **macrocycle** (usually 9-12 mo) is divided into mesocycles that last 3 to 4 mo. **Mesocycles** are subdivided into **microcycles** lasting 1 to 4 wk. Within and between cycles, training intensity increases as training volume decreases. For example, a 3 mo (12 wk) mesocycle can be divided into three 4 wk microcycles as follows: during weeks 1 through 4, three sets are performed at 12-RM or 70% 1-RM; during weeks 5 through 8, three sets are performed at 10-RM or 75% 1-RM; and during weeks 9 through 12, three sets are performed at 8-RM or 80% 1-RM (see "Sample Linear Periodized (LP) Resistance Training Program for Intermediate Lifter," p. 171).

Exercise Intensity and Recommended Rest Periods (Kraemer 2003)

Intensity	Length of rest
>13-RM ~<65% 1-RM	<1 min
11-RM to 13-RM ~65 to 74% 1-RM	1-2 min
8-RM to 10-RM ~75-80% 1-RM	2-3 min
5-RM to 7-RM ~76-87% 1-RM	3-5 min
<5-RM ~>87% 1-RM	>5 min

The training intensity increases from 70% 1-RM (12-RM) to 80% 1-RM (8-RM) while the training volume systematically decreases due to the progressive reduction in the number of repetitions (from 12 to 8) performed during each microcycle.

Reverse Linear Periodization Model

The **reverse linear periodization (RLP)** model reverses the progression of the LP training stimulus. Between and within cycles, training intensity decreases as training volume increases. The RLP configuration of the mesocycles and microcycles is as follows: weeks 1 through 4, three sets at 80% 1-RM (8-RM); weeks 5 through 8, three sets at 75% 1-RM (10-RM); and weeks 9 through 12, three sets at 70% 1-RM (12-RM). As you can see, the training intensity decreases from 80% to 70% 1-RM (8-RM to 12-RM) as the training volume increases (from 8 to 12 reps) during the three progressive microcycles.

Undulating Periodization Models

Compared to those in LP and RLP, the microcycles for **undulating periodization (UP)** are considerably shorter (biweekly, weekly, or even daily) so that they frequently change the training stimulus (intensity and volume). Your client may progress from high volume–low intensity to low volume–high intensity in the same week. For example, in a 3 days/wk UP program, the individual may perform three sets of 8-RM (high volume–low intensity) on day 1, three sets of 6-RM on day 2, and three sets of 4-RM on day 3 (low volume–high intensity). In subsequent microcycles (each week), this training stimulus could be repeated or could be varied to change the order of the training stimulus (e.g., day 1 = 4-RM, day 2 = 6-RM, and day 3 = 8-RM). One advantage of the UP program is that the training volume and intensity change frequently, subjecting the exercising muscles to a different training stimulus on a daily or weekly basis. As such, UP may avoid plateaus in training and maintain the client's interest and motivation for long-term resistance training.

Circuit Resistance Training

Circuit resistance training is a method of dynamic resistance training designed to increase strength, muscular endurance, and cardiorespiratory endurance (Gettman and Pollock 1981). Circuit resistance training compares favorably with the traditional resistance training programs for increasing muscle strength, especially if low-repetition, high-resistance exercises are used (Gettman et al. 1978; Wilmore et al. 1978).

A circuit resistance training program usually has 10 to 15 stations per circuit (see figure 7.1). The circuit is repeated two to three times so that the total time of continuous exercise is 20 to 30 min. At each exercise station, select a resistance that fatigues the muscle group in approximately 30 sec (as many repetitions as possible at approximately 40% to 55% of 1-RM). Include a 15 to 20 sec rest period between exercise stations. Circuit resistance training is usually performed 3 days/wk for at least 6 wk. This method of training is ideal for clients with a limited amount of time for exercise. As mentioned in chapter 5, you can add aerobic exercise stations to the circuit between each weightlifting station (i.e., super circuit resistance training) to obtain additional cardiorespiratory benefits.

Core Stability and Functional Training

Core stability training is widely promoted in fitness settings to improve functional capacity (activities of daily living and occupational tasks) and sport skills performance of healthy individuals. **Core stability** is the ability to maintain the ideal alignment of the neck, spine, scapulae, and pelvis while performing an exercise or a sport skill. For core stability training, resistance exercises are performed on unstable surfaces (e.g., wobble board, balance disc, and Swiss ball). Although exercising on unstable surfaces may challenge and motivate the client, most exercises performed on unstable devices dictate using lighter loads and movement velocities. As such, core stability training may be better suited for developing muscular endurance rather than muscle strength and power (Willardson 2008). The muscles and their functional contribution to core stability are presented in "Core Stability Muscles and Function."

For years, functional training has been widely used in physical rehabilitation programs to improve joint stability, neuromuscular control, flexibility, and muscular fitness (strength and endurance) of injured clients. Functional training programs typically include four types of exercise:

- Spinal stabilization exercises to improve stability of the spine during movement
- Proprioception and balance exercises to enhance neuromuscular coordination

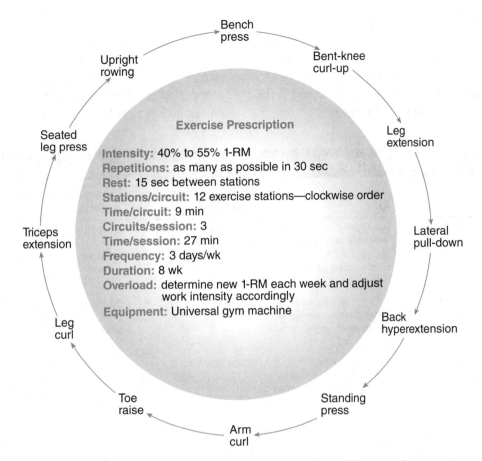

Exercise Prescription

Intensity: 40% to 55% 1-RM
Repetitions: as many as possible in 30 sec
Rest: 15 sec between stations
Stations/circuit: 12 exercise stations—clockwise order
Time/circuit: 9 min
Circuits/session: 3
Time/session: 27 min
Frequency: 3 days/wk
Duration: 8 wk
Overload: determine new 1-RM each week and adjust work intensity accordingly
Equipment: Universal gym machine

Figure 7.1   Sample circuit resistance training program. 1-RM = 1-repetition maximum.

- Resistance exercises to develop muscular fitness
- Flexibility exercises to regain range of movement

Functional training has gained popularity and recognition, especially in health and fitness clubs. Usually the goal of functional training is to train and develop muscles so that performing everyday activities is easier, safer, and more efficient (Yoke and Kennedy 2004). However, recent studies have examined the efficacy of functional training for improving sport performance (Thompson, Cobb, and Blackwell 2007).

Functional training is a system of exercise progressions for specific muscle groups that uses a

Core Stability Muscles and Function		
Muscles	**Location**	**Function**
Multifidus, rotators, intertransversalis, interspinalis	Between adjacent vertebrae	Maintain core stability by contracting in response to sudden changes in posture
Transversus abdominis, internal abdominal obliques, quadratus lumborum	Transverse processes of lumbar vertebrae	Stabilize the spine by drawing in umbilicus and increasing compressive forces between bodies of lumbar vertebrae
Rectus abdominis, external abdominal obliques, erector spinae, latissimus dorsi	Pelvic girdle and rib cage	Maintain core stability during performance of heavy ground-based movements with free weights (e.g., squats)
Hip flexors, extensors, adductors, and abductors	Pelvis and lumbar vertebrae to femur	Produce pelvic tilt that results in movement of lumbar spine affecting core stability

six-step approach developed by Yoke and Kennedy (2004). The difficulty (strength) and skill (balance and coordination) levels of specific exercises are rated, with 1 representing the least difficult exercises (requiring less strength and skill) and 6 the most difficult exercises (requiring more strength and skill). As the difficulty of the exercises progresses, greater strength, balance, core stability, and coordination are required. The hardest exercises (6 rating) require the most core stability. To maintain proper postural alignment, the strength of the core muscle groups (erector spinae and abdominal prime

Functional Exercise Progressions: Six-Step Approach and Example

Step	Aim	Body position, resistance	Example for knee extensors
1. Isolate and educate	Teach client to focus on individual muscle action and to selectively contract or isolate the specific muscle group	Lying supine or prone on bench or floor	Lying supine with knees bent, hips flexed to 45°, and arms at sides, client extends the knee one leg at a time.
2. Add resistance	Increase resistance by using exercise machines, longer lever length, or elastic tubing	Sitting on bench or floor	Sitting upright on a bench with elastic tubing attached to the ankle, client extends the knee one leg at a time.
3. Add functional training positions	Decrease supporting base to require greater use of stabilizing muscles	Sitting or standing	Supported at low back level by a stability ball pressed against the wall, with pelvis and spine in neutral position, feet shoulder-width apart and far enough away from wall so that knees flex no more than 90° during exercise, client squats, not allowing hips to drop below the knees.
4. Combine increased function with resistance	Overload core stabilizers in functional positions	Using exercise machines, free weights, or elastic exercise bands to increase resistance	With exercise band attached to ankles, client stands in upright, neutral spine position, balancing on support leg with exercise leg flexed at hip and knee slightly flexed. Client flexes the hip while extending the knee of the exercise leg.
5. Exercise multiple muscle groups with increased resistance and core challenge	Increase demand on strength, balance, coordination, and core stability	Using multijoint exercise machines to increase resistance	Using seated, lying, or standing leg press machine, client extends hips and knees simultaneously.
6. Add balance, increased function, speed, or rotation	Increase demand on balance, speed, and joint rotation	Using smaller or moving base of support such as stability balls and balance boards or discs; using free weights (barbells or dumbbells) to increase resistance	Standing in upright position with one hand on wall or support bar and holding dumbbell in other hand, client extends hip and places one leg on stability ball. Client rolls the back leg backward on the ball, flexing the knee (no more than 90°) of the opposite leg while keeping the pelvis and spine in a neutral position and the shoulders and hips squared. Client returns to starting position by extending the knee of exercising leg and rolling opposite leg forward on top of the ball.

movers and stabilizers) needs to be developed (**core strengthening**). Because core stability is dynamic, changing with body position during exercise, isolated core strengthening does not automatically increase core stability unless it is accompanied by motor skill training (Yessis 2003). Functional exercise progressions are designed to develop the strength and function of all muscle groups, not just core muscles. For an outline and example of functional exercise progressions, see "Functional Exercise Progressions: Six-Step Approach and Example," page 164.

It is not necessary for every client to progress to the most difficult levels (5 and 6) on the exercise continuum. Safety is of utmost importance. Be certain that your clients are able to perform exercises with proper form and postural alignment for the duration of the set before progressing to the next level. Your clients' ability to perform each level of exercise depends on their fitness and skill levels. Level 6 exercises are designed to challenge competitive athletes or very fit individuals with excellent balance, strength, motor skill, and core stability. Although functional training potentially adds variety and challenge to workouts, research is needed to compare its effectiveness to that of conventional strength and muscular endurance training. Improvements in strength, endurance, balance, flexibility, and coordination as well as in functional performance of everyday tasks need to be evaluated. For more information, detailed descriptions, and illustrations of functional exercise progressions for all muscle groups, see Yoke and Kennedy (2004).

Isokinetic Training

Isokinetic exercise combines the advantages of dynamic (full range of motion) and static (maximum force exerted) exercise. Since the resistance is accommodating, isokinetic training overcomes the problems associated with using either a constant- or variable-resistance exercise mode. You can use isokinetic training to increase strength, power, and muscular endurance. Isokinetic training involves dynamic, shortening contractions of the muscle group against an accommodating resistance that matches the force produced by the muscle group throughout the entire range of motion. The speed of the movement is controlled mechanically by the isokinetic exercise device. Isokinetic dynamometers are used for isokinetic training. If this equipment is not available, exercises can be done with a partner who offers accommodating resistance to the movement. The speed of the movement, however, is not precisely controlled.

Isokinetic training is done at speeds that vary between 24° and 300°·sec^{-1}, depending on the needs of the individual. The carryover effect appears to be greater when a person trains at faster speeds (180° to 300°·sec^{-1}) as compared to slower speeds (30° to 60°·sec^{-1}). In some studies, strength gains have been limited to velocities at or below the training velocity (Lesmes et al. 1978; Moffroid and Whipple 1970). Other researchers have reported significant strength gains at all testing velocities (30° to 300°·sec^{-1}) for high-velocity training groups (240° to 300°·sec^{-1}) (Coyle et al. 1981; Jenkins, Thackaberry, and Killian 1984). Additional research is needed to settle this issue. Table 7.7 presents general guidelines for designing isokinetic training programs for the development of strength and endurance.

A major advantage of isokinetic training over traditional forms of training is that little or no muscle soreness results because the muscles do not contract eccentrically. Isokinetic training is not the best choice, however, when the goal of training is an increase in muscle size. Eccentric contractions are apparently essential for muscle hypertrophy (Cote et al. 1988; Hather et al. 1991). Cote and colleagues (1988) reported no change in muscle fiber cross-sectional area during isokinetic training even though the strength of the quadriceps femoris increased 54%.

Table 7.7 Guidelines for Designing Isokinetic Training Programs

Type	Intensity	Repetitions	Sets	Speed	Frequency	Length of program
Isokinetic strength	Maximum contraction	2-15	3	24-180°·sec^{-1}	3-5 days/wk	6 wk or more
Isokinetic endurance	Maximum contraction	Until fatigued	1	≥180°·sec^{-1}	3-5 days/wk	6 wk or more

DEVELOPING RESISTANCE TRAINING PROGRAMS

Before designing a resistance training program for your client, review training principles and determine how each of these principles can be incorporated into your client's program. The training program needs to be individualized. By varying the combination of intensity, duration, and frequency of exercise, you can develop programs that meet the unique goals and needs of each client. Be sure to follow guidelines and recommendations for resistance training programs (see tables 7.2-7.5, pp. 157-158), as well as specific recommendations and precautions, when developing resistance training programs for children and older adults.

Application of Training Principles to Resistance Exercise

To develop effective resistance training programs, you must apply each of the training principles presented in chapter 3 (see pp. 47-48). This section reviews some of the more pertinent training principles and outlines how these principles are applied to the design of resistance training programs.

Specificity Principle

The development of muscular fitness is specific to the muscle group that is exercised, the type of contraction, and training intensity. To increase the dynamic strength of the elbow flexors, for example, you must select exercises that involve the concentric and eccentric contraction of that particular muscle group. For strength, the person performs exercises at a high intensity with low repetitions; exercising at a low intensity with high repetitions stimulates the development of muscular endurance.

Strength and endurance gains are also specific to the speed and range of motion used during the training. With isometric training, strength gains at angles other than the training angle are typically 50% less than those at the exercised angle. Similarly, as previously noted, strength gains in isokinetic training may be limited to velocities at or below the training velocity (Lesmes et al. 1978; Moffroid and Whipple 1970).

Overload Principle

To promote strength and endurance gains, it is necessary to exercise the muscle group at workloads that are greater than normal for the client. The exercise intensity should be at least 60% of maximum to stimulate the development of strength. Clients may achieve more rapid strength gains, however, by exercising the muscle at or near maximum (80% to 100%) resistance. To stimulate endurance gains, intensities as low as 30% of maximum may be used; however, at low intensities the muscle group should be exercised to the point of fatigue.

Progression Principle

Generally, throughout the resistance training program, you must periodically increase the training volume, or total amount of work performed, to continue overloading the muscle so that the person can make further improvements in strength and muscular endurance. The progression needs to be gradual because doing too much too soon may cause musculoskeletal injuries and excessive muscle soreness. Typically you progressively overload muscle groups by increasing the resistance or amount of weight lifted. As clients adapt to the training stimulus, they will be able to perform more repetitions at the prescribed resistance. Thus, the number of repetitions a client is able to perform will indicate when it is necessary to increase the resistance throughout the training program. In addition to increasing resistance, you may progressively overload muscle groups by increasing the total number of repetitions performed at a selected intensity, altering the speed of movement (slow, moderate, fast pace), and varying the duration of rest periods between sets of exercises (Ratamess et al. 2009).

Additional Principles

Individuals with lower initial strength will show greater relative gains and a faster rate of improvement in response to resistance training than those starting out with higher strength levels (principles of initial values and interindividual variability). However, the rate of improvement slows, and eventually plateaus, as clients progress through the program and move closer to their genetic ceiling (principle of diminishing returns). Also, when the individual stops resistance training, the physiological adaptations and improvements in muscle structure and function are reversed (principle of reversibility). Using periodization techniques (see "Periodization" on p. 161), you can lessen the effects of detraining on athletes and maintain strength gains during the competitive period by manipulating the intensity and volume of the resistance training exercise (see Wathen 1994b).

General Procedures and Sample Resistance Training Programs

After assessing your client's muscular fitness, you can individualize the resistance training exercise prescription to meet the client's individual needs and interests by using the steps outlined on this page.

The first example, on page 170, describes a beginning resistance training program developed for an older man (70 yr) with no previous weightlifting experience. The primary goal for this program is to develop adequate muscular fitness so that the client can retain functional independence. This program follows the guidelines suggested by ACSM (2010) for designing resistance training programs for older adults. During the first 4 wk of training, low-intensity (30% to 40% 1-RM), high-repetition (15 to 20 repetitions) exercises familiarize the client with weightlifting exercise and reduce the chance of injury and excessive muscle soreness. The client gradually increases the resistance so that by the end of this phase, the exercise intensity is 50% 1-RM.

After 8 wk, the intensity starts at 50% 1-RM and gradually increases to 75% 1-RM. The client does one or two sets of 10 to 15 repetitions for each exercise. To overload the muscles during this phase, he increases the resistance gradually, but only after he is able to complete 15 or more repetitions at the prescribed relative intensity. This program includes multijoint exercises using exercise machines only (no free weights). The client exercises two times a week, allowing at least 2 days of rest between each workout.

The second program (see p. 171) is for a 25 yr old woman whose primary goal is to improve muscle strength. This client is an experienced weightlifter. Results from her 1-RM tests indicated that her upper body strength (particularly the shoulder flexor and forearm flexor muscle groups) is below average. Therefore, two exercises are prescribed for each of the weaker muscle groups. The strength of all other muscle groups is average or above average; therefore, only one exercise is prescribed for each of these muscle groups. Given her initial strength levels and weightlifting experience, the prescription is for three sets of each exercise; and the exercise intensity is set at 70% to 80% 1-RM to maximize the development of strength. The client completes about eight repetitions at the prescribed intensity for each microcycle. She devotes 50 to 60 min, 3 days/wk, to her workouts.

STEPS FOR DEVELOPING A RESISTANCE TRAINING PROGRAM

The following steps, used to design the sample dynamic resistance training programs on pages 170-173, provide an outline of how you should proceed.

1. In consultation with your clients, identify the primary goal of the program (i.e., strength, muscular endurance, muscle size, or muscle toning) and ask clients how much time they are willing to commit to this program.

2. Based on your client's goal, time commitment, and access to equipment, determine the type of resistance training program (i.e., dynamic, static, or isokinetic).

3. Using results from your client's muscular fitness assessment, identify specific muscle groups that need to be targeted in the exercise prescription.

4. In addition to core exercises for the major muscle groups, select exercises for those muscle groups targeted in step 3.

5. For novice weightlifters, order the exercises so the same muscle group is not exercised consecutively.

6. Based on your client's goals, determine appropriate starting loads, repetitions, and sets for each exercise.

7. Set guidelines for progressively overloading each muscle group.

The third example (see p. 172) illustrates an advanced resistance training program developed for an experienced weightlifter (28 yr old male with superior strength) whose long-term goal is competitive bodybuilding. He engages in a high-volume undulating periodized training program. The intensity (70-85% 1-RM) and moderate repetitions (6 to 12 reps) vary systematically throughout each macro- and microcycle to maximize the development of muscle size. To achieve a high training volume, he performs three exercises for each muscle group and three or four sets of each exercise. To effectively overload the muscles, he performs three exercises for each muscle group consecutively (trisets) with little or no rest between the sets. He lifts weights 6 days/wk, splitting the routine so that he is not exercising the same muscle groups on consecutive days. With this routine, each muscle group is exercised two times a week.

Several excellent references deal with the design of advanced resistance training programs (Fleck and Kraemer 2004; Kraemer and Fleck 2007; National Strength and Conditioning Association 2008; Stone, Stone, and Sands 2007).

Designing Resistance Training Programs for Children

Children and adolescents can safely participate in resistance training if special precautions and recommended guidelines are carefully followed. Because children are anatomically and physiologically immature, high-resistance training programs are

YOUTH RESISTANCE TRAINING GUIDELINES

- Provide qualified instruction and supervision.
- Provide an exercise environment that is safe and free of hazards.
- Teach clients about the benefits and risks of strength training.
- Design a comprehensive program that focuses on developing muscular fitness and motor skills.
- Begin each workout with a 5 to 10 min warm-up.
- Select 8 to 12 multijoint exercises for major muscle groups; include exercises for the abdominal muscles and lower back.
- Use equipment that is appropriate for the size, strength, and maturity of the child.
- Start with one or two sets of 8 to 15 repetitions with light to moderate load (~60% 1-RM) for each exercise.
- Slowly progress to three or four sets at 60% to 80% 1-RM, or 8-RM to 15-RM, depending on the child's needs and goals; as strength improves, increase the number of repetitions before increasing resistance.
- Increase resistance gradually and only when the child can perform the specified number of repetitions with good form.

- Reduce the resistance for prepubescent children who cannot perform a minimum of eight repetitions with good form.
- Prescribe low-repetition (less than eight reps) exercises for mature adolescents only.
- Focus on correct exercise technique (slow and smooth movements and breathing) instead of amount of weight lifted.
- Train two or three times per week on nonconsecutive days.
- Closely supervise the child in the event of a failed repetition.
- Monitor progress (e.g., use workout logs), listen to the child's concerns, and answer questions.
- Systematically vary the training program to keep it fresh and challenging by adding new exercises, changing the number of sets and repetitions, and incorporating calisthenics as well as exercises using elastic tubing and fitness balls.
- Focus on participation and provide positive reinforcement.

Adapted from D.G. Behnm et al., 2008, "Canadian Society for Exercise Physiology position paper on resistance training for children and adolescents," *Applied Physiology, Nutrition, and Metabolism* 33: 547-561.

not typically recommended for them. Most experts agree that to lessen the risk of injury (e.g., epiphyseal growth plate fractures) to developing bones and joints, exercise intensity should not exceed 80% 1-RM, which equates to 8 to 15 repetitions per set. Faigenbaum and colleagues (1999) reported that high-repetition–moderate-intensity training (one set, 13-RM to 15-RM) was more effective than low-repetition–high-intensity training (one set, 6-RM to 8-RM) for improving the strength and muscle endurance of children (5-12 yr) during the initial training phase (8 wk). Strength gains in resistance-trained children result from neural adaptations (e.g., increased activation of motor units and coordination) rather than from hypertrophy (Guy and Micheli 2001). In addition, resistance training positively affects the bone mineral density of the femoral neck in adolescent girls ages 14 to 17 yr (Nichols, Sanborn, and Love 2001). There is no evidence that children lose flexibility when they resistance train (Guy and Micheli 2001). Resistance training is safe and beneficial for youth, especially when the established training guidelines are followed (see "Youth Resistance Training Guidelines"). These guidelines are based primarily on recommendations outlined in the Canadian Society for Exercise Physiology position paper on resistance training for children and adolescents (Behm et al. 2008).

Designing Resistance Training Programs for Older Adults

Resistance training provides many health benefits, especially for older adults. The primary goal of the resistance training program is to develop sufficient muscular fitness so that older adults may carry out activities of daily living without undue stress or fatigue and may retain their functional independence.

In addition to increasing strength and muscular endurance, resistance training may improve the performance of functional tasks such as lifting and reaching, rising from the floor or a chair to a standing position, stair climbing, and walking (Henwood and Taaffe 2003; Messier et al. 2000; Schot et al. 2003; Vincent et al. 2002). Also, the postural sway and balance of older, osteoarthritic adults were improved by participation in either long-term resistance training or aerobic walking (Messier et al. 2000). Improved strength and balance may help prevent falls and injuries in older adults.

The ACSM (2010) recommends moderate-intensity (rating of perceived exertion [RPE] = 5-6) to vigorous-intensity (RPE = 7-8) exercise at least 2 days/wk to improve the muscular fitness of older adults; prescribe at least one set of 10 to 15 repetitions for 8 to 10 different exercises each workout. Vincent and colleagues (2002) noted long-term (6 mo) improvements in the strength and muscular endurance of older adults (60-83 yr) who participated in either a low-intensity (one set at 50% 1-RM) or a high-intensity (one set at 80% 1-RM) resistance training program 3 days/wk. Likewise, Hunter and colleagues (2001) reported that isometric and dynamic muscle strength gains are similar for older adults (>60 yr) engaging in either a nonperiodized, high-intensity program (two sets at 80% 1-RM, 3 days/wk) or an undulating periodized (UP) program varying training volume each day (two sets at 50%, 65%, or 80% 1-RM, 3 days/wk). Some evidence suggests that training 1, 2, or 3 days a week at 80% 1-RM produces similar strength gains in older (65-79 yr) adults (Taaffe et al. 1999).

In addition to the general guidelines for designing resistance training programs for healthy adults (see table 7.2), the following guidelines and precautions are recommended for older adults:

- During the first 8 wk of training, use minimal resistance for all exercises.
- Instruct older adults about proper weightlifting and breathing techniques.
- Trained exercise leaders who have experience working with older adults should closely supervise and monitor the client's weightlifting techniques and resistance training program during the first few exercise sessions.
- Prescribe multijoint, rather than single-joint, exercises.
- Use exercise machines to stabilize body position and control the range of joint motion. Avoid using free weights with older adults.
- Each exercise session should be approximately 20 to 30 min and should not exceed 60 min.
- Older adults should rate their perceived exertion during exercise. Ratings of perceived exertion should be 5 or 6 (moderate) or 7 or 8 (vigorous).

Client data

Age	70 yr	Intensity	30-50% 1-RM for first 8 wk; 50-75% 1-RM thereafter
Gender	Male		
Body weight	160 lb (72.7 kg)	Frequency	2 days/wk; at least 48 hr between workouts
Program goal	Muscle fitness and functional independence		
		Duration	16 wk or longer
Time commitment	20-30 min per workout	Overload	Increase reps first; increase resistance only when able to complete >15 reps
Equipment	Exercise machines		
		Rest	2-3 min between exercises

Exercise[a]	1-RM (lb)*	Weeks[b]	Intensity[c] (%1-RM)	Weight (lb)	Repetitions	Sets	Muscle groups
Leg press (seated)	180	1-4	30-40	55-70	15-20	1	Hip extensors
		5-8	40-50	72-90	15-20	1	Knee extensors
		9-12	50-60	90-110	10-15	1	
		13-16	60-75	110-135	10-15	1	
Chest flys (seated)	90	1-4	30-40	30-36	15-20	1	Shoulder horizontal flexors
		5-8	40-50	36-45	15-20	1	Elbow extensors
		9-12	50-60	45-54	10-15	1	
		13-16	60-75	54-68	10-15	1	
Leg curl (seated)	45	1-4	30-40	13-18	15-20	1	Knee flexors
		5-8	40-50	18-22	15-20	1	
		9-12	50-60	22-27	10-15	1	
		13-16	60-75	27-34	10-15	1	
Lat pull-down	100	1-4	30-40	30-40	15-20	1	Shoulder extensors
		5-8	40-50	40-50	15-20	1	Elbow flexors
		9-12	50-60	50-60	10-15	1	
		13-16	60-75	60-75	10-15	1	
Shoulder press (seated)	50	1-4	30-40	15-20	15-20	1	Shoulder flexors and adductors
		5-8	40-50	20-25	15-20	1	
		9-12	50-60	25-30	10-15	1	
		13-16	60-75	30-38	10-15	1	
Heel (calf) raises (seated)	90	1-4	30-40	27-36	15-20	1	Ankle plantar flexors
		5-8	40-50	36-45	15-20	1	
		9-12	50-60	45-54	10-15	1	
		13-16	60-75	54-68	10-15	1	
Abdominal curl	–	1-4	–	Body weight	5-10	1-2	Trunk flexors
		5-8			10-15	1-2	
		9-12			15-20	1-2	
		13-16			20-25	1-2	

[a]Multijoint exercise machines are used for most exercises. Seated and lying (instead of standing) positions are recommended to stabilize the body while lifting. Do exercises in the order listed.

[b]During first 2 wk, closely monitor and supervise workouts. Initial training phase lasts 8 wk.

[c]Intensity is gradually increased every 2 wk, only after client is able to do more than the prescribed number of repetitions at each target intensity.

*1 lb = 0.45 kg

Sample Linear Periodized (LP) Resistance Training Program for Intermediate Lifter

Client data

Age	25 yr	Cycles	3; each microcycle = 4 wk
Gender	Female	Intensity	70-80% 1-RM
Body weight	155 lb (70.4 kg)	Repetitions	8-12
Program goal	Muscle strength	Sets	3
Time commitment	50-60 min per workout	Rest	1-2 min for 70% 1-RM; 2-3 min for 75-80% 1-RM
Equipment	Variable resistance machines and free weights	Frequency	3 days/wk, alternate days
		Duration	12 wk or longer

LP training program

Exercise[a]	1-RM (lb)[b]	Cycle 1 wk 1-4			Cycle 2 wk 5-8			Cycle 3 wk 9-12			Sets	Muscle groups
		Int	Wt[b]	Rep	Int	Wt[b]	Rep	Int	Wt[b]	Rep		
Leg press	200	70	140	12	75	150	10	80	160	8	3	Hip extensors, knee extensors
Bench press*	100	70	70	12	75	75	10	80	80	8	3	Shoulder flexors and adductors, elbow extensors
Leg curl (lying)	80	70	55	12	75	60	10	80	65	8	3	Knee flexors
Lat pull-down	140	70	100	12	75	105	10	80	110	8	3	Shoulder extensors and adductors, elbow flexors
Dumbbell fly* (flat bench)	40	70	25	12	75	30	10	80	35	8	3	Shoulder flexors and adductors
Heel (calf) raise (standing)	160	70	110	12	75	120	10	80	130	8	3	Ankle plantar flexors
Abdominal curl	—									25	3	Trunk flexors
Arm curl* (incline bench)	40	70	25	12	75	30	10	80	35	8	3	Elbow flexors
Lateral raise (dumbbell)	25	70	15	12	75	15-20	10	80	20	8	3	Shoulder abductors
Triceps press-down	60	70	40	12	75	45	10	80	50	8	3	Elbow extensors
Hammer curl* (dumbbells)	40	70	25	12	75	30	10	80	35	8	3	Elbow flexors

Int = %1-RM; Wt = weight lifted; Rep = number of repetitions.

[a]Do exercises in order listed, using larger muscle groups first. Perform multijoint exercises before single-joint exercises. Other exercises that work the same muscle groups may be substituted to add variety to the program (see appendix C.4, "Dynamic Resistance Training Exercises," p. 355).

[b]1 lb = 0.45 kg; weight is to nearest 5 lb increment for most exercises.

*Two exercises are prescribed for each of the weaker muscle groups (shoulder flexors and elbow flexors) identified from client's strength assessment.

Client data

Age	28 yr	Mesocycles	4; each mesocycle = 1 mo
Gender	Male	Microcycles	4; each microcycle = 1 wk
Body weight	190 lb (86.2 kg)	Intensity	70-85% 1-RM
Program goal	Hypertrophy	Repetitions	6-12
Time commitment	90 min per workout	Sets	3-4
Equipment	Free weights and exercise machines	Rest	1 min between tri-sets
		Frequency	6 days/wk, split routine
		Duration	24 wk or longer

UP mesocycles and microcycles

	Intensity	Volume
Month 1		
Week 1	70% 1-RM	3-4 sets; 12 reps
Week 2	75% 1-RM	3-4 sets; 10 reps
Week 3	80% 1-RM	3-4 sets; 8 reps
Week 4	85% 1-RM	3-4 sets; 6 reps
Month 2		
Week 1	75% 1-RM	3-4 sets; 10 reps
Week 2	80% 1-RM	3-4 sets; 8 reps
Week 3	85% 1-RM	3-4 sets; 6 reps
Week 4	70% 1-RM	3-4 sets; 12 reps
Month 3		
Week 1	80% 1-RM	3-4 sets; 8 reps
Week 2	85% 1-RM	3-4 sets; 6 reps
Week 3	70% 1-RM	3-4 sets; 12 reps
Week 4	75% 1-RM	3-4 sets; 10 reps
Month 4		
Week 1	85% 1-RM	3-4 sets; 6 reps
Week 2	80% 1-RM	3-4 sets; 8 reps
Week 3	75% 1-RM	3-4 sets; 10 reps
Week 4	70% 1-RM	3-4 sets; 12 reps

Split routine using tri-sets

Exercises	1-RM (lb)[c]	Muscles
Monday and Thursday[a]		
Chest[b]		
Flat bench press (barbell)	250	Pectoralis major (midsternal portion); triceps brachii
Incline dumbbell fly	80	Pectoralis major (clavicular portion); anterior deltoid
Decline bench press (barbell)	180	Pectoralis major (lower sternal portion)
Shoulders[b]		
Upright row (barbell)	140	Middle deltoid
Front dumbbell raises	80	Anterior deltoid
Posterior cable pull (horizontal plane)	100	Posterior deltoid

Exercises	1-RM (lb)[c]	Muscles
Tuesday and Friday[a]		
Hips and thighs[a]		
First tri-set		
Squats (Smith machine)	300	Gluteus maximus; quadriceps femoris; upper hamstrings
Leg extension (machine)	150	Quadriceps femoris
Leg curl (standing, unilateral, machine)	90	Hamstrings (mid-to-lower portions)
Second tri-set		
Leg press (seated)	400	Gluteus maximus; quadriceps femoris; upper hamstrings
Leg curl (lying)	130	Hamstrings (mid-to-lower portions)
Glut-ham raise	—	Gluteus maximus; hamstrings
Leg and calves[b]		
Standing calf (heel) raise	250	Gastrocnemius; soleus
Ankle flexion exercise (seated)	90	Tibialis anterior
Seated calf raise	180	Soleus; gastrocnemius
Wednesday and Saturday[a]		
Back[b]		
Lat pull-down (wide grip)	225	Latissimus dorsi (lateral portions); biceps brachii; brachialis
Seated row (narrow grip)	240	Latissimus dorsi (midportion); biceps brachii; brachialis
Dumbbell row	90	Latissimus dorsi (midportions); biceps brachii; brachialis
Elbow flexors[b]		
Standing barbell curl	130	Biceps brachii; brachialis; brachioradialis
Preacher curl (dumbbells)	100	Biceps brachii (mid portion); brachialis
Hammer curl (dumbbells)	80	Brachioradialis; brachialis
Elbow extensors[b]		
Lying triceps extension (barbell)	120	Triceps brachii (long head)
Triceps push-down (cables)	150	Triceps brachii (short and lateral heads)
Triceps pull-down with lateral flair (cables)	130	Triceps brachii (lateral head)

[a]Other exercises that work same muscles may be substituted on the second day to add variety to the program (see appendix C.4, "Dynamic Resistance Training Exercises," p. 355).

[b]For tri-sets, the three exercises listed are performed consecutively without rest; then the tri-set is repeated for the prescribed number of sets for that muscle group (1 min rest between sets).

[c]1 lb = 0.45 kg.

- Prescribe at least one set of 10 to 15 repetitions for 8 to 10 different exercises for the major muscle groups.
- Train at least 2 days/wk, allowing at least 48 hr of rest between the exercise workouts.
- Discourage clients with arthritis from lifting weights when they are actively experiencing joint pain or inflammation.
- When clients are returning to resistance training following a layoff of more than 3 wk, they should start with a low resistance that is less than 50% of the weight they were lifting prior to the layoff.

COMMON QUESTIONS ABOUT RESISTANCE TRAINING

Because of the popularity of resistance training, there is an overwhelming amount of information about the subject in professional journals as well as in popular magazines and newspapers. This section presents common questions that exercise professionals may have about designing resistance training programs and addresses questions and concerns that your clients may pose.

Program Design

■ *Which resistance training method, nonperiodized or periodized, is better?*

The answer depends on your client's initial training status and goals. During the first stage (4 wk) of resistance training, both nonperiodized and periodized multiple-set programs increase the muscular fitness of untrained and novice lifters (Baker, Wilson, and Carlyon 1994); however, a varied training stimulus is needed for continued improvements in muscle strength and endurance during long-term (>4 wk) training (Fleck 1999; Marx et al. 2001). Periodized training is highly recommended for intermediate and advanced lifters; nonperiodized training may be more appropriate for clients just starting a weightlifting program or primarily interested in maintaining strength and muscle tone. Varying workouts daily (undulating periodized training) helps prevent boredom and maintain exercise compliance.

■ *Which periodization model is best?*

The answer depends on your client's training goal. One research team conducted two studies to assess the effectiveness of different types of periodized programs (LP, RLP, and daily UP) for increasing the strength and local muscular endurance of young, resistance-trained women and men (Rhea et al. 2002, 2003b). The researchers reported that daily UP was superior to LP for developing the strength of young men who trained 3 days/wk for 12 wk. For endurance gains, there were no statistically significant differences in LP, RLP, and daily UP training. Analysis of effect sizes, however, indicated that RLP was more effective than either LP or daily UP for increasing the muscular endurance of women and men who trained 2 days/wk for 15 wk.

■ *Is single-set training as effective as multiple-set training?*

Some research suggests that single-set training is as effective as multiple-set training for increasing the strength of untrained individuals during the initial stage of resistance training. For long-term training, however, multiple sets elicit greater strength gains for trained men and women (Marx et al. 2001; Wolfe, LeMura, and Cole 2004). For a comprehensive quantitative meta-analysis of studies comparing single- and multiple-set programs, see Wolfe and colleagues (2004). Paulsen, Myklested, and Reestad (2003) noted that the best method depends on the muscle groups exercised. They reported that multiple sets were superior to single sets for increasing leg strength, whereas the two types of programs were equally effective for increasing the upper body strength of untrained men during the initial phase (6 wk) of training.

■ *Is it better to train using fixed-form or free-form exercise machines?*

Both fixed-form and free-form resistance exercise machines may be used to improve muscular fitness. Fixed-form devices limit the range of motion and plane of motion during the resistance exercise (e.g., a leg extension machine that allows flexion/extension in sagittal plane only). In contrast, free-form exercise machines allow movement in multiple planes (e.g., chest fly machine that allows press or fly movements in horizontal and oblique planes). One study compared the effects of 16 wk of fixed-form training and free-form training on strength and balance of sedentary men and women (Spennewyn 2008). The improvement in overall strength of the free-form training group (116%) was significantly greater than that of the fixed-form training group (58%). Also, overall balance performance improved 245% and 49%, respectively, for the free-form and fixed-form training groups. Additional research is needed to substantiate these preliminary findings.

■ *Are abdominal training devices more effective than traditional calisthenic exercises for strengthening abdominal muscles?*

Currently, there is little scientific evidence justifying manufacturers' claims that abdominal training devices improve strength more effectively than simply performing calisthenic exercises without these devices (e.g., curl-ups). These devices purportedly overload the abdominal muscles by adding resistance (e.g., abdominal belts) and isolate the abdominal musculature by supporting the head, neck, or back. However, studies using electromyography (EMG) show that exercising with these devices does not increase the muscle activity of the abdominal prime movers (rectus abdominis and external abdominal oblique muscles) more than exercising without the devices (American Council on Exercise 1997; Demont et al. 1999; Francis et al. 2001). Although research does not support the use of abdominal trainers, they can add variety to conventional abdominal exercises and may even improve some clients' adherence to the abdominal exercise regimen.

To progressively overload (increase the training stimulus of) the abdominal muscles, you can have your client modify body position (e.g., perform abdominal curls on a decline bench rather than on a flat bench), hold a weight across the chest, or change arm positions. Abdominal exercises become more difficult as the arms move from along the sides to behind the head to overhead.

■ *How can stability balls, medicine balls, and resistance bands be used to improve a client's fitness?*

Stability balls, medicine balls, and resistance bands can be used in a variety of ways to improve muscular strength, power, core stability, flexibility, and static and dynamic balance. Calisthenic exercises such as abdominal crunches and back extensions can be performed while clients are lying on the ball; dumbbell exercises can be performed while they are lying supine or prone or sitting on the ball. Stability and medicine ball exercises are used to train the body as a linked system, starting with the core muscle groups. Use of resistance bands and tubing allows the individual to train the muscles with exercises that simulate the movement patterns of a specific sport. For more information about stability ball, medicine ball, and resistance band training, see Goldenberg and Twist (2007) and Page and Ellenbecker (2005).

■ *Does performing the curl-up on a labile (movable) surface increase the challenge for the abdominal muscles?*

Another way to increase the training stimulus for developing abdominal muscular fitness is to perform curl-up exercises on a labile surface. Vera-Garcia, Grenier, and McGill (2000) studied the EMG activity of the abdominal muscles (upper and lower rectus abdominis and internal and external abdominal oblique muscles) during four types of curl-ups: curl-ups on a stable bench, curl-ups on a gym ball with feet flat on the floor, curl-ups on a gym ball with feet on a bench, and curl-ups on a wobble board. Curl-ups performed on labile surfaces (gym ball and wobble board) doubled the EMG activity of the rectus abdominis and quadrupled the activity of the external oblique muscles. In terms of maintaining whole-body stability, the curl-up on the gym ball with the feet flat on the floor was the most demand-

ing, as evidenced by increased EMG activity in all the abdominal muscles. Curl-ups with the upper body supported on the wobble board produced the most EMG activity in the upper rectus abdominis. Although exercising on a labile surface increases abdominal muscle activity and coactivation, it also increases loads on the spine. In rehabilitation programs, curl-ups on movable surfaces should be used only with clients who can tolerate higher spinal loads (Vera-Garcia, Grenier, and McGill 2000).

Client Concerns

■ *Is it OK to lift weights every day?*

During weightlifting, you are exercising your muscles at greater than normal workloads, producing microscopic tears in the muscle cells and connective tissues. Your body responds by producing new muscle proteins, which causes muscle growth and increased strength. For these changes to occur, you need to rest the exercised muscles between workouts. Most people show substantial improvements in strength when they lift weights every other day, just two or three times a week. If you lift weights every day, you run the risk of overtraining your muscles. Overtraining may cause muscle strains, tendinitis, bursitis, and other muscle and joint injuries. Experienced weightlifters who work out every day split their exercise routine so that they do not exercise the same muscle groups on consecutive days. A split routine reduces the risk of excessive muscle soreness and overuse injuries if you lift weights every day.

■ *Can I use calisthenic exercises like push-ups and pull-ups to improve my strength?*

You can use calisthenic exercises to increase your strength. Exercise professionals often prescribe push-ups and pull-ups in addition to free-weight and machine exercises to strengthen the chest, arm, and back muscles. When you do calisthenics, your body weight provides the resistance. If you are unable to lift your body weight, you will need to modify the calisthenic exercise. For example, doing push-ups with your body weight supported by your knees and hands is easier than doing standard push-ups with your body fully extended and your weight supported by your hands and feet. As your strength improves, you may increase the difficulty of the push-up by placing your hands wider than shoulder-width apart.

If you are unable to lift your body weight, you can modify pull-ups by using a spotter. As you pull up, assist your movement by extending your knees as the spotter supports your lower legs or ankles. To increase the difficulty of a pull-up, place your hands wider than shoulder-width apart and use an overhand (pronated) grip instead of an underhand (supinated) grip.

■ *I have followed my exercise prescription closely, but over the last several weeks I haven't seen any change in my strength. What should I do?*

At the beginning of your program, your strength gains were dramatic and rapid because your initial strength level was less than it is now. As your muscles adapt to the training stimulus, you may reach a plateau, or a point where you can't seem to improve further. It may be helpful if you periodically alter the training stimulus more frequently (weekly or even daily) by changing your combination of intensity, repetitions, and sets (ask your personal trainer about a periodized program). For example, if you are presently doing high-intensity–low-repetition exercises during each workout, you may want to decrease your intensity (from 80% to 70% 1-RM) and increase your repetitions (from 6-8 to 10-12) for several days. Selecting different exercises for the muscle groups may also help.

■ *Will I become muscle bound and lose flexibility if I lift weights?*

It is a common misconception that resistance training decreases joint flexibility. Studies of elite bodybuilders and powerlifters indicate that these athletes have excellent flexibility. Also, one study showed that resistance training actually increased the flexibility of elderly women. The key to remaining flexible during resistance training is to perform each exercise throughout the entire range of motion. Also, statically stretching the muscle groups after each workout may help you maintain flexibility.

■ *Will resistance training help me lose weight and fat?*

Resistance training positively alters your body composition and preserves your lean body tissues. Although your body weight may not change, your lean body mass (muscle and bone) increases and your body fat decreases. Given that muscle tissue is more metabolically active (burns more calories)

than fat tissue, the increase in muscle size and lean body mass helps maintain your resting metabolic rate when you are on a weight loss diet. Exercise science and nutrition professionals recommend using resistance training combined with aerobic exercise to maximize the loss of body fat and to maintain lean body tissues.

■ *Will my strength improve if I train aerobically at the same time that I am resistance training?*

If you concurrently participate in aerobic and resistance training, your muscle growth and strength improvement may be lessened because of the increased energy demands and protein requirements of endurance training. Although this possibility is an important consideration for competitive bodybuilders and power athletes, your decision to participate in both forms of training depends on your overall exercise program goal. If your goal is improved health or weight loss, experts recommend including both aerobic and resistance training in your program.

■ *Are protein and amino acid supplements necessary to maximize muscle growth and strength during resistance training?*

Although the protein needs of resistance-trained individuals (1.6-1.8 g·kg^{-1} each day) are higher than the recommended dietary allowance for inactive individuals (0.8 g·kg^{-1} each day), for most individuals a well-balanced diet containing 12% to 25% protein will meet increased protein needs during resistance training. Recently, Verdijk and colleagues (2009) studied the effects of timed protein supplementation immediately before and after exercise on muscle mass and strength gains of healthy, older men after 12 wk of resistance training. Results showed that in older men who regularly consume adequate amounts of dietary protein, timed protein supplementation does not further augment gains in muscle mass or strength produced by resistance training alone.

However, if your goal is to augment muscle hypertrophy and strength gains beyond those produced from resistance training alone, whole protein or amino acid supplementation, consumed close to the time you engage in resistance exercise, may dramatically enhance the acute anabolic response to the exercise (Hayes and Cribb 2008). Protein supplementation promotes muscle hypertrophy in the following ways:

- Supplementing protein close to the time of resistance exercise ensures a greater stimulation of anabolic activity in the muscles.

- Supplementing between meals may promote additional stimulation of protein synthesis and net gain in muscle protein.

- The acute anabolic response to meals diminishes with aging; however, strategic supplementation with proteins rich in essential amino acids, especially leucine, may help to restore the anabolic response to meals.

Amino acid supplementation is especially popular among strength-trained athletes. Studies show that ingesting amino acids or a protein–carbohydrate supplement (e.g., 6 g of essential amino acids and 35 g sucrose) immediately before and after exercise stimulates protein synthesis and maximizes the anabolic (protein building) response of skeletal muscle tissue to resistance training (Ratamess et al. 2003). Tipton and colleagues (2001) noted that ingesting an amino acid–carbohydrate supplement immediately before resistance exercise is more effective than ingesting the supplement immediately after exercise in terms of increasing the net protein balance in skeletal muscle. In a study of elderly men who resistance trained over 12 wk, it was noted that those who took a protein–carbohydrate supplement immediately after exercise (within 5 min) had greater gains in muscle hypertrophy, lean body mass, and muscular strength than those who ingested the supplement 2 hr after the training session (Esmarck et al. 2001). These studies show that the timing of amino acid supplementation is critical in optimizing muscle growth in response to resistance training.

■ *What types of protein and amino supplements are most effective for augmenting muscle and strength development in response to resistance training?*

The type of protein consumed may influence the anabolic response to resistance training. Whey protein supplements (i.e., >80% protein concentrates or >90% protein isolates) are widely used among athletes to increase muscle mass. Whey protein supplements are the richest source of branched-chain amino acids, particularly leucine, which is a regulator of muscle protein synthesis (Hayes and Cribb 2008). In a study comparing the effects of whey protein and casein supplements in athletic individuals engaging in a 10 wk resistance training program, the group taking whey protein isolates ($1.5 \text{ g·kg}^{-1}\text{·day}^{-1}$) had a fivefold better gain in fat-free mass and better gains in strength compared to the group taking an equivalent daily dose of casein supplements (Cribb et al. 2006). To enhance muscle hypertrophy and strength gains during resistance training, whey protein isolates should be consumed immediately before and after exercise (Hayes and Cribb 2008).

■ *Will creatine supplements enhance strength and muscle size during resistance training?*

Over 300 studies have tested the effects of creatine supplementation on performance. Overall, the data suggest that creatine supplementation can improve the performance of high-intensity exercise lasting less than 30 sec (Branch 2003; Rawson and Clarkson 2003). Studies demonstrate that creatine supplementation combined with resistance training increases muscular strength, body mass, fat-free mass, muscle fiber size, and training volume in healthy young adults as well as in older women and men (Brose, Parise, and Tarnopolsky 2003; Cribb et al. 2007; Nissen and Sharp 2003). However, differences in skeletal muscle morphology may affect hypertrophy responses (i.e., changes in lean body mass, fiber-specific hypertrophy, and contractile protein content) to resistance training (Cribb et al. 2007). Creatine supplements increase muscle creatine; but, there is much interindividual variability in the response (Rawson and Clarkson 2003). Theoretically, an increase in muscle creatine enhances training volume and decreases the amount of recovery time needed between sets and exercises. The increased training stimulus improves the physiological adaptation to resistance training for some individuals (i.e., they experience a greater gain in muscle mass and strength).

In addition, researchers have compared the separate and combined effects of creatine monohydrate (CrM) and whey protein supplementation on strength and muscle hypertrophy improvements with resistance training. After 10 or 11 wk of resistance training, both CrM and whey protein supplements resulted in significant improvements in strength compared to values in a control group. However, the addition of creatine monohydrate (0.1-$0.3 \text{ g·kg}^{-1}\text{·day}^{-1}$) to the whey protein supplement (1.5

g·kg⁻¹·day⁻¹) produced much greater gains in body weight, lean body mass, and muscle hypertrophy than whey protein alone (Cribb, Williams, and Hayes 2007; Cribb et al. 2007). Thus, if the goal of the resistance training program is to maximize gains in muscle mass and body weight along with strength improvement, the addition of CrM to a whey protein supplement is recommended (Hayes and Cribb 2008).

■ Is it safe to take creatine supplements?

Although there are anecdotal reports associating creatine supplementation with muscle cramping, gastrointestinal distress, and soft tissue injuries (Poortmans and Francaux 2000), short-term and long-term creatine supplementation does not appear to adversely affect kidney, liver, or cardiovascular function (Volek 1999) or markers of health status such as muscle and liver enzymes, lipid profiles, and electrolytes (Kreider et al. 2003).

One reported side effect of creatine supplementation is increased stiffness in the musculotendinous unit, which theoretically predisposes individuals to muscle strains and tears. To address this concern, Watsford and colleagues (2003) studied changes in stiffness following 28 days of creatine supplementation and reported that creatine ingestion does not increase the stiffness of the series elastic components in the musculotendinous unit of the triceps surae (the gastrocnemius and soleus). These findings suggest that the muscle strains and tears reportedly associated with creatine supplementation are not caused by a change in the elasticity (stiffness) of the musculotendinous system. Also, when compared to a placebo group, subjects taking creatine supplements showed no differences in markers of exercise-induced muscle damage following eccentric exercise (Rawson, Gunn, and Clarkson 2001).

■ Do β-hydroxy-β-methylbutyrate (HMB) supplements increase lean body mass and muscle strength?

In a meta-analysis of dietary supplements, Nissen and Sharp (2003) reported that **β-hydroxy-β-methylbutyrate (HMB)** is one of only two supplements (the other being creatine) that significantly increases the lean body mass and muscular strength of individuals engaging in resistance training. Analysis of nine studies that used control groups to assess HMB supplementation (3 g·day⁻¹) indicated that, on average, lean body mass and muscular strength

increased 0.28% and 1.40% per week, respectively, for the treatment groups. The effect sizes for net gains in lean body mass (ES = 0.15) and strength (ES = 0.19) were significant. HMB supplementation during 3 to 8 wk of resistance training did not adversely affect hematology or liver and kidney function but positively affected cardiovascular risk factors (decreased total cholesterol, low-density lipoprotein cholesterol, and systolic blood pressure) (Nissen and Sharp 2003).

EFFECTS OF RESISTANCE TRAINING PROGRAMS

Resistance training improves muscular fitness by increasing both strength and muscular endurance. This section addresses the morphological, neurological, and biochemical effects of resistance training.

Morphological Effects of Resistance Training on the Musculoskeletal System

Resistance training leads to morphological adaptations in skeletal muscles and bone. Structural changes in muscle fibers account for a large portion of the strength gains resulting from resistance training. Increases in bone mineral content and bone density improve bone health. The following questions deal with these adaptations.

■ What is exercise-induced muscle hypertrophy?

One effect of strength training is an increase in the size of the muscle tissue. This adaptation, known as **exercise-induced hypertrophy**, results from an increase in the total amount of contractile protein, the number and size of myofibrils per fiber, and the amount of connective tissue surrounding the muscle fibers (Goldberg et al. 1975).

■ Is it possible to increase the number of muscle fibers by resistance training?

Heavy resistance training has been reported to produce an increase in the number of muscle fibers (i.e., hyperplasia) in animals due to longitudinal splitting and satellite cell proliferation (Antonio and Gonyea 1993; Edgerton 1970; Gonyea, Ericson, and Bonde-Petersen 1977). Such processes, however, have not been clearly demonstrated in human skeletal muscle tissue (Taylor and Wilkinson

1986; Tesch 1988). Although some data suggest that human skeletal muscle has the potential to increase muscle fiber number (Alway et al. 1989; Sjostrom et al. 1992), hyperplasia probably contributes less than 5% to overall muscle growth in response to heavy resistance training (Kraemer, Fleck, and Evans 1996). The major factor contributing to exercise-induced hypertrophy for humans apparently is an increase in the size of existing muscle fibers.

■ Does resistance training alter muscle fiber type from slow-twitch to fast-twitch?

Although strength training produces greater hypertrophy in fast-twitch (type II) muscle fibers than in slow-twitch (type I) fibers (Tesch 1988; Thorstensson et al. 1976), there is no evidence to support the conversion of slow-twitch to fast-twitch fibers (Costill et al. 1979; Dons et al. 1979; Mikesky et al. 1991). Resistance training does not alter the percentage of type I and II muscle fibers. However, heavy resistance training affects the proportion of fibers comprising subgroups of type II muscle fibers, increasing the percentage of type IIB (fast-twitch—glycolytic) muscle fibers while decreasing the percentage of type IIA (fast-twitch—oxidative) fibers in both men and women (Deschenes and Kraemer 2002; Kraemer et al. 1995; Staron et al. 1994).

■ Is the relationship between muscle size and strength the same for men and women?

Muscle strength is directly related to the cross-sectional area of the muscle tissue. Ikai and Fukunaga (1968) noted that the static strength per unit of cross-sectional area of the elbow flexors was similar for young men and women. These values ranged between 4.5 and 8.9 kg·cm^2; average values were 6.2 and 6.7 kg·cm^2 for women and men, respectively. Cureton and colleagues (1988) also reported that the dynamic strength per unit of cross-sectional area (CSA) was similar for men and women. Posttraining ratios of elbow flexor/extensor strength to upper arm CSA were 1.65 kg·cm^2 and 1.85 kg·cm^2, respectively, for men and women. Likewise, the posttraining ratios for leg strength to thigh CSA were 1.10 kg·cm^2 for men and 0.90 kg·cm^2 for women.

■ How much do women's muscles hypertrophy in response to resistance training?

In the past, it was believed that resistance training produced less muscle hypertrophy in women than in men even though their relative strength gains were similar, but muscle hypertrophy was assessed indirectly using anthropometric and body composition measures. Cureton and colleagues (1988), however, using computerized tomography to directly assess muscle hypertrophy in a heavy resistance training program (70% to 90% 1-RM, 3 days/wk for 16 wk), found significant increases in CSA of the upper arms of women (5 cm^2 or 23%) as well as men (7 cm^2 or 15%). Although absolute change in muscle volume was greater in men, the relative degree of hypertrophy (% change) was similar for men and women (Cureton et al. 1988). Research confirms this observation. Walts and colleagues (2008) reported that 10 wk of strength training resulted in similar relative gains in muscle volume of the knee extensors of Caucasian and African American men (9%) and women (7.5%).

Today experts agree that the relative increases in fiber size are similar for women and men when the training stimulus is the same (Deschenes and Kraemer 2002). In addition, periodized resistance training is particularly effective for increasing muscle size in women. Kraemer and colleagues (2004) compared the effects of total and upper body periodized training programs on muscle hypertrophy in young women. Over 6 mo of training, the total body periodized program produced greater and more consistent gains in overall (upper and lower body) muscle size compared to upper body periodized training. An intensity range of 3-RM to 8-RM produced greater muscle hypertrophy than did a range of 8-RM to 12-RM.

■ Is it possible for older adults to increase the size of their muscles by resistance training?

Electromyographic evidence led Moritani and deVries (1979) to conclude that increased strength in older men who engaged in resistance training was highly dependent on neural changes, such as increased frequency of motor neuron discharge and recruitment of motor units. Because of studies such as this, it was long believed that strength gains from resistance training in older individuals were due primarily to neural adaptation rather than muscle hypertrophy.

However, Frontera and colleagues (1988) reported that resistance training produces muscle hypertrophy in men ages 60 to 72 yr. The men trained in a high-intensity program for the knee extensors and flexors (three sets at 80% 1-RM) for

12 wk. Computerized tomography revealed significant increases in total thigh area (4.8%), total muscle area (11.4%), and quadriceps area (9.3%). The relative increase in total muscle area was similar to values reported for young men (Luthi et al. 1986). Research also shows significant increases in muscle size in older women, as well as in very old (87 to 96 yr) men and women, due to high-intensity (80% 1-RM) resistance training (Charette et al. 1991; Fiatarone et al. 1991).

Exercise-induced hypertrophy appears to be an important mechanism underlying strength gains in older women and men. This implies that older adults can effectively counter age-related loss in muscle mass by participating in a vigorous resistance training program.

■ *Does resistance training improve bone health and joint integrity?*

Resistance training has beneficial effects on bone health that may decrease the risk of osteoporosis and bone fractures, particularly in women. This form of training may help to achieve the highest possible peak bone mass in premenopausal women and may aid in maintaining and increasing bone in postmenopausal women and older adults (Layne and Nelson 1999). Bone mineral density of the lumbar spine and femur in premenopausal women significantly increased after 12 to 18 mo of strength training (Lohman et al. 1995). Also, lumbar bone mineral density of early-postmenopausal women was improved following 9 mo of strength training (Pruitt et al. 1992). However, in a study of older women (65 to 79 yr), 12 mo of high-intensity (80% 1-RM) and low-intensity (40% 1-RM) resistance training did not significantly improve the bone mineral density of the lumbar spine and hip (Pruitt, Taaffe, and Marcus 1995). Still, evidence suggests that resistance training and higher-intensity weight-bearing activities (not walking) may slow the decline in bone loss even if there is no significant increase in bone mineral density. Improvements in bone mineral density appear to be site specific; the greater changes occur in bones to which the exercising muscles attach. Experts agree that resistance training has a more potent effect on bone health than do weight-bearing aerobic exercises such as walking and jogging (Layne and Nelson 1999).

Resistance training also improves the size and strength of ligaments and tendons (Edgerton 1973;

Summary of Effects of Resistance Training

Morphological Factors

- Muscle hypertrophy due to increase in contractile proteins, number and size of myofibrils, connective tissues, and size of type II muscle fibers
- No change in relative amounts of type I and II muscle fibers
- Little or no change in the number of muscle fibers (<5%)
- Increase in size and strength of ligaments and tendons
- Increase in bone density and bone strength
- Increase in muscle capillary density

Neural Factors

- Increase in motor unit activation and recruitment
- Increase in discharge frequency of motor neurons
- Decrease in neural inhibition

Biochemical Factors

- Minor increase in ATP and CP stores
- Minor increase in creatine phosphokinase (CPK), myosin adenosine triphosphatase (ATPase), and myokinase activity
- Decrease in mitochondrial volume density
- Increase in testosterone, growth hormone, insulin-like growth factor (IGF-I), and catecholamines during resistance training exercises
- Enhanced fat oxidation and fat availability during submaximal cycle ergometer exercise following resistance exercise

Additional Factors

- Little or no change in body mass
- Increase in fat-free mass
- Decrease in fat mass and relative body fat
- Improved bone health increases with exercise intensity

Fleck and Falkel 1986; Tipton et al. 1975). These changes may increase joint stability, thereby reducing the risk of sprains and dislocations.

Biochemical Effects of Resistance Training

The morphological changes in skeletal muscles due to resistance training are caused by hormones. This section addresses questions regarding hormonal responses to resistance exercise, as well as changes in the metabolic profile of skeletal muscles.

■ *What causes the increase in muscle size with resistance training?*

Exercise-induced hypertrophy occurs through hormonal mechanisms. Anabolic (protein building) hormones such as testosterone, growth hormone, and insulin-like growth hormone increase in response to heavy resistance exercise and interact to promote protein synthesis. The magnitude of testosterone and growth hormone release, however, appears to be related to the size of the muscle groups used, the exercise intensity (%1-RM), and the length of rest between sets, with larger increases observed for high-intensity (5- to 10-RM) exercise and short (1 min) rest periods involving large muscle groups (Kraemer et al. 1991). In men, high-intensity resistance training produces significant increases in testosterone and growth hormone, but testosterone appears to be the principal muscle-building hormone (Deschenes and Kraemer 2002). Levels of catecholamines (norepinephrine, epinephrine, and dopamine), which augment the release of testosterone and insulin-like growth factor, also increase in men in response to heavy resistance exercise (Kraemer et al. 1987). In women, growth hormone is likely the most potent muscle-building hormone (Deschenes and Kraemer 2002).

■ *Does resistance training alter the metabolic profile of skeletal muscles?*

Although high-intensity resistance training results in substantial increases in muscle proteins, it appears to have little or no effect on muscle substrate stores and enzymes involved with the generation of adenosine triphosphate (ATP). Although stores of ATP and creatine phosphate (CP) may increase significantly in response to strength training (MacDougall et al. 1979), the changes are not large enough to have practical significance.

Strength training produces only minor alterations in myosin adenosinetriphosphatase (ATPase) activity (Tesch 1992) and other ATP turnover enzymes, such as creatine phosphokinase (CPK), in response to strength training (Costill et al. 1979; Komi et al. 1978; Thorstensson et al. 1976). Strength training using heavy resistance and explosive exercises results in decreased activities for hexokinase, myofibrillar ATPase, and citrate synthase (Tesch 1988).

■ *Does resistance training decrease aerobic capacity and endurance performance?*

The mitochondrial volume density following heavy resistance training has been reported to decrease as a consequence of a disproportionate increase of contractile protein in comparison with mitochondria. In theory, this could be detrimental to aerobic capacity and endurance performance. A review of studies of this phenomenon, however, concluded that participation in heavy resistance training does not negatively affect aerobic power (Dudley and Fleck 1987; Sale et al. 1987). Also, capillary density has been shown to increase, which in turn enhances the potential to remove lactate produced by the muscles during moderate-intensity, high-volume resistance exercise (Kraemer et al. 1996).

In fact, Goto and colleagues (2007) reported that resistance exercise performed 20 min before a submaximal (50% $\dot{V}O_2$max) exercise bout significantly improved fat availability and fat oxidation during a 60 min aerobic exercise bout on a cycle ergometer. Resistance exercise also increased norepinephrine, growth hormone, glycerol concentrations, and blood lactate levels prior to the aerobic exercise bout.

However, Nader (2006) concluded that endurance training may potentially interfere with strength improvements due to resistance training when individuals engage in both forms of training concurrently. The interference may be caused by changes in protein synthesis induced by endurance exercise or by too-frequent training sessions. Endurance exercise activates adenosine monophosphate kinase (AMPK), which in turn may inhibit muscle protein synthesis. Nader presents a working model of how molecular mechanisms may inhibit strength gains with concurrent strength and endurance training.

Neurological Effects of Resistance Training

In addition to muscle hypertrophy, neural adaptations significantly contribute to strength gains, especially during the initial stages of resistance training. This section addresses questions regarding neural adaptations to short- and long-term resistance training.

■ *What changes in neural function occur in response to resistance training?*

The nervous system responds to resistance training by increasing the activation and recruitment of motor units (the alpha motor neuron and all of the muscle fibers it innervates) and by decreasing the cocontraction of antagonistic muscle groups (Sale 1988). Recruiting additional motor units as well as increasing the frequency of firing results in greater muscular force production. Some evidence suggests that the central drive from higher neural centers (e.g., motor cortex of brain) changes and that the amounts of neurotransmitters and postsynaptic receptors at the neuromuscular junction increase (Deschenes and Kraemer 2002). These changes facilitate the activation and recruitment of additional motor units, thereby increasing force production.

■ *At what stage during resistance training does neural adaptation occur?*

In the past, it was believed that neural adaptations are primarily responsible for strength gains only during the initial stage (first 2-8 wk) of resistance training. At about 8 to 10 wk of resistance training, muscle hypertrophy contributes more than neural adaptation to strength gains, but hypertrophy eventually levels off (Sale 1988). Evidence suggests that muscle hypertrophy is finite and may be limited to no more than 12 mo (Deschenes and Kraemer 2002). Given that long-term resistance training (>6 mo) continues to increase strength without hypertrophy, experts now believe that a secondary phase of neural adaptation is most likely responsible for strength gains occurring between 6 and 12 mo of training (Deschenes and Kraemer 2002).

■ *What role do neural factors play in age-related loss of muscle strength?*

Over the past decade, the term **sarcopenia**, or an age-related loss in muscle mass, has also been used to define age-related loss in muscle strength.

This implies that changes in muscle mass are fully responsible for changes in strength. According to a recent report by Clark and Manini (2008), longitudinal studies indicate that age-related changes in muscle mass account for less than 5% of the change in strength with aging. Changes in muscle mass and strength do not follow the same time course, suggesting that neural factors, along with changes in muscle factors (e.g., muscle architecture, fiber type transformations, and electro-contractile coupling), may modulate age-related loss of strength. They recommend using the term **dynapenia** to refer to age-related loss in strength. Although it is difficult to identify specific neural mechanisms associated with dynapenia, changes in supraspinal drive, coactivation of antagonist muscles, muscle synergism, and maximal spinal cord output may mediate strength loss with aging (Clark and Manini 2008).

■ *Is vibration training an effective way to increase the muscular strength of my clients?*

Vibration loading has been used to prevent bone mineral loss in astronauts and to enhance the rehabilitation of injuries such as sprains and tendinitis. With vibration loading, a power-plate vibration machine applies a low-amplitude, high-frequency (25-40 Hz) current to a platform on which the client stands erect, relaxed, on heels, shifting weight from one leg to the other, or performs exercises such as push-ups, triceps dips, squats, light jumping, and static stretching.

The potential of using whole-body mechanical vibration as a method (**vibration training**) for increasing strength, balance, and bone integrity and for attenuating muscle soreness due to eccentric exercise has been investigated (Bakhtiary, Safavi-Farokhi, and Aminian-Far 2007; Roelants et al. 2004; Torvinen et al. 2002). Research has demonstrated that whole-body vibration improves the explosive power of physically active individuals (Bosco et al. 1999), the balance of older adults (Runge, Rehfeld, and Resnicek 2000), bone formation of postmenopausal women (Rubin et al. 1998), and the activation and coactivation of the biceps and triceps of young adults during isometric flexion and extension of the elbow (Mischi and Cardinale 2009). Also, applying vibration to the quadriceps, hamstrings, and calf muscles prior to eccentric exercise on a treadmill significantly reduced the degree of muscle soreness 24 hr postexercise (Bakhtiary, Safavi-Farokhi, and Aminian-Far 2007).

Vibration loading produces small changes in muscle length that stimulate a **tonic vibration reflex.** This reflex activates muscle spindles and alpha motor neurons, causing the muscles to contract (Torvinen et al. 2002). Torvinen and colleagues examined the long-term (4 mo) effects of vibration training combined with unloaded static and dynamic exercises on strength, power, and balance. They noted that the greatest relative gains in isometric leg extension strength and in leg power (measured by the vertical jump) occurred after the first 2 mo of training. Gains in strength and power during the last 2 mo of training were minimal. Thus, it appears that vibration training elicits a neural response and adaptation (recruitment of motor units through the activation of muscle spindles) similar to that observed during the early stages of conventional resistance training. When compared to a standard fitness program (combined aerobic and resistance training) and to conventional resistance training (exercise machines) in women, vibration training during unloaded static and dynamic exercises produced similar gains in isometric, isokinetic, and dynamic strength over 3 to 4 mo (Delecluse, Roelants, and Verschueren 2003; Roelants et al. 2004). However, Abercromby and colleagues recently reported that more than 10 min a day of whole-body vibration training may have adverse health effects (Abercromby et al. 2007). Vibration training warrants further study, especially to determine its applicability in improving strength, flexibility, and possibly even balance in elderly individuals in order to prevent falls, as well as to identify any long-term potential health hazards for this form of training.

MUSCULAR SORENESS

Muscular soreness may develop as a result of resistance training because isolated muscle groups are being overloaded beyond normal use. **Acute-onset muscle soreness** occurs during or immediately following the exercise and is usually caused by ischemia and the accumulation of metabolic waste products in the muscle tissue. The pain and discomfort may persist up to 1 hr after the cessation of the exercise.

In **delayed-onset muscle soreness (DOMS),** the pain occurs 24 to 48 hr after exercise. Although the causes of DOMS are not known (Armstrong 1984; Smith 1991), it appears to be related to the type of muscle contraction. Eccentric exercise produces a greater degree of delayed muscular soreness than either concentric or isometric exercise (Byrnes, Clarkson, and Katch 1985; Schwane et al. 1983; Talag 1973). Little or no muscular soreness occurs with isokinetic exercise (Byrnes, Clarkson, and Katch 1985). This most likely reflects the fact that isokinetic exercise devices offer no resistance to the recovery phase of the movement and therefore the muscle does not contract eccentrically.

Theories of Delayed-Onset Muscle Soreness

Although the precise causes of DOMS remain unclear, several theories have been proposed. The more widely recognized theories suggest that exercise, particularly eccentric exercise, causes damage to skeletal muscle cells and connective tissues, producing an acute inflammation.

Connective Tissue Damage

Abraham (1977) extensively studied the factors related to DOMS produced by resistance training. He suggested that DOMS most likely results from disruption in the connective tissue of the muscle and its tendinous attachments. Abraham noted that urinary excretion of hydroxyproline, a specific by-product of connective tissue breakdown, was higher in subjects who experienced muscular soreness than in those who did not. Because a significant rise in urinary hydroxyproline levels indicates an increase in both collagen degradation and synthesis, he concluded that more strenuous exercise damages the connective tissue, which increases the degradation of collagen and creates an imbalance in collagen metabolism. To compensate for this imbalance, the rate of collagen synthesis increases.

Skeletal Muscle Damage

Researchers have assessed skeletal muscle damage induced through exercise. **Exercise-induced muscle damage (EIMD)** may occur when individuals engage in novel exercise, eccentric exercise, or exercise to which they are unaccustomed. The muscle damage results in decreased force production and increased passive tension, as well as increased muscle soreness, swelling, and intramuscular proteins in the blood (Howatson and van Someren 2008). Much of the research on EIMD has focused on the effects of eccentric exercise on muscle damage and soreness. Regardless of the speed or intensity of contraction, eccentric exercise injures both the contractile and cytoskeletal components of myofibrils as well as the excitation coupling system; this is especially true for novel exercise (Howatson and van Someren 2008). Friden, Sjostrom, and Ekblom (1983) observed structural damage to myofibrillar Z bands resulting from eccentric exercise. Proske and Morgan (2001) pointed out that disruption of the sarcomere organization within the skeletal muscle is most likely the cause of the decreased active tension and force production that follows a series of intense eccentric contractions. Recently, Mackey and colleagues (2008) reported that electrically stimulated isometric contractions may also produce muscle damage at the sarcomere level. Z-line disruption and microphage infiltration provided direct evidence of damage to myofibers and sarcomeres. More research is needed to assess the effects of various types of muscle contraction, as well as high- and low-impact eccentric exercise (e.g., downhill running and eccentric cycle exercise), on muscle damage (Friden 2002).

Researchers also have examined markers of muscle damage such as serum CPK, lactate dehydrogenase, and myoglobin. Schwane and colleagues (1983) noted a significant increase in plasma CPK levels produced by downhill running. They suggested that the mechanical stress from eccentric exercise causes cellular damage resulting in an enzyme efflux. Clarkson and colleagues (1986) reported similar increases in serum CPK levels following concentric (37.6%), eccentric (35.8%), and isometric (34%) arm curl exercises. They concluded that muscle damage occurred with all three types of contraction; however, the subjects perceived greater muscle soreness with eccentric and isometric exercises. Likewise, Byrnes and colleagues (1985) observed that both concentric and eccentric resistance training elevated serum CPK levels but that individuals who trained concentrically did not develop DOMS.

Armstrong's Model of Delayed-Onset Muscle Soreness

On the basis of an extensive literature review, Armstrong (1984) proposed the following model of the development of DOMS:

1. The structural proteins in muscle cells and connective tissue are disrupted by high mechanical forces produced during exercise, especially eccentric exercise.

2. Structural damage to the sarcolemma alters the permeability of the cell membrane, allowing a net influx of calcium from the interstitial space. Abnormally high levels of calcium inhibit cellular respiration, thereby lessening the cell's ability to produce ATP for active removal of calcium from the cell.

3. High calcium levels within the cell activate a calcium-dependent proteolytic enzyme that degrades Z discs, troponin, and tropomyosin.

4. This progressive destruction of the sarcolemma (postexercise) allows intracellular components to diffuse into the interstitial space and plasma. These substances attract monocytes and activate mast cells and histocytes in the injured area.

5. Histamine, kinins, and potassium accumulate in the interstitial space because of the active phagocytosis and cellular necrosis. These substances, as well as increased tissue edema and temperature, may stimulate pain receptors resulting in the sensation of DOMS.

Acute Inflammation Theory

Smith (1991) suggested that acute inflammation, in response to muscle cell and connective damage caused by eccentric exercise, is the primary mechanism underlying DOMS. Many of the signs and symptoms of acute inflammation, such as pain, swelling, and loss of function, are also present with DOMS. On the basis of research about acute inflammation and DOMS, Smith proposed the following sequence of events:

1. Connective tissue and muscle tissue disruption occurs during eccentric exercise, especially when the individual is not accustomed to eccentric exercise.

2. Within a few hours, neutrophils in the blood are elevated and migrate to the site of injury for several hours postinjury.

3. Monocytes also migrate to the injured tissues at 6 to 12 hr postinjury.

4. Macrophages synthesize prostaglandins (series E).

5. The prostaglandins sensitize type III and IV pain afferents, resulting in the sensation of pain in response to intramuscular pressure caused by movement or palpation.

6. The combination of increased pressure and hypersensitization produces the sensation of DOMS.

Prevention of Exercise-Induced Muscle Damage and Muscular Soreness

Given that eccentric muscle contraction is an integral part of human locomotion, physical activities, and sport, researchers have explored myriad intervention strategies to lessen the negative effects of eccentric muscle actions and to treat EIAD. These approaches include nutritional (e.g., antioxidants, carbohydrate–protein supplements, and β-hydroxy-β-methylbutyrate) and pharmacological strategies (e.g., aspirin, ibuprofen, and naproxen), manual (e.g., massage and cryotherapy) and electrical (e.g., transcutaneous electrical nerve stimulation [TENS] and ultrasound) therapies, and exercise (e.g., prior bouts of eccentric exercise and stretching). Of these approaches, a single bout of low-volume, high-intensity eccentric exercise has been consistently shown to have a positive effect on reducing EIMD. Howatson and van Someren (2008) provide an excellent review of research dealing with the prevention and treatment of EIAD.

For many years, slow static stretching exercises were recommended to warm up major muscle groups at the start of the resistance training workout. It was believed that this form of stretching prevented muscle injury and soreness (deVries 1961). However, evidence suggests that stretching prior to physical activity does not prevent injury (Pope et al. 2000) or muscle soreness (Herbert and de Noronha 2007); and in fact, stretching prior to resistance exercise may actually decrease strength and force production (Rubini, Costa, and Gomes 2007). Therefore, stretching immediately prior to resistance exercise is not recommended. Instead of performing static stretching, your client should warm up by completing 5 to 10 repetitions of the exercise at a low intensity (e.g., 40% 1-RM). Law and Herbert (2007) reported that low-intensity exercise (i.e., warm-up) prior to unaccustomed eccentric exercise (e.g., walking backward downhill on an inclined treadmill for 30 min) reduced muscle soreness up to 48 hr after exercise. In contrast, neither low-intensity, cool-down exercise nor stretching after exercise reduces muscle soreness (Herbert and de Noronha 2007; Law and Herbert 2007).

Using a gradual progression of exercise intensity at the beginning of a resistance training program also may help to prevent muscular soreness. Some experts suggest using 12- to 15-RM during the beginning phases of strength training. Make sure that your clients gradually increase exercise intensity throughout the resistance training program. Avoiding eccentric contractions during dynamic resistance training also may lessen the chance of muscular soreness. An assistant or exercise partner should return the weight to the starting position.

KEY POINTS

- The specificity principle states that muscular fitness development is specific to the muscle group, type of contraction, training intensity, speed, and range of movement.

- The overload principle states that the muscle group must be exercised at greater than normal workloads to promote muscular strength and endurance development.

- For nonperiodized resistance training programs, the training volume must be progressively increased to overload the muscle groups for continued gains in strength and muscular endurance.

- In most programs, resistance training exercises should be ordered so that successive exercises do not involve the same muscle group. For advanced programs, however, exercises for the same muscle group should be done consecutively.

- Dynamic resistance training can be used to develop muscular strength, power, size, or endurance by modifying the intensity, repetitions, sets, and frequency of the exercise.

- Periodization programs can result in greater changes in strength than nonperiodized resistance training programs.

- Strength and endurance gains resulting from resistance training are due to morphological, neurological, and biochemical changes in the muscle tissue.

- Eccentric exercise produces a greater degree of DOMS than either concentric, isometric, or isokinetic exercise.

- Little or no muscular soreness is produced by isokinetic training.

- The precise cause of DOMS is unknown; however, connective tissue and muscle damage, as well as acute inflammation, have been proposed as possible causes.

KEY TERMS

Learn the definition of each of the following key terms. Definitions of terms can be found in the glossary on page 411.

acute-onset muscle soreness	muscle balance
β-hydroxy-β-methylbutyrate (HMB)	periodization
compound sets	pyramiding
core stability	repetition maximum (RM)
core strengthening	repetitions
delayed-onset muscle soreness (DOMS)	reverse linear periodization (RLP)
dynapenia	sarcopenia
exercise-induced hypertrophy	set
exercise-induced muscle damage (EIMD)	split routine
functional training	supersetting
high intensity–low repetitions	tonic vibration reflex
linear periodization (LP)	training volume
low intensity–high repetitions	tri-sets
macrocycle	undulating periodization (UP)
mesocycle	vibration training
microcycle	

REVIEW QUESTIONS

In addition to being able to define each of the key terms, test your knowledge and understanding of the material by answering the following review questions.

1. What are the health benefits of resistance training?

2. Name three general types of resistance training. Which one is best suited for physical therapy rehabilitation programs?

3. What is the major advantage of isokinetic training compared to traditional forms of resistance training?

4. Describe the ACSM guidelines for designing resistance training programs for healthy adults. What modifications are necessary when you are planning resistance training programs for children and older adults?

5. Describe how the basic exercise prescriptions for strength training and muscular endurance training programs differ.

6. Describe how you can increase training volume for advanced strength training and hypertrophy programs.

7. Describe two methods of varying sets for advanced strength training programs.

8. Explain two methods that an advanced weightlifter can use to completely fatigue a targeted muscle group.

9. Describe three periodization models. How do they differ?

10. Explain how the specificity, overload, and progression principles are applied in the design of resistance training programs.

11. Explain what causes the exercise-induced hypertrophy resulting from resistance training. In the time course of a resistance training program, when is this morphological adaptation most likely to occur?

12. Define sarcopenia and dynapenia. Identify muscle morphological and neurological mechanisms responsible for dynapenia.

13. What neural adaptations account for initial strength gains during resistance training? When are these changes most likely to be observed during the time course of resistance training?

14. Describe the potential effects of resistance training on bone health.

15. Describe one theory of DOMS. What can you instruct your clients to do to help prevent and relieve muscle soreness caused by resistance training?

16. What will you tell your clients if they ask about supplementing their resistance training with creatine?

chapter

8

Assessing Body Composition

KEY QUESTIONS

- Why is it important to measure body composition, and how are body composition measures used by health and fitness professionals?
- What are the standards for classifying body fat levels?
- What is the difference between two-component and multicomponent body composition models?
- What are the guidelines and limitations of the hydrostatic weighing method?
- Is air displacement plethysmography as accurate as hydrostatic weighing?
- Is dual-energy X-ray absorptiometry considered a "gold standard" method for measuring body composition?
- What are the guidelines, limitations, and sources of measurement error for the skinfold method?
- What is bioelectrical impedance analysis? What factors affect the accuracy of this method?
- Can circumferences and skeletal diameters be used to accurately assess body composition?
- What anthropometric indices can be used to identify at-risk individuals?
- Is near-infrared interactance a viable alternative to skinfolds and bioimpedance analysis for measuring body composition in field settings?

Body composition is a key component of an individual's health and physical fitness profile. Obesity is a serious health problem that reduces life expectancy by increasing one's risk of developing coronary artery disease, hypertension, type 2 diabetes, obstructive pulmonary disease, osteoarthritis, and certain types of cancer. Too little body fat also poses a health risk because the body needs a certain amount of fat for normal physiological functions. Essential lipids, such as phospholipids, are needed for cell membrane formation; nonessential lipids, like triglycerides found in adipose tissue, provide thermal insulation and store metabolic fuel (free fatty acids). In addition, lipids are involved in the transport and storage of fat-soluble vitamins (A, D, E, and K) and in the functioning of the nervous system, the menstrual cycle, and the reproductive system, as well as in growth and maturation during pubescence. Thus, too little body fatness, as found in individuals with eating disorders (e.g., anorexia nervosa), exercise addiction, and certain diseases such as cystic fibrosis, can lead to serious physiological dysfunction.

This chapter describes standardized testing procedures for reference (hydrostatic weighing, air displacement plethysmography, and dual X-ray absorptiometry) and field (skinfold, bioimpedance, and anthropometry) methods for assessing body composition. For each method, you will learn to identify potential sources of measurement error, as well as ways to minimize these errors.

CLASSIFICATION AND USES OF BODY COMPOSITION MEASURES

To classify level of body fatness, the **relative body fat (%BF)** is used. Table 8.1 presents recommended %BF standards for men, women, and children, as well as physically active adults. The minimal, average, and obesity fat values vary with age, gender, and activity status. For example, the average or median %BF values for adult men and women (18 to 34 yr) are 13% for men and 28% for women; the minimal fat values are 8% and 20%, respectively; and the standard for obesity is >22% BF for men and >35% BF for women.

In addition to classifying your client's %BF and disease risk, body composition measures are useful for

- estimating a healthy body weight and formulating nutritional recommendations and exercise prescriptions (see chapter 9);

- estimating competitive body weight for athletes participating in sports that use body weight classifications for competition (e.g., wrestling and bodybuilding);

- monitoring the growth of children and adolescents and identifying those at risk because of under- or overfatness; and

- assessing changes in body composition associated with aging, malnutrition, and certain diseases, and assessing the effectiveness of nutrition and exercise interventions in counteracting these changes.

BODY COMPOSITION MODELS

In order to make the most valid assessment of body composition for your client, it is necessary to understand the underlying theoretical models. You may recall that the body is composed of water, protein, minerals, and fat. The two-component model of

Table 8.1 Percent Body Fat Standards for Adults, Children, and Physically Active Adults

| | NR* | RECOMMENDED %BF LEVELS FOR ADULTS AND CHILDREN | | | |
		Low	Mid	High	Obesity
Males					
6-17 years	<5	5-10	11-25	26-31	>31
18-34 years	<8	8	13	22	>22
35-55 years	<10	10	18	25	>25
55+ years	<10	10	16	23	>23
Females					
6-17 years	<12	12-15	16-30	31-36	>36
18-34 years	<20	20	28	35	>35
35-55 years	<25	25	32	38	>38
55+ years	<25	25	30	35	>35

| | RECOMMENDED %BF LEVELS FOR PHYSICALLY ACTIVE ADULTS | | |
	Low	Mid	Upper
Males			
18-34 years	5	10	15
35-55 years	7	11	18
55+ years	9	12	18
Females			
18-34 years	16	23	28
35-55 years	20	27	33
55+ years	20	27	33

*NR = not recommended; %BF = percent body fat.

Data from Lohman, Houtkooper, and Going 1997.

body composition (Brozek et al. 1963; Siri 1961) divides the body into a fat component and a **fat-free body (FFB)** component. The FFB consists of all residual chemicals and tissues including water, muscle (protein), and bone (mineral). The **two-component model** of body composition makes the following five assumptions:

1. The density of fat is 0.901 $g \cdot cc^{-1}$.
2. The density of the FFB is 1.100 $g \cdot cc^{-1}$.
3. The densities of fat and the FFB components (water, protein, mineral) are the same for all individuals.
4. The densities of the various tissues composing the FFB are constant within an individual, and their proportional contribution to the lean component remains constant.
5. The individual being measured differs from the reference body only in the amount of fat; the FFB of the reference body is assumed to be 73.8% water, 19.4% protein, and 6.8% mineral.

This two-component model has served as the foundation for the **hydrodensitometry** (underwater weighing) method. With use of the assumed proportions of water, mineral, and protein and their respective densities, equations were derived to convert the individual's total body density (Db) from hydrostatic weighing into relative body fat proportions (%BF). Two commonly used equations are the Siri (1961) equation, %BF = (4.95 / Db – 4.50) × 100, and the equation of Brozek and colleagues (1963), %BF = (4.57 / Db – 4.142) × 100. These two equations yield similar %BF estimates for body densities ranging from 1.0300 to 1.0900 $g \cdot cc^{-1}$. For example, if a client's measured Db is 1.0500 $g \cdot cc^{-1}$, the %BF estimates obtained by plugging this value into the Siri and Brozek equations are 21.4% and 21.0%, respectively.

Generally, two-component model equations provide accurate estimates of %BF as long as the basic assumptions of the model are met. However, there is no guarantee that the FFB composition of an individual within a certain population subgroup will exactly match the values assumed for the reference body. Researchers have reported that FFB density varies with age, gender, ethnicity, level of body fatness, and physical activity level, depending mainly on the relative proportion of water and mineral composing the FFB (Baumgartner et al. 1991; Williams et al. 1993a). For example, the average FFB density of black women and black men (~1.106 $g \cdot cc^{-1}$) is greater than 1.10 $g \cdot cc^{-1}$ because of their higher mineral content (~7.3% FFB) or relative body protein (or both) (Cote and Adams 1993; Ortiz et al. 1992; Wagner and Heyward 2001). Because of this difference in FFB density, the body fat of blacks will be systematically underestimated when two-component model equations are used to estimate %BF. In fact, negative %BF values were reported for professional football players whose measured Db exceeded 1.10 $g \cdot cc^{-1}$ (Adams et al. 1982). Likewise, the FFB density of white children is estimated to be only 1.086 $g \cdot cc^{-1}$ because of their relative lower mineral (5.2% FFB) and higher body water values (76.6% FFB) compared to the reference body (Lohman, Boileau, and Slaughter 1984). Also, the average density of the FFB of elderly white men and women is 1.098 $g \cdot cc^{-1}$ because of the relatively low body mineral value (6.2% FFB) in this population (Heymsfield et al. 1989). Thus, the relative body fat of children and persons who are elderly will be systematically overestimated using two-component model equations.

For certain population subgroups, therefore, scientists have applied **multicomponent models** of body composition based on measured total body water and bone mineral values. With the multicomponent approach, you can avoid systematic errors in estimating body fat by replacing the reference body with population-specific reference bodies that take into account the age (e.g., for children, for persons who are elderly), gender, and ethnicity of the individual. Table 8.2 provides population-specific formulas for converting Db to %BF. You will note that population-specific conversion formulas do not yet exist for all age groups within each ethnic group. You may have to use the age-specific conversion formula developed for white males and females in these cases. Also, you can use the population-specific conversion formulas for anorexic and obese females only when it is obvious that your client is either anorexic or obese.

REFERENCE METHODS FOR ASSESSING BODY COMPOSITION

In many laboratory and clinical settings, **densitometry** and dual-energy X-ray absorptiometry are used to obtain reference measures of body composition. For densitometric methods, total **body density (Db)** is estimated from the ratio of body mass to

Table 8.2 Population-Specific Two-Component Model Formulas for Converting Body Density to Percent Body Fat

Population	Age (yr)	Gender	%BF[a]	FFB_d (g·cc^{-1})*
Race or ethnicity				
African American	9-17	Female	(5.24 / Db) − 4.82	1.088
	19-45	Male	(4.86 / Db) − 4.39	1.106
	24-79	Female	(4.85 / Db) − 4.39	1.106
American Indian	18-62	Male	(4.97 / Db) − 4.52	1.099
	18-60	Female	(4.81 / Db) − 4.34	1.108
Asian				
Japanese Native	18-48	Male	(4.97 / Db) − 4.52	1.099
		Female	(4.76 / Db) − 4.28	1.111
	61-78	Male	(4.87 / Db) − 4.41	1.105
		Female	(4.95 / Db) − 4.50	1.100
Singaporean (Chinese, Indian, Malay)		Male	(4.94 / Db) − 4.48	1.102
		Female	(4.84 / Db) − 4.37	1.107
White	8-12	Male	(5.27 / Db) − 4.85	1.086
		Female	(5.27 / Db) − 4.85	1.086
	13-17	Male	(5.12 / Db) − 4.69	1.092
		Female	(5.19 / Db) − 4.76	1.090
	18-59	Male	(4.95 / Db) − 4.50	1.100
		Female	(4.96 / Db) − 4.51	1.101
	60-90	Male	(4.97 / Db) − 4.52	1.099
		Female	(5.02 / Db) − 4.57	1.098
Hispanic		Male	NA	NA
	20-40	Female	(4.87 / Db) − 4.41	1.105
Athletes				
Resistance trained	24 ± 4	Male	(5.21 / Db) − 4.78	1.089
	35 ± 6	Female	(4.97 / Db) − 4.52	1.099
Endurance trained	21 ± 2	Male	(5.03 / Db) − 4.59	1.097
	21 ± 4	Female	(4.95 / Db) − 4.50	1.100
All sports	18-22	Male	(5.12 / Db) − 4.68	1.093
	18-22	Female	(4.97 / Db) − 4.52	1.099
Clinical populations				
Anorexia nervosa	15-44	Female	(4.96 / Db) − 4.51	1.101
Obesity	17-62	Female	(4.95 / Db) − 4.50	1.100
Spinal cord injury (paraplegic or quadriplegic)	18-73	Male	(4.67 / Db) − 4.18	1.116
		Female	(4.70 / Db) − 4.22	1.114

FFB_d = fat-free body density; Db = body density; %BF = percent body fat; NA = no data available for this population subgroup.

[a]Multiply value by 100 to calculate %BF.

*FFB_d based on average values reported in selected research articles.

Reprinted, by permission, from V. Heyward and D. Wagner, 2004, *Applied body composition assessment,* 2nd ed. (Champaign, IL: Human Kinetics), 9.

body volume (Db = BM / BV). Body volume can be measured using either hydrostatic weighing or air displacement plethysmography.

Hydrostatic Weighing

Hydrostatic weighing (HW) is a valid, reliable, and widely used laboratory method for assessing total Db. Hydrostatic weighing provides an estimate of total **body volume (BV)** from the water displaced by the body's volume. According to **Archimedes' principle,** weight loss under water is directly proportional to the volume of water displaced by the body volume. For calculating Db, body mass is divided by body volume. The total Db is a function of the amounts of muscle, bone, water, and fat in the body.

Using Hydrostatic Weighing

Determine BV by totally submerging the body in an underwater weighing tank or pool and measuring the **underwater weight (UWW)** of the body. To measure UWW, you can use either a chair attached

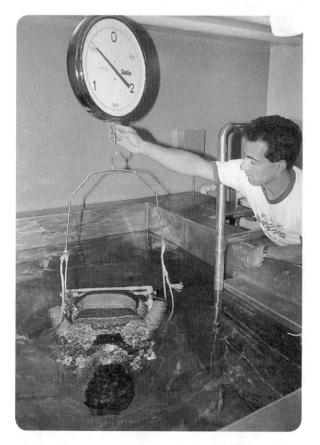

Figure 8.1 Hydrostatic weighing using scale and chair.

to an HW scale (see figure 8.1) or a platform attached to load cells (see figure 8.2). Given that the weight loss under water is directly proportional to the volume of water displaced by the body's volume, the BV is equal to the body mass (BM) minus the UWW (see figure 8.3). The net UWW is the difference between the UWW and the weight of the chair or platform and its supporting equipment (i.e., tare weight). The BV must be corrected for the volume of air remaining in the lungs after a maximal expiration (i.e., **residual volume** or **RV**), as well as the volume of air in the gastrointestinal tract (GV). The GV is assumed to be 100 ml.

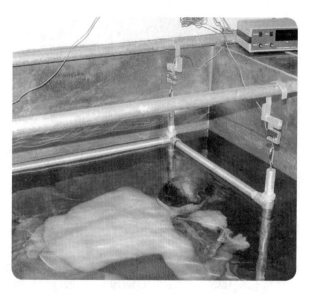

Figure 8.2 Hydrostatic weighing using load cells and platform.

The RV is commonly measured using helium dilution, nitrogen washout, or oxygen dilution techniques. The RV is measured in liters and must be converted to kilograms (kg) in order to correct UWW. This is easy to do because 1 L of water weighs approximately 1 kg; therefore, the water weight per liter of RV is 1 kg. To correct the BV, you subtract the equivalent weight of the RV and the GV (100 ml or 0.1 kg). Since water density varies with water temperature, the BV is corrected for water density (see figure 8.3). Under normal circumstances, the water temperature of the underwater weighing tank or swimming pool will be between 34° and 36° C. The resulting equation for BV is

BV = [(BM – net UWW) / density of water] – (RV + GV)

Hydrostatic Weighing Data

Name _____   Date _____

Gender _____

Ethnicity _____

Body mass (BM) _____ lb _____ kg   Age _____

I. Measured RV:
    (average 2 trials within 100 ml)

    Estimated RV (select one equation from appendix D.1, p. 362):

    Trial 1 _____ Trial 2 _____ Trial 3 _____

    Average measured RV = _____ L   Estimated RV = _____ L

II. Water temperature _____ °C
    Water density _____ g·cc⁻¹

Temperature (°C)	Density (g·cc⁻¹)
33	0.9947
34	0.9944
35	0.9941
36	0.9937
37	0.9934

III. Gross underwater weight (in kg)

    Trial 1 _____   Trial 6 _____
    Trial 2 _____   Trial 7 _____
    Trial 3 _____   Trial 8 _____
    Trial 4 _____   Trial 9 _____
    Trial 5 _____   Trial 10 _____
    Average (3 trials within 0.1 kg)   _____ kg

IV. Tare weight (chair, platform, and supporting
    equipment)   _____ kg

V. Net underwater weight
    gross UWW _____ – tare weight _____ =   _____ kg

VI. Body volume (BV)
    [(BM in kg – net UWW in kg) / water density] – (RV + GV)
    Note: GV assumed value = 100 ml or 0.1 L   BV = _____ L

VII. Body density = BM (kg) / BV (L)
    (carry out to 5 or 6 decimal places) D_b = _____ g·cc⁻¹

VIII. Percent body fat (select conversion formula from table 8.2)   BF = _____ %

IX. Fat weight = BM × %BF (decimal)
    _____ × _____   FW = _____ kg

X. Fat-free mass = BM – FW
    _____ – _____   FFM = _____ kg

Comments and observations:

Figure 8.3 Hydrostatic weighing data collection form.

Calculate body density (Db in g·cc⁻¹) by dividing BM by BV: Db = BM / BV. After you calculate Db, you can convert it into **percent body fat (%BF)** by using the appropriate population-specific conversion formula (see table 8.2).

You should adhere to "Guidelines for Hydrostatic Weighing" when using the HW technique.

In addition to the HW testing guidelines, following the suggestions in "Tips for Minimizing Error in Hydrostatic Weighing" may improve the accuracy of your underwater weighing measurements.

Special Considerations

Some clients may have difficulty performing the HW test using these standardized procedures. Accurate test results are highly dependent on the client's skill, cooperation, and motivation. The following section addresses the use of modified HW procedures, as well as other questions and concerns about the use of this method.

Guidelines for Hydrostatic Weighing

Pretest Guidelines for Clients

■ Do not eat or engage in strenuous exercise for at least 4 hr before your scheduled appointment.

■ Avoid ingesting any gas-producing foods or beverages (e.g., baked beans, diet soda) for at least 12 hr before your test.

■ Bring a towel and a tight-fitting, lightweight swimsuit.

Testing Procedure Guidelines

■ Carefully calibrate the body weight scale and underwater weighing scale. To determine the accuracy of the autopsy scale, hang calibrated weights from the scale and check the corresponding scale values. To calibrate a load cell system, place weights on the platform and check the recorded values.

■ Measure the underwater weight of the chair or platform and of the supporting equipment and weight belt; the total is the **tare weight.**

■ Measure your client's dry weight (weight in air) to the nearest 50 g.

■ Check and record the water temperature of the tank just before the test; it should range between 34° and 36° C. Use the constant values in figure 8.3 (see p. 194) to determine the density of the water at that temperature.

■ Instruct your client to enter the tank slowly, so that the water stays calm. Have the client gently submerge without touching the chair or weighing platform and rub hands over the body to eliminate air bubbles from the swimsuit, skin, and hair.

■ Have the client kneel on the underwater weighing platform or sit in the chair. Your client may need to wear a scuba diving weight belt to facilitate the kneeling or sitting position. If RV is being measured simultaneously, insert the mouthpiece at this time. If RV is measured outside of the tank, administer the RV test before the client changes clothes and showers.

■ Have the client take a few normal breaths and then exhale maximally while slowly bending forward to submerge the head. Check to make certain that the client's head and back are completely underwater and that the arms and feet are not touching the sides or bottom of the tank. Instruct the client to continue exhaling until RV is reached. The client needs to remain as still as possible during this procedure. A relaxed and motionless state underwater will aid in an accurate reading of UWW.

■ Record the highest stable weight with the client fully submerged at RV; then signal to the client that the trial is completed.

■ Administer as many trials as needed to obtain three readings within ±100 g. Most clients achieve a consistent and maximal UWW in four or five trials (Bonge and Donnelly 1989). Average the three highest trials and record this value as the gross UWW.

■ Determine the net UWW by subtracting the tare weight from the gross UWW. The net UWW is used to calculate body volume (see figure 8.3, p. 194).

■ *What should I do when my client is unable to blow out all of the air from the lungs or remain still while under water?*

You will likely come across clients who are uncomfortable expelling all of the air from their lungs during HW. In such cases, you can weigh these individuals at functional residual capacity (FRC) or total lung capacity (TLC) instead of RV. Thomas and Etheridge (1980) underwater-weighed 43 males, comparing the body densities measured at FRC (taken at the end of normal expiration while the person was submerged) and at RV (at the end of maximal expiration). The two methods yielded similar results. Similarly, Timson and Coffman (1984) reported that Db measured by HW at TLC (vital capacity + RV) was similar (less than 0.3% BF difference) to that measured at RV if TLC was measured in the water. However, when the TLC was measured out of the water, the method significantly overestimated Db. When using these modifications of the HW method, you must still measure RV in order to calculate the FRC or TLC of your client. Also, be certain to substitute the appropriate lung volume (FRC or TLC) for RV in the calculation of BV.

Because of their lower Db, clients with greater amounts of body fat are more buoyant than leaner individuals; therefore, they have more difficulty remaining motionless while under the water. To correct this problem, place a weighted scuba belt around the client's waist. Be certain to include the weight of the scuba belt when measuring and subtracting the tare weight of the HW system.

■ *What should I do when my clients are afraid to put their face in the water or are not flexible enough to get their backs and heads completely submerged?*

Occasionally, you will encounter clients who are extremely fearful of being submerged, who dislike facial contact with water, or who are unable to bend forward to assume the proper body position for HW. In such cases, a satisfactory alternative would be to weigh your clients at TLC while their heads remain above water level. Donnelly and colleagues (1988) compared this measure (i.e., TLCNS or total lung capacity with head not submerged) to the criterion Db obtained from HW at RV for 75 men and 67 women. Vital capacity was measured with the subject submerged in the water to shoulder level. Regression analysis yielded the following equations for predicting Db at RV, using the Db determined at TLCNS as the predictor:

Tips for Minimizing Error in Hydrostatic Weighing

- Make sure that your clients adhere to all pretesting guidelines.

- Before each test session, check the calibration of the BW and UWW scales or load cells and carefully calibrate the gas analyzers used to measure RV.

- Precisely measure BW to ±50 g, UWW to ±100 g, and RV to ±100 ml.

- Coach the client to maximally exhale and remain motionless under the water.

- Steady the underwater weighing apparatus as the client submerges, but remove your hand from the scale before actually reading the UWW.

- If possible, use a load cell system and measure RV and UWW simultaneously.

- Carry the calculated Db value out to five decimal places. Rounding off a Db of 1.07499 g·cc^{-1} to 1.07 g·cc^{-1} corresponds to a difference of 2.2% BF when converted with the Siri (1961) two-component model formula.

- If you are estimating %BF from Db with a two-component model, use the appropriate population-specific conversion formula (see table 8.2).

Males

Db at RV = 0.5829(Db at TLCNS) + 0.4059

$r = 0.88$, $SEE = 0.0067$ g·cc^{-1}

Females

Db at RV = 0.4745(Db at TLCNS) + 0.5173

$r = 0.85$, $SEE = 0.0061$ g·cc^{-1}

The correlations (*r*) between the actual Db at RV and the predicted Db at RV were high, and the standard errors of estimate (*SEE*) were within acceptable limits. These equations were cross-validated for an independent sample of 20 men and 20 women. The differences between the Db from HW at RV and the predicted Db from weighing at TLCNS were quite small (less than 0.0014 g·cc^{-1} or 0.7% BF). This method may be especially useful for HW of older adults, obese individuals with limited flexibility, and people with physical disabilities.

■ *Will the accuracy of the HW test be affected if I estimate RV instead of measuring it?*

Several prediction equations have been developed to estimate RV based on the individual's age, height, gender, and smoking status (see appendix D.1, "Prediction Equations for Residual Volume" p. 362). However, these RV prediction equations have large prediction errors (*SEE* = 400 to 500 ml). When RV is measured, the precision of the HW method is excellent (≤1% BF). However, this precision error increases substantially (±2.8% to 3.7% BF) when RV is estimated (Morrow et al. 1986). Therefore, always measure RV when you are using the HW method.

■ *When is the best time during the menstrual cycle to hydrostatically weigh my female clients?*

Some women, particularly those whose body weight fluctuates widely during their menstrual cycles, may have significantly different estimates of Db and %BF when weighed hydrostatically at different times in their cycles. Bunt, Lohman, and Boileau (1989) reported that changes in total body water values due to water retention during the menstrual cycle partly explain the differences in body weight and Db during a menstrual cycle. On the average, the relative body fat of the women was 24.8% BF at their lowest body weights, compared to an average of 27.6% BF at their peak body weights during their menstrual cycles. Because their low and peak body weights occurred at different times during the menstrual cycle (varied from 0 to 14 days prior to the onset of the next menses), the effect of total body water fluctuations cannot be routinely controlled by using the same day of the menstrual cycle for all women. However, when you are monitoring changes in body composition over time or establishing healthy body weight for a female client, it is recommended that you hydrostatically weigh her at the same time within her menstrual cycle and outside of the period of her perceived peak body weight.

Air Displacement Plethysmography

Air displacement plethysmography (ADP) is a method used to measure body volume and density that uses air displacement instead of water displacement to estimate volume. Because ADP is quick

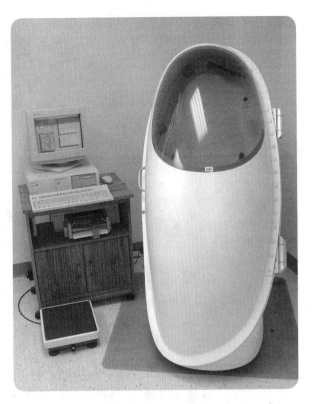

Figure 8.4 Air displacement plethysmograph.

(usually 5-10 min) and requires minimal client compliance and minimal technician skill, it may prove to be an alternative to hydrostatic weighing. The ADP method requires a whole-body plethysmograph such as the Bod Pod. The Bod Pod is a large, egg-shaped fiberglass chamber that uses air displacement and pressure–volume relationships to measure body volume (see figure 8.4).

The Bod Pod system consists of two chambers: a front chamber in which the client sits during the measurement and a rear reference chamber. A molded fiberglass seat forms the wall between the two chambers, and a moving diaphragm mounted in this wall oscillates during testing (figure 8.5). The oscillating diaphragm creates small volume changes between the two chambers. These changes are equal in magnitude but opposite in sign, and they produce small pressure fluctuations. The pressure–volume relationship is used to calculate the volume of the front chamber when it is empty and when the client is sitting in it. Body volume is calculated as the difference in the volume of the chamber with and without the client inside.

The principle underlying ADP centers on the relationship between pressure and volume. At

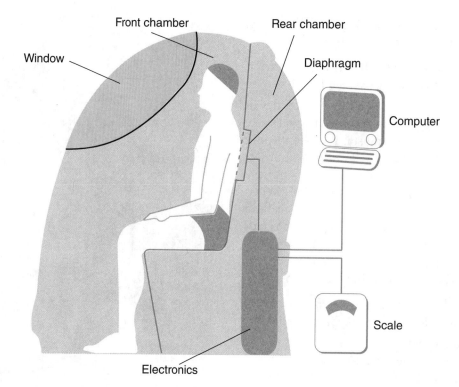

Figure 8.5 Two-chamber Bod Pod system.

a constant temperature (isothermal condition), volume (V) and pressure (P) are inversely related. According to **Boyle's law,**

$$P_1 / P_2 = V_2 / V_1,$$

where P_1 and V_1 represent one paired condition of pressure and volume and P_2 and V_2 represent another paired condition. P_1 and V_1 correspond to the pressure and volume of the Bod Pod when it is empty; P_2 and V_2 represent the pressure and volume of the Bod Pod when the client is in the chamber.

One assumption of the ADP method is that the Bod Pod controls the isothermal effects of clothing, hair, thoracic gas volume, and body surface area in the enclosed chamber. Bod Pod clients are tested while wearing minimal clothing (a swimsuit) and a swim cap to compress the hair. An estimate of the **body surface area**, calculated from the height and weight of the client, is used to correct for the isothermal effects at the body's surface. **Thoracic gas volume (TGV)** is the volume of air in the lungs (functional residual capacity) at midexhalation. The TGV is either directly measured or estimated by the Bod Pod to account for the isothermal conditions in the lungs. The Bod Pod software calculates the functional residual capacity at end exhalation by subtracting one-half of the exhaled tidal volume from the FRC measured at midexhalation.

Numerous studies have assessed the accuracy of the Bod Pod for measuring Db. Several researchers reported only small differences in average Db (≤ 0.002 g·cc^{-1}) measured by the Bod Pod and HW (Fields et al. 2001; Vescovi et al. 2001; Yee et al. 2001). Some studies have reported slightly higher and statistically significant differences (0.003-0.007 g·cc^{-1}) in adults (Collins et al. 1999; Demerath et al. 2002; Dewit et al. 2000; Millard-Stafford et al. 2001; Wagner, Heyward, and Gibson 2000). In high school male athletes and collegiate track and field female athletes, the Bod Pod significantly underestimated average body density (Bentzur, Kravitz, and Lockner 2008; Moon et al. 2008).

Several studies, however, showed "good" group prediction errors (*SEE* ≤ 0.008 g·cc^{-1}) for adults (Fields, Hunter, and Goran 2000; Nunez et al. 1999; Wagner et al. 2000). Compared to multicomponent body composition models, the Bod Pod and HW methods have similar predictive accuracy (Fields et al. 2001). Because the Bod Pod is more accommodating than HW, there is much interest in establishing the validity of the ADP method for estimating %BF in clinical populations and special populations such as children and older adults (Heyward and Wagner 2004).

Using the ADP Method

The Bod Pod is user friendly, providing computer prompts for each step of the procedure. Air displacement plethysmography is faster and easier than HW; researchers reported better compliance with ADP and a preference for ADP over HW among participants, including among children (Demerath et al. 2002; Dewit et al. 2000; Lockner et al. 2000). Before the scheduled appointment, give your client pretesting instructions. These instructions are the same as those for HW (see p. 195) except for the addition of bringing a swim cap. For step-by-step instructions for Bod Pod testing, see "Testing Procedures for the Bod Pod."

Special Considerations for the ADP Method

Accurate test results from the Bod Pod depend on a number of factors. The following questions address these factors.

■ *How will the test results be affected if my client has excess body hair?*

As mentioned earlier, isothermal air trapped in body hair may affect test results. For clients with beards, %BF may be underestimated by 1%; when scalp hair is exposed (no swim cap), relative body fat is underestimated by about 2.3% BF (Higgins et al. 2001). Wearing a tight-fitting swim cap and shaving excess facial and body hair ensure the most accurate estimate of body volume and Db.

■ *Can I use the Bod Pod to measure the body composition of children?*

During the 20 sec test, the client must remain very still, as the body volume estimate from the ADP method can vary if the client moves during testing. Fields and Goran (2000) commented that it took twice as long to measure children compared to adults, primarily because children move during the test. As a result, the test–retest reliability of the Bod Pod is lower in children ($r = 0.90$) than in adults ($r = 0.96$) (Demerath et al. 2002).

Also, several researchers commented that body size may affect Bod Pod estimates, with the largest effects seen in the smallest clients (Demerath et al. 2002; Lockner et al. 2000; Nunez et al. 1999). The ideal chamber-to-client volume ratio may be exceeded for clients who have a small body, especially children (Fields and Goran 2000). This area requires further investigation.

■ *Is it absolutely necessary that my client wear a swimsuit and swim cap during the Bod Pod test?*

The original investigators of the Bod Pod recognized that the isothermal effect of clothing leads to an underestimation of body volume; they

---

Testing Procedures for the Bod Pod

- Instruct the client to change into a swimsuit and to completely void the bladder and bowels.

- Measure the client's height to the nearest centimeter and body weight to the nearest 5 g using the Bod Pod scale. These measures are used to calculate body surface area.

- Perform the two-point calibration: (a) baseline calibration with the chamber empty and (b) phantom calibration with a 50 L calibration cylinder. Be careful when handling the calibration cylinder; a dent in the cylinder alters its volume.

- Instruct your client to sit in the chamber and close the door tightly. During this 20 sec test, ask your client to breathe normally.

- Open the door and then close it tightly; repeat the 20 sec test. If the two tests disagree by more than 150 ml, perform additional tests until two results agree within 150 ml; average these and use them to calculate raw BV.

- Open the door and connect the client to the system's breathing circuit to begin the TGV measurement.

- Close the door. After a few tidal volume (normal) breathing cycles, the airway is occluded by the Bod Pod. Instruct your client to perform the puffing maneuver. If the computer-calculated figure of merit (indicating similar pressure signals in the airway and chamber) is not met, repeat this step.

recommended that clients wear only a swimsuit and swim cap during testing to minimize this effect (Dempster and Aitkens 1995; McCrory et al. 1995). More clothing leads to a larger layer of isothermal air and a greater underestimation of body volume. For example, wearing a hospital gown instead of a swimsuit lowers %BF by about 5% (Fields et al. 2000). Thus, the clothing recommendation needs to be followed.

■ Do I need to measure my client's TGV or can I use a predicted TGV?

Although McCrory and colleagues (1998) reported an insignificant difference (54 ml) between measured and predicted TGV, the *SEE* was large (442 ml). Some researchers have reported larger mean differences (344-400 ml) and *SEE*s (650 ml) (Collins et al. 1999; Lockner et al. 2000). Given that only 40% of the TGV value is used to calculate body volume, using a predicted TGV has a relatively smaller effect on Db and %BF compared to using a predicted RV for the HW method. Nevertheless, a measured TGV maximizes accuracy.

■ Does the Bod Pod yield a valid and reliable measure of functional residual capacity?

Davis and colleagues (2007) compared FRC measures obtained from the Bod Pod and traditional gas dilution techniques in healthy males and females (18-50 yr). The FRC at midexpiration as measured by the Bod Pod was corrected to an end-exhalation volume by subtracting approximately one-half of the measured tidal volume. The mean difference between FRC from the Bod Pod and gas dilution FRC measures was –32 ml for males ($r = 0.925$; *SEE* = 0.246 L) and –23 ml for females ($r = 0.917$; *SEE* = 0.216 L). The test–retest reliability of the Bod Pod FRC was excellent ($r = 0.95$ to 0.97). These results suggest that the Bod Pod provides a valid and reliable measure of FRC in healthy adults.

■ If I use both hydrostatic weighing and the Bod Pod to measure my client's body composition, which test should I give first?

The Bod Pod manufacturer recommends testing clients under resting conditions and when the body is dry. Although there are no published studies indicating the amount of error that may occur if these guidelines are violated, experts suggest adhering to these recommendations (Fields, Goran, and McCrory 2002). Thus, if a test battery includes both

HW and ADP, administer the Bod Pod test first. If doing so is not possible, make certain that your client is completely dry and fully recovered from the HW test before you administer the Bod Pod test.

■ Which model and equation should I use to convert Db to %BF?

Using a multicomponent model and a population-specific conversion formula increases the group and individual accuracy of %BF estimates. The default equation in the Bod Pod software is the Siri (1961) two-component model formula for non-black adults. A formula for blacks is also available. In field settings, these two-component conversion formulas may be appropriate for some clients with certain demographic characteristics. For other clients you may need to select an appropriate population-specific, two-component model formula (see table 8.2, p. 192).

Dual-Energy X-Ray Absorptiometry

Dual-energy X-ray absorptiometry (DXA) is gaining recognition as a reference method for body composition research (see figure 8.6). This method yields estimates of bone mineral, fat, and lean soft tissue mass. Dual-energy X-ray absorptiometry is an attractive alternative to HW because it is safe and rapid (a total body scan takes 10-20 min), requires minimal client cooperation, and, most importantly, accounts for individual variability in bone mineral content.

The basic principle underlying DXA technology is that the attenuation of X rays with high and low photon energies is measurable and dependent on the thickness, density, and chemical composition of the underlying tissue. The **attenuation**, or weakening, of X rays through fat, lean tissue, and bone varies due to differences in the densities and chemical compositions of these tissues. The attenuation ratios for the high and low X-ray energies are thought to be constant for all individuals (Pietrobelli et al. 1996).

It is difficult to assess the validity of the DXA method because each of the three manufacturers of DXA instruments (see "Sources for Equipment," p. 227) has developed its own models and software over the years. As many researchers and some clinicians have discovered, body composition results vary with manufacturer, model, and software version. Thus, some of the variability reported in DXA validation studies may be due to the different DXA scanners and software versions. Thus experts who

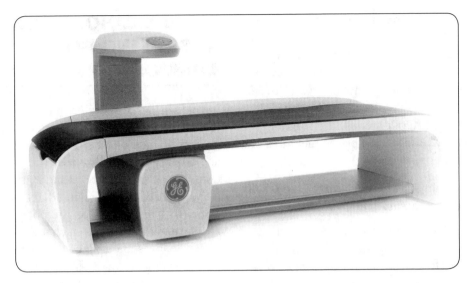

Figure 8.6 Dual-energy X-ray absorptiometer.
© 2006 General Electric Company.

have reviewed DXA studies have called for more standardization among manufacturers (Genton et al. 2002; Lohman 1996).

Some researchers have reported that the predictive accuracy of DXA is better than that of HW (Fields and Goran 2000; Friedl et al. 1992; Prior et al. 1997; Wagner and Heyward 2001; Withers et al. 1998). However, the opposite finding (that HW is more accurate than DXA) has also been reported (Bergsma-Kadijk et al. 1996; Goran, Toth, and Poehlman 1998; Millard-Stafford et al. 2001). In a review of the DXA studies using recently developed software, Lohman and colleagues concluded that DXA estimates of %BF are within 1% to 3% of multicomponent model estimates (Lohman et al. 2000). Although some body composition prediction equations have been developed and validated with DXA as the reference method, further research is needed before DXA can be firmly established as the best reference method. Still, the DXA method is widely used in light of its availability, ease of use, and low radiation exposure (Yee and Gallagher 2008).

Using the DXA Method

The DXA method requires minimal client cooperation and minimal technical skill. However, to use the scanner to get precise and accurate DXA scans, proper training is essential. Also, many states require that a licensed X-ray technician perform the scan. For general procedures for DXA testing, see "Basic Testing Procedures for DXA."

Basic Testing Procedures for DXA

- Before testing, calibrate the DXA scanner with a calibration marker provided by the manufacturer.
- Measure your client's height and weight with the client wearing minimal clothing and no shoes.
- Carefully place the client in a supine position on the scanner bed for a head-to-toe, anteroposterior scan.
- Use a skeletal anthropometer to accurately determine body thickness (see "Sagittal Abdominal Diameter" on p. 222).
- Set the scanner for a whole-body scan at medium speed, which usually takes about 20 min. For clients with sagittal abdominal diameters exceeding 27 cm (10.6 in.), use a slow scan, which typically takes 40 min.

Special Considerations

The accuracy of DXA results depends on a number of factors. The following questions address some of these factors.

■ **Will my client's body size and hydration state affect the test results?**

The DXA method should not be used to assess the body composition of clients whose body dimensions exceed the length or width of the scanning bed. Research has shown that normal fluctuations in hydration have little effect on DXA estimates (Lohman et al. 2000). However, the measurement error of DXA for lean tissue mass was higher in obese children compared to nonobese children (Wosje, Knipstein, and Kalkwarf 2006). Also, Williams and colleagues (2006) reported that in longitudinal studies, DXA may yield biased measures of changes in body composition.

■ *For client comfort and compliance, is DXA better than other reference methods?*

Compared to other reference methods, DXA requires little client participation. The client does not need to perform the breathing maneuvers that are required for measuring RV for hydrostatic weighing and TGV for air displacement plethysmography.

■ *How do the various DXA machines and software versions affect test results?*

As mentioned previously, variability among DXA technologies is a major source of error. Although all DXA equipment uses the same underlying physical principles, the instruments differ in their generation of the high- and low-energy beams (filter or switching voltage), imaging geometry (pencil beam or fan beam), X-ray detectors, calibration methodology, and algorithms (Genton et al. 2002). Updated software versions have improved the accuracy of DXA over that of the early 1990s (Kohrt 1998; Lohman et al. 2000; Tothill and Hannan 2000); however, the accuracy of updated DXA devices and software still needs to be determined (Genton et al. 2002). Because of technological differences, you should use the same DXA device and software version for longitudinal assessments or cross-sectional comparisons of body composition.

■ *Is the DXA method safe for my clients, given that it uses X rays to measure body composition?*

Dual-energy X-ray absorptiometry is considered safe for estimating body composition. The average skin dose of radiation is low, similar to a typical weekly exposure of environmental background radiation (Lukaski 1993). Still, DXA tests are not recommended for pregnant women.

FIELD METHODS FOR ASSESSING BODY COMPOSITION

In field settings, you can use more practical methods to estimate your client's body composition. Your choices include bioelectrical impedance, skinfold, and other types of anthropometric prediction equations. To use these methods and equations appropriately, you need to understand the basic assumptions and principles, as well as the potential sources of measurement error for each method. You must closely follow standardized testing procedures, and you must practice in order to perfect your measurement techniques for each method. For more detailed information about these field methods and how they are applied to various population subgroups, see Heyward and Wagner (2004).

Skinfold Method

A **skinfold (SKF)** indirectly measures the thickness of subcutaneous adipose tissue. When you use the SKF method to estimate total Db in order to calculate relative body fat (%BF), certain basic relationships are assumed:

■ **The SKF is a good measure of subcutaneous fat.** Research has demonstrated that the subcutaneous fat, assessed by SKF measurements at 12 sites, is similar to the value obtained from magnetic resonance imaging (Hayes et al. 1988).

■ **The distribution of fat subcutaneously and internally is similar for all individuals within each gender.** The validity of this assumption is questionable. There are large interindividual differences in the patterning of subcutaneous adipose tissue within and between genders (Martin et al. 1985). Older subjects of the same gender and Db have proportionally less subcutaneous fat than their younger counterparts. Also, lean individuals have a higher proportion of internal fat, and the proportion of fat located internally decreases as overall body fatness increases (Lohman 1981).

■ **Because there is a relationship between subcutaneous fat and total body fat, the sum of several SKFs can be used to estimate total body fat.** Research has established that SKF thicknesses at multiple sites measure a common body fat factor

(Jackson and Pollock 1976; Quatrochi et al. 1992). It is assumed that approximately one-third of the total fat is located subcutaneously in men and women (Lohman 1981). However, there is considerable biological variation in subcutaneous, intramuscular, intermuscular, and internal organ fat deposits (Clarys et al. 1987), as well as essential lipids in bone marrow and the central nervous system. Age, gender, and degree of fatness all affect variation in fat distribution (Lohman 1981).

■ **There is a relationship between the sum of SKFs (ΣSKF) and Db.** This relationship is linear for homogeneous samples (population-specific SKF equations) but nonlinear over a wide range of Db (generalized SKF equations) for both men and women. A linear regression line depicting the relationship between the ΣSKF and Db will fit the data well only within a narrow range of body fatness values. Thus, you will get an inaccurate estimate if you use a population-specific equation to estimate the Db of a client who is not representative of the sample used to develop that equation (Jackson 1984).

■ **Age is an independent predictor of Db for both men and women.** Using age and the quadratic expression of the sum of skinfolds (ΣSKF²) accounts for more variance in Db of a heterogeneous population than using the ΣSKF² alone (Jackson 1984).

Using the Skinfold Method

Skinfold prediction equations are developed using either linear (population specific) or quadratic (generalized) regression models. There are well over 100 population-specific equations for predicting Db from various combinations of SKFs, circumferences, and bony diameters (Jackson and Pollock 1985). These equations were developed for relatively homogeneous populations and are assumed to be valid only for individuals having similar characteristics, such as age, gender, ethnicity, or level of physical activity. For example, an equation derived specifically for 18 to 21 yr old sedentary men would not be valid for predicting the Db of 35 to 45 yr old sedentary men. Population-specific equations are based on a linear relationship between SKF fat and

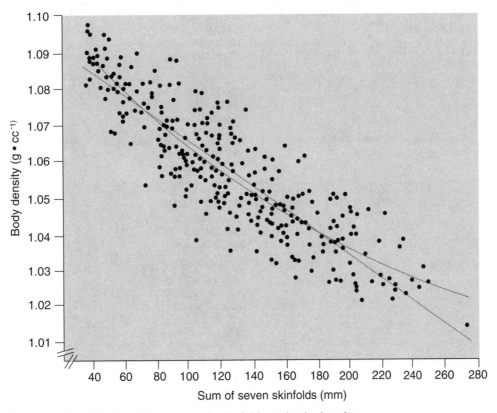

Figure 8.7 Relationship of sum of skinfolds to body density.

Db (linear model); however, research shows that there is a curvilinear relationship (quadratic model) between SKFs and Db across a large range of body fatness (see figure 8.7, p. 203). Population-specific equations will tend to underestimate %BF in fatter subjects and overestimate it in leaner subjects.

Using the quadratic model, Jackson and colleagues (Jackson and Pollock 1978; Jackson, Pollock, and Ward 1980) developed generalized equations applicable to individuals varying greatly in age (18 to 60 yr) and body fatness (up to 45% BF). These equations also take into account the effect of age on the distribution of subcutaneous and internal fat. An advantage of the generalized equations is that you can use one equation, instead of several, to accurately estimate your clients' %BF.

Given that these generalized SKF equations were developed on predominately white adults, Jackson and colleagues (2009) recently cross-validated the equations with samples of young white, Hispanic, and African American men and women (17-35 yr). The DXA method was used to obtain reference measures of %BF for 706 women and 423 men. Although the generalized SKF equations were highly correlated ($r = 0.91$) with $\%BF_{DXA}$, these equations lacked accuracy when applied to racially and ethnically diverse samples. New race-specific equations were developed and reported. Before these equations can be recommended, however, additional research is needed to establish the validity of DXA as a reference method.

Most equations use two or three SKFs to predict Db. Experts recommend using equations that have SKF measures from a variety of sites, including both upper and lower body sites (Martin et al. 1985). The Db is then converted to %BF using the appropriate population-specific conversion formula (see table 8.2). Table 8.3 presents commonly used

Table 8.3 Skinfold Prediction Equations

SKF sites	Population subgroups	Equation	Reference
Σ7SKF (chest + abdomen + thigh + triceps + subscapular + suprailiac + midaxilla	Black or Hispanic women, 18-55 yr	Db (g·cc^{-1})^a = 1.0970 − 0.00046971(Σ7SKF) + 0.00000056(Σ7SKF)^2 − 0.00012828(age)	Jackson et al. (1980)
	Black men or male athletes, 18-61 yr	Db (g·cc^{-1})^a = 1.1120 − 0.00043499(Σ7SKF) + 0.00000055(Σ7SKF)^2 − 0.00028826(age)	Jackson and Pollock (1978)
Σ4SKF (triceps + anterior suprailiac + abdomen + thigh)	Female athletes, 18-29 yr	Db (g·cc^{-1})^a = 1.096095 − 0.0006952(Σ4SKF) + 0.0000011(Σ4SKF)^2 − 0.0000714(age)	Jackson et al. (1980)
Σ3SKF (triceps + suprailiac + thigh)	White or anorexic women, 18-55 yr	Db (g·cc^{-1})^a = 1.0994921 − 0.0009929(Σ3SKF) + 0.0000023(Σ3SKF)^2 − 0.0001392(age)	Jackson et al. (1980)
Σ3SKF (chest + abdomen + thigh)	White men, 18-61 yr	Db (g·cc^{-1})^a = 1.109380 − 0.0008267(Σ3SKF) + 0.0000016(Σ3SKF)^2 − 0.0002574(age)	Jackson and Pollock (1978)
Σ3SKF (abdomen + thigh + triceps)	Black or white collegiate male and female athletes, 18-34 yr	%BF = 8.997 + 0.2468(Σ3SKF) − 6.343(gender^b) − 1.998(race^c)	Evans et al. (2005)
Σ2SKF (triceps + calf)	Black or white boys, 6-17 yr Black or white girls, 6-17 yr	%BF = 0.735(Σ2SKF) + 1.0 %BF = 0.610(Σ2SKF) + 5.1	Slaughter et al. (1988)

ΣSKF = sum of skinfolds (mm).

^{a}Use population-specific conversion formulas to calculate %BF (percent body fat) from Db (body density).

^{b}Male athletes = 1; female athletes = 0.

^{c}Black athletes = 1; white athletes = 0.

population-specific and generalized SKF prediction equations. Select the appropriate SKF equation and population-specific conversion formula in table 8.2 to estimate %BF based on physical demographics (e.g., age, gender, ethnicity, and physical activity level) of your client. Using these equations, you can accurately estimate the %BF of your clients within the recommended value, ±3.5% BF (Lohman 1992).

Alternatively, nomograms exist for some SKF prediction equations. The nomogram in figure 8.8

was specifically developed for the Jackson sum-of-three-SKFs equations. To use this nomogram, plot the sum of three skinfolds (Σ3SKF) and age in the appropriate columns and use a ruler to connect these two points. The corresponding %BF is read at the point where the connecting line intersects the %BF column on the nomogram.

Although nomograms are potential time-savers, you should be aware that this nomogram is based on a two-component body composition model,

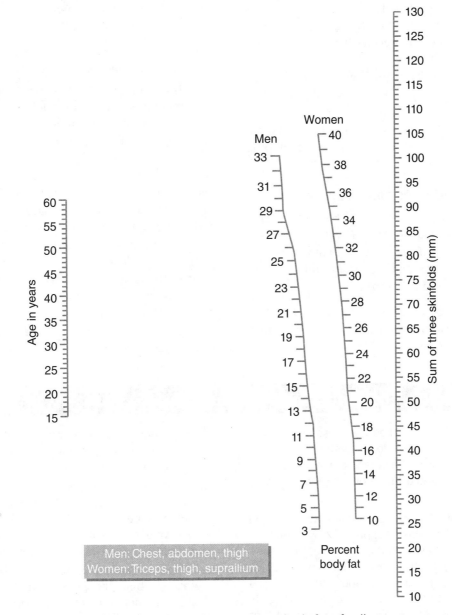

Figure 8.8 Nomogram to estimate percent body fat of college-age men and women using the Jackson sum-of-three-skinfolds equations.

From "A nomogram for the estimate of percent body fat from generalized equations," by W.B. Baun, M.R. Baun, and P.B. Raven, 1981, *Research Quarterly for Exercise and Sport,* 52(3), pg. 382. Copyright 1981 by American Alliance for Health, Physical Education, and Dance, 1900 Association Drive, Reston, VA 20191.

using the Siri equation to convert Db to %BF. In general, use this nomogram only to calculate %BF of clients with an estimated fat-free body density of 1.100 g·cc^{-1} (see table 8.2).

Skinfold Technique

It takes a great deal of time and practice to develop your skill as a SKF technician. Following standardized procedures (p. 207) will increase the accuracy and reliability of your measurements.

You will also be able to increase your skill as a SKF technician by following the recommendations (p. 207) made by experts in the field (Jackson and Pollock 1985; Lohman et al. 1984; Pollock and Jackson 1984).

In addition to perfecting your technical skills, you should develop your interpersonal skills when administering SKF and other anthropometric tests. For suggestions about developing interpersonal skills (Habash 2002), see "Tips for Developing Interpersonal Skills."

Sources of Measurement Error

The accuracy and precision of SKF measurements and the SKF method are affected by the technician's skill, the type of SKF caliper, and client factors. The following questions and responses address these sources of measurement error.

■ *Is there high agreement among SKF values when the measurements are taken by two different technicians?*

A major source of measurement error is differences between SKF technicians. Objectivity, or between-technician reliability, is improved when SKF technicians follow standardized testing procedures, practice taking SKFs together, and mark the SKF site (Pollock and Jackson 1984). A major cause of low intertester reliability is improper location and measurement of the SKF sites (Lohman et al. 1984). The amount of between-technician error depends on the SKF site, with larger errors reported for the abdomen (8.8%) and thigh (7.1%) sites than for the triceps (~3.0%), subscapular (~3.0-5.0%), and suprailiac (~4%) sites (Lohman et al. 1984).

■ *Are the anatomical descriptions for specific SKF sites the same for all SKF equations?*

In the past, for some SKF sites, the anatomical location and direction of the fold have varied. For example, Behnke and Wilmore (1974) recommend measuring the abdominal SKF using a horizontal fold adjacent to the umbilicus; Jackson and Pollock (1978), however, recommend measuring a vertical fold taken 2 cm (0.8 in.) lateral to the umbilicus. Inconsistencies such as this have led to confusion and lack of agreement among SKF technicians. As a result, groups of experts in the field of anthropometry have developed standardized testing procedures and detailed descriptions for identification and measurement of SKF sites (Harrison et al. 1988; Ross and Marfell-Jones 1991). Appendix D.2, "Standardized Sites for Skinfold Measurements" (p. 363), summarizes some of the most commonly used sites

---

Tips for Developing Interpersonal Skills

■ Before the scheduled test session, instruct your clients to wear loose clothing that allows easy access to the measurement sites, such as shorts and a T-shirt or two-piece exercise gear.

■ Often clients are apprehensive about having their SKFs measured, particularly when they are meeting you for the first time. During the testing, put your client at ease by establishing good rapport (e.g., talk about some unrelated topic), projecting a sense of relaxed confidence, and creating a test environment that is friendly, private, safe, and comfortable.

■ Perform the test in an uncluttered private room that holds a small table for calipers,

pens, and clipboards and a chair for clients who are unstable standing or need to rest during the testing.

■ Some clients feel more comfortable having their SKFs measured by a technician of the same gender. If this is not feasible, you could ask your clients if they would like another person of the same gender to observe the test.

■ Educate your clients about the SKF test by talking about the purpose and use of the measurements, pointing to the SKF sites on your body, and demonstrating on yourself how the SKF is measured.

■ Limit your verbal and facial reactions while collecting SKF data.

STANDARDIZED PROCEDURES FOR SKINFOLD MEASUREMENTS

1. Take all SKF measurements on the right side of the body.

2. Carefully identify, measure, and mark the SKF site, especially if you are a novice SKF technician (see appendix D.2, "Standardized Sites for Skinfold Measurements," p. 363).

3. Grasp the SKF firmly between the thumb and index finger of your left hand. Lift the fold 1 cm (0.4 in.) above the site to be measured.

4. Lift the fold by placing the thumb and index finger 8 cm (~3 in.) apart on a line that is perpendicular to the long axis of the SKF. The long axis is parallel to the natural cleavage lines of the skin. For individuals with extremely large SKFs, you will need to separate your thumb and finger more than 8 cm in order to lift the fold.

5. Keep the fold elevated while you take the measurement.

6. Place the jaws of the caliper perpendicular to the fold, approximately 1 cm below the thumb and index finger and halfway between the crest and the base of the fold. Release the jaw pressure slowly.

7. Take the SKF measurement 3 sec after the pressure is released. The American College of Sports Medicine (ACSM 2010) recommends that you wait only 1 to 2 sec before reading the caliper.

8. Open the jaws of the caliper to remove it from the site. Close the jaws slowly to prevent damage or loss of calibration.

---

as described in the *Anthropometric Standardization Reference Manual*.

Although the objective is to have all SKF technicians follow standardized procedures and recommendations for site location and SKF measurements, you may not be able to do so under all circumstances. For example, if you are using the generalized equations of Jackson and Pollock (1978) and Jackson and colleagues (1980), the chest, midaxillary, subscapular, abdominal, and suprailiac SKFs will be located at sites that differ from those described in the *Anthropometric Standardization Reference Manual*. The descriptions for the sites used in these equations are presented in appendix D.3, "Skinfold Sites for Jackson's Generalized Skinfold Equations," page 368.

RECOMMENDATIONS FOR SKINFOLD TECHNICIANS

- Be meticulous when locating the anatomical landmarks used to identify the SKF site, when measuring the distance, and when marking the site with a surgical marking pen.

- Read the dial of the caliper to the nearest 0.1 mm (Harpenden or Holtain), 0.5 mm (Lange), or 1 mm (plastic calipers).

- Take a minimum of two measurements at each site. If values vary from each other by more than ±10%, take additional measurements.

- Take SKF measurements in a rotational order (circuits) rather than taking consecutive readings at each site.

- Take the SKF measurements when the client's skin is dry and lotion free.

- Do not measure SKFs immediately after exercise because the shift in body fluid to the skin tends to increase the size of the SKF.

- Practice taking SKFs on 50 to 100 clients.

- Avoid using plastic calipers if you are an inexperienced SKF technician. Instead use metal calipers.

- Train with skilled SKF technicians and compare your results.

- Use a SKF training videotape that demonstrates proper SKF techniques (Lohman 1987; Human Kinetics 1995).

- Seek additional training through workshops held at state, regional, and national conferences or through distance education courses (Human Kinetics 1999).

■ *How many measurements do I need to take at each SKF site?*

A lack of intratechnician reliability or consistency of measurements by the SKF technician is another source of error for the SKF method. You need to practice your SKF technique on 50 to 100 clients to develop a high degree of skill and proficiency (Jackson and Pollock 1985). Take a minimum of two measurements at each site using a rotational order. If values vary from each other by more than ±10%, take additional measurements and average the two trials that meet this criterion. Use this average value in the SKF prediction equation. The ±10% value for duplicate measurements at each site is recommended as the standardized procedure in the *Anthropometric Standardized Reference Manual.*

However, if you are preparing to take an ACSM certification examination, you will need to modify this standardized procedure slightly by using the ACSM-recommended criterion for duplicate SKF measurements. The ACSM (2010) also suggests taking at least two measurements at each site in rotational order; however, these two measurements at a given site need to be within 1 to 2 mm of each other. If you take more than two measurements to meet this criterion, average the two trials that are within ±1 to 2 mm of each other and use this value in the prediction equation to estimate Db and %BF. On the other hand, some researchers suggest taking three SKF measurements at each site and using the median (middle score) instead of the mean (average) (Ward and Anderson 1998).

■ *What types of SKF calipers are available and how do they differ?*

There is a variety of high-quality metal and plastic calipers for measuring SKF thickness (see figure 8.9). When choosing a caliper, you need to consider factors such as cost, durability, accuracy, and precision as well as consider which type of caliper was used for developing a specific SKF equation. Table 8.4 and figure 8.10 compare some of the basic characteristics of selected SKF calipers.

High-quality metal calipers are accurate and precise throughout the range of measurement. The Harpenden, Lange, Holtain, and Lafayette calipers exert constant pressure (~7-8 g/mm²) over their range (0-60 mm). Calipers should not have tension that varies by more than 2.0 g/mm² throughout the range of measurement or exceeds 15 g/mm² (Edwards et al.

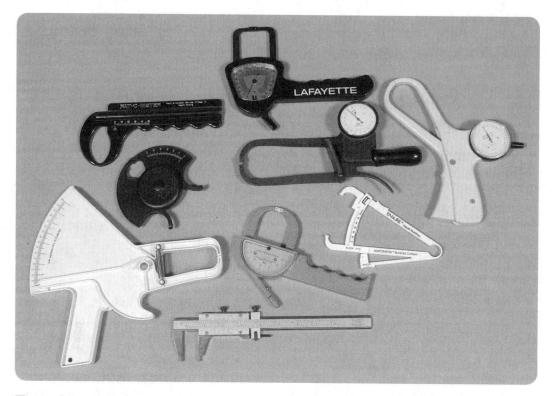

Figure 8.9 Skinfold calipers.

Table 8.4 Comparison of High-Quality Metal Calipers and Plastic SKF Calipers

Caliper type	Average pressure (g/mm²)	Range (mm)	Scale precision (mm)	Accuracy	Durability	Relative cost[c]	Unique features	Supplier[d]
METAL								
Harpenden (HA)	8.2	0-55	0.2	HA < LNG[a]	Excellent	$$$		Creative Health Products
Lange (LNG)	8.4	0-60	0.5	LNG > HA[a]	Excellent	$$		Creative Health Products
Lafayette (LF)	7.5	0-100	0.5	LF > LNG[a]	Excellent	$$$	Measurement range 0-100 mm	Creative Health Products
Skyndex (SKN)	7.3		0.5	SKN < LNG[a]; SKN ≈ HA[a]	Excellent	$$$	Skyndex I: built-in computer, Durnin and Womersley and Jackson and Pollock equations; Syndex II: digital readout but no computer	Creative Health Products
Holtain (HO)			0.2	HO < HA, LNG[b]	Excellent	$$$		Hotain, Ltd.
PLASTIC								
Accu-Measure (AM)	NR	0-60	1.0	NR	Fair	$	Can be used for self-assessment of body fat	Accu-Measure
Body Caliper (BC)	NR	0-60	1.0	BC ≈ HA[b]	Good	$$	Measurement scale on both sides of caliper; suitable for right- or left-handed technician	The Caliper Company
Fat-O-Meter (F)	5.6	0-40	2.0	F ≈ LNG[b]	Poor	$		Creative Health Products
Fat Track (FT)	NR	0-60	0.1	NR	Good	$$	Can be used for self-assessment of body fat; digital readout; Jackson and Pollock equations	Accu-Measure
McGaw (MG)	12.0	0-40	2.0	MG ≈ HA[b]; MG < LNG[b]	Fair	$		None available
Ross Adipometer (RA)	12.0	0-60	2.0	RA ≈ HA[b]; RA < LNG[b]	Fair	$		Ross Products Division
Slim Guide (SG)	7.5	0-80	1.0	SG ≈ HA ≈ SKN[a]; SG < LNG[a]	Good	$		Creative Health Products

[a]Determined by comparing dynamic compression of foam rubber models of human skinfolds.

[b]Determined by comparing skinfold thicknesses of individuals measured by a technician; thus, any differences include not only instrument error but also error associated with technician skill and client factors.

[c]Cost: $ = <$25; $$ = $50-$200; $$$ = >$200.

[d]For supplier's address, see list on page 228.

NR = not reported; ≈ approximately equal.

1955). Excessive tension and pressure cause client discomfort (pinching sensation) and significantly reduce the SKF measurement (Gruber et al. 1990). High-quality calipers also have excellent scale precision (e.g., 0.2 and 1.0 mm, respectively, for Harpenden and Lange).

Although the Harpenden and Lange SKF calipers have similar pressure characteristics, a number of researchers reported that SKFs measured with Harpenden calipers are significantly smaller than those measured with Lange calipers (Gruber et al. 1990; Lohman et al. 1984; Schmidt and Carter 1990). This difference translates into a systematic underestimation (~1.5% BF) of average %BF by the Harpenden calipers (Gruber et al. 1990). Even though the pressure is similar for the Lange (8.37 g/mm²) and Harpenden (8.25 g/mm²) calipers (Schmidt and Carter 1990), researchers noted that opening the jaws of the Harpenden caliper requires three times more force. Therefore, it is likely that the Harpenden compresses adipose tissue to a greater extent, resulting in SKF measurements smaller than those that the Lange caliper yields.

■ *Are plastic SKF calipers as accurate as high-quality metal calipers?*

Compared to high-quality calipers, some plastic calipers have less scale precision (~2 mm), do not exert constant tension throughout the range of measurement, and have a smaller range of measurement (0-40 mm). Despite these differences, some plastic calipers compare well (see table 8.4) with more expensive, high-quality metal calipers (Cataldo and Heyward 2000). Given that the type of caliper is a potential source of measurement error, follow these suggestions to minimize error:

■ Use the same caliper when monitoring changes in your client's SKF thicknesses.

■ Use the same type of caliper as was used in the development of the specific SKF prediction equation you have selected. If the same type of caliper is not available, use one that gives similar readings (see figure 8.10).

■ Periodically check the accuracy of your caliper and calibrate if needed.

■ *Will my client's hydration level affect the SKF measurements?*

Skinfold measurements may also be affected by compressibility of the adipose tissue and hydration

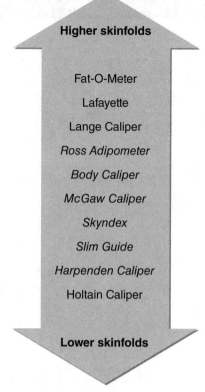

Figure 8.10 Relative ranking of values measured by various types of skinfold calipers. Calipers in italics give similar skinfold readings.

levels of your clients (Ward, Rempel, and Anderson 1999). Martin, Drinkwater, and Clarys (1992) reported that variation in SKF compressibility may be an important limitation of the SKF method. In addition, an accumulation of extracellular water (edema) in the subcutaneous tissue—caused by factors such as peripheral vasodilation or certain diseases—may increase SKF thicknesses (Keys and Brozek 1953). This suggests that you should not measure SKFs immediately after exercise, especially in hot environments. Also, most of the weight gain experienced by some women during their menstrual cycles is caused by water retention (Bunt et al. 1989). This theoretically could increase SKF thicknesses, particularly on the trunk and abdomen, but there are no empirical data to support or refute this hypothesis.

■ *Should SKFs be measured on the right or left side of the body?*

There are only small differences (1 to 2 mm) between SKF thicknesses on the right and left sides of the body for the typical individual. The standard practice in the United States, as well as in European and developing countries, however, is to take SKF measurements on the right side of the body, as recommended in the *Anthropometric Standardization Reference Manual* (Lohman, Roche, and Martorell 1988) and by the International Society for the Advancement of Kinanthropometry (Norton et al. 2000).

■ *Should I use SKFs to measure the body fat of obese clients?*

It is difficult, even for highly skilled SKF technicians, to measure the SKF thickness of extremely obese individuals accurately. Sometimes the client's SKF thickness exceeds the maximum aperture of the caliper, and the jaws of the caliper may slip off the fold during the measurement, resulting in a potentially embarrassing and awkward situation for you and your client. Therefore, avoid using the SKF method to measure body fat of extremely obese clients.

Bioelectrical Impedance Method

Bioelectrical impedance analysis (BIA) is a rapid, noninvasive, and relatively inexpensive method for evaluating body composition in field settings. With this method, a low-level electrical current is passed through the client's body, and the **impedance (Z)**, or opposition to the flow of current, is measured with a BIA analyzer. You can estimate the individual's total body water (TBW) from the impedance measurement because the electrolytes in the body's water are excellent conductors of electrical current. When the volume of TBW is large, the current flows more easily through the body with less resistance (R). The resistance to current flow is greater in individuals with large amounts of body fat, since adipose tissue, with its relatively low water content, is a poor conductor of electrical current. Because the water content of the FFB component is relatively large (~73% water), **fat-free mass (FFM)** can be predicted from TBW estimates. Individuals with large FFM and TBW have less resistance to current flowing through their bodies than those with a smaller FFM.

Bioelectrical impedance indirectly estimates FFM and TBW. Therefore, the following assumptions are made about the geometric shape of the body and the relationship of impedance to the length and volume of the conductor.

■ **The human body is shaped like a perfect cylinder with a uniform length and cross-sectional area.** Of course, this assumption is not entirely true. Because the body segments are not uniform in length or cross-sectional area, resistance to the flow of current through these body segments will differ.

■ **Assuming that the body is a perfect cylinder, at a fixed signal frequency (e.g., 50 kHz) the impedance (Z) to current flow through the body is directly related to the length (L) of the conductor (height) and inversely related to its cross-sectional area [Z = ρ(L/A), where ρ is the specific resistivity of the body's tissues and is assumed to be constant].** To express this relationship in terms of Z and the body's volume, instead of its cross-sectional area, the equation is multiplied by L/L: $Z = \rho(L/A)(L/L)$. A × L is equal to volume (V), so rearranging this equation yields $V = \rho L^2 / Z$. Thus, the volume of the FFM or TBW of the body is directly related to L^2, or height squared (ht^2), and indirectly related to Z.

■ **Biological tissues act as conductors or insulators, and the flow of current through the body will follow the path of least resistance.** Because the FFM contains large amounts of water (~73%) and electrolytes, it is a better conductor of electrical current than fat. Fat is anhydrous and a poor conductor of electrical current. The total body impedance, measured at the constant frequency of 50 kHz, primarily reflects the volumes of the water and muscle compartments composing the FFM and the extracellular water volume (Kushner 1992).

■ **Impedance is a function of resistance and reactance, where $Z = \sqrt{(R^2 + X_c^2)}$.** Resistance (R) is a measure of pure opposition to current flow through the body; **reactance (X_c)** is the opposition to current flow caused by capacitance produced by the cell membrane (Kushner 1992). R is much larger than X_c (at a 50 kHz frequency) when whole-body impedance is measured; therefore, R is a better predictor of FFM and TBW than Z (Lohman 1989). For these reasons, the **resistance index (ht^2/R)**, instead of ht^2/Z, is often used in BIA models to predict FFM or TBW.

Using the Bioelectrical Impedance Analysis Method

The traditional BIA method measures whole-body resistance using a tetrapolar wrist-to-ankle electrode configuration at a single frequency for estimating

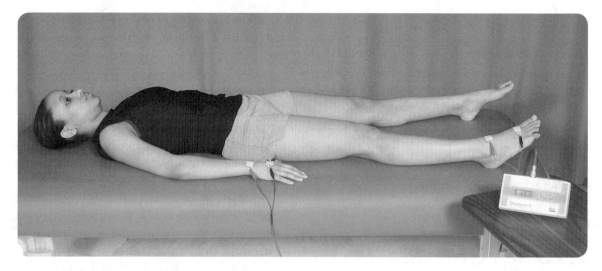

Figure 8.11 Bioelectrical impedance analysis electrode placement and client positioning.

TBW or FFM (figure 8.11). However, technological advances and changes in theoretical modeling have led to a number of variations in the traditional BIA method. These variations use sophisticated models to assess segmental body composition and fluid subcompartments, thereby improving the clinical usefulness of BIA. Also, user-friendly BIA analyzers designed for home use and individual monitoring of health and fitness use upper or lower body impedance measures to estimate body composition (figure 8.12).

Whole-body bioimpedance measures (Z, R, and X_c) are used in BIA prediction equations to estimate TBW and FFM. These prediction equations are based on either population-specific or generalized models. A population-specific equation is valid for only those individuals whose physical characteristics match the sample from which the equation was derived. Researchers have developed equations specific to age (Deurenberg et al. 1990; Lohman 1992), ethnicity (Stolarczyk et al. 1994), body fatness (Gray et al. 1989; Segal et al. 1988), and level of physical activity (Houtkooper et al. 1989). Alternatively, generalized BIA equations have been developed for heterogeneous populations varying in age, gender, and body fatness (Deurenberg et al. 1990; Gray et al. 1989; Kyle et al. 2001; Kushner and Schoeller 1986; Lukaski and Bolonchuk 1988; Van Loan and Mayclin 1987).

Inexpensive lower body (foot-to-foot) and upper body (hand-to-hand) BIA devices are available and have been marketed for home use. The Tanita ana-

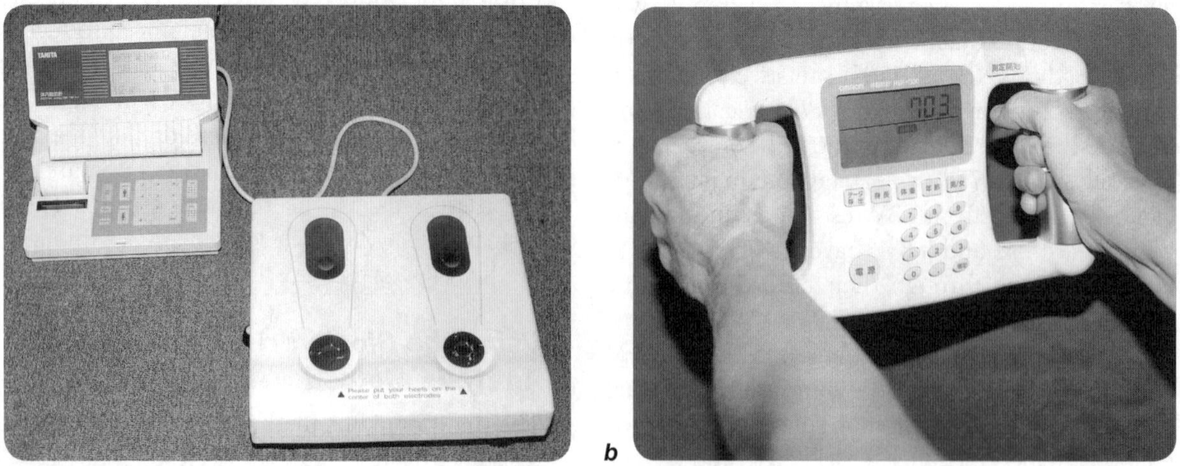

a

b

Figure 8.12 (a) Tanita and (b) Omron bioelectrical impedance analyzers.

lyzers measure lower body impedance between the right and left legs as the individual stands on the analyzer's electrode plates (see figure 8.12a). The Omron Body Logic analyzer, which is handheld, measures upper body impedance between the right and left arms (see figure 8.12b). The Tanita and Omron analyzers estimate %BF and FFM using proprietary equations developed by the manufacturers. Typically, it is not possible to obtain impedance (resistance and reactance) data from these analyzers. However, they do provide the general public with an inexpensive, simple, and reasonably accurate means of self-assessing body fat.

Table 8.5 presents commonly used population-specific and generalized BIA equations. With these equations, you can accurately estimate the FFM of your clients within the recommended values, ±2.8 kg for women and ±3.5 kg for men (Lohman 1992). To use these equations, obtain R and X_c directly from your BIA analyzer. Estimate the %BF of your client by determining the **fat mass (FM)** (FM = BM – FFM) and dividing FM by the client's body mass [%BF = (FM / BM) × 100].

Experts recommend not using the FFM and %BF estimates obtained directly from your BIA analyzer (e.g., BMR, Holtain, RJL, or Valhalla) unless you know for sure which equations are programmed in the analyzer's computer software, obtain information from the manufacturer regarding the validity and accuracy of these equations, and determine that these equations are applicable to your clients.

Although the relative predictive accuracy of the BIA method is similar to that of the SKF method, BIA may be preferable in some settings for the following reasons:

- It does not require a high degree of technician skill.
- It is generally more comfortable and does not intrude as much upon the client's privacy.
- It can be used to estimate body composition of obese individuals.

Bioelectrical Impedance Analysis Technique

Bioelectrical impedance analysis accuracy highly depends on controlling the factors that may increase measurement error. Regardless of the BIA method (whole, upper, or lower body) being used, your client must adhere to the "BIA Pretesting Client Guidelines," which are designed to control fluctuations in hydration status.

Table 8.5 Bioelectrical Impedance Analysis Prediction Equations

Population subgroup	%BF level[a]	Equation	Reference
American Indian, black, Hispanic, or white men, 17-62 yr	<20% BF	FFM (kg) = 0.00066360(ht^2) – 0.02117(R) + 0.62854(BM) – 0.12380(age) + 9.33285	Segal et al. (1988)
	≥20%	FFM (kg) = 0.00088580(ht^2) – 0.02999(R) + 0.42688(BM) – 0.07002(age) + 14.52435	Segal et al. (1988)
American Indian, black, Hispanic, or white women, 17-62 yr	<30%	FFM (kg) = 0.000646(ht^2) – 0.014(R) + 0.421(BM) + 10.4	Segal et al. (1988)
	≥30%	FFM (kg) = 0.00091186(ht^2) – 0.01466(R) + 0.29990(BM) – 0.07012(age) + 9.37938	Segal et al. (1988)
White boys and girls, 8-15 yr	NA	FFM (kg) = 0.62(ht^2/ R) + 0.21(BM) + 0.10(X_c) + 4.2	Lohman (1992)
White boys and girls, 10-19 yr	NA	FFM (kg) = 0.61(ht^2/ R) + 0.25(BM) + 1.31	Houtkooper et al. (1992)
Female athletes, 18-27 yr	NA	FFM (kg) = 0.282(ht) + 0.415(BM) – 0.037(R) + 0.096(X_c) – 9.734	Fornetti et al. (1999)
Male athletes, 19-40 yr	NA	FFM (kg) = 0.186(ht^2/ R) + 0.701(BM) + 1.949	Oppliger et al. (1991)

NA = not applicable.

[a]For clients who are obviously lean, use the <20% BF (men) and <30% BF (women) equations. For clients who are obviously obese, use the ≥20% BF (men) and ≥30% BF (women) equations. For clients who are not obviously lean or obese, calculate their FFM using both the lean and obese equations and then average the two FFM estimates.

%BF = percent body fat; FFM = fat-free mass (kg); BM = body mass (kg); R = resistance (Ω); X_c = reactance (Ω); ht = height (cm).

BIA Pretesting Client Guidelines

- No eating or drinking within 4 hr of the test.

- No moderate or vigorous exercise within 12 hr of the test.

- Void completely within 30 min of the test.

- Abstain from alcohol consumption within 48 hr of the test.

- Do not ingest diuretics, including caffeine, before the assessment unless they are prescribed by a physician.

- If you are in a stage of your menstrual cycle during which you perceive you are retaining water, postpone testing (female clients).

Use standardized testing procedures to minimize error in the BIA method (see "Standardized Procedures for the Whole-Body BIA Method").

Sources of Measurement Error

The accuracy and precision of the BIA method are affected by instrumentation, client factors, technician skill, environmental factors, and the prediction equation used to estimate FFM. The following questions address sources of BIA measurement error.

■ *Can different types of whole-body BIA analyzers be used interchangeably?*

Research demonstrates significant differences in whole-body resistance when different brands of single-frequency analyzers are used (Graves et al. 1989; Smye, Sutcliffe, and Pitt 1993). For example, Smye and colleagues (1993) reported lower resistances (6% or 32-36 Ω) for the Holtain device compared to the Bodystat, RJL, and EZcomp analyzers. Graves and colleagues (1989) noted that the correlation between resistance values measured with the Valhalla and Bioelectrical Sciences (BES) analyzers was only $r = 0.59$; the average %BF estimated for men from one BIA equation differed by 6.3% using the resistances from these two instruments. Although there is a high correlation ($r = 0.99$) between resistances measured with the Valhalla and RJL analyzers, the Valhalla analyzer produces significantly higher resistances for men (~16 Ω) and women (~19 Ω), corresponding to a systematic underestimation of FFM in men

(~1.3 kg) and women (~1.0 kg) (Graves et al. 1989). Also, differences may exist within a given model of analyzer. The Z values from three RJL (model 101) analyzers differed by 7 to 16 Ω, causing a difference in FFM of 2.1 kg for some individuals (Deurenberg, van der Kooy, and Leenan 1989).

■ *Do upper and lower body BIA analyzers accurately estimate body composition?*

The Tanita Corporation now markets about 20 different models of lower body analyzers that vary in weight capacity, software and memory, and data output. Compared to two-component model estimates of FFM obtained from underwater weighing, Tanita analyzer estimates of the average FFM of heterogeneous adult samples are reasonably good (*SEE* = 3.5-3.7 kg) (Cable et al. 2001; Utter et al. 1999). Estimates by Tanita analyzers also agree well with SKF estimates of %BF in collegiate wrestlers (Utter et al. 2001) and with DXA estimates of FFM in children (Sung et al. 2001; Tyrrel et al. 2001). Compared to UWW estimates of FFM of high school wrestlers, the prediction error for the Tanita analyzer (TBF-300WA) was larger than that of the SKF method (3.64 kg vs. 1.97 kg). Utter and colleagues (2005), therefore, recommend using the leg-to-leg Tanita analyzer only when trained SKF technicians are not available.

In the late 1990s, Omron Healthcare developed a low-cost, hand-to-hand BIA analyzer for home use. Omron's proprietary equation was developed and cross-validated on a large heterogeneous sample from three laboratories using HW to obtain two-component model reference measures of %BF and FFM (Loy et al. 1998). The group predictive accuracy (*SEE*) for estimating FFM was 3.9 kg for men and 2.9 kg for women. In an independent cross-validation of the Omron analyzer, Gibson and colleagues (2000) reported slightly smaller prediction errors (*SEE* = 2.9 kg for men and 2.2 kg for women). Loy and colleagues (1998) noted that the average FFM estimates from the Omron device are similar to values obtained with whole-body (RJL and Valhalla) analyzers. Lastly, in a study of Japanese men, the accuracy of upper body (Omron, HBF-300), lower body (Tanita, TBF-102), and whole-body (Selco, SIF-891) analyzers was compared to two-component model reference measures of %BF obtained from HW. The average difference between reference and predicted %BF values was slightly smaller for the

Standardized Procedures for the Whole-Body BIA Method

- Take bioimpedance measures on the right side of the body with the client lying supine on a nonconductive surface in a room with normal ambient temperature (~25° C).

- Clean the skin at the electrode sites with an alcohol pad.

- Place the sensor (proximal) electrodes on (a) the dorsal surface of the wrist so that the upper border of the electrode bisects the head of the ulna and (b) the dorsal surface of the ankle so that the upper border of the electrode bisects the medial and lateral malleoli (see figure 8.11). You can use a measuring tape and surgical marking pen to mark these points for electrode placement.

- Place the source (distal) electrodes at the bases of the second or third metacarpophalangeal joints of the hand and foot (see figure 8.11). Make certain there is at least 5 cm (~2 in.) between the proximal and distal electrodes.

- Attach the lead wires to the appropriate electrodes. Red leads are attached to the wrist and ankle, and black leads are attached to the hand and foot.

- Make certain that the client's legs and arms are comfortably abducted, at about a 30° to 45° angle from the trunk. Ensure that there is no contact between the arms and trunk and between the thighs, as contact will short-circuit the electrical path, dramatically affecting the impedance value.

Omron (2.2% BF) than for the whole-body (3.3% BF) and lower body (3.2% BF) analyzers (Demura et al. 2002). However, estimation errors from the Omron and Tanita devices tended to be greater at the lower and upper extremes of the %BF distribution.

Omron also developed BIA prediction equations to estimate the body composition of physically active adults. These equations are programmed in the HBF-306 Omron analyzer along with prediction equations for nonactive adults and children. The predictor variables in the manufacturer's equation for this unit are upper body impedance, age, gender, height, weight, and level of physical activity (i.e., athlete or nonathlete). The prediction errors for athletes (SEE = 3.8% and 3.6% BF for male and female athletes, respectively) were somewhat less than those for nonathletes (SEE = 4.5% BF) (K. Yamanoto, personal communication).

The Omron (HBF-306) model has been tested on ethnically diverse samples of European and Asian populations. Generally the group predictive accuracy is good for these subgroups, but individual prediction errors can be high (Deurenberg-Yap et al. 2001; Deurenberg and Deurenberg-Yap 2002). Deurenberg-Yap and colleagues (2001) noted that Omron data misclassified (gave false negatives) for 24% of the obese females and 44% of the obese males in their study. When the Omron estimates of %BF were compared with those of a multicom-

ponent model, the SEE was 4.5% BF; the error in estimating %BF using the Omron analyzer was related to the age, body fatness, and arm span-to-height ratio of the subjects (Deurenberg and Deurenberg-Yap 2002).

■ *Compared to handheld and leg-to-leg BIA analyzers, does octapolar bioimpedance spectroscopy (BIS) provide a better estimate of body composition?*

New **bioimpedance spectroscopy (BIS)** analyzers combine upper body, lower body, and whole-body bioimpedance to estimate FFM and %BF. The octapolar (four pairs of electrodes) system of the InBody 720 and InBody 320 BIS analyzers has electrodes embedded into the analyzers' handles (thumb and arm) and floor scale (ball of foot and heel). Comparing estimates from the BIS analyzers to multicomponent model estimates of relative body fat, Gibson and colleagues (2008) reported large prediction errors for samples of Hispanic, black, and white men (SEE = 5.2% BF) and women (SEE = 4.8% BF). The average %BF of the women was significantly overestimated by 2.5% to 3.0% BF for both BIS analyzers.

■ *How does my client's hydration level affect the accuracy of bioimpedance measures?*

A major source of error with the BIA method is intraindividual variability in whole-body resistance due to factors that alter the client's hydration.

Between 3.1% and 3.9% of the variance in resistance may be attributed to day-to-day fluctuations in body water (Jackson et al. 1988). Factors such as eating, drinking, dehydrating, and exercising alter the hydration state, thereby affecting total body resistance and the estimate of FFM. Measuring resistance 2 to 4 hr after a meal decreases R as much as 13 to 17 Ω and likely overestimates the FFM of your client by almost 1.5 kg (Deurenberg et al. 1988). Likewise, Gallagher and colleagues (1998) found a significant decrease in impedance 2 hr following breakfast, and this effect lasted for 5 hr after consumption. In contrast to these studies, at only 1 hr postmeal, there appear to be greater individual variability and smaller changes in R (Fogelholm et al. 1993). Kushner, Gudivaka, and Schoeller (1996) concluded that eating or drinking minimally influences whole-body Z within 1 hr following consumption but is likely to decrease Z (<3%) at 2 to 4 hr. Dehydration has the opposite effect: R increases (~40 Ω), leading to a 5.0 kg underestimation of FFM (Lukaski 1986).

How does exercise affect bioimpedance measures?

Kushner and colleagues (1996) suggested three ways in which exercise may influence BIA measurements:

- Increased blood flow and warming of skeletal muscle tissue reduce Z and the specific resistivity (ρ) of muscle.
- Increased cutaneous blood flow, skin temperature, and sweating lower Z.
- Fluid loss due to exercise increases Z.

The effect of aerobic exercise on resistance measurements partially depends on exercise intensity and duration. Jogging and cycling at moderate intensities (~70% $\dot{V}O_2max$) for 90 to 120 min substantially decreased R (by 50-70 Ω), resulting in a large overestimation of FFM (~12 kg) (Khaled et al. 1988; Lukaski 1986). In contrast, cycling at lower intensities (100 and 175 W) for 90 min had a much smaller effect on R (1-9 Ω) (Deurenberg et al. 1988). Liang and Norris (1993) reported a decrease in R of about 3% immediately after 30 min of moderate-intensity exercise, but R returned to normal 1 hr postexercise with water ad libitum. The decrease in R following strenuous exercise most likely reflects a relatively greater loss of body water in the sweat and expired air compared to the loss of electrolytes. This difference leads to a higher electrolyte concentration in the body's fluids, thereby lowering R (Deurenberg et al. 1988).

The BIA method was found to adequately predict changes in TBW after heat-induced dehydration and glycerol-induced hyperhydration but not after exercise-induced dehydration; thus, factors other than just total fluid volume affect BIA measures following exercise (Koulmann et al. 2000). Researchers hypothesized that the redistribution of body fluids to active muscles during exercise, which relatively increases hydration in these segments (legs), might partially conceal the decreased fluid volumes in less active segments (trunk and arms).

Can I measure bioimpedance at any time during my client's menstrual cycle?

Although the menstrual cycle alters TBW, the ratio of extracellular to intracellular water, and body weight, researchers found only small differences in bioimpedance measures (Z and R) between the follicular and premenstrual stages (~5-8 Ω) and between menses and the follicular stage (~7 Ω) (Deurenberg et al. 1988; Gleichauf and Rose 1989). However, the average body weight of the women studied was stable (<0.2 kg difference) during the menstrual cycle. In women experiencing relatively large body weight gains (2-4 kg or 4.4-8.8 lb) during the menstrual cycle, a large part of the gain is due to an increase (1.5 kg or 3.3 lb on average) in TBW (Bunt et al. 1989). Until there are more conclusive data on this issue, you should take BIA measurements at a time during the menstrual cycle when the client perceives that she is not experiencing a large weight gain. This practice should minimize error and more accurately estimate FFM for your clients.

Is there high agreement between bioimpedance values measured by two different technicians?

Technician skill is not a major source of BIA measurement error. There is virtually no difference in R measurements taken by different technicians, provided that standardized procedures for electrode placement and client positioning are closely followed (Jackson et al. 1988). The proximal electrodes in particular need to be correctly positioned at the wrist and ankle, as a 1 cm (0.4 in.) displacement may result in a 2% error in R (Elsen et al. 1987). Lukaski (1986) reported a 16% increase in R (~79 Ω) due to improper electrode placement.

■ How does body position affect bioimpedance measures?

Proper positioning of the client is important for an accurate measurement. As a standard practice, whole-body resistance is measured with the client lying in a supine position. Changes in body position alter Z values as much as 12% (Lozano, Rosell, and Pallas-Areny 1995); moving from a standing to supine position immediately increases Z by about 3% because of fluid shifts (Kushner et al. 1996). Also, the amount of time that the client lies supine before Z is recorded needs to be standardized; in the supine position Z gradually increases over several hours (Kushner et al. 1996). Experts recommend having your client lie supine for at least 10 min before BIA measurement (Ellis et al. 1999). In addition, make sure that your client's arms are abducted (30°-45°) from the trunk and that the thighs are not touching each other. Crossing the limbs short-circuits the electrical path, dramatically affecting bioimpedance values.

■ Should I measure whole-body bioimpedance on the right or left side of the body?

The standard practice is to measure whole-body bioimpedance on the right side of the body. The differences between R measurements using ipsilateral (right arm–right leg or left arm–left leg) and contralateral (right arm–left leg or left arm–right leg) electrode placements are generally small (Graves et al. 1989; Lukaski et al. 1985).

■ How does temperature affect bioimpedance?

Bioimpedance measurements should be made with the client lying supine on a nonconductive surface (e.g., stretcher bed or mat) in a room at normal ambient temperature (25° C [77° F]). Researchers have demonstrated that ambient temperature affects skin temperature, and R varies inversely with skin temperature (Caton et al. 1988; Gudivaka, Schoeller, and Kushner 1996; Liang, Su, and Lee 2000). Cool ambient temperatures (~14° C) drop skin temperature (24° C compared to 33° C under normal conditions), significantly increasing total body R (by 35 Ω, on average) and decreasing estimated FFM (by ~2.2 kg) (Caton et al. 1988). Liang and colleagues (2000) reported a slightly greater difference in R (46 Ω) between cold (17° C ambient temperature and 28.7° C skin temperature) and hot (35° C ambient and 35.8° C skin temperature) conditions.

Other Anthropometric Methods

Anthropometry refers to the measurement of the size and proportion of the human body. Body weight and stature (standing height) are measures of body size, whereas ratios of weight to height represent body proportion. Circumferences, SKF thicknesses, skeletal diameters, and segment lengths may be used to assess the sizes and proportions of body segments. A **circumference (C)** is a measure of the girth of a body segment such as the arm, thigh, waist, or hip. A **skeletal diameter (D)** is a measure of bony width or breadth (e.g., of the knee, ankle, or wrist).

Anthropometric measures such as circumferences, SKFs, and skeletal diameters have been used to assess total and regional body composition. Also, anthropometric indices such as body mass index (BMI), waist-to-hip circumference ratio (WHR), waist circumference, and sagittal abdominal diameter (SAD) are used to identify individuals at risk for disease. Compared to SKFs, other anthropometric measures are relatively simple and inexpensive, and they do not require a high degree of technical skill and training. They are well suited for large epidemiological surveys and for clinical purposes.

The basic principles underlying the use of anthropometric measures such as circumference, skeletal diameter, and BMI to estimate body composition are as follows:

■ Circumferences are affected by fat mass, muscle mass, and skeletal size; therefore, they are related to fat mass and lean body mass. Jackson and Pollock (1976) reported that circumference and bony diameter are markers of lean body mass (muscle mass and skeletal size); however, some circumferences are also highly associated with body fat. These findings confirm that circumferences reflect both fat and fat-free components of body composition.

■ Skeletal size directly relates to lean body mass. Behnke (1961) proposed that lean body mass could be accurately estimated from skeletal diameters and developed equations for doing so. Cross-validation of these equations yielded a moderately high (r = 0.80) relationship and closely estimated average lean body mass values obtained from hydrodensitometry (Wilmore and Behnke 1969, 1970). Behnke's hypothesis was also supported by the observation that skeletal diameters, along with circumferences, are strong markers of lean body mass (Jackson and Pollock 1976).

■ **To estimate total body fat from weight-to-height indices, the index should be highly related to body fat but independent of height.** On the basis of data from two large-scale epidemiological surveys (National Health and Nutrition Examination Surveys I and II), Micozzi and colleagues (1986) reported that BMI (body weight divided by height squared) is not significantly related to the height of men ($r = -0.06$) and women ($r = -0.16$). However, BMI is not totally independent of height, especially in younger children (<15 yr). Although BMI was directly related to SKF thickness and the estimated fat area of the arm ($r = 0.72$ to 0.80) (Micozzi et al. 1986), the relationship of BMI to body fat varied with age, gender, and ethnicity (Deurenberg and Deurenberg-Yap 2001; Deurenberg, Yap, and van Staveren 1998; Gallagher, Walker, and O'Dea 1996; Rush et al. 1997; Wang et al. 1994).

Using the Anthropometric Method to Estimate Body Composition

Although some anthropometric prediction models use SKFs, circumferences, and skeletal diameters to estimate body composition, only those equations using circumferences and diameters are addressed in this chapter, for the following reasons:

- The predictive accuracy of anthropometric (circumference and diameter) equations is not greatly improved by the addition of SKF measures.

- Anthropometric equations using only circumferences estimate the body fatness of obese individuals more accurately than SKF prediction equations (Seip and Weltman 1991).

- Compared to SKFs, circumferences and skeletal diameters can be measured with less error (Bray and Gray 1988a).

- Some practitioners may not have access to SKF calipers.

Anthropometric prediction equations estimate total body density (Db), relative body fat (%BF), and fat-free mass (FFM) from combinations of body weight, height, skeletal diameters, and circumferences. Generally, equations using only skeletal measures have larger prediction errors than those using both circumferences and bony diameters. Like SKF and BIA equations, anthropometric equations are based on either population-specific or generalized models.

Population-specific anthropometric equations are valid only for individuals whose physical characteristics (age, gender, ethnicity, and level of body fatness) are similar to those of the specific population. For example, anthropometric equations developed to estimate the body composition of obese individuals (Weltman et al. 1988, 1987) should not be applied to nonobese individuals.

On the other hand, generalized equations, applicable to individuals of various age and body fatness, have been developed for heterogeneous populations of women (15-79 yr; 13%-63% BF) and men (20-78 yr; 2%-49% BF) (Tran and Weltman 1988, 1989). The predictive accuracy of these generalized equations for estimating the %BF of obese men and women was similar to that of fatness-specific (obese) equations (Seip and Weltman 1991). Typically, generalized equations include body weight or height, along with two or three circumferences, as predictors of Db or %BF. As in generalized SKF models, the relationship between some circumference measures and Db is curvilinear (Tran and Weltman 1988, 1989). Also, age has been shown to be an independent predictor of Db for women (Tran and Weltman 1989). Table 8.6 provides anthropometric prediction equations for various population subgroups.

Using Anthropometric Indices to Classify Disease Risk

Anthropometric measures have other uses besides estimating body composition. In large-scale epidemiological surveys and clinical settings, indirect anthropometric indices such as BMI, WHR, waist circumference, and SAD are used to assess regional fat distribution (upper and lower body fat) and to identify at-risk individuals.

Body Mass Index

The body mass index is used to classify individuals as obese, overweight, and underweight; to identify individuals at risk for obesity-related diseases; and to monitor changes in the body fatness of clinical populations (U.S. Department of Health and Human Services 2000; World Health Organization 1998). Body mass index is a significant predictor of cardiovascular disease and type 2 diabetes (Janssen

Table 8.6 Circumference Prediction Equations

Population subgroup	Equation	Reference
White women, 15-79 yr	$Db (g \cdot cc^{-1})^a = 1.168297 - 0.002824(abdom\ C^b) + 0.0000122098(abdom\ C^b)^2 - 0.000733128(hip\ C) + 0.000510477(ht) - 0.00021616(age)$	Tran and Weltman (1989)
White men, 15-78 yr	$\%BF = -47.371817 + 0.57914807(abdom\ C^b) + 0.25189114(hip\ C) + 0.21366088(iliac\ C) - 0.35595404(BM)$	Tran and Weltman (1988)
White, obese women, 20-60 yr	$\%BF = 0.11077(abdom\ C^b) - 0.17666(ht) + 0.14354(BM) + 51.033$	Weltman et al. (1988)
White, obese men, 24-68 yr	$\%BF = 0.31457(abdom\ C^b) - 0.10969(BM) + 10.834$	Weltman et al. (1987)

[a]Use population-specific conversion formula to calculate %BF from Db.

[b]abdom C (cm) is the average abdominal circumference measured at two sites: (1) anteriorly midway between the xiphoid process of sternum and the umbilicus and laterally between the lower end of the rib cage and iliac crests; (2) at the umbilicus level.

Db = body density; %BF = percent body fat; BM = body mass (kg); ht = height (cm).

et al. 2002). Because of this association and the fact that BMI is easily calculated (BMI = body weight / height squared), BMI is widely used in population-based and prospective studies to identify at-risk individuals.

Body mass index, however, is limited as an index of obesity (body fatness) because it does not account for the composition of body weight. In addition, factors such as age, ethnicity, body build, and frame size affect the relationship between BMI and %BF. Thus, using BMI as an index of obesity may result in misclassifications of underweight, overweight, and obese. Also, because BMI is a better measure of nonabdominal and abdominal subcutaneous fat than of visceral fat (Janssen et al. 2002), other anthropometric indices need to be used to assess fat distribution.

Body mass index (BMI) is the ratio of body weight to height squared: BMI (in kg/m^2) = wt (in kilograms) / ht^2 (in meters). To calculate BMI, measure the body weight in kilograms and convert the height from centimeters to meters (m = cm / 100). Alternatively, you can use a nomogram (see figure 8.13) to calculate your client's BMI (Bray 1978). To use this nomogram, plot your client's height and body weight in the appropriate columns and connect the two points with a ruler. Read the corresponding BMI at the point where the connecting line intersects the BMI column.

Table 8.7 describes standards for classifying BMI values. The World Health Organization (1998) defines obesity as a BMI of 30 kg/m^2 or more, overweight as a BMI between 25 and 29.9 kg/m^2, and underweight as a BMI of less than 18.5 kg/m^2. These

suggested cutoffs are based on the relationship between BMI and morbidity and mortality reported in observational studies in Europe and the United States. The use of BMI in health risk appraisals assumes that people who are disproportionately heavy are so because of excess fat mass. However, controversy exists concerning the most appropriate cutoff for designating obesity (Deurenberg 2001).

The relationship between BMI and %BF is affected by age, gender, ethnicity, and body build (Deurenberg et al. 1998; Snijder, Kuyf, and Deurenberg 1999). For a given BMI value, older individuals have a greater %BF compared to their younger counterparts, and young adult males have a lesser %BF than young adult females. Also, for a given %BF, age- and gender-matched whites have a higher BMI (1.3-4.6 kg/m^2) compared to other ethnic groups

Table 8.7 Classification of Overweight and Obesity Based on Body Mass Index (BMI)

Classification	BMI value
Underweight	<18.5
Normal weight	18.5-24.9
Overweight	25.0-29.9
Obesity	
Class I	30.0-34.9
Class II	35.0-39.9
Class III	≥40.0

Data from WHO Report, 1998, Obesity: Preventing and managing the global epidemic. *Report of a WHO Consultation of Obesity.* Geneva: World Health Organization.

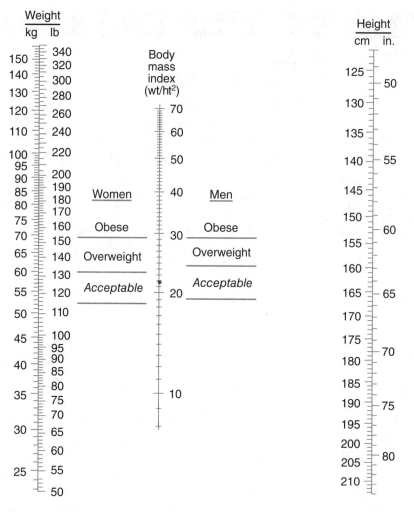
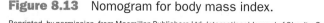

Figure 8.13 Nomogram for body mass index.

Reprinted, by permission, from Macmillan Publishers Ltd. *International Journal of Obesity*, G.A. Bray, "Definitions, measurement, and classifications of the syndromes of obesity," 2(2): 99-112. Copyright 1978.

(e.g., African Americans, Chinese, Indonesians, Ethiopians, and Polynesians) (Deurenberg et al. 1998). These findings suggest that using a universal BMI cutoff to define obesity (≥30 kg/m²) may not be appropriate. Ethnic-specific cutoff values need to be established that account for the relationship between BMI and %BF and for the morbidity and mortality risks in relation to BMI for specific ethnic groups (Deurenberg 2001).

Waist Circumference

Waist circumference is gaining support as a measure of regional adiposity (i.e., abdominal obesity) and as a predictor of obesity-related cardiometabolic disease (Moore 2009). Waist circumference coupled with BMI predicts health risk better than BMI alone, especially for white men (Ardern, Katzmarzyk, and Ross 2003; Zhu et al. 2004). However, some stud-

ies showed that waist circumference alone predicts obesity-related health risk even better than the combination of BMI and waist circumference (Janssen, Katzmarzyk, and Ross 2004; Zhu et al. 2005). The National Cholesterol Education Program (NCEP 2001) recommends using waist circumference cut-offs of >102 cm (40 in.) for men and >88 cm (34.6 in.) for women to evaluate obesity as a risk factor for cardiovascular and metabolic diseases. However, Zhu and colleagues (2005) proposed using waist circumference cutoffs of >100 cm (39 in.) for men and >95 cm (47.4 in.) for women to identify individuals with a high risk for cardiovascular disease. These cutoffs apply to black, Mexican American, and white adults (Zhu et al. 2005). Selection of the most appropriate waist circumference cut-points is complex given that age, sex, race-ethnicity, and BMI influence these values; optimum waist circumference cut-points will likely vary according to health outcomes and the population studied (Klein et al. 2007).

Waist-to-Hip Ratio

The waist-to-hip ratio (WHR) is an indirect measure of lower and upper body fat distribution. Upper body obesity, or central adiposity, measured by the WHR moderately relates ($r = 0.48$ to 0.61) to risk factors associated with cardiovascular and metabolic diseases in men and women (Ohrvall, Berglund, and Vessby 2000). Young adults with WHR values in excess of 0.94 for men and 0.82 for women are at high risk for adverse health consequences (Bray and Gray 1988b).

Although the WHR has been used as an anthropometric measure of central adiposity and visceral fat, it has certain limitations:

■ The WHR of women is affected by menopausal status (Svendsen et al. 1992; Weits et al. 1988). Postmenopausal women show more of a male pattern of fat distribution than do premenopausal women (Ferland et al. 1989).

■ The WHR is not valid for evaluating fat distribution in prepubertal children (Peters et al. 1992).

■ The accuracy of the WHR in assessing visceral fat decreases with increasing fatness.

■ Hip circumference is influenced only by subcutaneous fat deposition; waist circumference is affected by both visceral fat and subcutaneous fat depositions. Thus, the WHR may not accurately detect changes in visceral fat accumulation (Goran, Allison, and Poehlman 1995; van der Kooy et al. 1993).

To calculate the **waist-to-hip ratio (WHR)**, one divides waist circumference (in centimeters) by hip circumference (in centimeters). The measurement site for waist circumference, however, has not been universally standardized. The World Health Organization (1998) recommends measuring waist circumference midway between the lower rib margin and the iliac crest and measuring hip circumference at the widest point over the greater trochanters. In contrast, the *Anthropometric Standardization Reference Manual* (Callaway et al. 1988) recommends measuring the waist circumference

at the narrowest part of the torso and the hip circumference at the level of the maximum extension of the buttocks. The WHR norms (table 8.8) were established using the measurement procedures described in the *Anthropometric Standardization Reference Manual*. Instead of calculating the WHR by hand, you can use the WHR nomogram (figure 8.14) to obtain values for your clients. Plot the client's waist and hip circumferences in the corresponding columns of the nomogram and connect these points with a straight line. Read the WHR at the point where this line intersects the WHR column.

Waist-to-Height Ratio

The **waist-to-height ratio (WHTR)** (i.e., waist circumference/standing height) has been suggested as a better indicator of adiposity and health risks than waist circumference alone (Ashwell and Hsieh 2005; Hsieh, Yoshinaga, and Muto 2003). A cut-off

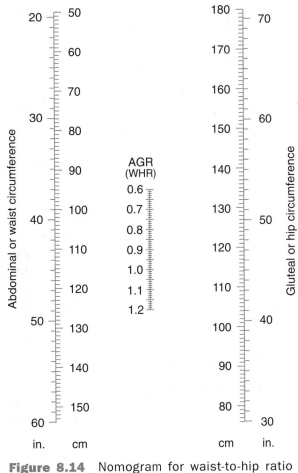

Figure 8.14 Nomogram for waist-to-hip ratio (WHR).

Reprinted, by permission of *The Western Journal of Medicine*, G.A. Bray and D.S. Gray, "Obesity: Part I - Pathogenesis," 1988b, 149: 432. © BMJ Publishing Group.

Table 8.8 Waist-to-Hip Circumference Ratio Norms for Men and Women

	Age	Low	Moderate	High	Very high
			RISK		
Men	20-29	<0.83	0.83-0.88	0.89-0.94	>0.94
	30-39	<0.84	0.84-0.91	0.92-0.96	>0.96
	40-49	<0.88	0.88-0.95	0.96-1.00	>1.00
	50-59	<0.90	0.90-0.96	0.97-1.02	>1.02
	60-69	<0.91	0.91-0.98	0.99-1.03	>1.03
Women	20-29	<0.71	0.71-0.77	0.78-0.82	>0.82
	30-39	<0.72	0.72-0.78	0.79-0.84	>0.84
	40-49	<0.73	0.73-0.79	0.80-0.87	>0.87
	50-59	<0.74	0.74-0.81	0.82-0.88	>0.88
	60-69	<0.76	0.76-0.83	0.84-0.90	>0.90

Adapted from Bray and Gray, 1988b, "Obesity - Part I - Pathogenesis," *The Western Journal of Medicine* 149: 432.

boundary value of WHTR >0.50 indicates an increased health risk for men and women, for people of different ethnic groups, and for children >5 yr of age (Ashwell and Hsieh 2005). As a rule, waist circumference should be less than half the height. Flegal and colleagues (2009) reported that WHTR, waist circumference, and BMI were highly related (r = 0.85 to 0.97) across age groups and genders. Although all three of these anthropometric indices performed similarly as indicators of body fatness, the relationship of WHTR with %BF was slightly higher (r = 0.66 to 0.87).

The Ashwell Shape Chart can be used to identify your client's health risk based on body shape (see appendix D.6, p. 371). To use this chart, measure your client's standing height and waist circumference at the umbilical level. Find the point corresponding to your client's height (y-axis of chart) and waist circumference (x-axis). This chart is applicable to adults from all race-ethnic groups, as well as children 5 yr of age or older.

Sagittal Abdominal Diameter

The **sagittal abdominal diameter (SAD)** is a measure of the anteroposterior thickness of the abdomen at the umbilical level. Research suggests that the SAD is an excellent indirect measure of visceral fat (Ohrvall et al. 2000; Zamboni et al. 1998). The SAD is strongly related to visceral adipose tissue in men (r = 0.82) and women (r = 0.76), even after adjusting for BMI (r = 0.66 and 0.63, respectively, for

men and women) (Zamboni et al. 1998). However, this relationship is stronger in lean or moderately overweight individuals than in obese individuals. Compared to waist circumference, WHR, and BMI, SAD is more strongly related to risk factors for cardiovascular and metabolic diseases in women and men (Ohrvall et al. 2000). The SAD is also associated with cardiovascular disease risk factors in older women (67-78 yr) (Turcato et al. 2000).

The procedures for measuring SAD have not been standardized. In most studies, SAD was measured while the client was lying supine, legs extended, on an examination table. A sliding-beam anthropometer is used to measure the vertical distance (to the nearest 0.1 cm) between the top of the table and the abdomen at the level of the umbilicus or iliac crests. In some studies, SAD was measured with the hips and legs flexed or with the client standing instead of lying supine.

Using Anthropometric Measures to Classify Frame Size

Skeletal diameters are used to classify frame size in order to improve the validity of height–weight tables for evaluating body weight. The rationale for including frame size is that skeletal breadths are important estimators of the bone and muscle components of fat-free mass. Estimating frame size allows you to differentiate between those who weigh more because of a large musculoskeletal mass and those who weigh more because of a large fat mass (Himes and Frisancho 1988). Since there are health implications for individuals who are overweight, a critical evaluation of body weight is important. You can classify frame size by using reference data for elbow breadth (see table 8.9). The anatomical landmarks for measurement are described in appendix D.5, "Standardized Sites for Bony Breadth Measurements," page 370.

Anthropometric Techniques

You must practice in order to become proficient in measuring skeletal diameters and circumferences. Following the standardized procedures (see p. 224) will increase the accuracy and reliability of your measurements (Callaway et al. 1988; Wilmore et al. 1988).

Sources of Measurement Error

The accuracy and reliability of anthropometric measures are potentially affected by equipment, technician skill, and client factors (Bray 1978; Callaway et al. 1988). The following questions and responses concern these sources of measurement error.

■ *What equipment will I need to measure bony widths?*

Use skeletal anthropometers and sliding or spreading calipers to measure bony widths and body breadths (see figure 8.15). The precision characteristics (0.05 to 0.50 cm) and range of measurement (0 to 210 cm) depend on the type of skeletal anthropometer or caliper you are using (Wilmore et al. 1988). The instruments must be carefully maintained and must be calibrated periodically so that their accuracy can be checked and restored.

■ *Can I use any type of tape measure to measure body circumferences?*

Use an anthropometric tape measure to measure circumferences (see figure 8.15). The tape measure should be made from a flexible material that does not stretch with use. You can use a plastic-coated tape measure if an anthropometric tape measure is not available. Some anthropometric tapes have a spring-loaded handle (i.e., Gulick handle) that allows a constant tension to be applied to the end of the tape during the measurement.

■ *How much skill and practice are required to ensure accurate circumference and skeletal diameter measurements?*

Technician skill is not a major source of measurement error for these methods compared to the SKF method. However, you need to practice in order to perfect the identification of the measurement sites and your measurement technique. Experts recommend practicing on at least 50 people and taking

Table 8.9 Elbow Breadth Norms (in cm) for Men and Women in the United States

	Age (yr)	Small	Medium	Large
			FRAME SIZE	
		Small	Medium	Large
Men	18-24	≤6.6	>6.6 and <7.7	≥7.7
	25-34	≤6.7	>6.7 and <7.9	≥7.9
	35-44	≤6.7	>6.7 and <8.0	≥8.0
	45-54	≤6.7	>6.7 and <8.1	≥8.1
	55-64	≤6.7	>6.7 and <8.1	≥8.1
	65-74	≤6.7	>6.7 and <8.1	≥8.1
Women	18-24	≤5.6	>5.6 and <6.5	≥6.5
	25-34	≤5.7	>5.7 and <6.8	≥6.8
	35-44	≤5.7	>5.7 and <7.1	≥7.1
	45-54	≤5.7	>5.7 and <7.2	≥7.2
	55-64	≤5.8	>5.8 and <7.2	≥7.2
	65-74	≤5.8	>5.8 and <7.2	≥7.2

STANDARDIZED PROCEDURES FOR ANTHROPOMETRIC MEASUREMENTS

1. Take all circumference and bony diameter measurements of the limbs on the right side of the body.

2. Carefully identify and measure the anthropometric site. Be meticulous about locating anatomical landmarks used to identify the measurement site (see appendix D.4, "Standardized Sites for Circumference Measurements," p. 369; and appendix D.5, "Standardized Sites for Bony Breadth Measurements," p. 370), and instruct your clients to relax their muscles during the measurement.

3. Take a minimum of three measurements at each site in rotational order.

4. To measure the breadth of smaller segments, like the elbow or wrist, use small sliding calipers (range of 30 cm or 11.8 in.) with greater scale precision instead of larger skeletal anthropometers (range of 60 to 80 cm or 23.6 to 31.5 in.).

5. Hold the skeletal anthropometer or caliper in both hands so the tips of the index fingers are adjacent to the tips of the caliper.

6. Place the caliper on the bony landmarks and apply firm pressure to compress the underlying muscle, fat, and skin. Apply pressure to a point where the measurement no longer continues to decrease.

7. Use an anthropometric tape to measure circumferences. Hold the zero end of the tape in your left hand, positioned below the other part of the tape that is held in your right hand.

8. Apply tension to the tape so that it fits snugly around the body part but does not indent the skin or compress the subcutaneous tissue.

9. For some circumferences (e.g., waist, hip, and thigh), you should align the tape in a horizontal plane, parallel to the floor.

---

a minimum of three measurements for each site in rotational order (Callaway et al. 1988). Closely follow standardized testing procedures for locating measurement sites, positioning the anthropometer or tape measure, and applying tension during the measurement. Appendix D.4 ("Standardized Sites for Circumference Measurements," p. 369) and appendix D.5 ("Standardized Sites for Bony Breadth Measurements," p. 370) describe some of the most commonly used circumference and skeletal diameter sites.

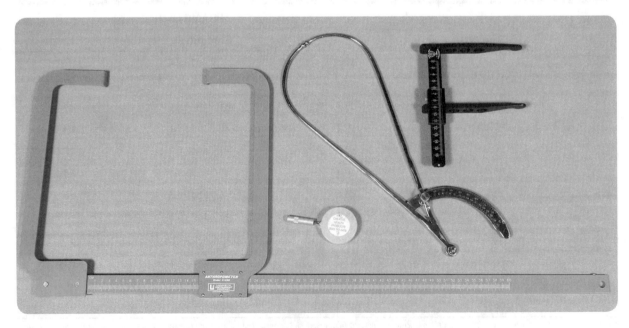

Figure 8.15 Skeletal anthropometers and anthropometric tape measure.

■ *Is there good agreement in circumference and skeletal diameter values when the measurements are taken by two different technicians?*

Variability in circumference measurements taken by different technicians is relatively small (0.2 to 1.0 cm), with some sites differing more than others (Callaway et al. 1988). Skilled technicians can obtain similar values even when measuring circumferences of obese individuals (Bray and Gray 1988a).

■ *Are the circumferences of obese clients more easily measured than SKFs?*

As with the SKF method, it is more difficult to obtain consistent measurements of circumference for obese compared to lean individuals (Bray and Gray 1988a). However, circumferences are preferable to SKFs for measuring obese clients, for several reasons:

■ You can measure circumferences of obese individuals regardless of their size, whereas the maximum aperture of the SKF caliper may not be large enough to allow measurement.

■ Measurement of circumferences requires less technician skill.

■ Differences between technicians are smaller for circumferences compared to SKF measurements (Bray and Gray 1988a).

■ *Is it possible to accurately measure bony widths of heavily muscled and obese clients?*

Accurate measurement of bony diameters in heavily muscled or obese individuals may be difficult because the underlying muscle and fat tissues must be firmly compressed. It may be difficult to identify and palpate bony anatomical landmarks, leading to error in locating the measurement site.

Near-Infrared Interactance Method

Near-infrared interactance (NIR) is a method that indirectly assesses tissue composition (fat and water) by measuring optical density, or the amount of light absorbed and reflected at a specific body site (typically the biceps site). Near-infrared interactance has been commercially available for years as an alternative method for assessing body composition. Futrex, Inc. is the only manufacturer of a commercial NIR device that measures optical density values for estimating %BF. In the late 1990s,

Futrex developed a new line of NIR analyzers (the 1100, 5000/XL, and 6100/XL to replace the 1000, 5000, and 6000, respectively). Most of the upgrades in the Futrex models were designed to make the product more user friendly (e.g., ability to print in color and to download data to computers) rather than to change the way it measures optical density. All of the Futrex analyzers except the Futrex-6100/XL measure NIR light at two wavelengths. The Futrex-6100/XL measures NIR light at up to six wavelengths.

There are over 20 cross-validation studies of the manufacturer's equations for the Futrex NIR analyzers. With few exceptions, the prediction errors have been large (*SEE* >3.5% BF). In most cases, the Futrex-5000 equation underestimates %BF by 2% to 10% BF. The degree of underestimation appears to be directly related to the level of body fatness (Elia, Parkinson, and Diaz 1990; Heyward et al. 1992). Some studies noted large underestimations of average %BF when the Futrex-5000 equation was compared to multicomponent model estimates of %BF for obese women (Fuller, Sawyer, and Elia 1994) and for overweight arthritic patients (Heitmann et al. 1994). Thus, the Futrex-5000 manufacturer's equation is likely to yield gross underestimates of the %BF of fatter clients compared to estimates for leaner clients.

The vast majority of NIR research has been done on the Futrex-5000 analyzer; however, a few studies have used other models. The Futrex-1000 is a handheld, battery-operated device designed for home use. Studies including both the Futrex-5000 and the Futrex-1000 have reported lower validity coefficients and higher prediction errors for the Futrex-1000 (Smith et al. 1997; Stout et al. 1994a, 1994b, 1996). Even though the Futrex-5000A is marketed for use with children, Smith and colleagues (1997) observed that the Futrex-5000 more accurately estimates %BF for female gymnasts (13-17 yr) than the 5000A does. Likewise, Cassady and colleagues (1993) reported unacceptable %BF prediction errors when using the Futrex-5000A manufacturer's equation to assess the body composition of children. One study compared %BF estimates from the Futrex-6000 and from DXA. In this study of obese females, the mean difference between %BF$_{Futrex-6000}$ and %BF$_{DXA}$ was small (1.4% BF); however, the individual predictive accuracy for the Futrex-6000 was poor (–8.0% to 10.7% BF) (Panotopoulos et al. 2001). From these limited data, it appears that these models (Futrex-5000A and Futrex-6000) of analyzers are no better than the Futrex-5000 at estimating %BF and, in some cases, that they are even worse. Because many research studies have reported unacceptable prediction errors, the Futrex manufacturer's equations should not be used to assess the body fatness of your clients.

Sources for Equipment

Product	Supplier's Contact Information
Air displacement plethysmograph	
Bod Pod Body Composition System	Life Measurement, Inc. (800) 426-3763 www.bodpod.com
Anthropometers	
Spreading calipers Sliding calipers Standard skeletal anthropometer	Rosscraft Industries (604) 324-9400 www.Rosscraft.ca
Anthropometric tape measure	Country Technology, Inc. (608) 735-4718 www.fitnessmart.com
Bioimpedance analyzers	
Bio-Analogics	Bio-Analogics (800) 327-7953 www.bioanalogics.com
Biodynamics	Biodynamics Corp. (800) 869-6987 www.biodyncorp.com
Bioimpedance spectroscopy (BIS) analyzers (InBody 320 and 720 analyzers)	Biospace, Inc. (310) 358-0360 www.biospaceamerica.com
Bodystat	Bodystat (USA), Inc. (813) 258-3570 www.bodystat.com
Data-Input	Data-Input GmbH +49 6151 13613-0 www.b-i-a.de
Holtain	Holtain, Ltd. +44 (0) 1239-891656 www.fullbore.co.uk/holtain/medical
Impedimed (distributors of SEAC BIA analyzers)	Impedimed (877) 247-0111 www.impedimed.com
Maltron	Maltron International, Ltd. +44 (0) 1268-778251 www.maltronint.com

Product	Supplier's Contact Information
OMRON	OMRON Healthcare, Inc. (847) 680-6200 www.omronhealthcare.com
RJL	RJL Systems (800) 528-4513 www.rjlsystems.com
Tanita	Tanita Corp. of America, Inc. (847) 640-9241 www.tanita.com
Xitron Hydra ECF/ICF	Xitron Technologies, Inc. (858) 530-8099 www.xitrontech.com
Calibration instruments and supplies	
Skinfold calibration blocks (15 mm)	Creative Health Products (800) 742-4478 www.chponline.com
Standard calibration weights	Ohaus Scale Corp. (973) 377-9000 www.ohaus.com
Vernier caliper	L.S. Starrett Co. (978) 249-3551 www.lsstarrett.com
Dual-energy X-ray absorptiometers	
Hologic	Hologic, Inc. (781) 999-7300 www.hologic.com
Norland	Cooper Surgical (800) 243-2974 www.coopersurgical.com
Lunar	GE Lunar Medical Systems (608) 274-2663 www.gemedicalsystems.com
Near-infrared interactance analyzer	
Futrex NIR analyzers	Zelcore, Inc. (301) 791-9220 www.futrex.com
Scales	
Chatillon underwater weighing scale Detecto balance beam scale Health-O-Meter balance beam scale Health-O-Meter digital scale Seca digital scale	Creative Health Products (800) 742-4478 www.chponline.com

(continued)

Sources for Equipment *(continued)*

Product	Supplier's Contact Information
Skinfold calipers	
Accu-Measure	Accu-Measure, LLC (800) 866-2727 www.accumeasurefitness.com
Adipometer (plastic)	Ross Products Division/Abbott Laboratories (800) 344-9739 www.abbott.com
Body Caliper	The Caliper Company, Inc. (866) 207-6308 www.bodycaliper.com
Fat-Control (plastic) Fat-o-Meter Lafayette Skyndex Slim-Guide	Creative Health Products (800) 742-4478 www.chponline.com
Harpenden	Baty International +44 (0) 1444 235621 www.baty.co.uk
Holtain	Holtain, Ltd. +44 (0) 1239-891656 www.holtain.com
Lange	Cambridge Scientific Products (877) 873-3522 www.cambridgescientific.com
McGaw (plastic)	McGaw, Inc. (714) 660-2055 www.mcgaw.com
Stadiometers	
Harpenden	Baty International +44 (0) 1444 235621 www.baty.co.uk
Holtain	Holtain, Ltd. +44 (0) 1239-891656 www.holtain.com

KEY POINTS

- Body composition is a key component of health and physical fitness; total body fat and fat distribution are related to disease risk.
- Standards for percent body fat can be used to classify body composition.
- Average %BF and standards for obesity vary according to age, gender, and physical activity levels.
- Hydrostatic weighing is a valid and reliable reference method for assessing body composition.
- Air displacement plethsymography is used to measure body volume and body density.
- Dual-energy X-ray absorptiometry is gaining recognition as a reference method for assessing body composition.
- Population-specific conversion formulas, based on multicomponent models of body composition, should be used to convert Db into percent body fat.
- The SKF method is widely used in field and clinical settings.
- Generalized SKF equations for the prediction of Db are reliable and valid for a wide range of individuals.
- Bioelectrical impedance analysis is a viable alternative for assessing body composition of diverse population subgroups.
- Circumferences and skeletal diameters can be used to estimate body composition.
- Body mass index is a crude index of total body fatness.
- Waist-to-hip ratio, waist circumference, WHTR, and SAD are acceptable indices for identifying at-risk clients.

KEY TERMS

Learn the definition for each of the following key terms. Definitions of terms can be found in the glossary on page 411.

air displacement plethysmography (ADP)

anthropometry

Archimedes' principle

attenuation

bioelectrical impedance analysis (BIA)

bioelectrical spectroscopy (BIS)

body density (Db)

body mass index (BMI)

body surface area

body volume (BV)

Boyle's law

circumference (C)

densitometry

dual-energy X-ray absorptiometry (DXA)

fat-free body (FFB)

fat-free mass (FFM)

fat mass (FM)

hydrodensitometry

hydrostatic weighing (HW)

impedance (Z)

multicomponent model

near-infrared interactance (NIR)

optical density

percent body fat (%BF)

reactance (X_c)

relative body fat (%BF)

residual volume (RV)

resistance (R)

resistance index (ht^2/R)

sagittal abdominal diameter (SAD)

skeletal diameter (D)

skinfold (SKF)

tare weight

thoracic gas volume (TGV)

two-component model

underwater weight (UWW)

waist-to-height ratio (WHTR)

waist-to-hip ratio (WHR)

REVIEW QUESTIONS

In addition to being able to define each of the key terms, test your knowledge and understanding of the material by answering the following review questions.

1. Why is it important to assess the body composition of your clients?

2. What are the standards for classifying obesity and minimal levels of body fat for men and women?

3. What are the assumptions of the two-component model of body composition? Identify two commonly used two-component model equations for converting Db into %BF.

4. Explain how gender, ethnicity, and age affect FFB density and therefore two-component model estimates of %BF.

5. Name three methods that can be used to obtain reference measures of body composition. Which method is best? Explain your choice.

6. Identify two ways to measure (not estimate) your client's Db.

7. Distinguish between total Db and FFB density.

8. Describe how the HW method could be modified to test clients who are unable to be weighed underwater at RV.

9. Identify potential sources of measurement error for the SKF method.

10. In lay terms, explain the basic theory underlying the use of BIA.

11. To obtain accurate estimates of body composition using the BIA method, your client must adhere to pretesting guidelines. Identify these client guidelines.

12. Explain how BMI, WHR, WHTR, and waist circumference may be used to identify clients at risk due to obesity.

13. Identify suitable field methods and prediction equations (i.e., SKF, BIA, or other anthropometric methods) to estimate body composition for each of the following subgroups of the population: older adults, children, obese individuals, and athletes.

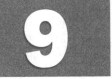
Designing Weight Management and Body Composition Programs

KEY QUESTIONS

- What is obesity and how prevalent is it worldwide?

- What are the health risks associated with having high or low levels of body fat?

- What are the primary causes of overweight and obesity?

- How is healthy body weight determined?

- What are the guidelines for a well-balanced diet? Are vitamin and mineral supplements necessary for most clients?

- What steps should I follow in planning a weight management program?

- What are the recommended guidelines for weight loss and weight gain programs?

- Why is exercise important for weight management?

- What types of exercise are best for weight loss?

- Does exercising without dieting improve body composition?

Health and longevity are threatened when a person is either overweight or underweight. Overweight and obesity increase one's risk of developing serious cardiovascular, pulmonary, and metabolic diseases and disorders. Likewise, individuals who are underweight may have a higher risk than others of cardiac, musculoskeletal, and reproductive disorders. Thus, healthy weight is key to a healthy and longer life.

As a health and fitness professional, you have an enormous challenge and responsibility to help determine a healthy body weight for your clients and to provide scientifically sound weight management programs for them. This chapter presents guidelines and techniques for determining healthy body weight. You will learn about weight control principles and practices, as well as guidelines for designing exercise programs for weight loss, weight gain, and body composition change.

OBESITY, OVERWEIGHT, AND UNDERWEIGHT: DEFINITIONS AND TRENDS

Individuals with body fat levels falling at or near the extremes of the body fat continuum are likely to have serious health problems that reduce life expectancy and threaten their quality of life. Obese individuals have a higher risk of cardiovascular disease, dyslipidemia, hypertension, glucose intolerance, insulin resistance, diabetes mellitus, obstructive pulmonary disease, gallbladder disease, osteoarthritis, and certain types of cancer (U.S. Department of Health and Human Services 2000b). The prevalences of hypercholesterolemia, hypertension, and type 2 diabetes are, respectively, 2.9, 2.1, and 2.9 times greater in overweight than non-overweight persons (National Institutes of Health Consensus Development Panel 1985). Obesity is independently associated with coronary heart disease (CHD), heart failure, cardiac arrhythmia, stroke, and menstrual irregularities (Pi-Sunyer 1999).

At the opposite extreme, underweight individuals with too little body fat tend to be malnourished. These people have a relatively higher risk of fluid–electrolyte imbalances, osteoporosis and osteopenia, bone fractures, muscle wasting, cardiac arrhythmias and sudden death, peripheral edema, and renal and reproductive disorders (Fohlin 1977; Mazess, Barden, and Ohlrich 1990; Vaisman et al. 1988a). One disease associated with extremely low body fat levels is anorexia nervosa. **Anorexia nervosa,** an eating disorder found primarily in females, is characterized by excessive weight loss. Anorexia nervosa afflicts approximately 1% of the female population in the United States (Hudson et al. 2007). Compared to normal women, those with anorexia have extremely low body fat (8% to 13% body fat), signs of muscle wasting, and less bone mineral content and bone density (Mazess et al. 1990; Vaisman et al. 1988b).

Definitions of Obesity, Overweight, and Underweight

Obesity is an excessive amount of body fat relative to body weight and is not synonymous with overweight. In many epidemiological studies, overweight is defined as a body mass index (BMI) between 25 and 29.9 kg/m²; obesity is defined as a BMI of 30 kg/m² or more; and underweight is defined by a BMI of less than 18.5 kg/m² (U.S. Department of Health and Human Services 2000b). To identify children and adolescents who are overweight, the 85th and 95th percentile cutoffs for age and sex developed from the Centers for Disease Control and Prevention growth charts are commonly used in the United States. Children with a BMI greater than the 95th percentile for their age and sex are categorized as overweight; those with BMI values between the 85th and 94th percentiles are categorized as **at risk for overweight.** However, these definitions are not universally accepted. Pooled international data for BMI have been used to develop international standards for evaluating

childhood overweight and obesity. These standards are based on growth curves that relate the cutoff points for BMI of different age–gender groups (2-18 yr) to the adult categories for overweight (BMI ≥25 kg/m²) and obesity (BMI ≥30 kg/m²) (see Cole et al. 2000). Because these criteria do not take into account the composition of the individual's body weight, they are limited as indexes of obesity and may result in misclassifications of underweight, overweight, and obesity. There is considerable variability in body composition for any given BMI. Some individuals with low BMIs may have as much relative body fat as those with higher BMIs. Older people have more relative body fat at any given BMI than younger people (Baumgartner, Heymsfield, and Roche 1995). Thus, the prevalence of obesity could be worse than currently thought.

Trends in Overweight and Obesity

Globally, the prevalence of overweight and obesity has reached epidemic proportions. The World Health Organization (2007) reported that more than 1.6 billion adults are overweight and over 400 million are obese. The World Health Organization estimates that by the year 2015 the number of overweight people globally will increase to 2.3 billion; more than 700 million will be obese (American Heart Association [AHA] 2009).

The prevalence of overweight and obesity in adults varies among countries, depending in part on the nation's level of industrialization (see table 9.1). In the European Union, Greece and Germany have the highest prevalence of overweight and obesity; almost 3 out of 4 adults are either overweight or obese (see table 9.1). In the United States, 34% of adults are obese (BMI >30 kg/m²), and 2 out of 3 adults are overweight (BMI = 25-29.9 kg/m²). On average, France, Italy, Switzerland, and the Scandinavian countries (e.g., Denmark and Norway) have relatively low prevalence of adult obesity. It is projected that by the year 2025, the proportion of overweight and obese people will rise to 24% in India and to 37% to 40% in China (AHA 2009).

Childhood obesity is also a global problem. The prevalence of children and adolescents (6-19 yr) at risk for overweight (BMI = 85th-95th percentile) in Canada and the United States ranges from 29% to 35% (AHA 2009; Hedley et al. 2004; Ogden, Carroll, and Flegal 2008; Tremblay and Willms 2000). In comparison, children in Australia (~20%)

Table 9.1 Prevalence of Obesity and Overweight in Adults From Selected Countries

Country	Survey year	OBESITY Men (%)	OBESITY Women (%)	OVERWEIGHT AND OBESITY Men (%)	OVERWEIGHT AND OBESITY Women(%)
Armenia	2000/2001		14		
Australia	2004/2005	19	17	62	45
Austria	2005/2006	23	21	66	53
Azerbaijan	2001		12		
Belgium*	2004	12	13	63	41
Bosnia and Herzegovina	2002	17	25		
Canada	2007			40	40
Croatia	2003	22	23		
Cyprus	1999/2000	27	24	73	58
Czech Republic*	2002	14	16	73	58
Denmark*	2000	10	9	52	37
England	2004	23	24	67	58
Estonia*	2004	14	15	46	43
Finland	2000/2001	21	24	68	52
France	2006	12	13	47	26
Germany*	2002/2003	22	23	75	59
Greece	2004	26	18	73	46
Hungary*	2003/2004	17	18	63	49
Iceland*	2002	12	12		
Ireland*	2002	14	12	66	48
Israel	1999/2001	20	25		
Italy*	2003	9	9	51	34
Kazakhstan	1999		13		
Kyrgyzstan	1997		9		
Latvia*	2004	12	20	50	50
Lithuania*	2004	14	17	58	42
Macedonia, TFYR	1999		11		
Malta*	2002	25	21	69	51
Netherlands	1998/2001	10	12	54	39
Norway*	1998	7	6		
Poland	2000	16	20	56	48
Portugal	2003/2004	15	15	59	47
Romania	1997	9	19		
Serbia and Montenegro	2000	14	20		
Slovenia*	2001	17	14	57	45
Spain	2003	13	14	58	48
Sweden	2002/2003	15	11	58	38
Switzerland*	2002	8	8		
Turkey	1997	13	30		
Turkmenistan	2000		10		
United States	2006	33	35	67	67
Uzbekistan	2002	5	7		

*Estimate from self-reported data. Obesity is defined as body mass index (BMI) ≥30 kg/m²; overweight is defined as BMI between 25 and 29.9 kg/m².

Blank cells indicate insufficient data or data not available.

Data compiled from World Health Organization 2007, International Association for the Study of Obesity 2007, and Australian Bureau of Statistics 2008.

and Mexico (10.8%-19.1%) have a relatively lower prevalence of being at risk for overweight (del Rio-Navarro et al. 2004; Magarey, Daniels, and Boulton 2001). Since 1980 the number of overweight American children has doubled, and the number of overweight American adolescents has tripled (World Health Organization 2004b). Also, it is alarming that even for preschool children (2-5 yr), the prevalence of overweight and obesity ranges from 18% in Australia to 25.6% in Canada (Canning, Courage, and Frizzell 2004).

Because of the health risks and medical costs associated with obesity, the goal of the U.S. surgeon general is to reduce the prevalence of overweight in children and obesity in adults to no more than 5% and 15%, respectively, by the year 2010 (U.S. Department of Health and Human Services 2000b).

OBESITY: TYPES AND CAUSES

Combating obesity is not an easy task. Many overweight and obese individuals have incorporated patterns of overeating and physical inactivity into their lifestyles, while others have developed eating disorders, exercise addictions, or both. In an effort to lose weight quickly and to prevent weight gain, many are lured by fad diets and exercise gimmicks; some resort to extreme behaviors, such as avoiding food, bingeing and purging, and exercising compulsively. In a survey of weight control practices of adults in the United States, Weiss and colleagues (2006) reported that 48% of women and 34% of men were trying to lose weight by means of such practices as eating less food, eating less fat, choosing low-calorie foods, and exercising. Less common practices included drinking water, skipping meals, eating diet foods, taking special supplements or diet pills, joining weight loss programs, taking prescription diet pills, and taking laxatives. Only one-third of those trying to lose weight reported using the recommended method of restricting caloric intake and increasing physical activity to at least 150 min/wk; less than 25% combined caloric restriction with higher levels of physical activity (>300 min/wk).

In a report on leisure-time physical activity among overweight adults in the United States ("Prevalence of Leisure-Time Physical Activity" 2000), two-thirds of overweight adults reported

that they engaged in physical activity to try to lose weight; however, only 20% exercised at least 30 min a day at a moderate intensity on most days of the week. Although most of these individuals exercised 30 min or longer per session, only a minority exercised at least five times per week. Therefore, low frequency of physical activity was the main reason that the physical activity recommendation was not met.

Types of Obesity

The way in which fat is distributed in the body may be more important than total body fat for determining one's risk of disease. The waist-to-hip ratio (WHR) is strongly associated with visceral fat, and the impact of regional fat distribution on health is related to the amount of visceral fat located in the abdominal cavity. Abdominal fat is strongly associated with diseases such as CHD, diabetes, hypertension, and hyperlipidemia (Bjorntorp 1988; Blair et al. 1984; Ducimetier, Richard, and Cambien 1989).

The terms **android obesity** and **gynoid obesity** refer to the localization of excess body fat mainly in the upper body (android) or lower body (gynoid). Android obesity (apple shaped) is more typical of males; gynoid obesity (pear shaped) is more characteristic of females. However, some men may have gynoid obesity, and some women may have android obesity. Other terms are also used to describe types of obesity and regional fat distribution. Android obesity is frequently simply called **upper body obesity**, and gynoid obesity is often described as **lower body obesity**.

In field settings, you can assess regional fat distribution using the WHR. Chapter 8 presents measurement procedures (see p. 221) and WHR norms (see table 8.8, p. 222). Generally, young adults with WHR values in excess of 0.94 for men and 0.82 for women are at very high risk for adverse health consequences (Bray and Gray 1988b).

Causes of Overweight and Obesity

Many questions may arise in regard to overweight and obesity. This section addresses common questions relating to the causes of overweight and obesity.

■ *Why do people gain or lose weight?*

An energy imbalance in the body results in a weight gain or loss. There is an energy balance when the caloric intake equals the caloric expenditure.

A **positive energy balance** is created when the input (food intake) exceeds the expenditure (resting metabolism plus activity level). For every 3500 kcal of excess energy accumulated, 1 lb (0.45 kg) of fat is stored in the body. A **negative energy balance** is produced when the energy expenditure exceeds the energy input. People can accomplish this by reducing the food intake or increasing the physical activity level. A caloric deficit of approximately 3500 kcal produces a loss of 1 lb of fat.

■ *How are energy needs and energy expenditure measured?*

Energy need and expenditure are measured in kilocalories (kcal). A **kilocalorie** is defined as the amount of heat needed to raise the temperature of 1 kg (2.2 lb) of water 1° C. Direct calorimetry is used to measure the energy yield and caloric equivalent of various foods. These foods are burned in a closed chamber in the presence of oxygen, and the amount of heat liberated is measured precisely in kilocalories. Table 9.2 gives the energy yield and caloric equivalents for carbohydrate, protein, and fat.

The energy or caloric need is a function of an individual's metabolic rate and physical activity level. The **basal metabolic rate (BMR)** is a measure of the minimal amount of energy (kcal) needed to maintain basic and essential physiological functions such as breathing, blood circulation, and temperature regulation. Basal metabolic rate varies according to age, gender, body size, and body composition. For assessment of BMR, the individual needs to be rested and fasted and should be in a controlled environment. Since this is not always practical, we use the term **resting metabolic rate (RMR)**, or **resting energy expenditure (REE)**, to indicate the energy required to maintain essential physiological processes in a relaxed, awake, and reclined state. The RMR is approximately 10% higher than the BMR.

Total energy expenditure (TEE) is the sum of the energy expended for BMR or RMR, **dietary thermogenesis** (i.e., energy needed for digesting, absorbing, transporting, and metabolizing foods), and physical activity. The gold standard for measuring TEE is the doubly labeled water (with deuterium and oxygen-18) method. This method is expensive and requires considerable expertise as well as specialized equipment. Therefore, age- and gender-specific prediction equations have been developed to estimate TEE (see table 9.3).

Alternatively, energy expenditure during basal, resting, or activity states can be measured in laboratory settings through indirect calorimetry. In this case, the body's energy expenditure is estimated from oxygen utilization. Every liter of oxygen consumed per minute yields approximately 5 kcal (see table 9.2). For specific physical activities, energy expenditure is typically expressed in METs (see chapter 4 and appendix E.4) as a multiple of the RMR. One MET equals the relative rate of oxygen consumption of 3.5 ml·min^{-1} for each kilogram of body weight (3.5 ml·kg^{-1}·min^{-1}) or the relative rate of energy expenditure of 1 kcal·hr^{-1} for each kilogram of body weight (1 kcal·hr^{-1}·kg^{-1}).

The Western Human Nutrition Research Center of the U.S. Department of Agriculture developed a **digital activity log.** The digital activity log allows the client to record in a handheld computer the type and duration of physical activity performed during the day. The hours spent in various MET-level activities are calculated and used, along with RMR, number of waking hours, and estimated energy expenditure during sleep, to measure TEE. Validation studies showed that in women of normal weight, this method yields TEE values that are within 10% of reference measures (Kretsch et al. 2004).

■ *How is RMR regulated?*

Thyroxine is extremely important in regulating RMR. Inadequate levels of this hormone can be produced by thyroid tumors or lack of iodine in the diet. Underproduction of thyroxine can reduce RMR 30% to 50%. If energy input and expenditure

Table 9.2 Energy Yield and Caloric Equivalents for Macronutrients

Nutrient	Energy yield (kcal·g^{-1})	Caloric equivalents (kcal·L^{-1} O$_2$)
Carbohydrate	4.1	5.1
Protein	4.3	4.4
Fat	9.3	4.7

Table 9.3 Prediction Equations for Estimating TEE (kcal·day⁻¹) of Children and Adults

Gender and age	Equation	Physical activity coefficient (PA)
Male 3-18 yr	TEE = 88.5 − (61.9 × age) + PA [(26.7 × wt) + (903 × ht)]	1.00, if PAL ≥1.0 and <1.4 (sedentary)
		1.13, if PAL ≥1.4 and <1.6 (low)
		1.26, if PAL ≥1.6 and <1.9 (active)
		1.42, if PAL ≥1.9 and <2.5 (very active)
Male ≥19 yr	TEE = 662 − (9.53 × age) + PA [(15.9 × wt) + (540 × ht)]	1.00, if PAL ≥1.0 and <1.4 (sedentary)
		1.11, if PAL ≥1.4 and <1.6 (low)
		1.25, if PAL ≥1.6 and <1.9 (active)
		1.48, if PAL ≥1.9 and <2.5 (very active)
Female 3-18 yr	TEE = 135.3 − (30.8 × age) + PA [(10.0 × wt) + (934 × ht)]	1.00, if PAL ≥1.0 and <1.4 (sedentary)
		1.16, if PAL ≥1.4 and <1.6 (low)
		1.31, if PAL ≥1.6 and <1.9 (active)
		1.56, if PAL ≥1.9 and <2.5 (very active)
Female ≥19 yr	TEE = 354 − (6.91 × age) + PA [(9.36 × wt) + (726 × ht)]	1.00, if PAL ≥1.0 and <1.4 (sedentary)
		1.12, if PAL ≥1.4 and <1.6 (low)
		1.27, if PAL ≥1.6 and <1.9 (active)
		1.45, if PAL ≥1.9 and <2.5 (very active)

TEE = total energy expenditure in kcal·day⁻¹; PA = physical activity coefficient; wt = body weight in kilograms; ht = height in meters; PAL = physical activity level.

From Institute of Medicine 2002.

are not adjusted accordingly, the positive energy balance that is created results in a weight gain.

Growth hormone, epinephrine, norepinephrine, and various sex hormones may elevate RMR as much as 15% to 20%. These hormones increase during exercise and may be responsible for the elevation in RMR after cessation of exercise.

■ *Does weight gain increase both the number and size of fat cells?*

Obesity is associated with increases in both the number and size of fat cells. A normal-weight individual has 25 to 30 billion fat cells, whereas an obese person may have as many as 42 to 106 billion fat cells. Also, the adipose cell size of obese individuals is on the average 40% larger than that of nonobese persons (Hirsh 1971). An increase in fat cell number (**hyperplasia**) occurs rapidly during the first year of life and again during adolescence but remains fairly stable in adulthood, except in cases of morbid obesity. Epidemiological studies suggest that weight gain in the first 6 mo of life is primarily a gain in fat and that this time period is critical for development of obesity and cardiometabolic problems in adulthood (Gillman 2008).

Fat cells increase in size (**hypertrophy**) during the adolescent growth spurt and continue to grow when excess fat is stored in the cells as triglycerides. Weight gain in adults is typically characterized by the enlargement of existing fat cells rather than the creation of new fat cells. Also, caloric restriction and exercise are effective in reducing fat cell size but not the number of fat cells in adults (Hirsh 1971). Perhaps the key to preventing obesity is to closely monitor the dietary intake and energy expenditure, especially during the adolescent growth spurt and puberty. This could potentially retard the development of new fat cells and control the size of existing fat cells.

■ *What is the relative importance of genetics and environment in developing obesity?*

Scientists have debated the relative contributions of genetics and environment to obesity. Mayer (1968) observed that only 10% of children who had normal-weight parents were obese. Overweight adolescents have a 70% chance of becoming overweight adults; this probability increases to 80% if one parent or both parents are overweight or obese (U.S. Department of Health and Human Services

2007). Although these data suggest a genetic influence, they do not rule out environmental influences such as eating and exercise habits.

In a controlled study of long-term (100 days) overfeeding in identical twins, Bouchard and colleagues (1990) observed large individual differences in the tendency toward obesity and distribution of body fat, even within each pair of twins. Changes in body weight due to overfeeding of twins were moderately correlated ($r = 0.55$). Overall, increases in body weight, fat mass, trunk fat, and visceral fat were three times greater in high weight gainers compared to low weight gainers. These data suggest that genotype explains some, but not all, of a person's adaptation to a sustained energy surplus. Approximately 25% of the variability among individuals in absolute and relative body fat is attributed to genetic factors, and 30% is associated with cultural (environmental) factors (Bouchard et al. 1988).

Hill and Melanson (1999) suggested that the major cause of obesity in the United States is our environment. Over the past 30 yr, the U.S. population has been exposed to an environment that strongly promotes the consumption of high-fat, energy-dense foods (increased energy intake) and reliance on technology that discourages physical activity and reduces the amount of physical activity (decreased energy expenditure) needed for daily living.

WEIGHT MANAGEMENT PRINCIPLES AND PRACTICES

Proper nutrition (eating a well-balanced diet) and daily physical activity are key components of a weight management program. In weight management programs, most clients are interested in losing body weight and body fat, but some need to gain body weight. The basic principle underlying safe and effective weight loss programs is that weight can be lost only through a negative energy balance, which is produced when the caloric expenditure exceeds the caloric intake. The most effective way of creating a caloric deficit is through a combination of diet (restricting caloric intake) and exercise (increasing caloric expenditure). On the other hand, for weight gain programs, the caloric intake must exceed the caloric expenditure in order to create a positive energy balance. "Weight Management Principles" (p. 239) summarizes principles and practices underlying the design of weight management programs.

People can win the battle of controlling body weight and obesity by not only understanding why they eat and monitoring their food intake closely, but also by incorporating more physical activity into their lifestyles. The physically active lifestyle is characterized by

- daily aerobic exercise;
- strength and flexibility exercises;
- increased participation in recreational activities such as bowling, golf, tennis, and dancing; and
- increased physical activity in the daily routine at home and work through restricting use of labor-saving devices such as escalators, power tools, automobiles, and home and garden appliances.

In addition to these suggestions, you should encourage your clients to follow the *Dietary Guidelines for Americans 2005* (U.S. Department of Health and Human Services 2005a). New, updated dietary guidelines are scheduled for release in the fall of 2010.

Adequate Nutrients Within Calorie Needs

- Consume a variety of nutrient-dense foods within and among the basic food groups; choose foods that limit intake of saturated and trans fats, cholesterol, added sugars, and salt; and limit intake of alcohol.
- Meet recommended intakes within energy needs by adopting a balanced eating pattern.

Weight Management

- To maintain body weight in a healthy range, balance calories from foods and beverages with calories expended.
- To prevent gradual weight gain over time, make small decreases in food and beverage calories and increase physical activity.

Physical Activity

- To reduce risk of chronic disease in adulthood, engage in at least 30 min of moderate-intensity physical activity, above usual activity, at work or home on most days of the week.

- For most people, greater health benefits can be obtained by engaging in physical activity of more vigorous intensity or longer duration.

- To help manage body weight and prevent gradual, unhealthy body weight gain in adulthood, engage in approximately 60 min of moderate- to vigorous-intensity exercise on most days of the week while not exceeding caloric intake requirements.

- To sustain weight loss in adulthood, participate in at least 60 to 90 min of daily moderate-intensity physical activity while not exceeding caloric intake requirements. Some people may need to consult with a health care provider before participating in this level of activity.

- Achieve physical fitness by including cardiovascular conditioning, stretching exercises for flexibility, and resistance exercises or calisthenics for muscle strength and endurance.

Food Groups to Encourage

- Consume a sufficient amount of fruits and vegetables while staying within energy needs. Two cups of fruit and 2 1/2 cups of vegetables per day are recommended for a reference 2000-calorie intake, with higher or lower amounts depending on the calorie level.

- Choose a variety of fruits and vegetables each day. In particular, select from all five vegetable subgroups (dark green, orange, legumes, starchy vegetables, and other vegetables) several times a week.

- Consume 3 or more ounce equivalents of whole-grain products per day, with the rest of the recommended grains coming from enriched or whole-grain products. In general, at least half the grains should come from whole grains.

- Consume 3 cups per day of fat-free or low-fat milk or equivalent milk products.

Carbohydrates

- Choose fiber-rich fruits, vegetables, and whole grains often.

- Choose and prepare foods and beverages with little added sugars or caloric sweeteners.

- Reduce the incidence of dental caries by practicing good oral hygiene and consuming sugar- and starch-containing foods and beverages less frequently.

Sodium and Potassium

- Consume less than 2300 mg (approximately 1 tsp of salt) of sodium per day.

- Choose and prepare foods with little salt. At the same time, consume potassium-rich foods such as fruits and vegetables.

Alcoholic Beverages

- Those who drink alcoholic beverages should do so sensibly and in moderation—defined as the consumption of up to one drink per day for women and up to two drinks per day for men.

- Alcoholic beverages should not be consumed by individuals who cannot restrict their alcohol intake, women of childbearing age who may become pregnant, pregnant and lactating women, children and adolescents, individuals taking medications that can interact with alcohol, and those with specific medical conditions.

- Alcoholic beverages should be avoided by individuals engaging in activities that require attention, skill, or coordination such as driving or operating machinery.

WELL-BALANCED NUTRITION

Before you can help your clients with their weight management, you must understand good nutrition. A well-balanced diet should contain adequate amounts of protein, fat, carbohydrate, vitamins, minerals, and water. The Institute of Medicine (2002) recommends that adults seeking well-balanced nutrition get 45% to 65% of their calories from carbohydrates, 20% to 35% of their calories from fat, and 10% to 25% of their calories from protein.

Trends in the dietary intake of energy and macronutrients by U.S. adults (Wright et al. 2004) were evaluated through analysis of National Health and Nutrition Examination Survey (NHANES) data from 1971 (NHANES I) to 2000 (NHANES IV). Analysis showed that the average daily energy intake increased ~7% for men and 21% for women. This increase in calorie intake was attributed primarily to increases in the relative and absolute carbohydrate intake. The relative carbohydrate intake increased from 42% to 49% in men and from 45% to 51.6% in women. On average, the absolute

Weight Management Principles

Weight loss	Weight gain	Exercise
■ A well-balanced diet for good nutrition contains carbohydrate, protein, fat, vitamins, minerals, and water.	■ The dietary protein intake should be increased to 1.2 to 1.6 g·kg^{-1} body weight.	■ The major cause of obesity is lack of physical activity, not overeating.
■ The weight loss should be gradual—no more than 2 lb a week.	■ The weight gain should be gradual—no more than 2 lb a week.	■ For fat-weight loss, aerobic exercise should be performed daily or twice daily.
■ The caloric intake should be at least 1200 kcal·day^{-1}, and the caloric deficit should not exceed 1000 kcal·day^{-1}.	■ The daily caloric intake should exceed caloric needs by 400 to 500 kcal·day^{-1}.	■ Resistance exercise training is excellent for maintaining fat-free mass (for weight loss) and increasing FFM (for weight gain).
■ A caloric deficit of 3500 kcal is needed to lose 1 lb of fat.	■ A positive energy balance of 2800 to 3500 kcal is needed to gain 1 lb of muscle tissue.	■ For weight loss, exercise helps create a caloric deficit by increasing caloric expenditure.
■ Weight loss should be due to fat loss rather than lean body tissue.	■ Weight gain should be due to increased fat-free mass rather than fat mass.	■ Exercise is better than dieting for maximizing fat loss and minimizing lean tissue loss.
■ On the same diet, a taller, heavier person will lose weight at a faster rate than a shorter, lighter person due to a higher RMR.	■ The individual should eat three meals and two or three healthy snacks per day (e.g., dried fruits, nuts, seeds, and some liquid meals).	■ Compared to fat, muscle tissue is more metabolically active and uses more calories at rest.
■ Weight loss rate decreases over time, because the difference between the caloric intake and caloric needs gets smaller as one loses weight.	■ Protein powders are no more effective than natural protein sources (e.g., lean meats, skim milk, and egg whites).	■ Low-intensity, longer-duration exercise maximizes total energy expenditure better than high-intensity, shorter-duration exercise.
■ Men lose weight faster than women due to a higher RMR.	■ Amino acid supplements may promote muscle growth if taken immediately before or after exercise.	■ RMR remains elevated 30 min or longer after vigorous exercise.
■ The individual should eat at least three meals a day.	■ Vitamin B$_{12}$, boron, and chromium supplements do not increase fat-free mass.	■ At a given heart rate, the more physically fit individual expends calories at a faster rate than the less fit individual.
■ Quick weight loss diets, diet pills, and appetite suppressants should be avoided.		■ Exercise does not increase appetite.
■ Carnitine supplementation does not promote body fat loss.		■ Passive exercise devices (e.g., vibrators and sauna belts) do not massage away excess fat.
■ Compulsive eating behaviors should be identified and modified.		■ Spot reduction exercises do not preferentially mobilize subcutaneous fat stored near the exercising muscles.
		■ To increase caloric expenditure, avoid using labor-saving devices at home and work.

carbohydrate intake of men and women increased by 68 g and 62 g, respectively. In comparison, the relative intake of total fat decreased (from ~37% to ~33% for men and from 36% to ~33% for women). However, this relative decrease was attributed to the increase in total calorie intake. In fact, the average absolute amount of fat intake increased by 6.5 g for women but decreased by 5.3 g for men. The percentage of kilocalories obtained from protein slightly decreased for both men (from 16.5% to 15.5%) and women (from 16.9% to 15.1%).

Carbohydrates

Carbohydrates are grouped into two major categories—simple and complex. **Simple carbohydrates** consist of simple sugars (e.g., glucose and fructose) found in fruits, berries, some vegetables, table sugar, and honey. **Complex carbohydrates** are found in many plant-based foods, whole grains, and low-fat dairy products. The Institute of Medicine (2002) recommends that the largest proportion (45%-65%) of the daily calorie intake be in the form of carbohydrates. Experts recommend consuming a wide range of carbohydrates and emphasizing fruits, vegetables, whole grains, and low-fat dairy products. Foods with added sugars should be limited to no more than 25% of the total calories consumed; overweight people need much less. Carbohydrates provide an efficient source of energy (i.e., glucose) that the muscles and brain can directly use. The Institute of Medicine (2002) recommends a minimum daily intake of 130 g of carbohydrate to maintain proper brain function for children and adults. Also, many carbohydrates contain fiber; a high-fiber diet lowers the risk of heart disease, diabetes, and colon cancer (Harvard School of Public Health 2004).

Since 1981, the **glycemic index (GI)** has been used to classify carbohydrate-containing foods. The GI is a measure of the body's glycemic response (i.e., increase in blood glucose and insulin following consumption) to various foods. The GI rates the immediate effect of a specific food on blood glucose levels; to obtain the GI value of a food, the glycemic response of that food is compared with the glycemic response of glucose (GI = 100). The glycemic response of simple and complex carbohydrates varies greatly. Some complex carbohydrates are metabolized as rapidly as simple sugars. Generally, refined grain products and potatoes have a high GI (>60), legumes and unprocessed grains have a moderate GI (40-60), and nonstarchy fruits and vegetables have a low GI (<40). Lists of GI values for various foods may be found in nutrition books and journals and on Web sites (see Clark 2008; Foster-Powell and Miller 1995; Miller 2001).

Several popular diet books (e.g., *Sugar Busters, The Zone,* and *South Beach Diet*) advocate the consumption of low-GI foods. Although some international health organizations have endorsed the GI, its relevance to health and nutrition is controversial. For example, the AHA, American Diabetes Association, and American Dietetic Association do not endorse using the GI for disease prevention and treatment (Ludwig and Eckel 2002). In fact, Pi-Sunyer (2002) concluded that there is insufficient evidence to justify basing public health recommendations on the GI. Additional research is needed to assess the long-term effects of low-GI diets on the prevention and treatment of disease and obesity.

Recommendations for the dietary carbohydrate intake of athletes and physically active individuals depend on the intensity and duration of exercise. As intensity increases, the use of carbohydrates for energy increases and the proportion of energy coming from fat decreases. During extended exercise (lasting 1-2 hr), muscle glycogen is depleted, and the body must use blood glucose as a carbohydrate source for energy. Generally, a daily carbohydrate intake of 7 to 8 g·kg^{-1} of body weight is sufficient to maintain muscle glycogen stores day to day for individuals engaging in low-intensity, moderate-duration physical activity (American College of Sports Medicine [ACSM], American Dietetic Association, and Dietitians of Canada 2009). For those performing high-intensity or long-duration exercise, an intake of 7 to 12 g·kg^{-1} of body weight is recommended (Burke, Kiens, and Ivy 2004).

Protein

Approximately 10% to 25% of the daily caloric intake should be protein. The diet should include sources of the essential amino acids needed for protein synthesis. Lack of these essential amino acids may produce a loss of muscle tissue or prevent the synthesis of hormones, enzymes, and cellular structures. The amount of protein that the average individual needs to meet the daily protein requirements of the body is approximately 0.8 g·kg^{-1} of body weight, regardless of age or gender (Campbell et al. 2008). Experts agree that exercise increases the need for protein (American Dietetic Association 2000; Lemon 2000; Tipton and Wolfe 2004). The additional protein requirement depends on the type (resistance training or aerobic), intensity, and duration of exercise. The recommended daily protein intake for endurance athletes is 1.2 to 1.4 g·kg^{-1} of body weight, whereas strength-trained athletes may need as much as 1.7 g·kg^{-1} of body weight (ACSM et al. 2009; Lemon 2000). The diets of most athletes adequately meet these protein requirements, especially when the daily calorie intake is sufficient and the diet contains complete sources of protein such as meats, eggs, and fish (Campbell and Geik 2004; Manore 2004; Manore, Meyer, and Thompson 2009).

Amino acids are the building blocks of protein. Nine essential amino acids must be obtained through the diet because the body lacks the ability to synthesize them. Three essential amino acids—leucine, isoleucine, and valine—share a structural similarity and are known as branched-chain amino acids. Approximately 99% of the body's amino acids are incorporated into protein structures, and the remaining 1%, known as the free pool, can be found in the plasma and the intracellular and extracellular spaces. Amino acids enter the free pool through absorption of dietary protein, breakdown of tissue protein, and synthesis from carbohydrates or fat (Armsey and Grime 2002). Research suggests that muscle protein synthesis is regulated by levels of essential amino acids in the plasma rather than levels of intramuscular amino acids (Bohe et al. 2003). Leucine is one of the most important stimulators of skeletal muscle protein synthesis (Kimball and Jefferson 2002).

Excess protein cannot be stored in the body and is broken down into amino acids. Amino acids also cannot be stored and therefore will be used as fuel for energy. Too much protein in the diet causes dehydration due to excessive production of urea, which must be eliminated in the urine.

Fats

Fats and oils are part of a healthy diet and well-balanced nutrition. Some dietary fat is needed to supply fatty acids and to absorb fat-soluble vitamins. The omega-3 fatty acids (eicosapentaenoic acid [EPA] and docosahexanoic acid [DHA]) have a cardioprotective effect, reducing the risk of cardiovascular disease. In addition, free fatty acids are an important source of energy during aerobic exercise. Approximately 20% to 35% of the daily energy intake should come from fat; however, fats must be chosen wisely. To decrease their risk of elevated low-density lipo-protein cholesterol (LDL-C), most Americans need to decrease their intake of saturated fat, trans fatty acid, and cholesterol (U.S. Department of Health and Human Services 2004). Saturated fat should account for less than 10% of the daily calorie intake, and trans fatty acid consumption should be as low as possible, contributing to no more than 1% of the daily calorie intake. Dietary intake of cholesterol should be less than 300 mg per day for adults whose LDL-C is less than 130 $mg \cdot dl^{-1}$. For adults with elevated LDL-C (>130 $mg \cdot dl^{-1}$), dietary cholesterol should be limited to no more than 200 mg per day and saturated fat intake should not exceed 7% of total calorie intake. Also, consuming two servings of fish rich in EPA and DHA (e.g., salmon, trout, and light tuna) each week is recommended (U.S. Department of Health and Human Services 2004).

The National Cholesterol Education Program (2001) recommends a "Therapeutic Lifestyle Changes Diet" (table 9.4) to promote weight loss in those who are overweight and to reduce serum cholesterol levels. This diet limits dietary intakes of saturated fat and trans fatty acids (<7% of total calories), total fat (25% to 35% of total calories), and cholesterol (<200 mg per day).

Vitamins, Minerals, and Water

Micronutrients (vitamins and minerals) play an important role in energy production, maintenance of bone health, protection against oxidative damage,

Table 9.4 Nutrient Composition of the Therapeutic Lifestyle Changes Diet

Nutrient	Recommended intake
Saturated fat[a]	<7% of total calories
Polyunsaturated fat	Up to 10% of total calories
Monounsaturated fat	Up to 20% of total calories
Total fat	25-35% of total calories
Carbohydrate[b]	50-60% of total calories
Fiber	20-30 $g \cdot day^{-1}$
Protein	Approximately 15% of total calories
Cholesterol	<200 $mg \cdot day^{-1}$
Total calories[c]	Balance energy intake and expenditure to maintain desirable body weight or prevent weight gain

[a]Trans fatty acids are another low-density lipoprotein–raising fat that should be kept to a low intake.

[b]Carbohydrates should be derived predominantly from foods rich in complex carbohydrates including grains (especially whole grains), fruits, and vegetables.

[c]Daily energy expenditure should include at least moderate physical activity (contributing approximately 200 $kcal \cdot day^{-1}$).

Data from National Cholesterol Education Program, 2001, "Executive Summary of the Third Report of the National Cholesterol Education Program Expert Panel on Detection, Evaluation and Treatment of High Blood Cholesterol in Adults (Adult Treatment Panel III)," *Journal of the American Medical Association* 285 (1): 2490.

and synthesis and repair of muscle tissue during recovery from exercise. A well-balanced diet usually does not need to be supplemented to meet the minimum daily vitamin and mineral requirements of the body. Table 9.5 gives recommended dietary allowances (RDAs), adequate intakes (AIs), and upper intake levels (ULs) for vitamins and minerals.

Vitamins

Eating a well-balanced diet typically provides an individual's vitamin requirements. The body does not store the water-soluble vitamins (B complex and C); excessive amounts of these two vitamins are excreted in the urine. The excess accumulation of fat-soluble vitamins (A, D, E, and K) may produce

Table 9.5 Guidelines for Vitamin and Mineral Intakes: RDAs, AIs, and ULs* for Adults

	MEN AGE (YR)				WOMEN AGE (YR)				UL BOTH SEXES
	19-30	31-50	51-70	70+	19-30	31-50	51-70	70+	19-70+
VITAMINS									
A (µg RE)[a]	1000	1000	1000	1000	800	800	800	800	NA[c]
D (µg·day^{-1})	**5**	**5**	**10**	**15**	**5**	**5**	**10**	**15**	50
E (mg·day^{-1})	15	15	15	15	15	15	15	15	1000
K (µg)	70	80	80	80	60	65	65	65	NA
C (mg·day^{-1})	90	90	90	90	75	75	75	75	NA
Thiamin (mg·day^{-1})	1.2	1.2	1.2	1.2	1.1	1.1	1.1	1.1	NA
Riboflavin (mg·day^{-1})	1.3	1.3	1.3	1.3	1.1	1.1	1.1	1.1	NA
Niacin (mg·day^{-1})	1.6	1.6	1.6	1.6	1.4	1.4	1.4	1.4	35
B$_6$ (mg·day^{-1})	1.3	1.3	1.7	1.7	1.3	1.3	1.5	1.5	100
Folate (µg·day^{-1})	400	400	400	400	400	400	400	400	1000
B$_{12}$ (µg·day^{-1})	2.4	2.4	2.4	2.4	2.4	2.4	2.4	2.4	NA
Pantothenic acid (mg·day^{-1})	**5**	**5**	**5**	**5**	**5**	**5**	**5**	**5**	NA
Biotin (µg·day^{-1})	**30**	**30**	**30**	**30**	**30**	**30**	**30**	**30**	NA
Choline (mg·day^{-1})	**550**	**550**	**550**	**550**	**425**	**425**	**425**	**425**	3500
MINERALS									
Calcium (mg·day^{-1})	**1000**	**1000**	**1200**	**1200**	**1000**	**1000**	**1200**	**1200**	2500
Phosphorus (mg·day^{-1})[b]	700	700	700	700	700	700	700	700	3000-4000
Magnesium (mg·day^{-1})	400	420	420	420	310	320	320	320	350[d]
Fluoride (mg·day^{-1})	**4**	**4**	**4**	**4**	**3**	**3**	**3**	**3**	10
Iron (mg)	10	10	10	10	15	15	10	10	NA
Zinc (mg)	15	15	15	15	12	12	12	12	NA
Iodine (µg)	150	150	150	150	150	150	150	150	NA
Selenium (µg·day^{-1})	55	55	55	55	55	55	55	55	400

[a]Retinol equivalents: 1 RE = 1 µg retinol or 6 µg beta-carotene.

[b]3000 mg·day^{-1} for >70 yr; 4000 mg·day^{-1} for 19-70 yr.

[c]Not available.

[d]UL is for supplemental magnesium only.

*Recommended dietary allowances (RDAs) are in ordinary type, and adequate intakes (AIs) are in bold type. The RDA is the intake that meets the needs of almost all (97-98%) individuals in a group. The AI is believed to cover needs of all individuals in the group; however, sufficient scientific evidence is not available to estimate the RDA for this nutrient. The AI can be used to set goals for individuals. The tolerable upper intake level (UL) is the maximum amount of the nutrient that is unlikely to have adverse health effects in most healthy individuals.

Based on data from the National Academy of Sciences. National Academy Press, Washington, D.C. 2000.

decalcification of bones, headaches, nausea, diarrhea, and other toxic effects (Williams 1992).

According to the 2005 Dietary Guidelines Advisory Committee report (U.S. Department of Health and Human Services 2004), many Americans need to increase their intake of vitamins A, C, and E. Also, individuals older than 50 yr should eat foods fortified with vitamin B_{12} or take a vitamin B_{12} supplement daily. Elderly individuals and persons with dark skin may need more than the adequate intake recommendation (see table 9.5) for vitamin D (U.S. Department of Health and Human Services 2004). Some experts suggest that the current dietary reference intake of 200 and 600 IU per day for younger and older adults, respectively, needs to be increased to 1000 IU per day to achieve optimal health (Volpe 2009).

Vitamin deficiencies are uncommon in athletes and physically active individuals. However, athletes who restrict their food intake to maintain a low body weight or who engage in severe weight loss practices (e.g., wrestlers, dancers, and gymnasts) have a greater risk of vitamin deficiency (Manore 2004; Manore et al. 2009). Also, athletes who eat diets rich in fast foods or who do not eat a well-balanced diet may suffer from vitamin deficiencies, especially in B complex (B_6 and folate) and antioxidant (C, E, and beta-carotene) vitamins (Benardot et al. 2001). To be on the safe side, athletes and physically active individuals can take a multivitamin and mineral supplement daily or every other day. Vitamin supplementation improves sport performance only in athletes who are vitamin deficient (Benardot et al. 2001).

Minerals

The most common mineral deficiencies are of iron, zinc, and calcium. Physically active individuals, particularly those who choose to exclude meat from their diets, need to plan their diets carefully so that adequate amounts of iron and zinc are available. In some cases, it may be appropriate for you to recommend daily supplementation of iron, zinc, and calcium at 100% RDA in order to ensure adequate intake of these nutrients.

Iron is found in hemoglobin (in the red blood cells), which transports oxygen to exercising muscles. Iron deficiency has been frequently reported for both male and female athletes but is more common among women (Clarkson 1990). Iron requirements

for endurance athletes (e.g., distance runners) are increased by 70% (ACSM et al. 2009). Thus, iron supplementation may be warranted for some exercising individuals (Bonci 2009; Clark 2008; Rajaram et al. 1995).

Zinc plays an important role in energy metabolism (as a cofactor for enzymes), hormonal function, and the immune system. The average zinc intake of sedentary and athletic women in the United States is below the RDA (12 mg per day); for men, it typically exceeds the RDA (Clarkson and Haymes 1994). Zinc deficiency may result in decreased strength and endurance (Krotkiewski et al. 1982).

The recommended adequate intake (AI) for calcium is 1000 mg per day for men and women less than 51 yr of age and 1200 mg per day for older (51-70+ yr) adults. Most individuals can meet their calcium requirements by eating a well-balanced diet that contains milk products. When this is not possible, they should use calcium supplements. The recommended amounts of calcium and vitamin D for athletes with eating disorders, amenorrhea, and risk for early osteoporosis are 1500 mg of elemental calcium and 400 to 800 IU of vitamin D per day (ACSM et al. 2009).

Adequate dietary calcium intake and exercise are essential for bone mineralization and skeletal growth. Inadequate bone mineralization or excessive bone resorption results in bone loss and osteoporosis. In early-menopausal women, a high calcium intake (1500 mg per day), in combination with estrogen therapy, deterred bone loss. Calcium supplementation alone did not prevent bone loss in this group (Ettinger, Genault, and Cann 1987).

The recommended daily intake for magnesium is 320 mg for women and 420 mg for men. Magnesium is important in cellular metabolism and regulates neuromuscular, cardiovascular, immune, and hormonal functions. Magnesium deficiency may impair endurance performance. Supplementation may be recommended especially for athletes with inadequate dietary intakes.

The typical American diet contains more sodium than the recommended daily amount. The *Dietary Guidelines for Americans 2005* (U.S. Department of Health and Human Services 2005a) recommends limiting salt intake to less than 2300 mg per day (approximately 1 level tsp of salt). Excess salt (sodium chloride) intake may disrupt the electrolyte balance of the body and lead to increased fluid retention, hypertension, and calcium excretion. Thus, the amount of sodium in the diet should be restricted, especially for hypertensive or coronary-prone individuals. To counteract the effect of salt on blood pressure, foods rich in potassium are recommended; potassium lowers blood pressure.

Fraudulent claims sway many physically active individuals, particularly bodybuilders and strength-trained athletes, into believing that multivitamin and mineral supplements enhance muscle growth and exercise performance. Research suggests that long-term use of vitamin–mineral supplements does not increase strength or sport performance (Telford et al. 1992). Scientific studies (Williams 1993) demonstrate that

- vitamin B_{12} supplementation does not increase muscle growth or strength;

- carnitine (a vitamin-like compound) supplementation does not facilitate loss of body fat;

- chromium supplementation does not increase fat-free mass or decrease body fat;

- boron supplementation does not increase serum testosterone or fat-free mass; and

- magnesium supplementation does not improve muscle strength.

Water

The major sources of water for the body are fluid intake, food intake, and oxidation of foodstuffs by the body. Water is lost in urine, feces, perspiration, and expired air. During strenuous exercise, as much as 3 L of water may be lost through sweating. To prevent dehydration and electrolyte imbalances, athletes and physically active individuals need to hydrate before exercise, drink fluids during exercise, and rehydrate immediately after exercise. Although plain water is effective much of the time, carbohydrate sport drinks may also be used to maintain blood glucose levels and to replace fluids lost during exercise. The ideal fluid-replacement beverage contains some sodium to help maintain plasma osmolality and some glucose or sucrose to provide energy during exercise and to replenish muscle glycogen stores after exercise. Guidelines for maintaining hydration before, during, and after exercise have been developed by the ACSM (1996, 2009) and the National Athletic Trainers' Association (Casa et al. 2002):

- At least 4 hr before exercise, drink 5 to 7 ml·kg⁻¹ of body weight of water or a sport beverage.

- The amount and rate of fluid replacement depend on the athlete's sweat rate, exercise duration, and opportunities to drink. Do not restrict fluid intake during exercise; drink at least 150 to 350 ml (6-12 oz) of fluid every 15 to 20 min.

- Consume sport drinks containing carbohydrate (6-8%) and sodium when engaging in endurance exercise lasting 1 hr or more.

- After exercise, drink at least 16 to 24 oz (450-675 ml) of fluid for every pound (0.5 kg) of body weight lost during exercise.

DESIGNING WEIGHT MANAGEMENT PROGRAMS: PRELIMINARY STEPS

In designing weight management programs for weight loss or weight gain, you need to set body weight goals and assess the calorie intake and expenditure for your clients.

Setting Body Weight Goals

To set healthy body weight goals for your clients, you must first assess their present body weight, BMI, or body fat levels. You can easily measure the client's body weight by using a calibrated bathroom or physician's scale. Clients should wear indoor clothing but not shoes.

When you are evaluating your client's body weight, you should not use height–weight tables established by insurance companies These tables are limited for two reasons:

- The values represent height and weight with shoes and clothing. Whether individuals were measured with shoes and clothing was not standardized.

- Data were obtained from individuals who could afford life insurance; the data represent predominantly young to middle-aged white males and females and therefore are not representative of other population groups.

The *Dietary Guidelines for Americans 2005* (U.S. Department of Health and Human Services 2005a) recommends using BMI to determine a healthy body weight range. Use table 9.6 to determine if your client's BMI value falls within the healthy range. Individuals with a BMI from 18.5 up to 25 are considered to be at a **healthy body weight.**

Determining a healthy body weight from either BMI or any height–weight table alone may lead to invalid conclusions regarding your client's level of body fatness and health risk. These methods do not take into account the body composition of the individual. For example, with the use of BMI or height–weight tables, many mesomorphs having a large fat-free mass are classified as overweight, yet their body fat content may be lower than average. Similarly, individuals may be overfat or obese even though they are underweight according to the BMI and height–weight tables. Therefore, you should use the body composition technique to estimate a healthy body weight and body fat level for your clients.

When you use the body composition technique for estimating healthy body weight and body fat levels, assess the fat-free mass (FFM) and percent fat (%BF) using one of the methods described in chapter 8. A healthy body weight is based on the client's present FFM and %BF goal. Because some fat is needed for good health and nutrition, individuals should attempt to achieve a %BF somewhere between the low and upper values recommended in table 8.1 (see p. 190). Remember, minimal %BF depends on age and is estimated to be 5% to 10% for males and 12% to 15% for females. Cutoff values for obesity are also age dependent, ranging from >22% to >31% BF for males and >35% to >38% BF for

Table 9.6   Body Mass Index Chart

BMI[a]	NORMAL (HEALTHY) WEIGHT						OVERWEIGHT					OBESE					
	19	20	21	22	23	24	25	26	27	28	29	30	31	32	33	34	35
HEIGHT (IN.)	BODY WEIGHT (LB)																
58	91	96	100	105	110	115	119	124	129	134	138	143	148	153	158	162	167
59	94	99	104	109	114	119	124	128	133	138	143	148	153	158	163	168	173
60	97	102	107	112	118	123	128	133	138	143	148	153	158	163	168	174	179
61	100	106	111	116	122	127	132	137	143	148	153	158	164	169	174	180	185
62	104	109	115	120	126	131	136	142	147	153	158	164	169	175	180	186	191
63	107	113	118	124	130	135	141	146	152	158	163	169	175	180	186	191	197
64	110	116	122	128	134	140	145	151	157	163	169	174	180	186	192	197	204
65	114	120	126	132	138	144	150	156	162	168	174	180	186	192	198	204	210
66	118	124	130	136	142	148	155	161	167	173	179	186	192	198	204	210	216
67	121	127	134	140	146	153	159	166	172	178	185	191	198	204	211	217	223
68	125	131	138	144	151	158	164	171	177	184	190	197	203	210	216	223	230
69	128	135	142	149	155	162	169	176	182	189	196	203	209	216	223	230	236
70	132	139	146	153	160	167	174	181	188	195	202	209	216	222	229	236	243
71	136	143	150	157	165	172	179	186	193	200	208	215	222	229	236	243	250
72	140	147	154	162	169	177	184	191	199	206	213	221	228	235	242	250	258
73	144	151	159	166	174	182	189	197	204	212	219	227	235	242	250	257	265
74	148	155	164	171	179	186	194	202	210	218	225	233	241	249	256	264	272
75	152	160	168	176	184	192	200	208	216	224	232	240	248	256	264	272	279
76	156	164	172	180	189	197	205	213	221	230	238	246	254	263	271	279	287

[a]Body mass index (BMI) in kg/m^2; BMI <18.5 kg/m^2 is classified as underweight. To convert body weight in pounds to kilograms, divide body weight by 2.2; to convert height in inches to centimeters, multiply height by 2.54.

Instructions: Find your client's height (ht in inches) and body weight (in pounds). Read up the chart to find the corresponding BMI. If your client's BMI is classified as overweight or obese, use this chart to determine a healthy body weight for the client (i.e., a body weight corresponding to a BMI <25 kg/m^2).

Sample Calculation of Healthy Body Weight

Demographic Data

- Client: 31 yr old male
- Current body composition:
  - Body weight = 185 lb (84.1 kg)
  - Body fat = 20% BF
  - Fat-free mass (FFM) = 148 lb (67.3 kg)
- Goals: 12% BF and 88% FFM

Steps

1. Determine the client's present %BF using one of the body composition methods (see chapter 8).
2. Calculate the client's present FFM (in pounds): 185 lb × 0.80(current %FFM) = 148 lb (67.3 kg).
3. Set reasonable body composition goals for client: 12% BF and 88% FFM.
4. Divide the present FFM (in pounds) by the %FFM goal to obtain target body weight: 148 lb / 0.88 = 168 lb (76.4 kg).
5. Calculate weight loss by subtracting target body weight from present body weight: 185 − 168 = 17 lb (7.7 kg). Assuming that FFM is maintained, this client must lose 17 lb of fat to achieve his target body weight and body fat level.

---

females. For an example of how to calculate healthy body weight using the body composition technique, see "Sample Calculation of Healthy Body Weight."

With aging, there is a tendency to accumulate body weight and excess fat. Typically, adults may expect to gain 15 lb (9 kg) of fat weight and lose 5 lb (2.3 kg) of lean body mass per decade of life (Evans and Rosenberg 1992; Forbes 1976). This weight gain is primarily characterized by an increase in body fat and a decrease in muscle mass and is associated with declining physical activity levels with age. Each individual should attempt to maintain body weight and fatness at healthy levels.

Assessing Calorie Intake and Energy Expenditure

The second step in planning weight management programs is to assess the client's energy (calorie) intake and expenditure. You will use these baseline data to estimate the rate of weight loss or weight gain and the amount of time needed to achieve long-term goals of body composition and body weight.

Energy Intake

A food record (see appendix E.1, "Food Record and RDA Profile," p. 374) is used to determine an individual's daily caloric intake. The client keeps a record of the type and quantity of foods eaten each day for 3 to 7 days. Make certain that your client records all foods consumed; underreporting of food intake ranges from 10% to 45%. Use computer software to assess the average daily caloric intake and to compare average nutrient intakes to recommended amounts for each nutrient (see appendix E.2, "Sample Computerized Analysis of Food Intake," p. 376, for sample output). The food record also can help you analyze dietary patterns such as types of foods consumed, frequency of eating, and the caloric content of each meal.

Energy Expenditure

You can use either the factorial method or the TEE method to assess the energy needs of your clients. For the **factorial method,** RMR or REE and the additional calories expended during work, household chores, personal daily activities, and exercise are estimated. Various methods used to estimate RMR, and the additional energy requirements for occupational and physical activities are presented in this section. Although the factorial approach may reasonably estimate your client's energy expenditure, it is limited in that the equations used to estimate RMR have prediction errors and it is neither feasible nor practical to measure the wide range of activities performed throughout a normal day. Therefore, the TEE method for estimating total energy expenditure has been endorsed by the Institute of Medicine (2002). For the **total energy expenditure (TEE) method,** the individual's TEE

Methods of Estimating Resting Metabolic Rate (RMR)

Method	Equation
I. Body surface area (BSA)[a]	
Men	$RMR = BSA \times 38 \text{ kcal·hr}^{-1} \times 24 \text{ hr}$
Women	$RMR = BSA \times 35 \text{ kcal·hr}^{-1} \times 24 \text{ hr}$
II. A. Harris-Benedict equations[b]	
Men	$RMR = 66.473 + 13.751(BM) + 5.0033(ht) - 6.755(age)$
Women	$RMR = 655.0955 + 9.463(BM) + 1.8496(ht) - 4.6756(age)$
II. B. Mifflin et al. equations[b]	
Men	$RMR = [9.99(BM) + 6.25(ht) - 4.92(age)] + 5.0$
Women	$RMR = [9.99(BM) + 6.25(ht) - 4.92(age)] - 161$
III. Fat-free mass (FFM)	
Men and women	$RMR = 500 + 22(FFM \text{ in kg})$
IV. Quick estimate (from body mass)	
Men	$RMR = BM \text{ (in lb)} \times 11 \text{ kcal·lb}^{-1}$
	$RMR = BM \text{ (in kg)} \times 24.2 \text{ kcal·kg}^{-1}$
Women	$RMR = BM \text{ (in lb)} \times 10 \text{ kcal·lb}^{-1}$
	$RMR = BM \text{ (in kg)} \times 22.0 \text{ kcal·kg}^{-1}$

[a]Adjust RMR for age. RMR decreases 2% to 5% per decade after age 40.

[b]BM in kilograms; ht in centimeters; age in years.

is predicted using equations derived from doubly labeled water measures of TEE in free-living individuals (see table 9.3, p. 236).

Factorial Method: Estimation of Resting Metabolic Rate

Indirect calorimetry can be used to obtain reference measures of RMR or REE. Prediction equations are an inexpensive alternative to indirect calorimetry (see "Methods of Estimating Resting Metabolic Rate"). You can estimate body surface area (BSA) from height and weight using the nomogram in figure 9.1.

The average male or female between 20 and 40 yr of age burns 38 kcal·hr^{-1} and 35 kcal·hr^{-1}, respectively, for each square meter of BSA. For example, according to method I for estimating RMR, a 5 ft 2 in. (157.5 cm), 120 lb (54.5 kg) female has a BSA of 1.54 m^2 and a daily resting metabolic need of 1294 kcal (1.54 m^2 × 35 kcal·hr^{-1} × 24 hr).

You can obtain a quicker but less accurate estimate of RMR by multiplying the body weight by a factor of 10 (for BW measured in pounds) or 22 (for BW measured in kilograms) for women and a factor of 11 (for BW in pounds) or 24.2 (for BW

in kilograms) for men (see method IV). With this method, the RMR for the woman in our example is 1200 kcal (120 lb × 10).

Resting metabolic rate gradually decreases with age because the number of metabolically active cells is reduced. The RMR declines 2% to 5% during each decade of life after age 25 (Sharkey and Gaskill 2007). To prevent gradual weight gain with aging, people must reduce caloric intake or increase physical activity level. In the past, the Harris-Benedict (1919) equations (method II.A) were widely used to estimate RMR. However, the American Dietetic Association (2003) recommends using the equations of Mifflin and colleagues (1990) to estimate the RMR of healthy individuals (see method II.B). Both equations (Harris-Benedict and Mifflin) are gender specific and take into account not only height and weight but also age. Roza and Shizgal (1984) cross-validated the original Harris-Benedict equations, developed new equations using data from a large number of subjects, and concluded that the original equations published in 1919 yielded identical estimates of RMR. Also, the Harris-Benedict equations accurately estimated the REE of a large sample ($N = 2528$) of normal-weight, overweight,

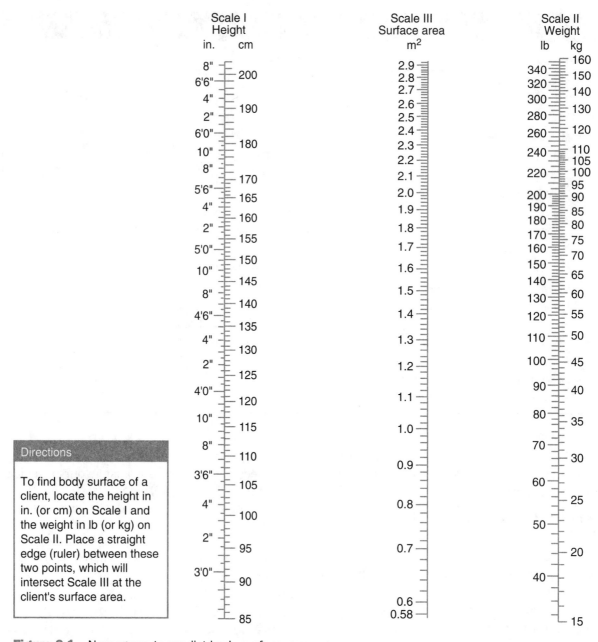

Figure 9.1 Nomogram to predict body surface area.

Reprinted, by permission, from W.E. Collins, 1967, *Clinical spirometry* (Braintree, MA: Warren E. Collins), 33. Copyright Warren E. Collins.

and obese individuals, but these equations tended to overestimate REE in underweight persons (Muller et al. 2004). In contrast, the American Dietetic Association (2003) reported that the Harris-Benedict equations generally overestimated RMR but that the equations of Mifflin and colleagues accurately estimated (within ±10%) the RMR for 80% of their sample. Compared to indirect calorimetry, both the Harris-Benedict equations and the equations of Mifflin and colleagues are more practical in terms of

effort and expense, and their accuracy is adequate for planning weight management programs.

In addition to body size and age, RMR is influenced by body composition. Muscular individuals have a higher RMR than fatter individuals of the same body weight because fat tissue is less metabolically active than muscle tissue. The RMRs of women are 5% to 10% lower than those of men (McArdle, Katch, and Katch 1996). This lower rate may be attributable to a greater relative fat content and lower FFM for women. To use method III (p. 247), you must measure the FFM of your client using one of the body composition methods suggested in chapter 8.

Factorial Method: Estimation of Additional Caloric Requirements

Resting metabolic rate accounts for 50% to 70% of total daily caloric needs, but this value depends on the activity level and occupation of the person. The percentage is greater for less active individuals, who require fewer calories above the resting level. For example, if a sedentary male office worker has a resting metabolic need of 1680 kcal, the additional caloric need as a consequence of the nature of his work is approximately 40% above resting level, or 672 kcal. Provided he performs no additional physical activities, his total daily caloric need is 2352 kcal. In this case, RMR accounts for 71% of his total daily caloric requirements. Table 9.7 presents additional caloric requirements for selected occupational activity levels.

After determining the daily energy needs of your clients from their RMR and occupation, you can estimate their additional calorie expenditure due to physical activity and exercise by using a physical activity log (appendix E.3, "Physical Activity Log," p. 381). The individual records every activity performed and the total amount of time spent in each activity. The estimated energy expenditure for a variety of activities is listed in appendix E.4, "Gross Energy Expenditure for Conditioning Exercises, Sports, and Recreational Activities," page 382. You can calculate the total caloric expenditure for each activity by converting the METs to kcal·kg^{-1}·hr^{-1} (1 MET = 1 kcal·kg^{-1}·hr^{-1}) and multiplying this value by the client's body weight (kg). This yields the total amount of kilocalories that the client expends per hour of that activity. You can determine the kcal·min^{-1} expenditure by dividing the kcal·hr^{-1} by 60 min. Calculate the TEE by multiplying the kcal·min^{-1} by the duration of the activity.

Keeping a physical activity log is a very time-consuming process for both you and your client, and it may not increase the accuracy of your estimate of additional caloric expenditure because many clients tend to overestimate the actual duration of their physical activity. It may be best to just ask your clients to list the frequency, intensity, and average time for the physical activities and sports that they perform on a regular basis; you can then determine their calorie expenditure for each activity as just described. Add these values to the daily caloric need estimated for the individual's RMR and occupation, and advise clients that on days they are active they can increase their calorie intake accordingly.

Total Energy Expenditure Method

For this method, the age- and gender-specific equations in table 9.3, page 236, are used to estimate your client's TEE. These equations predict TEE from

Table 9.7 Additional Energy Requirements for Selected Activity Levels

Occupational activity level*	PERCENTAGE ABOVE BASAL METABOLISM	
	Men	Women
Sedentary	15	15
Lightly active	40	35
Moderately active	50	45
Very active	85	70
Exceptionally active	110	100

*Examples for each occupational activity level are as follows:

Sedentary = inactive.

Lightly active = most professionals, office workers, shop workers, teachers, homemakers.

Moderately active = workers in light industry, most farm workers, active students, department store workers, soldiers not in active service, commercial fishing workers.

Very active = full-time athletes and dancers, unskilled laborers, forestry workers, military recruits and soldiers in active service, mine workers, steel workers.

Exceptionally active = lumberjacks, blacksmiths, female construction workers.

your client's age, body weight, height, and physical activity coefficient. The physical activity coefficient depends on your client's **physical activity level (PAL)**; given that energy expenditure is highly dependent on physical activity, PAL is commonly described as the ratio of TEE to BMR (PAL = TEE / BMR). The PAL categories were developed from doubly labeled water measures of TEE and BMR in normal, healthy individuals. Data from elite athletes and extremely active individuals (i.e., military personnel and astronauts) were not included (Brooks et al. 2004). Physical activity levels are classified as sedentary (1.0 to <1.4), low (1.4 to <1.6), active (1.6 to 1.9), and very active (1.9 to <2.5). To obtain a fairly good estimate of your client's PAL, you can use various tools such as self-reported physical activity questionnaires, physical activity diaries, pedometers, accelerometers, heart rate monitors, and digital activity logs (Keim, Blanton, and Kretsch 2004). For information about the validity and reliability of pedometers and accelerometers for monitoring physical activity levels, see chapter 3, pages 55-56. "Steps for Estimating TEE" illustrates how you can use the TEE equations to estimate your client's daily energy expenditure.

DESIGNING WEIGHT LOSS PROGRAMS

When the caloric expenditure exceeds the caloric intake, a negative energy balance or caloric deficit is created. The most effective way of producing this deficit is to use a combination of caloric restriction and exercise. Because a deficit of 3500 kcal is needed to lose 1 lb (0.45 kg) of fat, you can easily calculate the daily caloric deficit that is needed to result in the target weekly weight loss you set for your client. An average deficit of 500 kcal will produce a weekly weight loss of approximately 1 lb (0.45 kg), given that 500 kcal × 7 days = 3500 calories. An average deficit of 1000 will produce a weight loss of 2 lb (0.90 kg) a week (1000 kcal × 7 days, or 2 lb). The daily caloric deficit should not exceed 1000 kcal per day.

To ensure that the weight loss is a result of the loss of body fat rather than lean body tissue, you should

- use the body composition method to estimate the client's healthy body weight and fat loss;

Steps for Estimating TEE

To estimate your client's total energy expenditure (TEE) from age- and gender-specific TEE equations, follow these steps:

- Step 1: Determine the client's gender and age (50 yr male).
- Step 2: Measure the client's body weight and height (BW = 180 lb; ht = 70 in.). Convert body weight in pounds to body weight in kilograms: 180 lb / 2.204 = 81.7 kg. Convert height in inches to height in meters: 70 in × 0.0254 = 1.78 m.
- Step 3: Estimate your client's PAL (1.70, or active, from physical activity log).
- Step 4: Select the appropriate age- and gender-specific TEE prediction equation from table 9.3: for males ≥19 yr.

$$\text{TEE (kcal·day}^{-1}) = 662 - (9.53 \times \text{age}) + \text{PA} [(15.9 \times \text{wt}) + (540 \times \text{ht})]$$

- Step 5: Determine the physical activity coefficient corresponding to your client's PAL (1.25 for PAL = 1.70).
- Step 6: Substitute the values for age, body weight, physical activity, and height into the equation:

$$\text{TEE (kcal·day}^{-1}) = 662 - (9.53 \times 50 \text{ yr}) + 1.25 [(15.9 \times 81.7 \text{ kg}) + (540 \times 1.78 \text{ m})]$$

- Step 7: Calculate the estimated TEE (kcal·day^{-1}):

$$\text{TEE (kcal·day}^{-1}) = 662 - (9.53 \times 50 \text{ yr}) + 1.25 [(15.9 \times 81.7 \text{ kg}) + (540 \times 1.78 \text{ m})]$$
$$= 662 - (476.5) + [1.25 \times (1299 + 961)]$$
$$= 185.5 + 2260$$

$$\text{TEE} = 2445.7, \text{ or } 2446 \text{ kcal·day}^{-1}$$

- encourage daily participation in aerobic exercise and resistance training programs to enhance the loss of fat and to conserve FFM; and

- plan a diet that restricts calorie intake but contains adequate amounts of good sources of carbohydrate, protein, and fat. The diet should contain at least 130 g of carbohydrate per day and 0.8 g of protein per kilogram of body weight per day. Table 9.8 lists good sources of carbohydrate, protein, and fat rec-

ommended by the Harvard School of Public Health (2004).

When you design the weight loss program of diet and exercise, use descriptive data to help you set reasonable goals for your clients. These data include age, gender, height, body weight, relative body fat (%BF), %BF goal, average calorie intake, cardiorespiratory fitness level, and occupation. The steps to follow in designing a weight loss program are as follows:

Steps for Designing a Weight Loss Program

Summary of Client's Demographic Data

1. Client's age and gender (35 yr female)
2. Height (62 in. or 157.5 cm)
3. Body weight (131 lb or 59.55 kg)
4. Percent fat (26% BF); relative FFM (74%)
5. Percent fat goal (20% BF); relative FFM goal (80%)
6. Average daily calorie intake (2000 kcal)
7. Cardiorespiratory fitness level (below average)
8. Occupation (secretary)

Steps

1. Assess the body weight and body composition of the client.
2. Assess the daily calorie intake of the subject (use 3- or 7-day food records).
3. Estimate a healthy target body weight based on the client's percent fat goal.

    Present FFM = 96.9 lb (131 lb × 0.74) (relative FFM)

    Target body weight = 121 lb (96.9 lb / 0.80) (relative FFM goal)

4. Calculate the weight loss and total calorie deficit needed to achieve that weight loss.

    a. Weight loss = 10 lb (131 lb − 121 lb)

    b. Caloric deficit = 35,000 kcal (10 lb × 3500 kcal·lb^{-1})

5. Estimate the daily energy expenditure of the client from the equation: energy expenditure = RMR + daily activity level.

    a. RMR = 655.0955 + 9.463(59.55 kg) + 1.8496(157.5 cm) − 4.6756(35 yr) = 1346 kcal

    b. Daily occupational activity level: lightly active 35% above basal level (see table 9.7). Additional kcal = 1346 × 0.35 = 471 kcal

    c. Total energy expenditure = 1346 + 471 = 1817 kcal

6. Plan to produce a calorie deficit of 700 to 800 kcal per day by reducing the calorie intake by 500 kcal per day and increasing the calorie expenditure by 200 to 300 kcal per day through exercise. To calculate caloric expenditure during exercise, refer to appendix E.4. Multiply the calories burned per minute per kilogram of body weight by the duration of the activity and the client's body weight. Continue this program until the total calorie deficit of 35,000 kcal is reached.

(continued)

Steps for Designing a Weight Loss Program (continued)

Week 1	exercise = 100 kcal·day^{-1} × 7 days		=	700 kcal
	diet = 500 kcal·day^{-1} × 7 days		=	3500 kcal
		subtotal	=	4200 kcal
Week 2	exercise = 150 kcal·day^{-1} × 7 days		=	1050 kcal
	diet = 500 kcal·day^{-1} × 7 days		=	3500 kcal
		subtotal	=	4550 kcal
Weeks 3-4	exercise = 200 kcal·day^{-1} × 14 days		=	2800 kcal
	diet = 500 kcal·day^{-1} × 14 days		=	7000 kcal
		subtotal	=	9800 kcal
Weeks 5-6	exercise = 250 kcal·day^{-1} × 14 days		=	3500 kcal
	diet = 500 kcal·day^{-1} × 14 days		=	7000 kcal
		subtotal	=	10,500 kcal
Week 7	exercise = 300 kcal·day^{-1} × 7 days		=	2100 kcal
	diet = 500 kcal·day^{-1} × 7 days		=	3500 kcal
		subtotal	=	5600 kcal
		Total Weeks 1-7	**=**	**34,650 kcal**

In a little over 7 wk the client will lose approximately 10 lb (4.5 kg). This is a gradual average weight loss of 1 1/2 lb (0.7 kg) per week. Reassess the body composition to see if the percent fat goal was reached.

7. Put the client on a maintenance diet and exercise program.

   a. Calculate the total energy expenditure using an estimate of RMR based on the new body weight.

   RMR + activity level + exercise = total energy expenditure where:

   RMR = 1303 kcal (use Harris-Benedict formula substituting a body weight of 55 kg)

   Occupational activity level = 456 kcal (1303 × 0.35)

   Exercise = 300 kcal

   Total energy expenditure = 1303 + 456 + 300 = 2059 kcal

   b. Advise the client that if she continues to exercise daily, expending approximately 300 kcal per workout, she may increase her calorie intake to 2060 kcal per day. However, for days when she cannot exercise, the calorie intake must be restricted to 1760 kcal.

Weight Loss Diets

You may be overwhelmed by the vast amount of information about popular weight loss diets in magazines, newspapers, news shows, and scientific and professional journals. There is much controversy and hype about the effectiveness of low-carbohydrate, high-protein, or low-fat diets for weight loss. Also, in scientific journals it is possible to find arguments for or against any particular diet. According to a survey conducted by the Partnership for Essential Nutrition (2004), almost 50% of American adults believe that people can lose weight by cutting back on carbohydrates without cutting back on calories (a major premise of the popular Atkins diet). Studies show that high-protein or low-carbohydrate diets result in greater weight losses (~2.5-4.0 kg [5.5-8.8 lb]) over 3 to 6 mo than do low-fat diets (Foster et al. 2003; Samaha et al. 2003). These findings have led some researchers to question whether a calorie is a calorie or whether a calorie depends on the macronutrient composition of the diet (Buchholz and Schoeller 2004). Buchholz and Schoeller (2004) noted that increasing protein intake from 15% to between 30% and 35% increases resting and sleeping energy expenditure;

however, these changes account for only one-third of the difference in average weight loss between high-protein, low-carbohydrate diets and high-carbohydrate, low-fat diets. Also, the greater weight loss for high-protein diets cannot be explained by a greater loss of glycogen and water. Some evidence suggests that individuals on high-protein diets eat less (i.e., reduce their energy intake) over the long term and may be more compliant because protein increases satiety. In fact, comprehensive review articles and meta-analyses on this issue conclude that weight loss depends on calorie intake and not on the macronutrient composition (i.e., low carbohydrate, low fat, or high protein) of the diet (Bravata et al. 2003; Buchholz and Schoeller 2004; Ornish 2004; Seshadri 2004).

In addition to efficacy for weight loss, the long-term health benefits and risks of any diet that limits the intake of specific macronutrients should be assessed. Weight loss programs should help individuals lose weight in ways that promote health. To reduce chronic disease risk, the macronutrient content of the diet should be consistent with nutritional recommendations from health organizations. Recently, de Souza and colleagues (2008) evaluated the macronutrient content of the OmniHeart Study, Dietary Approaches to Stop Hypertension (DASH), Zone, Atkins, Mediterranean, South Beach, and Ornish diets. The OmniHeart diets were consistent with national guidelines to prevent cancer, diabetes and heart disease. With the exception of the Zone diet, most popular diets were unable to meet one or more of these guidelines.

Foster and colleagues (2003) conducted a 1 yr, multicenter, randomized control trial to compare the weight loss and health effects of a low-carbohydrate, high-protein, high-fat diet (i.e., Atkins diet) to those of a conventional high-carbohydrate, low-fat, energy-deficit diet. Results indicated that in the short term (up to 6 mo), the Atkins diet produces greater weight loss (~4%) in obese men and women (BMI ~34 kg/m^2); however, after 1 yr there was no statistically significant difference in the amount of weight loss between the groups. During the first 6 mo, the Atkins dieters had a greater energy deficit even though their protein and fat intake was not limited, and the energy intake of the conventional dieters was restricted. Thus, a greater calorie deficit, not the macronutrient composition of the diet, was most likely responsible for the greater weight

loss seen in the Atkins diet group. In terms of the overall long-term (1 yr) effect on CHD risk, the low-carbohydrate diet group showed greater relative improvements in some risk factors: triglycerides decreased 28% with the Atkins diet and increased 1.4% with the conventional diet, while high-density lipoprotein cholesterol (HDL-C) increased 18% with the Atkins diet but only 3.1% with the conventional diet. Changes in the other risk factors (blood pressure, insulin sensitivity, and LDL-C) were not statistically significant in either group. Given that the large amounts of saturated fats and small amounts of fruits, vegetables, and fiber in low-carbohydrate diets can independently increase the risk of CHD (Schaefer 2002), the authors concluded that there is insufficient information to determine whether the beneficial health effects of the Atkins diet (i.e., improvements in triglycerides and HDL-C) outweigh the potential adverse effects on CHD risk in obese individuals. Additional long-term studies are needed to evaluate the potential benefits and risks of low-carbohydrate and high-protein diets.

In the meantime, the optimal diet for health and long-term maintenance of weight loss may be one that not only restricts calorie intake but also contains adequate amounts of good sources of carbohydrate, protein, and fat (see table 9.8). An effective strategy for reducing energy intake is to eat less refined, processed food as well as less saturated and trans fat. The Healthy Eating Pyramid (see figure 9.2), a product of the Harvard School of Public Health, summarizes the best dietary information presently available. This pyramid has a foundation of daily physical activity and weight control and includes the following recommendations for food choices that promote health and weight control:

- **Whole grains.** The body needs carbohydrates for energy. Compared to highly processed carbohydrates such as white flour, whole grains have a lower glycemic index, allowing better control of blood glucose and insulin and reducing the risk of type 2 diabetes.

- **Plant oils.** When healthy unsaturated fats are eaten in place of highly processed carbohydrates, cholesterol levels improve and the risk of cardiac arrhythmias decreases.

- **Vegetables and fruits.** Diets rich in vegetables and fruits lower blood pressure and decrease the risk of heart attack, stroke, and certain cancers.

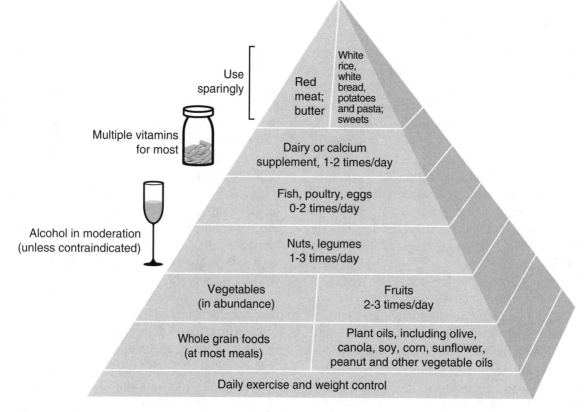

Figure 9.2 Harvard Medical School Healthy Eating Pyramid.

Reprinted with the permission of Simon & Schuster Adult Publishing Group from *Eat, Drink and Be Healthy: The Harvard Medical School Guide to Healthy Eating* by Walter C. Willett, MD. Copyright © 2001 by President and Fellows of Harvard College.

■ **Fish, poultry, and eggs.** These are good sources of protein. Chicken and turkey can be low in saturated fat. Eating fish can reduce the risk of CHD.

■ **Nuts and legumes.** These are excellent sources of protein, fiber, vitamins, and minerals; and many kinds of nuts contain healthy fats.

■ **Dairy products.** Nonfat or low-fat dairy products (e.g., milk, yogurt, and cheese) are an excellent source of calcium, which helps prevent osteopenia and osteoporosis. Two glasses of whole milk, however, contain as much saturated fat as eight slices of cooked bacon.

The apex of the pyramid lists foods that should be eaten sparingly. Red meats and butter contain saturated fat, which can increase total cholesterol and LDL-C levels. White rice, white bread, potatoes, pasta, and sweets should also be eaten sparingly because they are high-glycemic foods that can cause rapid increases in blood glucose levels and insulin resistance (which increases risk of type 2 diabetes), weight gain, and increased risk of developing CHD and other chronic disorders.

The *Dietary Guidelines for Americans 2005* (U.S. Department of Health and Human Services 2005a)

Table 9.8 Good Sources of Carbohydrate, Protein, and Fat

Macronutrient	Food sources
Carbohydrate	Whole grains, whole wheat bread, oatmeal, brown rice, fruits, vegetables
Protein	Fish, poultry, eggs, nuts, legumes, black beans, navy beans, garbanzo beans, nonfat or low-fat milk
Fat	Unsaturated plant oils such as olive, canola, soy, corn, sunflower, and peanut

and a revised U.S. food guide pyramid (see figure 9.3) describe a healthy diet as one that

- emphasizes fruits, vegetables, whole grains, and fat-free or low-fat milk and milk products;
- includes lean meats, poultry, fish, beans, eggs, and nuts; and
- is low in saturated fats, trans fats, cholesterol, salt (sodium), and added sugars.

The revised U.S. food guide pyramid has rainbow bands running from the tip to the base (U.S. Department of Health and Human Services 2005b). The color and width of the bands differ to indicate various food groups and the relative number of servings that should be eaten from each. Daily physical activity is represented by the figure of a person climbing steps. This new pyramid, called MyPyra-

mid, encourages Americans to use 1 of 12 models to customize their diet and exercise. The model selected varies with the client's age, gender, and level of daily physical activity. Figure 9.3 illustrates the recommended model for a moderately active 58 yr old female. To generate food guide pyramids for your clients, see www.MyPyramid.gov.

Other evidence-based food guides that depict healthy eating are the Asian, Latin American, Mediterranean, and Vegetarian pyramids (see appendix E.5, "Healthy Eating Pyramids," pp. 385-388). Each of these food guides has a foundation of daily physical activity and reflects traditional but healthy foods indigenous to the culture. For an overview and comparison of food guides from 12 different countries, see Painter, Rah, and Lee 2002.

It is strongly recommended that you work closely with a licensed nutritionist or registered dietitian

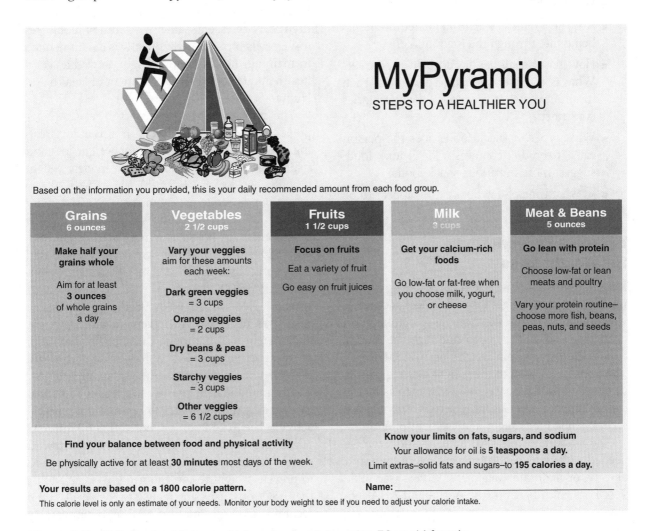

MyPyramid
STEPS TO A HEALTHIER YOU

Based on the information you provided, this is your daily recommended amount from each food group.

Grains 6 ounces	Vegetables 2 1/2 cups	Fruits 1 1/2 cups	Milk 3 cups	Meat & Beans 5 ounces
Make half your grains whole	Vary your veggies aim for these amounts each week:	Focus on fruits	Get your calcium-rich foods	Go lean with protein
Aim for at least **3 ounces** of whole grains a day	**Dark green veggies** = 3 cups **Orange veggies** = 2 cups **Dry beans & peas** = 3 cups **Starchy veggies** = 3 cups **Other veggies** = 6 1/2 cups	Eat a variety of fruit Go easy on fruit juices	Go low-fat or fat-free when you choose milk, yogurt, or cheese	Choose low-fat or lean meats and poultry Vary your protein routine— choose more fish, beans, peas, nuts, and seeds

Find your balance between food and physical activity — Be physically active for at least **30 minutes** most days of the week.

Know your limits on fats, sugars, and sodium — Your allowance for oil is **5 teaspoons a day.** Limit extras—solid fats and sugars—to **195 calories a day.**

Your results are based on a 1800 calorie pattern.

This calorie level is only an estimate of your needs. Monitor your body weight to see if you need to adjust your calorie intake.

Name: _____

Figure 9.3 U.S. food guide pyramid for a moderately active 58 yr old female.

U.S. Department of Agriculture and the U.S. Department of Health and Human Services or USDA and DHHS.

when planning diets for your clients. Food guides are useful tools for determining the recommended number of servings from each food group for healthy eating. When comparing your client's typical nutrient intake to recommended intakes, ask the following questions:

- How does the average caloric intake compare with the caloric needs and expenditure of the individual?
- What is the relative percentage of carbohydrate, protein, and fat in the diet?
- How much of the total fat intake is saturated fat and trans fat?
- Is the minimum daily protein requirement being met?
- What is the dietary cholesterol level?
- What is the sodium intake?
- Are the vitamin and mineral requirements being met through the food intake?
- How many meals per day does the person eat? What is the average caloric content of each meal? At what meal are most of the kilocalories consumed?
- What types of snack foods does the person eat? (If the diet contains a lot of junk food, suggest more nutritious snack foods.)
- At what time of day does eating appear to be a problem?

Exercise Prescription for Weight Loss

Exercise alone—without dieting—has only a modest effect on weight loss. The most successful weight loss programs, therefore, use a combination of dieting and exercising to optimize the energy deficit and to maintain weight loss (ACSM 2001). The exercise portion of the weight loss regimen is designed to produce a weight loss by increasing the calorie expenditure. Generally, aerobic activities are recommended for weight management programs.

The amount of physical activity and exercise needed to benefit health, prevent overweight and obesity, or maintain weight loss differs (see table 9.9). For health benefits, the ACSM and AHA recommend at least 30 min of moderate-intensity (3-6 METs) physical activity on a minimum of 5 days/wk or 20 min of vigorous-intensity (>6.0 METs)

activity on a minimum of 3 days/wk (ACSM 2008). Likewise, the 2008 "Physical Activity Guidelines for Americans" recommends 150 to 300 min/wk of moderate intensity (3-6 METs) or 75 to 150 min/wk of vigorous intensity or both (≥6.0 METs).

To prevent weight gain, the ACSM (2009a) recommends moderate-intensity physical activity between 150 and 250 min/wk. However, the International Association for the Study of Obesity (IASO) consensus statement suggests that 30 min of daily physical activity (210 min/wk) may be insufficient to prevent gaining weight or regaining weight after weight loss (Saris et al. 2003). To maintain weight and to prevent unhealthy weight gain and transition to overweight or obesity in adults, 45 to 60 min of moderate-to-vigorous activity (PAL = 1.7) on most, preferably all, days is recommended (Institute of Medicine 2002; U.S. Department of Health and Human Services 2005a; Saris et al. 2003). For children and adolescents, at least 60 min of moderate-to-vigorous physical activity daily is recommended to maintain healthy body weight as well as good health and fitness (U.S. Department of Health and Human Services 2007).

The optimal physical activity level (PAL) for preventing weight gain differs from that for creating a negative energy balance for weight loss and maintenance of weight loss. For a modest weight loss (i.e., 2-3 kg or 4.4-6.6 lb), the ACSM (2009a) recommends moderate-intensity physical activity between 150 and 250 min/wk; however, there is a dose effect for physical activity and weight loss, with >250 min/wk of physical activity associated with clinically significant (3% or greater) weight loss (ACSM 2009a).

The ACSM (2009a) acknowledges that physical activity is necessary to prevent regaining weight after weight loss. Although the specific amount of physical activity needed to prevent weight regain is uncertain at this time, some studies suggest that weight maintenance after weight loss is improved by engaging in more than 250 min/wk of physical activity. The ACSM (2009a) noted that 60 min/day of walking at a moderate intensity is associated with weight maintenance. To maintain weight loss and to prevent weight regain in formerly obese adults, the IASO consensus statement (see Saris et al. 2003) recommends a minimum of 60 min, but preferably 80 to 90 min, of moderate-intensity (2.8 to 4.3 METs) physical activity and exercise (e.g., walking or cycling) per day. This intensity and duration of physical activity approximately equals 35 min of vigorous activity (6 to 10 METs or PAL = 1.9 to 2.5).

Table 9.9 summarizes physical activity recommendations for health benefit, healthy weight loss, and weight management. The exercise prescription for weight loss and weight management will differ depending on your client's goal. You can use the information in table 9.9 to develop exercise prescriptions for weight loss, weight maintenance, and prevention of weight gain or regain.

Benefits of Exercise

This section highlights some common questions about the benefits of exercise in a weight loss program.

■ *Why is exercise an essential part of weight loss programs?*

A meta-analysis of studies comparing the effects of diet-only to diet plus physical activity (PA) interventions showed that the diet + PA programs resulted in a significantly greater weight loss (–1.1 kg) overall (Shaw et al. 2006). Curioni and Lourenco (2005) reported that diet + PA programs produced a 20% greater weight loss (–13 kg) compared to the diet-only (–9.9 kg) programs as well as a 20% greater sustained weight loss after 1 yr.

In addition to increasing energy expenditure and helping to create a negative energy balance for weight loss, adding exercise to dieting increases the amount of fat lost. Exercise also maintains or slows down the loss of FFM that occurs with dieting only and is important for maintaining weight loss after dieting.

Pavlou and colleagues (1985) studied the contribution of exercise to the preservation of FFM in mildly obese males on a rapid weight loss diet. The exercise group dieted and participated in an 8 wk walking-jogging program, 3 days/wk. The nonexercising group dieted only. Although the total weight loss of the exercise (–11.8 kg) and nonexercise (–9.2 kg) groups was similar, the composition of the weight loss differed significantly. The exercise group maintained FFM (–0.6 kg) while the nonexercise group lost a significant amount of FFM (–3.3 kg).

Table 9.9 Physical Activity and Exercise Recommendations for Health Benefit, Healthy Weight Loss, and Weight Management

Goal	Intensity	Duration	Frequency (days/wk)	Source*
Health benefit	Moderate[a] and/or	At least 30 min	5 minimum	ACSM and AHA
	Vigorous	20 min	3 minimum	
	Moderate	150-300 min/wk or		USDHHS
	Vigorous	75-150 min/wk		
Weight loss	Moderate	150-250 min/wk[c]		ACSM
Weight maintenance and prevention of weight gain	Moderate[a] (PAL ~1.7) to Vigorous[b] (PAL ~1.9-2.5)	45-60 min	5-7	IASO, IOM, and USDHHS
	Moderate	150-250 min/wk		ACSM
Prevention of weight regain	Moderate	60-90 min	7	USDHHS
	Moderate	At least 60 but preferably 80-90 min	7	IASO
	Vigorous	At least 35 min	7	IASO
	Moderate	>250 min/wk		ACSM

*ACSM = American College of Sports Medicine; AHA = American Heart Association; IASO = International Association for the Study of Obesity; IOM = Institute of Medicine (United States); USDHHS = U.S. Department of Health and Human Services; PAL = physical activity level.

[a]Moderate intensity ≅ 2.8 to 4.3 METs; PAL ≅ 1.7.

[b]Vigorous intensity ≅ 6 to 10 METs; PAL ≅ 1.9 to 2.5.

[c]Accumulate a total duration of activity of 150 min/wk, progressing to 200 to 250 min/wk; total weekly exercise energy expenditure ≥2000 kcal·wk^{-1}.

Also, the exercise group lost more fat (11.2 kg) than the nonexercise group (5.9 kg). In other words, for the nonexercising subjects, only 64% of the total weight loss was fat weight compared to 95% for the exercising subjects. The researchers concluded that the addition of aerobic exercise to the dietary regimen preserves existing FFM, increases fat utilization for energy production, and is more effective in reducing fat stores than diet alone.

Similarly, Kraemer and colleagues (1999b) compared the effects of a weight loss dietary regimen with and without exercise in overweight men. The diet-only group did not exercise; the exercise groups participated in either an aerobic exercise program or a combined aerobic and resistance training exercise program, 3 days·wk^{-1} for 12 wk. By the end of the program, all three groups lost a similar amount of body weight (~9 to 10 kg), but the composition of the weight loss differed significantly. For the diet-only group, only 69% of the total weight loss was fat weight compared to 78% for the diet plus aerobic exercise group and 97% for the diet and exercise (aerobic + resistance training) group. These results suggest that using a combination of aerobic and resistance training exercises in conjunction with dieting is more effective than dieting alone for preserving FFM and maximizing fat loss.

■ How does exercise promote fat loss and the preservation of lean body mass?

In response to aerobic and resistance training exercise, levels of growth hormone, epinephrine, and norepinephrine increase. These hormones stimulate the mobilization of fat from storage and activate the enzyme lipase, which breaks down triglycerides into free fatty acids. Free fatty acids are then metabolized and serve as an important energy source, especially during aerobic exercise. Heavy resistance training exercise also stimulates the release of anabolic hormones such as testosterone and growth hormone, resulting in increased protein synthesis, muscle growth, and FFM (Kraemer et al. 1991).

■ How does improved cardiorespiratory fitness help control body weight?

As the individual's cardiorespiratory fitness level increases through training, the amount of work that the person can accomplish at a given submaximal heart rate increases. Thus, the more fit individual expends calories faster than the less fit individual at a given exercise heart rate. For example, at a heart rate of 150 bpm, the rate of energy expenditure is approximately 10 and 15 kcal·min^{-1} for fair and superior fitness levels, respectively.

During high-intensity aerobic exercise, lactate production increases and inhibits fatty acid metabolism. However, endurance training increases the lactate threshold (point at which lactate accumulates significantly in the blood). In aerobically trained individuals, the percentage of the energy derived from the oxidation of free fatty acids during submaximal exercise is greater than that derived from glucose oxidation (Coyle 1995; Mole, Oscai, and Holloszy 1971). The reduction in muscle glycogen utilization is also associated with a greater rate of oxidation of intramuscular triglyceride (Coyle 1995).

In order to expend the amount of energy recommended to prevent weight regain after weight loss, cardiorespiratory fitness ($\dot{V}O_2max$) needs to increase. Therefore, weight reduction programs should increase cardiorespiratory fitness so that participants are able to reach this physical activity goal within a reasonable amount of time (Saris et al. 2003).

■ What effect does exercise have on the RMR?

Another reason for including exercise in the weight loss program is its positive effect on RMR. Research indicates that exercise may counter the reduction in RMR that usually occurs as a result of dieting (Thompson, Manore, and Thomas 1996). It is well known that the rate of weight loss declines in the later stages of dieting due to a decrease in RMR. The lowered RMR is an energy-conserving metabolic adaptation to prolonged periods of caloric restriction (Donahue et al. 1984). In a study of 12 overweight females, Donahue and colleagues (1984) reported that diet alone caused a 4.4% reduction in the relative RMR (RMR/BW). After the addition of 8 wk of aerobic exercise to the program, the relative RMR increased by 5%. The net effect of exercise was to offset the diet-induced metabolic adaptation and return the RMR to the normal, prediet level.

Exercise may also facilitate weight loss by causing an increase in postexercise RMR. Moderate- to high-intensity aerobic exercise increases the postexercise RMR by 5% to 16%, and the elevated RMR may persist for 12 to 39 hr postexercise (Bahr et al 1987; Bielinski, Schultz, and Jequier 1985; Sjodin et al.

1996). The postexercise elevation in RMR appears to be related to the exercise intensity and duration (Brehm 1988). Cycling at 70% $\dot{V}O_2$max for 20 min produced a 5% to 14% elevation in RMR for 12 hr in young, healthy men (Bahr et al. 1987). Although it is tempting to apply these findings to clients who are elderly or obese, it is not known whether the postexercise metabolic response of these individuals is similar to that of young men.

Types of Exercise

This section addresses common concerns regarding the types of exercise suitable for weight loss programs.

■ **Is aerobic exercise better than resistance exercise for weight loss?**

Most weight loss programs recommend energy restriction (diet) and increased physical activity to create an energy deficit. Evidence suggests a dose–response relationship for weight loss; individuals performing the greatest amount of physical activity achieve greater weight loss. Aerobic exercise (e.g., walking) is effective for weight loss, fat loss, and long-term weight control (Gordon-Larsen et al. 2009; Nelson and Folta 2009).

Although resistance training increases muscle mass and REE, this mode of training does not produce a clinically significant weight loss (~3% of body weight) and does not increase weight loss when combined with diet restriction. Resistance training, however, may increase the loss of fat mass when combined with aerobic exercise (ACSM 2009).

While aerobic exercise is more effective than resistance training for reducing body weight and fat mass, resistance training plays an important role in preserving FFM and increasing RMR, especially for individuals on a very low-calorie diet (Bryner et al. 1999).

■ **Is high-intensity exercise better than light- to moderate-intensity exercise for weight loss?**

An important reason for including exercise as part of a weight loss program is to maximize energy expenditure, thereby creating a larger negative energy balance. Weight loss and loss of fat mass are positively related to weekly energy expenditure (Ross and Janssen 2001). When the same amount of energy is expended, total fat oxidation is higher during low-intensity exercise than during high-intensity exercise. Close examination of energy expenditure during selected physical activities (appendix E.4, "Gross Energy Expenditure for Conditioning Exercises, Sports, and Recreational Activities," p. 382) reveals that increases in speed (intensity) of exercise produce only small increases in the rate of energy expenditure (METs). For example, if a 123 lb (56 kg) woman increases the speed of running from a slow (5.0 mph or 12 min·mi⁻¹) to a faster speed (7.0 mph or 8.5 min·mi⁻¹), the rate of expenditure increases only 3.2 kcal·min⁻¹. At the 8.5 min per mile pace, the woman expends 11.5 METs (11.5 kcal·kg⁻¹·min⁻¹ or 10.7 kcal·min⁻¹) and is able to run a maximum distance of 3 mi (4.8 km). The duration of the workout is 25.5 min (8.5 min·mi⁻¹ × 3 mi), and the total caloric expenditure is 274 kcal (25.5 min × 10.7 kcal·min⁻¹). When she reduces the exercise intensity by decreasing her speed to a 12 min per mile pace, her relative energy expenditure decreases (8 METs or 8 kcal·kg⁻¹·min⁻¹ or 7.5 kcal·min⁻¹), but she is able to run a distance of 4 mi (6.4 km). The duration of the workout increases to 48 min (12 min·mi⁻¹ × 4 mi), and the total caloric expenditure is increased (48 min × 7.5 kcal·min⁻¹ = 360 kcal). Thus, the duration of the exercise and total distance may be somewhat more important than the speed (intensity) of exercise for maximizing the energy expenditure.

Recently, Nicklas and colleagues (2009) reported that vigorous aerobic exercise (70-75% heart rate reserve [HRR]) and moderate-intensity aerobic exercise (45-50% HRR), combined with caloric restriction, produced similar amounts of weight loss and abdominal fat loss in overweight and obese women. Given that most obese individuals prefer to exercise at a slower pace and low-to-moderate intensity, it probably is not necessary to prescribe vigorous-intensity exercise as part of a weight loss program.

■ **Which aerobic exercise mode is best to maximize fat loss?**

In a meta-analysis of 53 studies dealing with the effects of exercise on body weight and composition, Ballor and Keesey (1991) reported that fat loss for males participating in aerobic exercise training was, on average, 1.9 kg for cycling (0.11 kg·wk⁻¹) and 1.6 kg for running and walking (0.12 kg·wk⁻¹). For resistance training, body weight increased an average of 1.2 kg, but fat mass was reduced by 1.0 kg. For females, fat mass decreased significantly (1.3

kg) for running and walking but not cycling. These studies suggest that in terms of fat loss, aerobic exercise modes are equally effective for men, but running and walking may be better than cycling for women.

■ *Are spot reduction exercises effective for decreasing body fat in localized regions of the body?*

Specific spot reduction exercises are no more effective than general aerobic exercise for changing limb and body girth measurements or for altering total body composition (Carns et al. 1960; Noland and Kearney 1978; Roby 1962; Schade et al. 1962). Katch and colleagues (1984) assessed changes in the diameter of adipose cells from the abdomen and gluteal and subscapular sites resulting from a 27-day training program in which each subject performed 5004 sit-ups. Although the training significantly reduced fat cell diameter, the effect was similar at all three sites: abdomen, –6.4%; gluteal, –5.0%; and subscapular, –3.7%. It appears that a sit-up exercise program does not preferentially reduce the fat in the abdominal region.

Despres and colleagues (1985) reported that a 20 wk cycling program significantly reduced %BF and body weight. Cycling affected trunk skinfolds (SKFs) (–22%) more than extremity SKFs (–12.5%). If fat was mobilized preferentially from subcutaneous stores near the exercising muscle mass, one would expect the lower extremity SKFs to be more affected by cycling than the trunk SKFs. Yet Despres and colleagues (1985) noted an 18% reduction in the suprailiac SKF compared to a 13% reduction in the thigh SKF. This suggests that subcutaneous fat cells in the abdomen are more sensitive to the lipolytic effect of catecholamines than subcutaneous fat cells in the thighs (Smith et al. 1979).

The enzyme lipoprotein-lipase is responsible for lipid accumulation. In women, lipoprotein-lipase activity is higher in the gluteofemoral region than in the abdominal region (Litchell and Boberg 1978). Estrogen and progesterone appear to enhance lipoprotein-lipase activity in women. Also, the lipolytic response to catecholamines is lower in the femoral than in the abdominal depots for both men and women (Rebuffe-Scrive 1985).

Thus, the regional distribution and mobilization of adipose tissue appear to follow a biologically selective pattern regardless of type of exercise. Even with weight reduction, the relative fat distribution remains stable as measured by the WHR; however, the waist-to-thigh ratio decreases, suggesting that the thigh region is slightly more resistant to fat mobilization in women (Ashwell et al. 1985).

In addition, upper body resistance training does not appear to preferentially reduce subcutaneous fat deposits in the upper arm. Kostek and colleagues (2007) reported that subcutaneous fat changes, measured by magnetic resonance imaging (MRI), in trained and untrained arms did not differ significantly following 12 wk of resistance training. These findings suggest that resistance training exercise does result in spot reduction.

DESIGNING WEIGHT GAIN PROGRAMS

Because genetics plays an important role in weight gain, some clients may have difficulty gaining weight, especially if they have inherited a high RMR. Before prescribing weight gain programs, you should rule out the possibility that diseases and psychological disorders associated with malnutrition (e.g., anorexia nervosa) are not causing your client to be underweight. For athletes who are competing in weight classes, Macedonio (2009) provides detailed information and suggestions for making weight.

The number of additional calories needed in order for a person to gain 1 lb (0.45 kg) of muscle tissue has not yet been firmly established. However, research suggests that an excess of 2800 to 3500 kcal is required. Thus, adding 400 to 500 kcal to the estimated daily caloric needs (RMR + occupational activity level) of the individual should produce a gradual weight gain of 1 lb per week (Williams 1992). The caloric intake must also be adjusted for additional calories expended during exercise.

Weight Gain Diets

Again, it is highly recommended that you consult with a trained nutrition professional when planning weight gain diets. When comparing your client's typical nutrient intakes to recommended dietary intakes, you should focus on the same questions as outlined for weight loss programs (see p. 256).

To ensure that your client's weight gain is due to increases in lean tissues rather than body fat, you should

- use the body composition method to estimate a healthy target body weight and gain in FFM;

- plan a high-calorie, well-balanced diet in which 60% to 65% of the total kilocalorie intake is derived from carbohydrate, 12% to 15% from protein, and 23% to 25% from fat;

- increase daily protein intake to 1.2 to 1.6 g per kilogram of body weight to increase muscle size; and

- monitor body composition regularly throughout the weight gain program using methods described in chapter 8.

Exercise Prescription for Weight Gain

As part of the weight gain program, you should prescribe resistance training to increase muscle size. A high-volume resistance training program is the best approach to maximize the development of muscle size. Because some clients may not be able to tolerate this volume of training at first, novice weightlifters should start slowly by performing only three sets of each exercise at the prescribed intensity and by reducing the number of exercises for each muscle group. Depending on your client's goal, this may be sufficient to increase FFM. For some clients, however, you may need to progressively increase the training volume in order to elicit further improvements in muscle size and FFM. Recommended guidelines for developing an exercise prescription for weight gain are as follows:

GUIDELINES FOR EXERCISE PRESCRIPTION FOR WEIGHT GAIN

- **Mode:** Resistance training
- **Intensity:** 70% to 75% 1-RM or 10- to 12-RM
- **Sets:** Three for novices; more than three for advanced weightlifters
- **Number of exercises:** One or two per muscle group for novices; three or four per muscle group for advanced weightlifters
- **Duration:** 60 min or longer
- **Frequency:** 3 days/wk for novices; 5 or 6 days/wk for advanced weightlifters
- **Length of program:** Dependent on desired weight gain

DESIGNING PROGRAMS TO IMPROVE BODY COMPOSITION

Some clients may wish to improve their body composition without changing their body weight. For these individuals, you can design exercise programs to decrease body fat, increase FFM, or both. Research has shown that regular participation in an exercise program may alter an individual's body composition. Aerobic exercise and resistance training are effective modes for decreasing SKF thicknesses, fat weight, and %BF of both women and men.

Questions About Exercise and Body Composition Changes

- *What is the effect of aerobic exercise training on body fat?*

Numerous studies have been conducted to determine the effect of aerobic exercise training on body composition. The modes of exercise include cycling, walking, jogging, running, and swimming. Wilmore and colleagues (1970) reported that a 10 wk jogging program (3 days/wk) produced a significant increase in body density of sedentary men. Because total body weight decreased and FFM remained stable, the increase in body density was attributed almost entirely to fat loss. Pollock and colleagues (1971) also noted that a 20 wk (4 days/wk) walking program produced a decrease in %BF and total body weight of men.

- *Which aerobic exercise mode is best for maximizing fat loss?*

One study compared cycling, running, and walking of equal frequency, duration, and intensity (Pollock et al. 1975). All three programs produced significant reductions in %BF and body weight. Also, Despres and colleagues (1985) reported that a 20 wk cycling program (four or five times a week) resulted in significant reductions in body weight, %BF, and fat cell weight in a group of sedentary men. On the basis of these studies it appears that aerobic exercise modes are equally effective in altering body composition.

■ *How many times a week should I exercise to maximize the loss of body fat?*

The frequency of the training program may affect the magnitude of the changes in body composition. Pollock and colleagues (1975) compared aerobic exercise programs consisting of 2, 3, or 4 days/wk. Even though the total mileage and caloric expenditure were the same, exercising 2 days/wk was not sufficient to produce significant alterations in body composition. The authors concluded that a 3 or 4 day a week program produces significant body composition changes, with 4 days/wk being superior to 3 days/wk.

■ *Does the intensity of aerobic exercise affect body composition changes?*

Irving and colleagues (2008) compared the effects of low-intensity (RPE ~10-11) and high-intensity (RPE ~12-15) exercise training on abdominal visceral fat and body composition of obese women with metabolic syndrome. Using computerized technology, they noted that high-intensity training produced significantly larger reductions in subcutaneous and visceral fat in the abdomen compared to low-intensity training.

■ *What effect does resistance training have on body fat and FFM?*

Although resistance training may increase body weight, it positively affects fat mass, %BF, and FFM (Ballor and Keesey 1991). Cullinen and Caldwell (1998) found that normal-weight women (19 to 44 yr) participating in a moderate-intensity resistance training program (2 days/wk for 12 wk) significantly increased FFM (~4.5%) and decreased %BF (~8.7%). In Wilmore's study (1974), subjects trained 2 days/wk for 10 wk. At each training session, they performed two sets of 7- to 9-RM for eight different weight training exercises. Men and women exhibited similar alterations in body composition. Although the total body weight remained stable, the FFM increased significantly for both sexes. As a result of resistance training, the relative body fat decreased 9.6% and 10.0% for women and men, respectively.

■ *How does exercise promote body composition changes?*

The significant loss of fat weight and %BF with aerobic exercise and resistance training is a func-

tion of hormonal responses to the exercise. Exercise increases the circulatory levels of growth hormone (GH), and the levels remain elevated for 1 to 2 hr after exercise (Hartley et al. 1972; Hartley 1975). Exercise also stimulates the release of catecholamines from the adrenal medulla. Both GH and catecholamines increase the mobilization of free fatty acids from storage (Hartley 1975). Eventually, the muscle may metabolize these free fatty acids during rest and low-intensity exercise.

The increase in FFM with resistance training may be due to muscle hypertrophy, increased protein content in the muscle, or increased bone density. Muscle hypertrophy and increased protein are mediated by changes in serum testosterone and GH levels in response to weightlifting. Immediately following heavy resistance weightlifting, serum testosterone levels are significantly elevated for men but not for women (Fahey et al. 1976; Weiss, Cureton, and Thompson 1983). Growth hormone levels in men are increased significantly for 15 min following a 21 min bout of high-intensity (85% of 1-RM) leg press exercises. However, low-intensity, high-repetition (28% of 1-RM, 21 reps per set) leg presses produced no significant change in GH even though the total amount of work and duration of exercise were equal. Thus, the intensity and number of repetitions play a role in GH release in response to weightlifting exercise (Vanhelder, Radomski, and Goode 1984).

In addition, resistance training has an effect on the hormonal profiles of younger (30 yr) and older (62 yr) men (Kraemer et al. 1999a). Following a 10 wk periodized strength–power training program, young men had significant increases in free testosterone at rest and in response to weightlifting exercise. Younger men also showed increases in resting levels of insulin-like growth factor-binding protein-3 after training. For the older men, training produced a significant increase in total testosterone in response to weightlifting exercise, as well as a significant reduction in resting cortisol levels.

Exercise Prescription for Body Composition Change

While light- to moderate-intensity aerobic exercise may be more beneficial for fat loss, high-intensity resistance training is better for FFM gain. Thus, combining aerobic and resistance training exercises may be the most effective way to alter body composition of nondieting individuals (Dolezal and Potteiger 1998). When designing exercise programs to promote changes in body composition, adhere to the following guidelines. Prescribe aerobic exercise to reduce body fat and resistance training exercise to increase FFM.

GUIDELINES FOR EXERCISE PRESCRIPTION FOR FAT LOSS

- **Goal:** Fat loss
- **Mode:** Type A and B aerobic activities (see p. 106)
- **Intensity:** Moderate to high (RPE 10-15)
- **Duration:** 30 to 45 min
- **Frequency:** Minimum of 3 days/wk
- **Length:** Minimum of 8 wk

GUIDELINES FOR EXERCISE PRESCRIPTION FOR FAT-FREE MASS GAIN

- **Goal:** Increase FFM and reduce body fat
- **Mode:** Dynamic resistance training
- **Intensity:** 70% to 85% 1-RM
- **Repetitions:** 6 to 12 reps
- **Sets:** Three sets
- **Frequency:** Minimum of 3 days/wk
- **Length:** Minimum of 8 wk

KEY POINTS

- Obesity is an excess of body fat that increases health risks.

- Two types of obesity are upper body (android) and lower body (gynoid) obesity.

- The number of fat cells in the body is determined primarily during childhood and adolescence.

- Weight gain in adults is associated with an increase in the size of existing fat cells (hypertrophy), rather than an increase in the number of fat cells (hyperplasia).

- Physical inactivity is a common cause of obesity.

- The body composition method provides a useful estimate of a healthy body weight.

- Well-balanced nutrition includes adequate amounts of carbohydrate, protein, fat, minerals, vitamins, and water.

- Weight loss depends on calorie intake, not on the macronutrient composition of the diet.

- Effective weight loss programs create a negative energy balance by restricting caloric intake and increasing physical activity and exercise; weight gain programs create a positive energy balance by increasing caloric intake.

- For weight loss programs, the combined daily caloric deficit due to calorie restriction and extra exercise should not exceed 1000 kcal; for weight gain programs, the daily caloric intake should exceed the energy need by no more than 400 to 500 kcal.

- Adding a combination of aerobic and resistance training exercises to the dieting regimen is an effective way to maximize fat loss and preserve FFM during weight loss.

- The optimal amount of physical activity for preventing weight gain differs from that needed to create a negative energy balance for weight loss and for maintenance of weight loss.

- For weight gain programs, resistance training will ensure that most of the weight gain is due to increases in lean body tissues.

- Aerobic exercise and resistance training are effective ways to improve body composition without changing body weight.

KEY TERMS

Learn the definition for each of the following key terms. Definitions of terms can be found in the glossary on page 411.

android obesity

anorexia nervosa

at risk for overweight

basal metabolic rate (BMR)

complex carbohydrates

dietary thermogenesis

digital activity log

factorial method

glycemic index (GI)

gynoid obesity

healthy body weight

hyperplasia

hypertrophy

kilocalorie

lower body obesity

negative energy balance

obesity

physical activity level (PAL)

positive energy balance

resting energy expenditure (REE)

resting metabolic rate (RMR)

simple carbohydrates

total energy expenditure (TEE)

total energy expenditure (TEE) method

underweight

upper body obesity

REVIEW QUESTIONS

In addition to being able to define each of the key terms, test your knowledge and understanding of the material by answering the following review questions.

1. Using BMI, what are the cutoff values for classification of obesity, overweight, healthy body weight, and underweight?

2. Describe how you can determine a healthy body weight for your client.

3. For typical weight loss programs, identify the minimal caloric intake per day and maximal caloric deficit (i.e., negative energy balance) per day. What is the best way to create this daily caloric deficit?

4. Explain why a taller, heavier person will lose weight at a faster rate than a shorter, lighter person when the two individuals are on the same diet.

5. For well-balanced nutrition, what are the recommended proportions of carbohydrate, fat, and protein in the diet?

6. Explain why exercise is an important component of weight loss and weight gain programs.

7. Describe two methods that you can use to estimate the energy needs of your clients.

8. Describe the optimal amount of physical activity (intensity, duration, and frequency) for health benefits, weight loss, weight maintenance, and prevention of weight regain.

9. Estimate the daily caloric intake for a 50 yr old, 150 lb (68 kg) female professor who is 5 ft 5 in. and who bikes a total of 60 min, 5 days/wk, to and from the university.

10. Describe the basic exercise prescriptions for weight loss and weight gain programs.

Assessing Flexibility

KEY QUESTIONS

- What is the difference between static and dynamic flexibility?
- What factors affect flexibility? How is flexibility assessed?
- Are indirect measures of flexibility valid and reliable?
- What are the general guidelines for flexibility testing?
- What test can I use to assess the flexibility of older adults?

Flexibility is an important, yet often neglected, component of health-related fitness. Adequate levels of flexibility are needed for maintenance of functional independence and performance of activities of daily living such as bending to pick up a newspaper or getting out of the backseat of a two-door car. Over the years, flexibility tests have been included in most health-related fitness test batteries, since it has been long thought that lack of flexibility is associated with musculoskeletal injuries and low back pain. However, compared to research on other physical fitness components, there are not many studies substantiating the importance of flexibility to health-related fitness.

Research suggests that individuals with too little (ankylosis) or too much (hypermobility) flexibility are at higher risk than others for musculoskeletal injuries (Jones and Knapik 1999), but there is limited evidence that a greater than normal amount of flexibility actually decreases injury risk (Knudson, Magnusson, and McHugh 2000). Also, research fails

to support an association between lumbar or hamstring flexibility and the occurrence of low back pain (Jackson et al. 1998; Plowman 1992). Still, flexibility should be included in health-related fitness test batteries to identify individuals at the extremes who may have a higher risk of musculotendinous injury.

This chapter describes direct and indirect methods for assessing flexibility. It presents guidelines for flexibility testing as well as norms for commonly used flexibility tests.

BASICS OF FLEXIBILITY

Flexibility and joint stability are highly dependent on the joint structure, as well as the strength and number of ligaments and muscles spanning the joint. To fully appreciate the complexity of flexibility, you should review the anatomy of joints and muscles. This section deals with the definitions and nature of flexibility and also presents factors influencing joint mobility.

Definitions and Nature of Flexibility

Flexibility is the ability of a joint, or series of joints, to move through a full range of motion (ROM) without injury. Static flexibility is a measure of the total ROM at the joint and is limited by the extensibility of the musculotendinous unit. Dynamic flexibility is a measure of the rate of torque or resistance developed during stretching throughout the ROM. Although dynamic flexibility accounts for 44% to 66% of the variance in static flexibility (Magnusson et al. 1997; McHugh et al. 1998), more research is needed to firmly establish the relationship between static and dynamic flexibility and to determine whether these two types of flexibility are distinct entities or two aspects of the same flexibility component (Knudson et al. 2000).

The ROM is highly specific to the joint (i.e., specificity principle) and depends on morphological factors such as the joint geometry and the joint capsule, ligaments, tendons, and muscles spanning the joint. The joint structure determines the planes of motion and may limit the ROM at a given joint. **Triaxial joints** (e.g., ball-and-socket joints of the hip and shoulder) afford a greater degree of movement in more directions than **nonaxial**, **uniaxial** or **biaxial joints** (see table 10.1).

The tightness of soft tissue structures such as muscle, tendons, and ligaments is a major limitation to both static and dynamic flexibility. Johns and Wright (1962) determined the relative contribution of soft tissues to the total resistance encountered by the joint during movement:

- Joint capsule—47%
- Muscle and its fascia—41%
- Tendons and ligaments—10%
- Skin—2%

The joint capsule and ligaments consist predominantly of collagen, a nonelastic connective tissue. The muscle and its fascia, however, have elastic connective tissue; therefore, they are the most important structures in terms of reducing resistance to movement and increasing dynamic flexibility.

The tension within the muscle–tendon unit affects both static flexibility (ROM) and dynamic flexibility (stiffness or resistance to movement). The tension within this unit is attributed to the **viscoelastic properties** of connective tissues, as well as to the degree of muscular contraction resulting from the stretch reflex (McHugh et al. 1992). Individuals with less flexibility and tighter muscles and tendons have a greater contractile response during stretching exercises and a greater resistance to stretching. The **elastic deformation** of the muscle–tendon unit during stretching is proportional to the load or tension applied, whereas the **viscous deformation** is proportional to the speed at which the tension is applied. When the muscle and tendon are stretched and held at a fixed length (e.g., during **static stretching**), the tension within the unit, or tensile stress, decreases over time (McHugh et al. 1992). This is called **stress relaxation**. A single static stretch sustained for 90 sec produces a 30% increase in viscoelastic stress relaxation and decreases muscle stiffness for up to 1 hr (Magnusson 1998). Thus, static stretching exercise is an excellent way to induce viscoelastic stress relaxation. Mahieu and associates (2007) reported that 6 wk static and ballistic stretching programs had different effects on passive resistive torque and tendon stiffness. Both forms of stretching increased ankle dorsiflexion ROM. Static stretching significantly reduced passive resistive torque of the calf muscles but had no effect on Achilles tendon stiffness, whereas ballistic stretching had the reverse effect—Achilles tendon stiffness decreased, but passive resistive torque of the plantar flexors was unchanged.

Factors Affecting Flexibility

Flexibility is related to body type, age, gender, and physical activity level. This section addresses some commonly asked questions about flexibility.

- *Does body type limit flexibility?*

Individuals with large hypertrophied muscles or excessive amounts of subcutaneous fat may score poorly on ROM tests because adjacent body segments in these people contact each other sooner

Table 10.1 Joint Classification by Structure and Function			
Type of joint	**Axes of rotation**	**Movements**	**Examples**
Gliding	Nonaxial	Gliding, sliding, twisting	Intercarpal, intertarsal, tarsometatarsal
Hinge	Uniaxial	Flexion, extension	Knee, elbow, ankle, interphalangeal
Pivot	Uniaxial	Medial and lateral rotation	Proximal radioulnar, atlantoaxial
Condyloid and saddle	Biaxial	Flexion, extension, abduction, adduction, circumduction	Wrist, atlanto-occipital, metacarpophalangeal, first carpometacarpal
Ball and socket	Triaxial	Flexion, extension, abduction, adduction, circumduction, rotation	Hip, shoulder

than in those with smaller limb and trunk girths. However, this does not necessarily mean that all heavily muscled or obese individuals have poor flexibility. Many bodybuilders and obese individuals who routinely stretch their muscles have adequate levels of flexibility.

■ Why do older individuals tend to be less flexible than younger people?

Inflexible and older individuals have increased muscle stiffness and a lower stretch tolerance compared to younger individuals with normal flexibility (Magnusson 1998). As muscle stiffness increases, static flexibility progressively decreases with aging (Brown and Miller 1998; Gajdosik, Vander Linden, and Williams 1999). A decline in physical activity and development of arthritic conditions, rather than a specific effect of aging, are the primary causes for the loss of flexibility as one grows older. Still, flexibility training can help to counteract age-related decreases in ROM. Girouard and Hurley (1995) reported significant improvements in shoulder and hip ROM of older men (50 to 69 yr) following 10 wk of flexibility training. Thus, older persons can benefit from flexibility training and should be encouraged to perform stretching exercises at least three times a week to counteract age-related decreases in ROM.

■ Are females more flexible than males?

Some evidence suggests that females generally are more flexible than males at all ages (Alter 1996; Payne et al. 2000). The greater flexibility of women is usually attributed to gender differences in pelvic structure and hormones that may affect connective tissue laxity (Alter 1996). However, the effect of gender on ROM appears to be joint and motion specific. Females tend to have more hip flexion and spinal lateral flexion than males of the same age. On the other hand, males have greater ROM in hip extension and spinal flexion and extension in the thoracolumbar region (Norkin and White 1995).

■ How do physical activity and inactivity affect flexibility?

Habitual movement patterns and physical activity levels apparently are more important determinants of flexibility than gender, age, and body type (Harris 1969; Kirby et al. 1981). Lack of physical activity is a major cause of inflexibility. It is well documented that inactive persons tend to be less flexible than active persons (McCue 1953) and that exercise increases flexibility (Chapman, deVries,

and Swezey 1972; deVries 1962; Hartley-O'Brien 1980). Disuse, due to lack of physical activity or immobilization, produces shortening of the muscles (i.e., contracture) and connective tissues, which in turn restricts joint mobility.

Moving the joints and muscles in a repetitive pattern or maintaining habitual body postures may restrict ROM because of the tightening and shortening of the muscle tissue. For example, joggers and people who sit behind a desk for long periods need to stretch the hamstrings and low back muscles to counteract the tautness developed in these muscle groups.

■ Does warming up affect flexibility?

Although active warm-up exercises such as walking, jogging, and stair climbing increase muscle temperature and decrease muscle stiffness, warming up alone does not increase ROM (deWeijer, Gorniak, and Shamus 2003; Shrier and Gossal 2000). Studies have shown that active warm-up combined with static stretching is more effective than static stretching alone in increasing the length of the hamstring muscles (deWeijer et al. 2003) and in improving ROM (Shrier and Gossal 2000). Therefore, when you administer flexibility (ROM) tests, make certain that your clients warm up and statically stretch the muscle groups before you measure them, and administer multiple trials for each test item.

■ Can you develop too much flexibility?

It is important to recognize that excessive amounts of stretching and flexibility training may result in hypermobility, or an increased ROM of joints beyond normal, acceptable values. Hypermobility leads to joint laxity (looseness or instability) and may increase one's risk of musculoskeletal injuries. For example, it is not uncommon for gymnasts and swimmers to experience shoulder dislocations because of joint laxity and hypermobility. As an exercise specialist, you need to be able to accurately assess ROM and to design stretching programs that improve your clients' flexibility without compromising joint stability.

ASSESSMENT OF FLEXIBILITY

Field and clinical tests are available for assessing static flexibility. Although ROM data are important, measures of dynamic flexibility (i.e., joint stiffness and resistance to movement) may be more meaningful in terms of physical performance. Dynamic flexibility tests measure the increase in resistance during muscle elongation; several studies have shown that less stiff muscles are more effective in using the elastic energy during movements involving the stretch–shortening cycle (Kubo et al. 2000, 1999). However, dynamic flexibility testing is limited to the research setting because the equipment is expensive. Typically, static flexibility is assessed in field and clinical settings by direct or indirect measurement of the ROM.

Direct Methods of Measuring Static Flexibility

To assess static flexibility directly, measure the amount of joint rotation in degrees using a goniometer, flexometer, or inclinometer. The following sections describe the procedures for these tests.

Universal Goniometer Test Procedures

The universal goniometer is a protractor-like device with two steel or plastic arms that measure the joint angle at the extremes of the ROM (see figure 10.1). The stationary arm of the goniometer is attached at the zero line of the protractor, and the other arm is movable. To use the goniometer, place the center of the instrument so it coincides

GENERAL GUIDELINES FOR FLEXIBILITY TESTING

To assess a client's flexibility, you should select a number of test items because of the highly specific nature of flexibility (Dickinson 1968; Harris 1969). Direct tests that measure the range of joint rotation in degrees are usually more useful than indirect tests that measure static flexibility in linear units. When administering these tests,

- have the client perform a general warm-up followed by static stretching prior to the test and avoid fast, jerky movements and stretching beyond the pain-free range of joint motion;
- administer three trials of each test item;
- compare the client's best score to norms in order to obtain a flexibility rating for each test item; and
- use the test results to identify joints and muscle groups in need of improvement.

with the fulcrum, or axis of rotation, of the joint. Align the arms of the goniometer with bony landmarks along the longitudinal axis of each moving

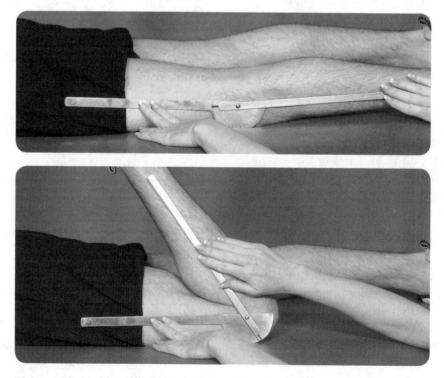

Figure 10.1 Measuring range of motion at knee joint using universal goniometer.

Table 10.2 Universal Goniometer Measurement Procedures

Joint	Body position	GONIOMETER POSITION			Stabilization	Special considerations
		Axis of rotation	Stationary arm	Moving arm		
Shoulder						
Extension	Prone	Acromion process	Midaxillary line	Lateral epicondyle of humerus	Scapula and thorax	Elbow is slightly flexed and palm of hand faces body.
Flexion	Supine	Same as extension	Same as extension	Same as extension	Scapula and thorax	Palm of hand faces body.
Abduction	Supine	Anterior axis of acromion process	Midline of anterior aspect of sternum	Medial midline of humerus	Scapula and thorax	Palm of hand faces anteriorly; humerus is laterally rotated; elbow is extended.
Medial/lateral rotation	Supine	Olecranon process	Perpendicular to floor	Styloid process of ulna	Distal end of humerus and scapula	Arm is abducted 90°; forearm is perpendicular to supporting surface in mid-pronated-supinated position; humerus rests on pad so that it is level with acromion process.
Elbow						
Flexion	Supine	Lateral epicondyle of humerus	Lateral midline of humerus	Lateral midline of radial head and styloid process	Distal end of humerus	Arm is close to body; pad is placed under distal end of humerus; forearm is fully supinated.
Forearm						
Pronation	Sitting	Lateral to ulna styloid process	Parallel to anterior midline of humerus	Lies across dorsal aspect of forearm, just proximal to styloid processes of radius and ulna	Distal end of humerus	Arm is close to body, elbow flexed 90°; forearm is midway between supination and pronation (thumb toward ceiling).
Supination	Sitting	Medial to ulna styloid process	Parallel to anterior midline of humerus	Lies across ventral aspect of forearm, just proximal to styloid processes of radius and ulna	Distal end of humerus	Testing position is same as for pronation of forearm.
Wrist						
Flexion and extension	Sitting	Lateral aspect of wrist over the triquetrum	Lateral midline of ulna, using olecranon and ulnar styloid processes for reference	Lateral midline of fifth metacarpal	Radius and ulna	Client sits next to supporting surface, abducts shoulder 90° and flexes elbow 90°; forearm is in mid-supinated-pronated position; palm of hand faces ground; forearm rests on supporting surface; hand is free to move.
Radial or ulnar deviation	Sitting	Middle of dorsal aspect of wrist over capitate	Dorsal midline of forearm, using lateral humeral epicondyle as reference	Dorsal midline of third metacarpal	Distal ends of radius and ulna	Same as for wrist flexion.

(continued)

Table 10.2 (continued)

Joint	Body position	GONIOMETER POSITION			Stabilization	Special considerations
		Axis of rotation	Stationary arm	Moving arm		
Hip						
Flexion and extension	Supine; prone	Lateral aspect of hip joint, using greater trochanter as reference	Lateral midline of pelvis	Lateral midline of femur, using lateral epicondyle for reference	Pelvis	Knee is allowed to flex as range of hip flexion is completed; knee is flexed during hip extension.
Abduction and adduction	Supine	Centered over anterior superior iliac spine	Horizontally align arm with imaginary line between anterior superior iliac spines	Anterior midline of femur, using midline of patella for reference	Pelvis	Knee is extended during abduction.
Medial/lateral rotation	Sitting	Centered over anterior aspect of patella	Perpendicular to floor	Anterior midline of lower leg, using crest of tibia and point midway between malleoli for reference	Distal end of femur; avoid rotation and lateral tilt of pelvis	Client sits on supporting surface, knees flexed 90°; place towel roll under distal end of femur; contralateral knee may need to be flexed so that hip being measured can complete full range of lateral rotation.
Knee						
Flexion	Supine	Over the lateral epicondyle of femur	Lateral midline of femur, using greater trochanter for reference	Lateral midline of fibula, using lateral malleolus and fibular head for reference	Femur to prevent rotation, abduction, and adduction	As knee flexes, the hip also flexes.
Ankle						
Dorsiflexion and plantar flexion	Sitting	Over the lateral aspect of lateral malleolus	Lateral midline of fibula, using head of fibula as reference	Parallel to lateral aspect of fifth metatarsal	Tibia and fibula	Client sits on end of table with knee flexed and ankle positioned at 90°.
Subtalar						
Inversion and eversion	Sitting	Centered over anterior aspect of ankle midway between malleoli	Anterior midline of lower leg, using the tibial tuberosity for reference	Anterior midline of second metatarsal	Tibia and fibula	Client sits with knee flexed 90° and lower leg over edge of supporting surface.
Lumbar spine						
Lateral flexion	Standing	Centered over posterior aspect of spinous process of S1	Perpendicular to the ground	Posterior aspect of spinous process of C7	Pelvis to prevent lateral tilt	Client stands erect with 0° of spinal flexion, extension, and rotation.
Rotation	Sitting	Centered over superior aspect of client's head	Parallel to imaginary line between tubercles of iliac crests	Imaginary line between two acromion processes	Pelvis to prevent rotation	Keep feet flat on floor to stabilize pelvis.

body segment. Measure the ROM as the difference between the joint angles (degrees) at the extremes of the movement.

Table 10.2 (p. 269) summarizes procedures for measuring ROM for various joints using a universal goniometer. The American College of Sports Medicine (ACSM 2010) recommends using goniometers to obtain precise measurement of joint ROM. For more detailed descriptions of these procedures, see Greene and Heckman 1994 and Norkin and White 1995. Table 10.3 presents average ROM values for healthy adults.

Flexometer Test Procedures

Another tool you can use to measure ROM is the Leighton flexometer (see figure 10.2). This device consists of a weighted 360° dial and weighted pointer. The ROM is measured in relation to the downward pull of gravity on the dial and pointer. To use this device, strap the instrument to the body segment, and lock the dial at 0° at one extreme of the ROM. After the client executes the movement, lock the pointer at the other extreme of the ROM. The degree of arc through which the movement takes place is read directly from the dial. Tests have been devised

to measure the ROM at the neck, trunk, shoulder, elbow, radioulnar, wrist, hip, knee, and ankle joints using the Leighton flexometer (Hubley-Kozey 1991; Leighton 1955).

Inclinometer Test Procedures

The inclinometer is another type of gravity-dependent goniometer (see figure 10.3). To use this device, hold it on the distal end of the body segment. The inclinometer measures the angle between the long axis of the moving segment and the line of gravity. This device is easier to use than the flexometer and universal goniometer because it is held by hand on the moving body segment during the measurement and does not have to be aligned with specific bony landmarks. Also, the American Medical Association (1988) recommends the double-inclinometer technique, using two inclinometers, to measure spinal mobility (see figure 10.3).

Validity and Reliability of Direct Measures

The validity and reliability of these devices for directly measuring ROM are highly dependent on the joint being measured and technician skill.

Table 10.3 Average Range-of-Motion (ROM) Values for Healthy Adults

Joint	ROM (degrees)	Joint	ROM
Shoulder		**Thoracic-lumbar spine**	
Flexion	150-180	Flexion	60-80
Extension	50-60	Extension	20-30
Abduction	180	Abduction	25-35
Medial rotation	70-90	Rotation	30-45
Lateral rotation	90	**Hip**	
Elbow		Flexion	100-120
Flexion	140-150	Extension	30
Extension	0	Abduction	40-45
Radioulnar		Adduction	20-30
Pronation	80	Medial rotation	40-45
Supination	80	Lateral rotation	45-50
Wrist		**Knee**	
Flexion	60-80	Flexion	135-150
Extension	60-70	Extension	0-10
Radial deviation	20	**Ankle**	
Ulnar deviation	30	Dorsiflexion	20
Cervical spine		Plantar flexion	40-45
Flexion	45-60	**Subtalar**	
Extension	45-75	Inversion	30-35
Lateral flexion	45	Eversion	15-20
Rotation	60-80		

Data from the American Academy of Orthopaedic Surgeons (Greene and Heckman 1994) and the American Medical Association 1988.

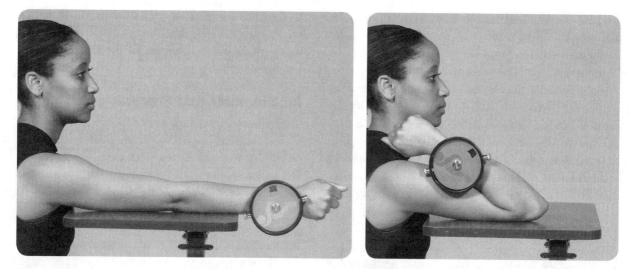

Figure 10.2 Measuring range of motion at elbow joint using Leighton flexometer.

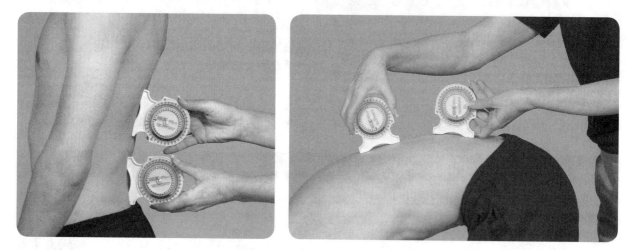

Figure 10.3 Measuring lumbosacral flexion using the double-inclinometer technique.

Radiography is considered to be the best reference method for establishing validity of goniometric measurements. Research shows high agreement between ROM measured by radiographs and universal goniometers for the hip and knee joints (Ahlback and Lindahl 1964; Enwemeka 1986). Mayer, Tencer, and Kristoferson (1984) reported no difference between radiography and the double-inclinometer technique for assessing spinal ROM of patients with low back pain.

The intratester and intertester reliabilities of goniometric measurements are affected by difficulty in identifying the axis of rotation and palpating bony landmarks. Measurements of upper extremity joints are generally more reliable than ROM measurements of the lower extremity joints (Norkin

and White 1995). Generally, the inclinometer reliably measures ROM at most joints; however, the intertester reliability of inclinometer measurements is variable and joint specific. Studies have reported reliability coefficients ranging from 0.48 for lumbar extension (Williams et al. 1993b) to 0.96 for subtalar joint position (Sell et al. 1994). Also, the intrarater reliabilities for inclinometer measurements of the flexibility of the iliotibial band (hip adduction), and for ROM measurements of the lumbar spine and lordosis, generally exceed 0.90 (Ng et al. 2001; Reese and Bandy 2003). In order to obtain accurate and reliable ROM measurements, you need a thorough knowledge of anatomy and of standardized testing procedures, as well as training and practice to develop your measurement techniques.

Indirect Methods of Measuring Static Flexibility

Because of the belief that lack of flexibility is associated with low back pain and musculoskeletal injuries, most health-related fitness test batteries include a sit-and-reach test to evaluate the static flexibility of the lower back and hamstring muscles (Payne et al. 2000). The sit-and-reach test provides an indirect, linear measurement of the ROM. Several sit-and-reach protocols have been developed using either a yardstick (meter stick) or a box, or both, to measure flexibility in inches or centimeters.

Although some fitness professionals assume the sit-and-reach to be a valid measure of low back and hamstring flexibility, research has shown that these tests are moderately related to hamstring flexibility ($r = 0.39$ to 0.89) but poorly related to low back flexibility ($r = 0.10$ to 0.59) in children (Patterson at al. 1996), adults (Hui et al. 1999; Hui and Yuen 2000; Jackson and Langford 1989; Martin et al. 1998; Minkler and Patterson 1994), and older adults (Jones et al. 1998). Moreover, in a prospective study of adults, Jackson and colleagues (1998) reported that the sit-and-reach test has poor criterion-related validity and is unrelated to self-reported low back pain. Likewise, Grenier, Russell, and McGill (2003) noted that sit-and-reach test scores do not relate to a history of low back pain or discomfort in industrial workers. Although sit-and-reach scores were moderately related ($r = 0.42$) to lumbar ROM in the sagittal plane, the sit-and-reach test could not distinguish between workers who had low back discomfort and workers who did not. The researchers concluded that standard fitness test batteries should include measures of lumbar ROM instead of the sit-and-reach test to assess low back fitness. Lumbar ROM in the sagittal plane can be measured directly with an inclinometer (double-inclinometer technique, see figure 10.3) or indirectly with the skin distraction test (see "Skin Distraction Test," page 276). Although research affirms that the sit-and-reach test does not validly measure low back flexibility, it may still be used to provide an indirect measure of hamstring length. Davis and colleagues (2008) reported that sit-and-reach scores were moderately related to other measures of hamstring length such as sacral angle ($r = 0.65$), knee extension angle ($r = 0.57$), and straight leg raise ($r = 0.65$). Sit-and-reach tests should be limited to identifying individuals at the extremes who may have a higher risk of muscle injury because of hypermobility or lack of flexibility in the hamstring muscles.

The following sections describe the protocols for various types of sit-and-reach tests, as well as the skin distraction test. Before clients take any of these tests, have them perform a general warm-up to increase muscle temperature, as well as stretching exercises for the muscle groups to be tested. Unless otherwise stated, have your clients remove their shoes for all sit-and-reach test protocols.

Standard Sit-and-Reach Test

The ACSM (2010) and the Canadian Society for Exercise Physiology (2003) recommend using the standard sit-and-reach test to assess low back and hamstring flexibility. This test uses a sit-and-reach box with a zero point at 26 cm. Have the client sit on the floor with her knees extended and the soles of her feet against the edge of the box. The inner edges of the soles of the feet must be 6 in. (15.2 cm) apart. Instruct the client to keep her knees fully extended, arms evenly stretched, and hands parallel with the palms down (fingertips may overlap) as she slowly reaches forward as far as possible along the top of the box. Have the client hold this position for ~2 sec. Advise your client that lowering the head maximizes the distance reached. The client's score is the most distant point along the top of the box that the fingertips contact. If the client's knees are flexed or motion is jerky or bouncing, do not count the score. Administer two trials and record the maximum score to the nearest 0.5 cm. Table 10.4 presents age–gender norms for this test.

V Sit-and-Reach Test

The V sit-and-reach, also known as the YMCA sit-and-reach test, uses a yardstick instead of a box. Secure the yardstick to the floor by placing tape (12 in. long) at a right angle to the 15 in. (38 cm) mark on the yardstick. The client sits, straddling the yardstick, with the knees extended (but not locked) and legs spread 12 in. (30.5 cm) apart. The heels of the feet touch the tape at the 15 in. mark. Instruct the client to reach forward slowly and as far as possible along the yardstick while keeping the two hands parallel (fingertips may overlap) and to hold this position momentarily (~2 sec). Make certain that the knees do not flex and that the client avoids

Table 10.4 Age–Gender Norms for Standard Sit-and-Reach Test[a]

	AGE (YR)					
	15-19	20-29	30-39	40-49	50-59	60-69
Men						
Excellent	≥39	≥40	≥38	≥35	≥35	≥33
Very good	34-38	34-39	33-37	29-34	28-34	25-32
Good	29-33	30-33	28-32	24-28	24-27	20-24
Fair	24-28	25-29	23-27	18-23	16-23	15-19
Needs improvement	≤23	≤24	≤22	≤17	≤15	≤14
Women						
Excellent	≥43	≥41	≥41	≥38	≥39	≥35
Very good	38-42	37-40	36-40	34-37	33-38	31-34
Good	34-37	33-36	32-35	30-33	30-32	27-30
Fair	29-33	28-32	27-31	25-29	25-29	23-26
Needs improvement	≤28	≤27	≤26	≤24	≤24	≤22

[a]Distance measured in centimeters using a sit-and-reach box with the zero point at 26 cm. If using a box with the zero point at 23 cm, subtract 3 cm from each value in this table.

The Canadian Physical Activity, Fitness & Lifestyle Approach: CSEP-Health & Fitness Program's Health-Related Appraisal and Counselling Strategy, 3rd Edition © 2003. Reprinted with permission of the Canadian Society for Exercise Physiology.

leading with one hand. The score (in centimeters or inches) is the most distant point on the yardstick contacted by the fingertips. Table 10.5 presents percentile ranks for the V sit-and-reach test.

Modified Sit-and-Reach Test

To account for a potential bias due to limb-length differences (i.e., individuals who have short legs relative to the trunk and arms may have an advantage when performing the standard sit-and-reach test),

Hoeger (1989) developed a modified sit-and-reach test that takes into account the distance between the end of the fingers and the sit-and-reach box and uses the finger-to-box distance as the relative zero point. This test uses a 12 in. (30.5 cm) sit-and-reach box (see figure 10.4). The client sits on the floor with buttocks, shoulders, and head in contact with the wall; extends the knees; and places the soles of the feet against the box. A yardstick is placed on top of the box with the zero end toward the client. Keep-

Table 10.5 Percentile Ranks for the V Sit-and-Reach Test*

Percentile rank	AGE (YR)											
	18-25		26-35		36-45		46-55		56-65		>65	
	M	F	M	F	M	F	M	F	M	F	M	F
90	22	24	21	23	21	22	19	21	17	20	17	20
80	20	22	19	21	19	21	17	20	15	19	15	18
70	19	21	17	20	17	19	15	18	13	17	13	17
60	18	20	17	20	16	18	14	17	13	16	12	17
50	17	19	15	19	15	17	13	16	11	15	10	15
40	15	18	14	17	13	16	11	14	9	14	9	14
30	14	17	13	16	13	15	10	14	9	13	8	13
20	13	16	11	15	11	14	9	12	7	11	7	11
10	11	14	9	13	7	12	6	10	5	9	4	9

*Sit-and-reach scores measured in inches.

Data from YMCA of the USA, 2000, YMCA fitness testing and assessment manual, 4th ed. (Champaign, IL: Human Kinetics).

ing the head and shoulders in contact with the wall, the client reaches forward with one hand on top of the other, and the yardstick is positioned so that it touches the fingertips. This procedure establishes the relative zero point for each client. As you firmly hold the yardstick in place, the client reaches forward slowly, sliding the fingers along the top of the yardstick. The score (in inches) is the most distant point on the yardstick contacted by the fingertips. Table 10.6 provides age–gender percentile norms for the modified sit-and-reach test.

Research comparing the standard and modified sit-and-reach test scores indicated that individuals with proportionally longer arms than legs (lower finger-to-box distance) had significantly better scores on the standard sit-and-reach test than those with moderate or high finger-to-box distances; in contrast, the modified sit-and-reach test scores did not differ significantly among the three groups (Hoeger et al. 1990; Hoeger and Hopkins 1992). However, Minkler and Patterson (1994) reported that the modified sit-and-reach test was only

Table 10.6   Percentile Ranks for the Modified Sit-and-Reach Test*

Percentile rank	WOMEN			MEN		
	≤35 yr	36-49 yr	≥50 yr	≤35 yr	36-49 yr	≥50 yr
99	19.8	19.8	17.2	24.7	18.9	16.2
95	18.7	19.2	15.7	19.5	18.2	15.8
90	17.9	17.4	15.0	17.9	16.1	15.0
80	16.7	16.2	14.2	17.0	14.6	13.3
70	16.2	15.2	13.6	15.8	13.9	12.3
60	15.8	14.5	12.3	15.0	13.4	11.5
50	14.8	13.5	11.1	14.4	12.6	10.2
40	14.5	12.8	10.1	13.5	11.6	9.7
30	13.7	12.2	9.2	13.0	10.8	9.3
20	12.6	11.0	8.3	11.6	9.9	8.8
10	10.1	9.7	7.5	9.2	8.3	7.8
5	8.1	8.5	3.7	7.9	7.0	7.2
1	2.6	2.0	1.5	7.0	5.1	4.0

*Sit-and-reach scores measured to the nearest 0.25 in.

From W.W.K. Haeger, 1989, *Lifetime physical fitness & wellness* (Englewood, CO: Morton Publishing Co.).

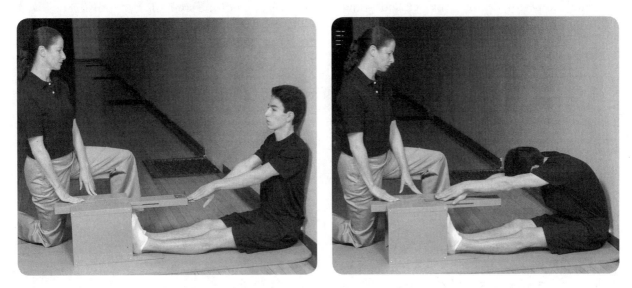

Figure 10.4   Modified sit-and-reach test.

moderately related to criterion measures of hamstring flexibility for women ($r = 0.66$) and men ($r = 0.75$) and poorly related to low back flexibility of women ($r = 0.25$) and men ($r = 0.40$). Similarly, Hui and colleagues (1999) compared the criterion-related validity of the standard and modified sit-and-reach tests and concluded that both tests were moderately valid measures of hamstring flexibility but poor measures of low back flexibility. Consequently, it appears that the validity of the modified sit-and-reach test is no better than that of the standard sit-and-reach test for assessing flexibility of the low back and hamstring muscle groups.

Back-Saver Sit-and-Reach Test

The standard, modified, and V sit-and-reach tests require the client to stretch the hamstring muscles of both legs simultaneously, causing some discomfort when the anterior portions of the vertebrae are compressed during the stretch. The back-saver sit-and-reach test was devised to relieve some of this discomfort by measuring the flexibility of the hamstring muscles one leg at a time. Instruct your client to place the sole of the foot of the extended (tested) leg against the edge of the sit-and-reach box and to flex the untested leg, placing the sole of that foot flat on the floor 2 to 3 in. (5 to 8 cm) to the side of the extended (tested) knee (see figure 10.5). Then follow the instructions for the standard sit-and-reach test to determine your client's flexibility score for each leg. Research suggests that the validity of this test ($r = 0.39$ to 0.71) is similar to that of the standard sit-and-reach test ($r = 0.46$ to 0.74) for assessing hamstring flexibility of men and women

(Hui and Yuen 2000; Jones et al. 1998). Norms for this test are available elsewhere (see Cooper Institute for Aerobics Research 1992).

Modified Back-Saver Sit-and-Reach Test

While performing the back-saver sit-and-reach test, some participants may complain about the uncomfortable position of the untested leg. Hui and Yuen (2000), therefore, modified this test by having the client perform a single-leg sit-and-reach on a 12 in. (30.5 cm) bench (see figure 10.6). Instruct the client to place the untested leg on the floor with the knee flexed at a 90° angle. Align the sole of the foot of the tested leg with the 50 cm mark on the meter rule. Then follow the instructions for the standard sit-and-reach test to determine your client's hamstring flexibility for each leg. Hui and Yuen (2000) reported that the validity of this test ($r = 0.50$ to 0.67) for assessing hamstring flexibility was similar to that of the standard ($r = 0.46$ to 0.53) and V ($r = 0.44$ to 0.63) sit-and-reach tests. The modified back-saver test, however, was rated as the most comfortable compared to the other test protocols. Norms for this test have not yet been established.

Skin Distraction Test

The modified Schober test (Mcrae and Wright 1969) or the simplified skin distraction test (Van Adrichem and van der Korst 1973) is useful in assessing low back flexibility. These field tests are reliable and have good agreement with radiographic measurements of spinal flexion and extension (Williams et al. 1993a). For the simplified skin distraction test,

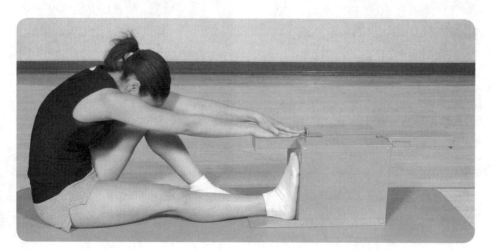

Figure 10.5 Back-saver sit-and-reach test.

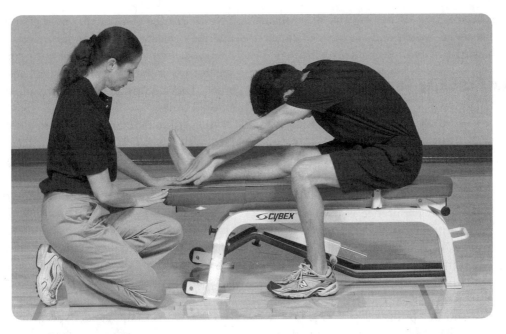

Figure 10.6 Modified back-saver sit-and-reach test.

place a 0 cm mark on the midline of the lumbar spine at the intersection of a horizontal line connecting the left and right posterior superior iliac spines while the client is standing erect. Place a second mark 15 cm (5.9 in.) superior to the 0 cm mark (see figure 10.7). As the client flexes the lumbar spine, these marks move away from each other; use an anthropometric tape measure to measure the new distance between the two marks. The lumbar flexion score is the difference between this measurement and the initial length between the skin markings (15 cm). In a group of 15 to 18 yr old subjects, the simplified skin distraction scores averaged 6.7 ± 1.0 cm in males and 5.8 ± 0.9 cm in females. However, normal values for other age groups are not yet available. You can also use this technique to measure lumbar spinal extension (simplified skin attraction test) by having the client

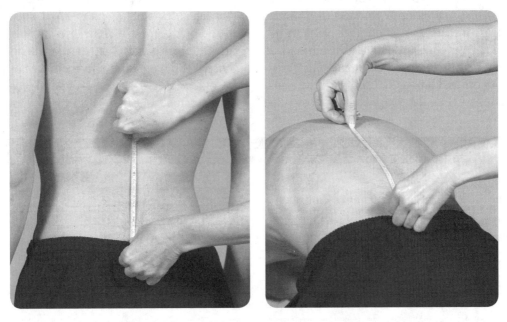

Figure 10.7 Measuring lumbosacral flexion using the simplified skin distraction test.

extend backward and measuring the difference between the initial length and the new distance between the superior and inferior skin markings.

Lumbar Stability Tests

Lumbar instability increases the risk of developing low back pain. The primary muscle groups responsible for stabilizing the lumbar spine are the trunk extensors (erector spinae), trunk flexors (rectus abdominis and abdominal oblique muscles), and lateral flexors (quadratus lumborum). Research indicates that muscle endurance is more protective than muscle strength for reducing low back injury (McGill 2001). To evaluate the balance in the isometric endurance capabilities of these muscle groups in healthy individuals, McGill, Childs, and Liebenson (1999) used three tests: trunk extension, trunk flexion, and side bridge.

To measure the isometric endurance of the trunk extensors, have your client lie prone with the lower body secured (use straps) to the test bed at the ankles, knees, and hips and with the upper body extended over the edge of the bed. The test bed should be approximately 25 cm (10 in.) above the surface of the floor. During the test, the client holds the upper arms across the chest, with the hands resting on the opposite shoulders. Instruct your client to assume and maintain a horizontal position above the floor for as long as possible. Use a stopwatch to record in seconds the time from which the client assumes the horizontal position until the time at which the upper body contacts the floor.

To measure the isometric endurance of the trunk flexors, have your client sit on a test bench with a movable back support set at a 60° angle. The client flexes the knees and hips to 90° and folds the arms across the chest. Use toe straps to secure the cli-

ent's feet to the test bench. Instruct your client to maintain this body position for as long as possible after you lower or remove the back support. End the test when the client's trunk falls below the 60° angle. Use a stopwatch to record in seconds the elapsed time.

To measure the isometric endurance of the lateral flexors, use the side bridge. Ask your client to assume a side-lying position on a mat, with his legs extended. Place the top foot in front of the lower foot for support. Instruct your client to lift his hips off the mat while supporting his body in a straight line on one elbow and the feet for as long as possible. He should hold the uninvolved arm across the chest. End the test when his hips return to the mat. Use a stopwatch to record in seconds the elapsed time. Administer this test for both the right and left sides of the body.

Table 10.7 contains gender-specific reference data for the isometric endurance of the trunk extensor, trunk flexor, and lateral flexor muscle groups. You can use these reference values to evaluate lumbar stability and to set training goals for your clients.

FLEXIBILITY TESTING OF OLDER ADULTS

Flexibility is an important component of the functional fitness of older individuals. Older adults need to perform activities of daily living (ADL) safely in order to maintain their functional independence as they age. Flexibility facilitates ADL such as getting in and out of a car or chair, dressing, and bathing. The Senior Fitness Test, developed by Rikli and Jones (2001), includes two measures of flexibility for older adults—the chair sit-and-reach and the back scratch tests.

Table 10.7 Reference Values for Isometric Lumbar Stabilization Tests in Healthy Adults

Test item	MEN		WOMEN	
	Endurance time (sec)	Ratio*	Endurance time (sec)	Ratio*
Trunk extension	146	1.00	189	1.00
Trunk flexion	144	0.99	149	0.79
Side bridge (right)	94	0.64	72	0.38
Side bridge (left)	97	0.66	77	0.40

*Ratio is calculated by dividing endurance time of each item by trunk extension endurance time.

Data from S.M. McGill, A. Childs, and D.C. Lieberson, 1999, "Endurance times for low back stabilization exercises: Clinical targets for testing and training from a normal database," *Archives of Physical Medicine and Rehabilitation* 80: 941-944.

Chair Sit-and-Reach Test
(Rikli and Jones 2001)

Many older individuals have difficulty performing sit-and-reach tests because functional limitations (e.g., low back pain and poor ROM) prevent them from getting down to and up from the floor. Jones and colleagues (1998) devised a chair sit-and-reach test that is similar to the back-saver protocol (see figure 10.6) in that it tests only one leg, thereby reducing stress on the spine and lower back. Compared to standard ($r = 0.71$ to 0.74) and back-saver ($r = 0.70$ to 0.71) sit-and-reach protocols, the chair test yielded similar criterion-related validity coefficients ($r = 0.76$ to 0.81) as a measure of hamstring flexibility in older (>60 yr) men and women. Table 10.8 presents age–gender norms for the chair sit-and-reach test.

Purpose: Assess lower body (hamstring) flexibility.

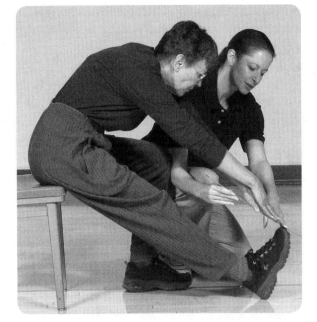

Figure 10.8 Chair sit-and-reach test.

Table 10.8 Chair Sit-and-Reach Test Norms*

Percentile rank	60-64 YR F	60-64 YR M	65-69 YR F	65-69 YR M	70-74 YR F	70-74 YR M	75-79 YR F	75-79 YR M	80-84 YR F	80-84 YR M	85-89 YR F	85-89 YR M	90-94 YR F	90-94 YR M
95	8.7	8.5	7.9	7.5	7.5	7.5	7.4	6.6	6.6	6.2	6.0	4.5	4.9	3.5
90	7.2	6.7	6.6	5.9	6.1	5.8	6.1	4.9	5.2	4.4	4.6	3.0	3.4	1.9
85	6.3	5.6	5.7	4.8	5.2	4.7	5.2	3.8	4.3	3.2	3.7	2.0	2.5	0.9
80	5.5	4.6	5.0	3.9	4.5	3.8	4.4	2.8	3.6	2.2	3.0	1.1	1.7	0.0
75	4.8	3.8	4.4	3.1	3.9	3.0	3.7	2.0	3.0	1.4	2.4	0.4	1.0	−0.7
70	4.2	3.1	3.9	2.4	3.3	2.4	3.2	1.3	2.4	0.6	1.8	−0.2	0.4	−1.4
65	3.7	2.5	3.4	1.8	2.8	1.8	2.7	0.7	1.9	0.0	1.3	−0.8	−0.1	−1.9
60	3.1	1.8	2.9	1.1	2.3	1.1	2.1	0.1	1.4	−0.8	0.8	−1.3	−0.7	−2.5
55	2.6	1.2	2.5	0.6	1.9	0.6	1.7	−0.5	1.0	−1.4	0.4	−1.9	−1.2	−3.0
50	2.1	0.6	2.0	0.0	1.4	0.0	1.2	−1.1	0.5	−2.0	−0.1	−2.4	−1.7	−3.6
45	1.6	0.0	1.5	−0.6	0.9	−0.6	0.7	−1.7	0.0	−2.6	−0.6	−2.9	−2.2	−4.2
40	1.1	−0.6	1.1	−1.1	0.5	−1.2	0.2	−2.3	−0.4	−3.2	−1.0	−3.5	−2.7	−4.7
35	0.5	−1.3	0.6	−1.8	0.0	−1.8	−0.3	−2.9	−0.9	−4.0	−1.5	−4.0	−3.3	−5.3
30	0.0	−1.9	0.1	−2.4	−0.5	−2.4	−0.8	−3.5	−1.4	−4.6	−2.0	−4.6	−3.8	−5.8
25	−0.6	−2.6	−0.4	−3.1	−1.1	−3.1	−1.3	−4.2	−2.0	−5.3	−2.6	−5.3	−4.4	−6.5
20	−1.3	−3.4	−1.0	−3.9	−1.7	−3.9	−2.0	−5.0	−2.6	−6.2	−3.2	−5.9	−5.1	−7.2
15	−2.1	−4.4	−1.7	−4.8	−2.4	−4.8	−2.8	−6.0	−3.3	−7.2	−3.9	−6.8	−5.9	−8.1
10	−3.0	−5.5	−2.6	−5.9	−3.3	−5.9	−3.7	−7.1	−4.2	−8.4	−4.8	−7.8	−6.8	−9.1
5	−4.0	−7.3	−3.9	−7.5	−4.7	−7.6	−5.0	−8.8	−5.0	−10.2	−6.3	−9.3	−7.9	−10.7

*Score is measured in inches.

F = females; M = males.

To convert inches to centimeters, multiply value in table by 2.54.

Adapted, by permission, from R. Rikli and C. Jones, 2001, *Senior fitness test manual* (Champaign, IL: Human Kinetics), 129.

Application: A measure of the ability to perform ADL such as climbing stairs and getting in and out of a car, chair, or bathtub.

Equipment: You will need a folding chair that has a seat height of 17 in. (43 cm) and that will not tip forward, as well as an 18 in. (46 cm or half a yardstick) ruler.

Test procedures: Place the folding chair against a wall for stability and have your client sit on the front edge of the seat. The client extends the leg being tested in front of the hip, with the heel on the floor and the ankle dorsiflexed approximately 90°. The client flexes the untested leg so that the sole of the foot is flat on the floor about 6 to 12 in. (15-30.5 cm) to the side of the body's midline. With the extended leg as straight as possible and the hands on top of each other (palms down), the client slowly bends forward at the hip joint, keeping the spine as straight as possible and the head in normal alignment (not tucked) with the spine (see figure 10.8). The client reaches down the extended leg, trying to touch the toes, and holds this position for 2 sec. Place the ruler parallel to your client's lower leg and administer two practice trials followed by two test trials.

Scoring: The middle of the big toe (medial aspect) at the end of the shoe represents a zero score. Reaches short of the toes are recorded as minus scores; reaches beyond the toes are recorded as plus scores. Record the best score to the nearest half inch and compare it to the norms in table 10.8.

Back Scratch Test (Rikli and Jones 2001)

Limited ROM in the upper body, especially in the shoulder joints, may cause painful movement and increase the chance of injury during performance of common tasks such as putting on and taking off clothes. The back scratch test appears to have good construct validity, as evidenced by its ability to detect declines in shoulder flexibility across age groups (60-90 yr) (Rikli and Jones 1999). Table 10.9 presents age–gender norms for the back scratch test.

Purpose: Assess upper body (shoulder joint) flexibility.

Application: A measure of the ability to perform ADL such as combing hair, dressing, and reaching for a seat belt.

Equipment: You will need an 18 in. (46 cm) ruler.

Test procedures: Ask your client to reach, with the preferred hand (palm down and fingers extended), over the shoulder and down the back while reaching around and up the middle of the back with the other hand (palm up and fingers extended) (see figure 10.9). Allow the client to choose the best, or preferred, hand through trial and error. Administer two practice trials followed by two test trials.

Scoring: Use the ruler to measure the overlap (plus score) or gap (minus score) between the middle fingers of each hand. If the fingers just touch each other, record a zero. Record the best score to the nearest half inch and compare this value to the norms in table 10.9.

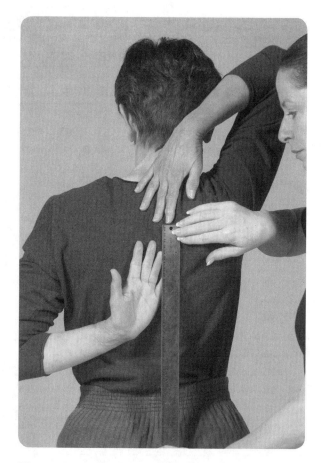

Figure 10.9 Back scratch test.

Table 10.9　Back Scratch Test Norms*

Percentile rank	60-64 YR		65-69 YR		70-74 YR		75-79 YR		80-84 YR		85-89 YR		90-94 YR	
	F	M	F	M	F	M	F	M	F	M	F	M	F	M
95	5.0	4.5	4.9	3.9	4.5	3.5	4.5	2.8	4.3	3.2	3.5	1.7	3.9	0.7
90	3.8	2.7	3.5	2.2	3.2	1.8	3.1	0.9	2.8	1.2	1.9	–0.1	2.2	–1.1
85	2.9	1.6	2.6	1.0	2.3	0.6	2.2	–0.3	1.8	–0.1	0.8	–1.2	0.9	–2.2
80	2.2	0.6	1.9	0.0	1.5	–0.4	1.3	–1.3	0.9	–1.2	–0.1	–2.2	–0.1	–3.2
75	1.6	–0.2	1.3	–0.8	0.8	–1.2	0.6	–2.2	0.2	–2.1	–0.9	–3.0	–1.0	–4.0
70	1.1	–0.9	0.7	–1.6	0.3	–2.0	0.0	–2.9	–0.4	–2.9	–1.6	–3.7	–1.8	–4.7
65	0.7	–1.5	0.2	–2.2	–0.2	–2.6	–0.5	–3.6	–1.0	–3.6	–2.1	–4.3	–2.5	–5.3
60	0.2	–2.2	–0.3	–2.9	–0.8	–3.3	–1.1	–4.3	–1.6	–4.3	–2.8	–5.0	–3.2	–6.0
55	–0.2	–2.8	–0.7	–3.5	–1.2	–3.9	–1.6	–4.9	–2.1	–5.0	–3.3	–5.6	–3.8	–6.6
50	–0.7	–3.4	–1.2	–4.1	–1.7	–4.5	–2.1	–5.6	–2.6	–5.7	–3.9	–6.2	–4.5	–7.2
45	–1.2	–4.0	–1.7	–4.7	–2.2	–5.1	–2.6	–6.3	–3.1	–6.4	–4.5	–6.8	–5.2	–7.8
40	–1.6	–4.6	–2.1	–5.3	–2.6	–5.7	–3.1	–6.9	–3.7	–7.1	–5.0	–7.4	–5.8	–8.4
35	–2.1	–5.3	–2.6	–6.0	–3.2	–6.4	–3.7	–7.6	–4.2	–7.8	–5.7	–8.1	–6.5	–9.1
30	–2.5	–5.9	–3.1	–6.6	–3.7	–7.0	–4.2	–8.3	–4.8	–8.5	–6.2	–8.7	–7.2	–9.7
25	–3.0	–6.6	–3.7	–7.4	–4.2	–7.8	–4.8	–9.0	–5.4	–9.3	–6.9	–9.4	–8.0	–10.4
20	–3.6	–7.4	–4.3	–8.2	–4.9	–8.6	–5.5	–9.9	–6.1	–10.2	–7.7	–10.2	–8.9	–11.2
15	–4.3	–8.4	–5.0	–9.2	–5.7	–9.6	–6.4	–10.9	–7.0	–11.3	–8.6	–11.2	–9.9	–12.2
10	–5.2	–9.5	–5.9	–10.4	–6.6	–10.8	–7.3	–12.1	–8.0	–12.6	–9.7	–12.3	–11.2	–13.3
5	–6.4	–11.3	–7.3	–12.1	–7.9	–12.5	–8.8	–14.0	–9.5	–14.6	–11.3	–14.1	–13.0	–15.1

*Score is measured in inches.

F = females; M = males.

To convert inches to centimeters, multiply value in table by 2.54.

Adapted, by permission, from R. Rikli and C. Jones, 2001, *Senior fitness test manual* (Champaign, IL: Human Kinetics), 130.

Sources for Equipment

Product	Supplier's address
Flexometer Inclinometer Sit-and-reach box Universal goniometer	Country Technology Inc. Phone: (608) 735-4718 www.fitnessmart.com

KEY POINTS

- Static flexibility is a measure of the total ROM at the joint.
- Dynamic flexibility is a measure of the rate of torque or resistance developed during movement through the ROM.
- Flexibility is highly joint specific, and the ROM depends, in part, on the structure of the joint.
- Lack of physical activity is a major cause of inflexibility.
- A universal goniometer, flexometer, or inclinometer can be used to obtain direct measures of ROM.

- A yardstick and anthropometric tape measure can be used to obtain indirect measures of ROM.
- Sit-and-reach tests measure flexibility of the hamstrings but not low back flexibility.
- The chair sit-and-reach and the back scratch tests can be used to assess flexibility of older adults.
- Lumbar instability increases risk of developing low back pain.
- Muscle endurance is more protective than muscle strength for reducing low back injury.

KEY TERMS

Learn the definition for each of the following key terms. Definitions of terms can be found in the glossary on page 411.

ankylosis	goniometer	static stretching
biaxial joints	hypermobility	stress relaxation
contracture	inclinometer	triaxial joints
dynamic flexibility	joint laxity	uniaxial joints
elastic deformation	nonaxial joints	viscoelastic properties
flexibility	range of motion (ROM)	viscous deformation
flexometer	static flexibility	

REVIEW QUESTIONS

In addition to being able to define each of the key terms, test your knowledge and understanding of the material by answering the following review questions.

1. Why are flexibility tests included in most health-related fitness test batteries?

2. Identify and explain how morphological factors affect range of joint motion.

3. How do age, gender, and physical activity (or lack thereof) affect flexibility?

4. Identify and briefly describe three direct methods for measuring static flexibility.

5. Do sit-and-reach tests yield valid measures of hamstring and low back flexibility? Explain.

6. Is the modified sit-and-reach test more valid than the standard sit-and-reach test for assessing hamstring and low back flexibility?

7. Describe three tests that can be used to evaluate lumbar stability.

8. Describe two tests that indirectly measure the flexibility of older adults.

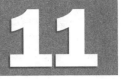

Designing Programs for Flexibility and Low Back Care

KEY QUESTIONS

- How do training principles apply to the design of flexibility training programs?
- Are all methods of stretching safe and effective for improving flexibility?
- What are the recommended guidelines for designing a stretching program?
- How do you individualize flexibility programs to meet the goals and abilities of each client?
- How often does a client need to exercise to improve flexibility?
- Is there an optimal combination of stretch duration and repetitions for improving range of motion?
- Can low back syndrome be prevented?
- What exercises are recommended for low back care?

Flexibility training is a systematic program of stretching exercises designed to progressively increase the range of motion (ROM) of joints over time. It is well documented that stretching improves flexibility and ROM. Generic exercise prescriptions for improving flexibility are not recommended; flexibility programs should be individualized to address the needs, abilities, and physical activity interests of

each client. Your client's flexibility assessment (see chapter 10) can help you focus on joints and muscle groups needing improvement. Lifestyle assessments (see appendix A.5, p. 326) can help identify muscle groups and body parts with limited joint mobility caused by habitual body postures (e.g., sitting at a desk for long times at work) or repetitive movement patterns during exercise (e.g., jogging).

This chapter presents guidelines for designing flexibility programs. Basic training principles are applied to developing flexibility programs. The chapter compares various methods of stretching and addresses questions about the flexibility exercise prescription. In addition, it presents approaches and recommendations for designing low back care programs.

TRAINING PRINCIPLES

The principles of overload, specificity, progression, and interindividual variability (see chapter 3, p. 47) apply to flexibility programs. Flexibility is joint specific (Cotten 1972; Harris 1969; Munroe and Romance 1975); to increase the ROM of a particular joint, select exercises that stretch the appropriate muscle groups (i.e., apply the specificity principle). Review your anatomy and kinesiology, particularly muscle origins and insertions, joint structures and functions, and agonist–antagonist muscle pairs. For excellent anatomical illustrations of muscles stretched during the performance of a variety of flexibility exercises, see Nelson and Kokkonen (2007). To improve ROM at a joint, your client must overload the muscle group by stretching the muscles beyond their normal resting length but not beyond the pain-free ROM. The pain-free ROM varies among individuals (interindividual variability principle), depending on their stretch tolerance (the amount of resistive force to stretch within target muscles that a person can tolerate before experiencing pain) and their perception of stretch and pain (Magnusson 1998; Shrier and Gossal 2000). Periodically your client will need to increase the total time of stretching by increasing the duration or number of repetitions of each stretch in order to ensure the overload required for further ROM improvements (progression principle).

STRETCHING METHODS

Traditionally, three stretching methods have been used to improve ROM: ballistic, slow static, and proprioceptive neuromuscular facilitation. **Ballistic stretching** uses jerky, bouncing movements to lengthen the target muscle, whereas **static stretching** uses slow, sustained muscle lengthening to increase ROM. Commonly used **proprioceptive neuromuscular facilitation (PNF)** stretching techniques involve maximal or submaximal contractions (isometric or dynamic) of target (agonist) and opposing (antagonist) muscle groups followed by passive stretching of the target muscles (Chalmers 2004). Stretching techniques are classified as active, passive, or active-assisted. In **active stretching**, the client moves the body part without external assistance (i.e., voluntarily contracts the muscle). In **passive stretching**, the client relaxes the target muscle group as the body part is moved by an assistant (e.g., partner, personal trainer, physical therapist, or athletic trainer). In **active-assisted stretching**, the client moves the body part to the end of its active ROM and the assistant then moves the body part beyond its active ROM. Table 11.1 summarizes the advantages and disadvantages of stretching methods. The following questions address issues that you should consider when selecting a stretching method for your client's flexibility program.

■ *Which method of stretching is best for improving ROM?*

All three stretching methods (ballistic, slow static, and PNF) produce acute and chronic gains in flexibility and ROM at the knee, hip, trunk, shoulder, and ankle joints (Thacker et al. 2004; Mahieu et al. 2007). Although slow static stretching is considered safer than ballistic or PNF stretching and is easier to perform because it does not require special equipment or an assistant, each stretching method has its proponents. Studies generally indicate that PNF stretching improves ROM more effectively than either slow static or ballistic stretching (Anderson and Burke 1991; Etnyre and Abraham 1986; Holt, Travis, and Okita 1970; Shrier and Gossal 2000; Wallin et al. 1985), but this finding has not been consistent (Thacker et al. 2004). Proprioceptive neuromuscular facilitation stretching is frequently used in sport and rehabilitation settings.

As mentioned in chapter 10, Mahieu and associates (2007) reported that both static and ballistic stretching programs increase ankle dorsiflexion ROM; but each mode of stretching has different effects on passive resistive torque and tendon stiff-

Table 11.1 Comparison of Stretching Techniques

Factor	Ballistic	Slow static	PNF[a]
Risk of injury	High	Low	Medium
Degree of pain	Medium	Low	High
Resistance to stretch	High	Low	Medium
Practicality (time and assistance needed)	Good	Excellent	Poor
Efficiency (energy consumption)	Poor	Excellent	Poor
Effective for increasing ROM[b]	Good	Good	Excellent

[a]Proprioceptive neuromuscular facilitation.

[b]Range of motion.

ness. Static stretching significantly reduced passive resistive torque of the calf muscles but had no effect on Achilles tendon stiffness, whereas ballistic stretching had the reverse effect—Achilles tendon stiffness decreased, but passive resistive torque of the plantar flexors was unchanged. These findings suggest that both types of stretching should be considered for training and rehabilitation programs. Therefore, choose a method that meets your client's specific abilities (e.g., stretch tolerance and pain threshold), needs, and long-term goals.

▪ *What are some of the commonly used PNF stretching techniques and how are they performed?*

Various PNF techniques use different combinations of dynamic (concentric and eccentric) and isometric contraction of target and opposing muscle groups. The **contract-relax (CR)** and **contract-relax agonist contract (CRAC)** techniques are common PNF procedures. In the CR technique, your client first isometrically contracts the target muscle group; this is immediately followed by slow, passive stretching of the target muscle group. The first two steps of the CRAC and CR techniques are identical except that the client assists the CRAC stretching phase by actively contracting the opposing muscle group. For example, to stretch the pectoral muscles, the client sits on the floor and extends the arms horizontally. The client isometrically contracts the pectoral muscles as the partner offers resistance to horizontal flexion. Following the isometric contraction, the partner slowly stretches the pectorals as the client actively contracts the horizontal extensors in the upper back (see figure 11.1). For detailed explanations and illustrations of PNF and facilitated stretching techniques, see Alter (2004) and McAtee and Charland (2007).

▪ *What are the general recommendations for performing PNF stretches?*

The following steps are recommended for performing PNF stretches to increase ROM:

- Stretch the target muscle group by moving the joint to the end of its ROM.
- Isometrically contract the stretched muscle group against an immovable resistance (such as a partner or wall) for 5 to 10 sec.
- Relax the target muscle group as you stretch it actively or passively (with a partner) to a new point of limitation.

- For the CRAC technique, contract the opposing muscle group submaximally for 5 or 6 sec to facilitate further stretching of the target muscle group.

▪ *Which is best—the CR or CRAC procedure?*

It has been reported that the CRAC technique improves ROM more effectively (Alter 2004; Moore and Hutton 1980). Moore and Hutton compared the relative levels of muscle relaxation during CR and CRAC stretching. Contract-relax agonist contract produced larger gains in hip flexion, but it also produced greater electromyographic activity in the hamstring muscle group and was ranked as more uncomfortable than CR in terms of perceived pain. Therefore, you need to consider your client's stretch tolerance when selecting a PNF stretching technique.

▪ *Is PNF stretching always superior to slow static stretching?*

A major disadvantage of the PNF technique is that most of the exercises cannot be performed alone. An assistant is needed to resist movement during the isometric contraction phase and to apply external force during the stretching phase. Overstretching may cause injury, especially if the assistant has not been carefully trained in the correct PNF procedures. Assisted stretching procedures such as PNF should be carefully performed by trained clients or exercise professionals who understand the correct procedures and the risks of incorrect stretching (Knudson, Magnusson, and McHugh 2000).

▪ *Why is slow static stretching safer than ballistic stretching?*

Many exercise professionals recommend slow static stretching over ballistic stretching because there is less chance of injury and muscle soreness resulting from jerky, rapid movements. Mahieu and associates (2007) observed that a 6 wk slow static stretching program produced a significant increase in ankle dorsiflexion ROM resulting from a significant decrease in passive resistive torque of the calf muscles. Ballistic stretching, however, had no effect on passive resistance but produced a significant decrease in the stiffness of the Achilles tendon. Ballistic stretching uses relatively fast bouncing motions to produce stretch. The momentum of the moving body segment rather than external force

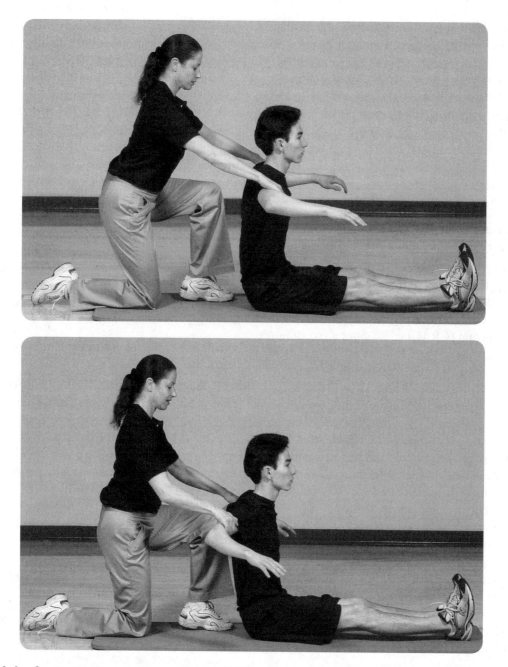

Figure 11.1 Contract-relax agonist contract (CRAC) proprioceptive neuromuscular facilitation stretching technique for the shoulder horizontal flexors.

pushes the joint beyond its present ROM. This technique appears counterproductive for increasing muscle relaxation and stretch. During the movement, the muscle spindles signal changes in both muscle length and contraction speed. The spindle responds more (due to a lower threshold) to the speed of the movement than to the length or position of the muscle. In fact, muscle spindle activity is directly proportional to the speed of movement. Thus, ballistic stretching evokes the stretch reflex,

producing more contraction and resistance to stretch in the target muscle group. Also, the muscle has viscous properties. The viscous material resists elongation more when the stretch is applied rapidly (Taylor et al. 1990). Therefore, ballistic stretching places greater strain on the muscle and may cause microscopic tearing of muscle fibers and connective tissues.

In slow static stretching, your client stretches the target muscle group when the joint is at the end of its

ROM. While maintaining this lengthened position, the client slowly applies torque to the target muscle group to stretch it further. Because the dynamic portion of the muscle spindle rapidly adapts to the lengthened position, spindle discharge decreases. This decrease lessens the reflex contraction of the target muscle group and allows the muscle to relax and be stretched even further. The force needed to lengthen a muscle is affected by the rate of stretching and by the duration over which the target muscle group is held at a specific length (Taylor et al. 1990). Resistance to elongation is greater for rapid (e.g., ballistic) stretching than for slow static stretching. Also, the resistance produced by the viscous properties of the muscle decreases over time as the target muscle is held at its stretched length. The resulting stress relaxation allows further elongation of the target muscle group (Chalmers 2004).

■ What are the physiological mechanisms underlying the increased ROM produced by the PNF method?

The mechanisms responsible for gains in ROM from PNF stretching are controversial. Two suggested hypotheses are the neurophysiological and the viscoelastic hypotheses (Burke, Culligan, and Holt 2000). Traditionally in the PNF literature, increases in ROM were explained by neurophysiological modifications such as inhibition of the spinal reflexes (e.g., stretch reflex and Golgi tendon organ, or GTO, reflex) in target muscles. These modifications are caused by decreased muscle spindle discharge during slow static stretching (i.e., less spindle activity leads to less reflex contraction and more muscle relaxation) and by increased GTO activity during isometric contraction (i.e., greater GTO activation leads to reflex relaxation). Also, voluntary contraction of opposing muscle groups during CRAC stretching was simply explained by reciprocal inhibition (as the opposing muscle group is voluntarily contracted, the target muscle group is reflexively inhibited).

The neuromuscular mechanisms underlying muscle stretch are extremely complicated and not fully understood. Simple explanations of the role of reciprocal inhibition during muscle stretching are inadequate. For example, recurrent collateral pathways from motor neurons of the opposing muscle group inhibit interneurons that reduce the excitation of alpha motor neurons of the target muscle group, thereby blocking inhibitory input to target muscle groups (Hultborn, Illert, and Santini 1974). In addition, presynaptic inhibition can modify transmission from sensory neurons, and interneurons can receive input from more than one sensory receptor as well as from multiple descending tracts in the central nervous system. For example, the interneuron activated by the sensory signals of GTOs in a target muscle group also receives input from many sensory and descending tracts. This input potentially modifies the simple spinal reflex pathway (Chalmers 2004).

Obviously, neurophysiological mechanisms such as muscle spindle and GTO reflexes do not singularly explain how PNF stretching improves ROM. Therefore, other mechanisms such as changes in the viscoelastic properties of stretched muscle (viscoelastic hypothesis) and the ability to tolerate stretch have been suggested. In light of the viscoelastic changes accompanying slow static stretching, ROM improvements from PNF stretching may also be partly explained by greater elastic deformation (proportional to the tension applied during stretching) and viscous deformation (proportional to the speed at which the tension is applied during stretching), as well as enhanced viscoelastic stress relaxation over time (Burke et al. 2000; Chalmers 2004). In addition, long-term PNF stretching enhances stretch tolerance because of the analgesic effect of stretching. As a result, more force can be applied to the muscle before the individual feels pain (Shrier and Gossal 2000).

■ During PNF stretches, what is the recommended duration of the isometric contraction phase to maximize long-term gains in ROM?

Traditionally, isometric contractions of 5 to 10 sec are recommended for PNF stretching programs; however, there is a lack of research justifying these durations or documenting their continued effectiveness for improving ROM during training. One study (Rowlands, Marginson, and Lee 2003) compared chronic gains in passive flexibility between two CRAC stretching programs with different durations of isometric contraction (5 sec vs. 10 sec). Training consisted of performing three repetitions of two different passive stretching exercises twice per week over 6 wk. Compared to a control group that did not stretch, both training groups experienced significant increases in hip flexion. However, greater gains in hip flexion resulted from 10 sec isometric contraction compared to 5 sec contraction. The authors concluded that the 10 sec isometric contraction allowed more time for changes in viscoelastic properties and therefore allowed greater relaxation of the target muscle group. They suggested that more research is needed comparing different PNF training programs and quantifying the roles of the neurophysiological and viscoelastic mechanisms underlying chronic gains in both active and passive flexibility.

DESIGNING FLEXIBILITY PROGRAMS: EXERCISE PRESCRIPTION

After assessing your client's flexibility, you must identify the joints and muscle groups needing improvement and select an appropriate stretching method and the specific exercises for the exercise prescription. Appendix F.1, "Selected Flexibility Exercises," on page 390 illustrates flexibility exercises for various regions of the body. For additional stretching exercises, see Anderson 1980, Alter 2004, McAtee and Charland 2007, and Nelson and Kokkonen 2007. Follow the guidelines (see "Guidelines for Designing Flexibility Programs" and "Client Guidelines for Stretching Programs" on p. 291) and be sure to address the following questions regarding your client's exercise prescription.

■ *How many exercises should be included in a flexibility program?*

A well-rounded program includes at least one exercise for each of the major muscle groups of the body including the neck, shoulders, upper and lower back, pelvis, hips, and legs. It is especially important to select exercises for problem areas such as the lower back, hips, and posterior thighs and legs. Use the results of the flexibility tests to identify specific muscle groups with relatively poor flexibility, and include more than one exercise for these muscle groups. The workout should take 15 to 30 min depending on the number of exercises to be performed.

■ *Are some stretching exercises safer than others?*

Some stretching exercises are not recommended for flexibility programs because they create excessive stress, thereby increasing your client's chance of musculoskeletal injuries—especially to the knee joints and low back region. Appendix F.2, "Exercise

Do's and Don'ts," page 399, illustrates exercises that are contraindicated for flexibility programs and suggests alternative exercises that you can prescribe to increase the flexibility of specific muscle groups. For detailed analysis of risk factors and options for minimizing risk for certain stretching exercises, see Alter (2004).

■ *What is a safe intensity for stretching exercises?*

The intensity of the exercise for the slow static stretching and PNF stretching exercises should always be below the pain threshold of the individual. Some mild discomfort will occur, especially during the PNF exercises when the target muscle is contracted isometrically. However, the joint should not be stretched beyond its pain-free ROM (American College of Sports Medicine [ACSM] 2010).

■ *How long does each stretch need to be held?*

To date there is a limited amount of research concerning the optimal time that a static stretch should be sustained to improve ROM. In the past, some experts have suggested varying lengths of static stretch, ranging from 10 to 60 sec (Beaulieu 1980). The ACSM (2010) recommends holding the stretched position 15 to 60 sec.

Borms and colleagues (1987) compared the effects of 10, 20, and 30 sec of static stretching on hip flexibility of women engaging in a 10 wk (two sessions a week) static flexibility training program. They reported similar improvements in hip flexibility for all three groups, suggesting that a duration of 10 sec of static stretching is sufficient for improving hip flexibility.

Another study compared the effect of three static stretching durations (15, 30, and 60 sec) on the hip flexibility of men and women with "tight" hamstring muscles (Bandy and Irion 1994). The subjects participated in a 6 wk static flexibility training program, stretching five times a week. The authors noted that 30 and 60 sec of static stretching were more effective than stretching 15 sec for increasing hip flexibility. They observed no significant difference between stretching for 30 sec and for 60 sec, indicating that a 30 sec stretch of the hamstring muscles was as effective as the longer-duration stretch.

Some research suggests that the total stretching time in a workout may be more important than the duration of each stretch (Cipriani, Abel, and Pirrwitz 2003; Roberts and Wilson 1999). Roberts and Wilson (1999) compared the effects of stretching 5 or 15 sec on active and passive ROM in the lower extremity. The treatment groups participated in a static stretching program three times a week for a 5 wk period. The investigators controlled the total amount of time spent stretching (45 sec) by having the 5 sec group perform nine repetitions and the 15 sec group perform three repetitions for each exercise. The improvement in passive ROM was similar for the 5 and 15 sec groups; however, the 15 sec group showed significantly greater improvement in active ROM.

Similarly, Cipriani and colleagues (2003) compared two stretching protocols that controlled for total stretch time (10 sec × 6 reps vs. 30 sec × 2 reps). Stretching was performed twice daily for a total workout duration of 2 min/day for 6 wk. The resulting gains in passive ROM at the hip joint were equal for these two protocols. The findings from these two studies have implications for designing flexibility programs. For clients with a low stretch tolerance, you can prescribe shorter stretch duration (e.g., 10 sec) and more repetitions; for those who can tolerate longer stretch durations (30 sec or more), you can prescribe fewer repetitions.

In light of these findings, you should consider having your clients perform each stretching exercise for a total of 45 sec to 2 min. The combination of duration and repetitions used to reach this recommended total should be individualized to your client's tolerance for the sensation of stretching. For short durations, the stretch should be sustained at least 10 to 15 sec. As flexibility improves, you can progressively overload the target muscle groups by changing either the stretch duration (10-30 sec) or the number of repetitions so that the total time the stretched position is held gradually increases. As your client's stretch tolerance improves, consider increasing the duration and decreasing the number of repetitions of each stretch. Remember that you must gradually increase the total stretching time for each exercise in order to ensure overload and further improvements in ROM.

▪ How many repetitions of each exercise should be performed?

The ACSM (2010) recommends at least four repetitions of each stretching exercise. As flexibility improves during the training program, the number of repetitions of each flexibility exercise may be gradually increased to five to progressively overload the muscle group.

▪ How often should flexibility exercises be performed?

"Physical Activity Guidelines for Americans" states that all adults should stretch to maintain flexibility for physical activity and performance of activities for daily living (U.S. Department of Health and Human Services 2008). Flexibility exercises should be performed a minimum of 2 or 3 days a week for at least 10 min (ACSM 2010) but preferably daily (Knudson et al. 2000). Flexibility exercises should be performed after moderate or vigorous physical activity and are often an integral part of the cool-down segments of aerobic exercise and resistance training workouts.

▪ Does stretching prevent injury and improve physical performance?

For years clinicians, coaches, and exercise practitioners have recommended stretching as part of the warm-up. Because an active warm-up prevents injury and because stretching is commonly included in the warm-up, one could easily but mistakenly conclude that stretching prevents injury. However, there is a lack of scientific evidence supporting the long-held belief that stretching before physical activity prevents injury (Pope et al. 2000; Shrier 1999; Thacker et al. 2004; Weldon and Hill 2003). Theories based on research data and clinical observations have been proposed to explain why stretching does not reduce the risk of injury:

- ▪ The ability of muscles to absorb energy is not related to flexibility. No scientific evidence supports the idea that more compliant (i.e., more flexible) muscles and connective tissues have a greater ability to absorb energy and are thus less likely to sustain injury (Shrier 1999).
- ▪ Even mild stretching can cause damage at the cellular level (Shrier 2000).
- ▪ The analgesic effect of stretching increases pain tolerance (Shrier and Gossal 2000).

Experts agree that there is insufficient evidence to endorse routine stretching for preventing injuries among competitive and recreational athletes (Herbert and Gabriel 2002; Thacker et al. 2004). To resolve this issue, additional research, particularly well-controlled randomized trials, is needed.

Also, some evidence suggests that stretching may be detrimental to strength performance. Several studies reported strength reductions after only 30 to 60 sec of stretching (Brandenburg 2006; Kay and Blazevich 2008; Knudson and Noffal 2005). Also, intense, prolonged stretching may create a strength deficit for up to 1 hr afterward (Fowles, Sales, and MacDougall 2000). To reach peak tension during contraction, stretched muscles need time to take up the slack in the musculotendinous unit produced by stretching. Therefore, stretching immediately before performance may impair strength and performance, especially when the muscle is not allowed enough time to take up slack (Bracko 2002). Knudson (1999) recommended stretching during the warm-up only for those engaging in activities that require extreme ROM, such as dancing, diving, and gymnastics.

■ Can vibration-aided static stretching increase flexibility?

Preliminary data suggest that vibration may be a promising method for increasing ROM beyond what is obtainable with static stretching. One study compared the effects of vibration-aided static stretching to static stretching alone in highly trained male gymnasts performing a forward split (Sands et al. 2006). The athletes stretched forward and rear legs to a point of discomfort for 10 sec followed by 5 sec of rest. They repeated this four times on each leg for a total stretching duration of 4 min. The experimental group performed this protocol with the vibration device turned on; the control received no vibration. The vibration-aided group showed dramatic increases in forward split flexibility for both legs; in a 4 wk follow-up test, the right rear leg continued to sustain a significant increase in ROM.

Similarly, Kinser and associates (2008) reported that the combination of vibration and static stretching resulted in significant increases in flexibility of young, competitive female gymnasts performing forward splits. In comparison, static stretching alone did not improve performance. Vibration (30 Hz with 2 mm displacement) was applied for 10 sec to four sites and repeated four times. In addition, there was no significant difference between the pre- and posttest explosive strength of the participants in the vibration-only, stretching-only, and simultaneous vibration and stretching groups.

■ Does the flexibility exercise prescription need to be adapted for older individuals?

Range of motion decreases with age due to disuse, changes in tissue viscoelasticity, and diseases such as arthritis. However, stretching improves ROM in older adults (Feland et al. 2001; Ferber, Osternig, and Gravelle 2002). There is a lack of research addressing optimal stretching methods and durations for older adults. Ferber and colleagues (2002) compared the effects of three stretching methods—static stretching, contract-relax (CR) PNF stretching, and agonist contract-relax (ACR) PNF stretching—on knee joint ROM in older adults (50-75 yr). The ACR technique produced greater gains in ROM (29% and 34%) than did the static stretching and CR methods, even though the ACR technique produced more electromyographic activity in the target muscles.

Feland and colleagues (2001) studied the effects of 15, 30, and 60 sec of static stretching on the rate of ROM improvement in older adults (65-97 yr) with tight hamstrings. The subjects trained five times a week for 6 wk, and knee extension ROM was measured weekly. The group that stretched for 60 sec had a greater rate of improvement ($2.4°\cdot wk^{-1}$) than those stretching for 30 sec ($1.3°\cdot wk^{-1}$) and 15 sec ($0.6°\cdot wk^{-1}$). Although these findings suggest that 60 sec is optimal for improving flexibility in older adults, the total time of stretching was not controlled in this study (i.e., the total time of stretching was 30 min for the 60 sec group and only 15 min and 7.5 min for the 30 sec and 15 sec groups, respectively). The difference in total time most likely explains why the 60 sec stretch duration was superior.

Swank and colleagues (2003) assessed the effectiveness of adding light wrist and ankle weights to a low-intensity, rhythmic movement program (the Body Recall Program) designed to improve and maintain the strength and flexibility of older adults. Compared to a control group and a group that participated only in the Body Recall Program, the group that added weights to the Body Recall Program showed significantly greater improvements in ROM at the neck (cervical rotation), hip (extension), and ankle (plantar flexion). Thus, adding weights may enhance the effectiveness of rhythmic movement and stretching programs designed to improve the flexibility of older adults.

Given the limited number of studies dealing with flexibility in older adults, at this time it is not possible to firmly recommend how to change program guidelines when designing flexibility programs for older adults. However, if you use the PNF method with older adults, take care that you do not exceed the stretch tolerance of your clients. The stretch tolerance of older adults is reduced due to age-related changes in the viscoelastic properties of muscle and connective tissue.

You can use the general guidelines presented in this section as a starting point for designing flexibility programs. You should individualize programs to take into account client factors such as tolerance to stretch and pain, needs, and long-range goals. For example, shorter-duration– higher-repetition static stretching may be more appropriate for clients with low stretch tolerance, whereas longer-duration PNF stretching may be more suitable for athletes or for clients in injury rehabilitation programs. Also, the optimal duration, frequency, and total time of stretching may vary among muscle groups because their viscoelastic properties and response to the stretch stimulus may differ (Shrier and Gossal 2000). See page 292 for a sample program for a 35 yr old woman who wants to improve her overall flexibility. Note that this program includes more than one exercise for muscle groups with poor-to-fair flexibility ratings.

GUIDELINES FOR DESIGNING FLEXIBILITY PROGRAMS

- **Mode:** Static or PNF stretching for most clients; ballistic stretching may be useful for clients engaging in sports that involve ballistic movements
- **Number of exercises:** 10 to 12
- **Frequency:** Minimum of 2 to 3 days a week, preferably daily
- **Intensity:** Slowly stretch the muscle to a position of mild discomfort
- **Duration of stretch:** 10 to 30 sec for static stretching; 5 to 10 sec contraction, followed by 10 to 30 sec of assisted stretching for PNF
- **Repetitions:** Four to six for each exercise so that the total duration of each stretching exercise is 45 to 120 sec
- **Time:** 15 to 30 min per session

Instruct clients who are engaging in stretching programs to adhere to the following guidelines (Kravitz and Heyward 1995; ACSM 2010):

CLIENT GUIDELINES FOR STRETCHING PROGRAMS

- Perform a general warm-up before stretching to increase body temperature and to warm the muscles to be stretched.
- Stretch all major muscle groups, as well as opposing muscle groups.
- Focus on the target muscles involved in the stretch, relax the target muscle, and minimize the movement of other body parts.
- Hold the stretch for 10 to 60 sec.
- Stretch to the limit (end point) of the movement, not to the point of pain.
- Keep breathing slowly and rhythmically while holding the stretch.
- Stretch the target muscle groups in different planes to improve overall ROM at the joint.
- Although stretching may not prevent injury or reduce muscle soreness, it is a reasonable practice to include stretching exercises following an active warm-up and as part of the cool-down phase of your exercise program (ACSM 2010).

DESIGNING LOW BACK CARE EXERCISE PROGRAMS

Low back pain frequently causes activity restrictions for middle-aged and older adults, disabling 3 to 4 million people each year. Chronic low back pain is the number one cause of disability in the working population (Carpenter and Nelson 1999). The safest and most effective way to prevent and rehabilitate low back injuries remains controversial. This section describes two approaches for low back care programs. The approach you select depends on your client's needs, health and fitness status, and training objective (e.g., reducing low back pain, lowering the risk of low back injury, or maximizing athletic performance).

Sample Flexibility Program

Client data

Age	35 yr	Duration of stretch	10 sec
Gender	Female	Repetitions	4-6 per exercise
Body weight	140 lb (63.6 kg)	Total stretch time	50-120 sec per exercise
Program goal	Improve overall flexibility	Frequency	Daily
Time commitment	20-30 min per workout	Overload	Gradually increase stretch duration or repetitions up to a maximum of 2 min per exercise
Number of exercises	12		
Method	Static stretching		
Intensity	Just below pain threshold		

Exercise[a]	Week	Duration (sec)	Reps	Total time (sec)	Muscle groups
Quad stretch (side-lying)	1-3	10	5	50	Quadriceps femoris
	4-6	12	5	60	
	7-9	15	6	90	
Half-straddle stretch*	1-3	10	5	50	Hamstrings; trunk extensors (low back)
	4-6	12	5	60	
	7-9	15	6	90	
Double knee to chest (supine)*	1-3	10	6	60	Hamstrings; trunk extensors (low back)
	4-6	15	6	90	
	7-9	20	6	120	
Butterfly stretch (seated)	1-3	10	5	50	Hip adductors
	4-6	10	6	60	
	7-9	12	6	72	
Trunk flex (hands and knees)*	1-3	15	5	75	Trunk extensors (low back)
	4-6	20	5	100	
	7-9	20	6	120	
Crossed-leg trunk rotation	1-3	10	5	50	Hip abductors; trunk rotators
	4-6	15	5	75	
	7-9	15	6	90	
Achilles (calf) stretch	1-3	10	5	50	Ankle plantar flexors
	4-6	12	5	60	
	7-9	15	5	75	
Pelvic tilt	1-3	15	5	75	Abdominal muscles
	4-6	20	5	100	
	7-9	30	4	120	
Towel stretch (standing)	1-3	10	5	50	Shoulder extensors
	4-6	12	5	60	
	7-9	15	5	75	
Towel stretch (kneeling prone)	1-3	12	5	60	Shoulder flexors
	4-6	15	5	75	
	7-9	20	5	100	
Triceps stretch	1-3	10	5	50	Elbow extensors
	4-6	12	5	60	
	7-9	15	5	75	
Neck rotation	1-3	12	5	60	Neck flexors; neck lateral flexors; neck rotators
	4-6	12	6	72	
	7-9	15	5	75	

[a]For descriptions of exercises, see appendixes F.1 and F.3, pages 390 and 404.

*Two or more exercises are included for the muscle groups with poor flexibility—the hamstrings and trunk extensors (low back).

Traditional Approach

Traditionally, low back care programs have been designed to correct improper alignment and support of the spinal column and pelvis. Generally, a combination of stretching and strengthening exercises is prescribed to increase (a) the ROM of the hip flexors, hamstrings, and low back extensor muscles and (b) the strength of the abdominal muscles.

Exercise professionals have focused primarily on strengthening the abdominal muscles in order to prevent low back pain and injury, giving little or no attention to the low back muscles. Research, however, suggests that low back strengthening programs are effective for relieving and preventing low back pain and injury (Carpenter and Nelson 1999). A current practice in some low back care programs is to include exercises to increase the strength and endurance of both the abdominal and low back extensor muscles.

To strengthen the low back (lumbar extensor) muscles, **pelvic stabilization** is a key requirement. If the pelvis is not stabilized during extension of the trunk, the hip extensor muscles rotate the pelvis (~110°), and the lumbar vertebrae maintain their relative position to each other (do not extend). On the other hand, when the pelvis is immobilized, the lumbar vertebrae extend (~72°) as the low back extensor muscles contract (Carpenter and Nelson 1999). Most calisthenic-type floor exercises do not isolate the low back muscles because the pelvis is free to move. Using a lumbar extension machine, with thigh and femur restraints to stabilize the pelvis, prevents hip extension and isolates the low back muscles during the movement. Exercising on a lumbar extension machine with a minimal training volume (one set of 8 to 15 repetitions of lumbar extension exercise to fatigue per week) significantly improves lumbar muscle strength and bone mineral density (Graves et al. 1994; Pollock, Garzarella, and Graves 1992) and reduces the incidence of back injuries (Mooney et al. 1995). Individuals with chronic low back pain who participate in this type of low back strengthening program can expect significant improvements in joint mobility and muscular strength and endurance, as well as relief from pain (Carpenter and Nelson 1999).

To strengthen the abdominal muscles, select exercises that maximize the activation of the abdominal muscles but minimize the compression (load) of the lumbar vertebrae (i.e., a high challenge:compression ratio). Since the psoas muscle (prime mover for hip flexion) is a major source of spinal loading, choose exercises that minimize the activation of this muscle, such as bent-knee curl-ups (feet free or anchored), dynamic cross-knee curl-ups (curl-ups with a twist), isometric side support (side bridge), and dynamic sideward curl exercises (Axler and McGill 1997; Juker et al. 1998; Knudson 1999). The bent-knee curl-up exercise emphasizes the rectus abdominis, while the isometric side support emphasizes the abdominal oblique and quadratus lumborum muscles. Because of their low challenge-to-compression ratios, the following abdominal exercises are not recommended: straight leg or bent-knee sit-ups, supine straight leg raises, and hanging bent-knee raises (Axler and McGill 1997).

Using the traditional approach, the following exercises are recommended for low back care. Some of these exercises are described and illustrated in appendix F.3, "Exercises for Low Back Care," page 404.

- Pelvic tilt (supine-lying position) to stretch the abdominal muscles
- Knee-to-chest (supine-lying position) to stretch the hamstring, buttock, and low back muscles
- Trunk flex (on hands and knees) to stretch the back, abdominal, and hamstring muscles
- Lumbar extension exercises with pelvic stabilization (on machine) to strengthen the low back extensors
- Curl-ups, dynamic cross-knee curl-ups, and isometric side-support exercises to strengthen the abdominal and quadratus lumborum muscles
- Single-leg extension (prone-lying position) to strengthen the hamstring and buttock muscles and to stretch the hip flexor muscles

Alternative Approach

Studies suggest that the major cause of low back injury during exercise or performance of activities of daily living is lumbar instability, rather than improper alignment of the spinal column and pelvis per se (McGill 2001). Research also indicates that muscle *endurance* is more protective than muscle *strength* for reducing low back injury, and that greater lumbar mobility (ROM) actually increases one's risk of low back injury (McGill 1998, 2001, 2007). Thus, sufficient stability of the lumbar spine (i.e., **lumbar stabilization**) is the major emphasis in this new approach to low back care. To measure lumbar stability, see "Lumbar Stability Tests" in chapter 10, page 278. For detailed discussion and suggestions for applying the concept of lumbar stabilization to low back care programs, see Bracko (2004) and Norris (2000).

To develop and maintain lumbar stability, experts (McGill 2001) recommend the following:

- "Bracing" the lumbar spine during activity by isometrically cocontracting the abdominal wall and low back muscles

- Maintaining a "neutral" spine (i.e., the natural lordotic curve in the lumbar spine while standing upright) during activity

- Avoiding end ROM positions (fully flexed or extended) of the trunk while lifting or exercising

- Performing exercises that emphasize the development of muscle endurance rather than strength

The following sequence of exercises is specifically recommended for beginners who are starting a low back care program. These exercises are illustrated in appendix F.3, "Exercises for Low Back Care," page 404.

- Cat-camel exercise to slowly and dynamically move through the full range of spinal flexion and extension, with emphasis on spinal mobility rather than pressing and holding the trunk position at the ends of the ROM (usually five to six cycles of this exercise are sufficient)

- Stretching exercises to increase mobility at the hip and knee joints

- Curl-ups with one leg flexed and hands placed underneath the lumbar spine to help in maintaining a neutral spine

- Isometric side-support (side bridge) exercises for the quadratus lumborum and abdominal oblique muscles

- Single-leg extension holds (modified bird dog exercises) while on hands and knees for the low back and hip extensor muscles

- Isometric stabilization exercises requiring simultaneous contraction of the abdominal muscles to generate an abdominal "brace" during performance of other exercises

- Dynamic "hollowing" or drawing of the navel toward the spine for the deeper abdominal wall muscles (i.e., transverse abdominis and internal obliques)

The North American Spine Society (2009) recommends stretching, core strengthening, and resistance training exercises to prevent back pain and to maintain a healthy back. To view images for each of these exercises, go online to www.spine.org/Pages/ConsumerHealth/SpineHealthAndWellness/PreventBackPain.

- Neck, inner thigh, and hamstring stretches
- Shoulder rolls and frontal core stretches
- Backward bending
- Standing thread the needle
- Doorway chest stretch
- Wall wash
- Transverse and sagittal core strengthening
- Abdominal crunch and other abdominal exercises
- Neck press
- Side bridge
- Prone bridge/plank

KEY POINTS

- The specificity, overload, progression, and interindividual variability principles should be applied to designing flexibility programs.
- Three methods of stretching are static, ballistic, and PNF.
- Typically, larger gains in ROM result from PNF stretching than from ballistic or static stretching.
- The contract-relax (CR) and contract-relax agonist contract (CRAC) are common PNF stretching techniques.
- Ballistic stretching is not generally recommended because of its high risk for injury and muscle soreness.
- For static stretching programs, gains in ROM are related to the total time the stretch is sustained; total time of stretching is a function of stretch duration and the number of repetitions of the exercise.
- A well-rounded flexibility program includes at least one exercise for each major muscle group.
- Muscle groups should not be stretched beyond the pain-free ROM.
- Typically, the duration of the stretch should be 10 to 15 sec for beginners and no more than 60 sec for more advanced clients.
- Beginners should start with four to six repetitions of each exercise.
- Flexibility exercises should be performed a minimum of 2 to 3 days/wk, but preferably daily.
- To progressively overload the target muscle group, gradually increase the total time of the stretch (45-120 sec) by increasing the duration of stretch (10-60 sec) and the number of repetitions (four to six repetitions).
- Stretching does not prevent injury or improve physical performance.
- Lumbar instability is a major cause of low back problems.
- Exercises that develop and maintain lumbar stability are recommended for low back care programs.
- Exercises developing muscle endurance may be more effective than exercises developing muscle strength for the prevention and treatment of low back injuries.

KEY TERMS

Learn the definition of each of the following key terms. Definition of terms can be found in the glossary on page 411.

active-assisted stretching

active stretching

ballistic stretching

contract-relax agonist contract (CRAC) technique

contract-relax (CR) technique

flexibility training

lumbar stabilization

passive stretching

pelvic stabilization

proprioceptive neuromuscular facilitation (PNF)

reciprocal inhibition

static stretching

stress relaxation

stretch tolerance

REVIEW QUESTIONS

In addition to being able to define each of the key terms, test your knowledge and understanding of material by answering the following review questions.

1. Explain why ballistic stretching is not usually recommended for flexibility programs.

2. Identify two sensory receptors of the musculotendinous unit and explain how each receptor is affected by slow static stretching.

3. What are the physiological mechanisms responsible for gains in ROM from PNF stretching?

4. Identify three high-risk flexibility exercises and suggest safe alternatives.

5. What are the advantages and disadvantages of slow static and PNF stretching?

6. Describe the basic guidelines for designing flexibility programs. Explain how the specificity and overload training principles apply.

7. Explain why stretching does not prevent injury.

8. Describe three abdominal exercises that have high challenge-to-compression ratios.

9. What are the similarities and differences between the traditional and alternative approaches to low back care programs?

10. Describe the recommended sequence of exercises for starting a low back care program.

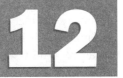

Assessing Balance and Designing Balance Programs

- What are static and dynamic balance?
- What factors affect balance?
- How is balance assessed?
- What are general guidelines for balance testing?
- What is balance training?
- What types of exercise are best suited for improving balance?
- What are the general recommendations for designing balance training programs?

Although balance is not generally included in health-related physical fitness test batteries, it is gaining recognition as a key component of functional fitness. In the past, balance was viewed primarily as a performance-based measure, with balance training geared toward improving sport performance. In a worldwide survey of fitness trends for 2009, balance training emerged as one of the top 10 trends, along with Pilates, stability ball exercise, and special exercise programs for older adults (Thompson 2008).

Balance is an especially important component of functional fitness for older adults in terms of preventing falls, performing activities of daily living, and maintaining functional independence. In the United States, more than one-third of older adults (65 yr or older) fall each year; falling is the leading cause of injury deaths among older adults (Centers for Disease Control and Prevention 2009). Over the past decade, the rate of fall-related deaths rose significantly in this population (Stevens 2006). To reduce the risk of falling, older adults are encouraged to exercise regularly and to engage in physical activity modes that improve strength and balance. The most recent "Physical Activity Guidelines for Americans" recommends that older adults participate in balance activities 3 or more days a week (U.S. Department of Health and Human Services 2008). Also, the American College of Sports Medicine (ACSM) and American Heart Association recommend balance exercises for those at risk for falls (Haskell et al. 2007).

This chapter presents definitions and theoretical frameworks for balance and describes tools and tests for assessing balance. Guidelines for balance testing are presented along with norms for selected balance tests, and suggestions for designing training programs to improve balance are provided.

DEFINITIONS AND NATURE OF BALANCE

Balance is the ability to keep the body's center of gravity within the base of support when one is maintaining a static position, performing voluntary movements, or reacting to external disturbances. Clinically, balance is commonly thought as static or dynamic. **Static balance** is the ability to maintain the center of gravity within the supporting base while standing or sitting, whereas **dynamic balance** refers to maintaining an upright position while the center of gravity and base of support are moving and the center of gravity is moving outside of the supporting base (e.g., walking). Postural stability and equilibrium are terms often used to refer to the construct of balance. **Functional balance** refers to the ability to perform daily movement tasks requiring balance such as picking up an object from the floor, dressing, and turning to look at something behind you.

Balance is a complex construct involving multiple biomechanical, neurological, and environmental systems. Over the years, the theoretical frameworks dealing with balance have moved from reflex and hierarchical perspectives to a dynamic systems model that describes how these systems function and interact to achieve balance and postural control. The reflex model assumes that sensory input controls motor output; the hierarchical model is based on control of movement by higher brain centers (e.g., cortex and midbrain). The dynamic systems model describes balance control as adaptive and functional, providing multiple solutions for accomplishing a movement goal. In this model, the higher brain centers work in conjunction with lower centers rather than controlling them. The visual, somatosensory (proprioception), and vestibular (inner ear) systems interact to maintain balance. The visual system provides information about the body's location relative to its environment; the somatosensory system discerns position and movements of body parts; the vestibular system provides information about head position in relation to gravity and senses how fast and in what direction the head is accelerating. In addition, internal factors such as muscle tone, strength, and range of motion, as well as environmental factors, contribute to balance.

FACTORS AFFECTING BALANCE AND RISK OF FALLING

Balance is related to age, gender, body size, and physical fitness level. This section addresses some commonly asked questions about balance and the risk of falling.

■ *How does body size affect balance?*

The height of the body's center of gravity relative to the supporting base affects balance. The higher the center of gravity is from the base of support, the lower the stability. Shorter individuals have a lower center of gravity and therefore potentially greater stability compared to taller individuals. Both height and body weight are predictors of postural sway.

■ *Does foot size affect balance?*

There is a direct relationship between the size of the supporting base and stability; the larger the supporting base, the greater the stability. A larger base of support allows the vertical projection of the body's center of gravity (i.e., **line of gravity**) to move a greater distance before falling outside of the supporting base and losing balance. This explains why it is more difficult to maintain your balance while standing on the tips of your toes compared to standing on both feet. Foot size (length and width) may affect balance especially when one is performing tasks that require standing on one leg.

■ *Do women have better static balance than men?*

Gender differences in skeletal structure (e.g., shape of pelvis) and body shape (apple vs. pear shaped) affect the location of the center of gravity within the body. Typically in women, the relative height of the center of gravity from the supporting base during standing tends to be lower than that of men (~55% and 57% of standing height, respectively) due to the wider pelvic structure of women and their tendency to be pear shaped. Therefore, one might hypothesize that static balance ability of women may be somewhat better than that of men. However, Springer and colleagues (2007) reported no gender differences in the unipedal or one-leg stance performance with eyes open and closed for adults 18 to 99 yr of age.

■ *What types of physical activities can be used to improve balance?*

Given that balance performance is affected by muscle strength and flexibility, resistance training and stretching programs may be useful for maintaining and improving balance. In addition to increasing strength and range of motion, Pilates, yoga, and tai chi are suitable activities for improving balance. Balance discs, foam pads and rollers, balance boards, and stability balls are tools that may add variety and challenge to balance training programs.

■ *Does regular exercise reduce the risk of falling?*

Regular exercise may be one way to prevent falls and fall-related fractures. Carter and associates (2001) reported that impairments in muscle and joint function, vestibular system, vision, proprioception, cognition, static and dynamic balance, and gait predispose individuals to falls and fractures. Balance, resistance, and flexibility training programs were more effective than endurance training for reducing risk of falling (Province et al. 1995). Although regular exercise can modify fall risk factors, the optimal exercise prescription to prevent falls has not been determined (Carter et al. 2001).

ASSESSMENT OF BALANCE

Field and clinical tests are available for assessing static and dynamic balance, as are tests of functional balance using indirect measures. For detailed descriptions and illustrations for static and dynamic balance field tests, see Reiman and Manske (2009). Because balance is complex, most balance test batteries are comprehensive and include multiple test items to assess both static and dynamic balance. A single, simple test such as the one-leg stance may be limited in that it measures only a few of the components composing the construct of balance. In addition to field test batteries, direct measures of balance may be obtained using computerized force plate devices to assess the adaptive functioning of the sensory, motor, and biomechanical components in accordance with the dynamic systems model of balance (see p. 306).

Assessing Static Balance Using Indirect Measures

As early as the mid-1800s, Romberg developed tests to measure static balance with a narrowed base of support during standing. The following sections describe the protocols for various types of static balance tests that may be easily used in field or clinical settings.

Romberg Tests

The Romberg tests measure static balance during standing with eyes open and eyes closed. For the original Romberg test, the client stands barefooted with arms folded across the chest and the feet close together in the frontal plane (Romberg test = feet side by side). For the modified Romberg test, the client stands barefooted using a tandem (feet positioned heel to toe) stance with eyes open and eyes closed. These tests are scored objectively; the number of seconds the client maintains a steady position without swaying, up to a maximum of 60 sec, is recorded.

The side-by-side and tandem stance tests were primarily developed to discriminate between poor and acceptable balance in elderly individuals. The test–retest reliability of the tandem stance test ranges from 0.76 (eyes closed) to 0.91 (eyes open) (Franchignoni et al. 1997). Shubert and colleagues (2006) reported that the tandem stance test is moderately related to walking speed ($r = 0.50$) and dynamic balance ($r = 0.46$) of older adults (65 yr and older) who are able to walk independently. Pajala and associates (2008) noted that the inability to complete the tandem stance is a significant predictor of fall risk. However, other researchers observed that the side-by-side and tandem stance tests have poor validity for predicting falls in older adults (Yim-Chiplis and Talbot 2000) and do not discriminate between individuals on the lower and higher ends of the balance spectrum (Curb et al. 2006).

Unipedal Stance Test

The unipedal stance or timed one-leg stance test also provides a simple measure of static balance performance. The validity of this test has been demonstrated by its relationship with gait performance, risk of falling, and ability to perform activities of daily living (ADL) for older adults (Bohannon 2006a). The test–retest reliability of the one-leg stance ranges from 0.74 (eyes closed) to 0.91 (eyes open) (Whitney, Poole, and Cass 1998). This widely used test provides a reliable measure of static balance for children and adults (Emery 2003; Emery et al. 2005).

For this test, the client stands on one leg with eyes open and closed. The test is scored as the number of seconds the client is able to maintain balance on the dominant leg. In a meta-analysis, Bohannon (2006b) reported that testing procedures for the one-leg stance test are not standardized. The following are some of the testing procedures that varied:

■ Client was barefoot or wearing shoes.

■ Dominant, nondominant, or both legs were tested.

- Maximum duration of the test varied between 5 and 60 sec.

- Number of trials varied from one to five.

- Dependent measure was either best score or average of the trials.

The test duration most frequently reported in the 22 studies that Bohannon reviewed was 30 sec. The average single-leg stance (eyes open) time for apparently healthy older adults declined across age groups: 27.0 sec for 60 to 69 yr, 17.2 sec for 70 to 79 yr, and 8.5 sec for 80 to 99 yr. Springer and colleagues (2007) developed age–gender norms for the unipedal stance test (eyes open and closed) for adults 18 yr to 99 yr (see table 12.1). To use these norms, be certain to follow testing procedures in "Test Procedures for Unipedal Stance Test."

Clinical Test of Sensory Integration of Balance

The clinical test of sensory integration of balance was designed to evaluate the contributions of the visual, proprioception, and vestibular sensory systems to balance. To study the role of these sensory systems on balance performance, you can modify the Romberg static balance tests by having clients stand on foam pads with eyes open or closed (Shumway-Cook and Horak 1986). The high-density foam pad reduces the individual's ability to use touch and proprioception in making postural adjustments to maintain balance during the test. Closing the eyes or being blindfolded eliminates the influence of vision on balance. For National Health and Nutrition Examination Survey IV (Centers for Disease Control and Prevention 2005), the balance

---

Test Procedures for Unipedal Stance Test

1. Determine clients' dominant leg by having them kick a ball.

2. Prior to raising one leg off the floor, clients fold their arms across the chest.

3. The client stands barefooted on dominant leg and raises the other foot near to but not touching the ankle of the stance limb. Start the stopwatch as soon as client lifts the foot off the floor

4. For the eyes-open test, the client focuses on a spot on the wall at eye level throughout the test.

5. Terminate the test when the client does any of the following:

   - Uncrosses or uses arms to maintain balance

   - Moves the raised foot away from the standing limb or touches the floor with raised foot

   - Moves the weight-bearing foot to maintain balance

   - Exceeds maximum duration of 45 sec

   - Opens eyes during the eyes-closed one-leg stance test

6. Administer three trials and use the best score.

Table 12.1 Age–Gender Norms for the Unipedal (One-Leg) Stance Test[a]

Age group (yr)	EYES OPEN (SEC)[b]		EYES CLOSED (SEC)[b]	
	Females	Males	Females	Males
18-39	45.1	44.4	13.1	16.9
40-49	42.1	41.6	13.5	12.0
50-59	40.9	41.5	7.9	8.6
60-69	30.4	33.8	3.6	5.1
70-79	16.7	25.9	3.7	2.6
80-99	10.6	8.7	2.1	1.8

[a]Maximum test duration is 45 sec.

[b]Use best of three trials.

Data from B.A. Springer et al., 2007, "Normative values for the unipedal stance test with eyes open and closed," *Journal of Geriatric Physical Therapy* 30: 8-15.

test battery consisted of the standard Romberg test with eyes open and closed (maximum duration = 15 sec) followed by the modified Romberg tests, standing on a foam pad, with the eyes open and closed (maximum duration = 30 sec). Of these tests, standing on the foam pad with eyes closed was most difficult. Curb and colleagues (2006) reported that of these four test items, only standing on the foam pad with eyes open has acceptable test–retest reliability ($r = 0.71$) and is reasonably able to discriminate between good and excellent balancing ability in younger and older adults. However, Emery and colleagues (2005) noted that the one-leg stance on a foam pad with eyes closed, up to a maximum duration of 180 sec, provided a reliable measure of balance for adolescent males and females 14 to 19 yr.

Assessing Dynamic Balance With Indirect Measures

Dynamic balance is the ability to maintain postural stability while moving. Dynamic balance involves completing functional tasks without compromising the base of support while moving; it is important for preventing falls, especially in older adults and children, and for preventing sport injuries in athletes and physically active individuals. This section describes field tests and clinical protocols for tests of dynamic balance of children, older adults, and athletes.

Functional Reach Tests

A functional reach test was developed to measure dynamic balance of adults by determining the maximum distance an individual can reach beyond arm's length without losing balance or moving the feet (Duncan et al. 1990). The validity of this test is good, with concurrent validity coefficients ranging between 0.64 (one-leg stance test) and 0.71 (center-of-pressure excursion). The test–retest reliability was $r = 0.86$ to 0.88 (Franchignoni et al. 1998; Whitney, Poole, and Cass 1998).

For this test, a yardstick or meter stick is attached to the wall, parallel to the floor, at the height of the client's acromion process. The client stands with the lateral aspect of the shoulder parallel to the wall, makes a fist with the right hand, and raises the right arm with elbow extended until the fist is at the height of the yardstick. The initial measure is the point along the measuring stick corresponding to the distal end of the third metacarpal. The client is instructed to reach forward as far as possible

without falling or taking a step, and the farthest distance reached along the stick is recorded (figure 12.1). The functional reach score is the difference between the two recorded distances, measured to the nearest 0.5 cm (0.25 in.). After one practice trial, three trials are administered, and scores are averaged. Scores on the functional reach test are used to classify older individuals into fall risk categories: low risk = >24.4 cm (>10 in.); moderate risk = 15.24 to 25.4 cm (6 to 10 in.); high risk = <15.24 cm (<6 in.); very high risk = unable to reach (Duncan et al. 1990, 1992).

The functional reach test has been used to assess the dynamic balance of children and adolescents, 5 to 15 yr, with test–retest reliability coefficients ranging from $r = 0.64$ to 0.75 (Donahue, Turner, and Worrell 1994). In this study, gender, height, body weight, and arm length did not predict functional reach performance. Conversely, Habib and Westcott (1998) reported that 17% of the variance in functional reach scores of children is attributed to age, and 15% of the variance may be attributed to height, body weight, and base of support (i.e., length of the feet). Recently, Norris and associates (2008) noted that only body weight ($r = 0.34$) was significantly related to functional reach scores of children 3 to 5 yr.

The functional reach test has been modified to measure upward reach during standing with reach distance normalized for foot length and stature. Row and Cavanaugh (2007) stated that the standing upward reach test posed a greater challenge to dynamic balance for both younger and older individuals compared to the forward functional reach test. In addition, the reach strategy (i.e., whether or not the heels were raised from the floor during the test) accounted for differences in reach performances of older adults.

Thompson and Medley (2007) proposed a variation of the functional reach test to assess the forward and lateral reach of adults 21 to 97 yr while sitting in a chair. This modification of the functional reach test can be used to assess the dynamic balance and risk of falling for individuals who use wheelchairs or frail older adults who cannot perform the standing functional reach test. The researchers reported that sitting reach scores of older adults are significantly less than those of younger and middle-aged adults. In addition, length of the arms did not affect performance.

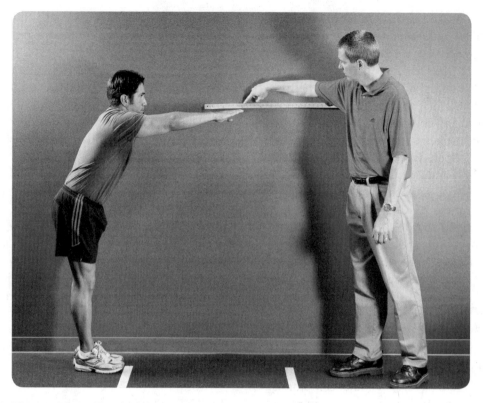

Figure 12.1 The functional reach balance test.

Reprinted, by permission, from M.P. Reiman, 2009, *Functional testing in human performance* (Champaign, IL: Human Kinetics), 110.

Timed Up and Go Tests

Timed up and go tests are used to assess dynamic balance and agility. These performance attributes are related to functional abilities such as getting up from a seated position to answer the phone or doorbell in a timely manner; therefore, this test is typically included in balance test batteries for older adults. Podsiadlo and Richardson (1991) described the timed up and go test as the amount of time needed to rise from an armchair, walk to a line 3 m (10 ft) away, turn, and return to a seated position in the chair. The timed up and go test has excellent test–retest reliability (r = 0.99), and test scores are related to gait speed, stair climbing, and risk of falling (Bohannon 2006a; Shumway-Cook, Brauer, and Woollacott 2000). Pondal and del Ser (2008) reported that approximately 26% of the variance in timed up and go scores of older adults (71-99 yr) without gait disturbances is explained by age, gender, body weight, nutritional status, and cognitive impairment.

The testing procedures for the timed up and go test vary among studies. In some studies, chairs differ in terms of seat height (40-50 cm) and style

(armchair or armless chair). Although almost all studies have the clients walking a distance of 10 ft (3 m), Rikli and Jones (2001) provide performance norms for an 8 ft (2.44 m) up and go test for older adults. Also, instructions for this test vary from walking at a normal pace to walking as quickly as possible. Usually more than one trial is administered (Bohannon 2006a). Each of these factors affects performance scores. Therefore, when using norms to evaluate your client's performance on this test, make certain you administer the test in the same manner and with the same instructions used to develop the test norms.

On the basis of a meta-analysis of 21 studies that included 4395 older adults (60-99 yr), Bohannon (2006a) concluded that timed up and go scores exceeding 9.0 sec for 60 to 69 yr, 10.2 sec for 70 to 79 yr, and 12.7 sec for 80 to 99 yr are considered to be worse than average for these age groups. Table 12.2 presents age–gender norms for older (>70 yr) adults (Pondal and del Ser 2008). For this variation of the timed up and go test, an armless chair with a 40 to 45 cm (about 16 to 18 in.) seat height was used. At the signal to go, subjects were instructed

Table 12.2 Age–Gender Norms for the 3 m (10 ft) Timed Up and Go Test[a]

| | AGE GROUP (YR) | | | | | | | |
| | 71-75 | | 76-80 | | 81-85 | | 86-99 | |
Percentile	M	F	M	F	M	F	M	F
95	13.3	15.0	14.3	18.6	19.5	20.0	21.0	22.0
90	11.0	14.0	13.6	15.2	14.0	17.6	18.2	19.6
80	10.0	13.0	11.0	13.0	13.0	15.0	13.8	16.0
70	9.0	12.0	10.0	12.0	12.0	14.2	12.0	15.0
60	9.0	11.0	10.0	11.0	10.0	12.0	11.2	13.8
50	8.0	10.0	9.0	10.0	9.0	12.0	11.0	12.0
40	8.0	10.0	8.0	9.4	8.0	11.0	10.6	12.0
30	7.0	9.0	7.0	9.0	8.0	10.0	8.1	10.4
20	7.0	9.0	7.0	8.0	8.0	10.0	7.4	9.8
10	6.4	7.5	7.0	6.6	7.0	8.0	6.7	9.0
5	5.7	7.0	6.0	5.8	6.0	8.0	6.0	9.0
1	5.0	6.0	5.0	5.0	5.0	8.0	6.0	9.0

[a]Time in seconds.

Data from M. Pondal and T. del Ser, 2008, "Normative data and determinants for the timed "up and go" test in a population-based sample of elderly individuals without gait disturbances," *Journal of Geriatric Physical Therapy* 31(2): 57-62.

to stand up, walk toward the marker (10 ft or 3 m distance), turn around, walk back to the chair, and sit down again as quickly as possible.

As part of the Senior Fitness Test Battery, Rikli and Jones (2001) suggest the 8 ft (2.44 m) timed up and go test to assess the balance and agility of older adults. This test has excellent test–retest reliability ($r = 0.95$) and is able to discriminate among functional categories of older adults. Table 12.3 presents age–gender norms for the 8 ft up and go test.

Purpose: Assess dynamic balance and agility.

Application: A measure of the ability to perform ADL such as getting up quickly to answer the phone or go to the bathroom.

Equipment: You will need a folding chair that has a seat height of 17 in. (43 cm) and that will not tip forward, as well as a measuring tape and cone marker.

Test procedures: Place the folding chair against a wall for stability and have your client sit in the middle of the chair, with hands on thighs, one leg slightly ahead of the other, and body leaning slightly forward. On the signal "go," have the client get up from the chair, walk as quickly as possible around a cone placed 8 ft (2.44 m) away, and return to the chair (figure 12.2). Administer one practice trial followed by two test trials.

Scoring: Start the stopwatch exactly on the signal to "go," and stop it at the exact time the client sits in the chair. Record the score to the nearest tenth of a second. Use the best score of the two trials and compare this value to the norms in table 12.3.

Star Excursion Balance Test

The star excursion balance test is a measure of dynamic balance that provides a significant challenge to athletes and physically active individuals. For this test, the individual must maintain a base of support on one leg while maximally reaching in different directions in a star pattern with the opposite leg. The goal of the test is to minimize displacement of the center of pressure and to maximize reach distance while maintaining unilateral support. The star excursion balance test is useful for screening deficits in dynamic postural control due to musculoskeletal injuries (e.g., ankle instability) and during the rehabilitation of orthopedic injuries in otherwise healthy, physically active adults (Olmsted et al. 2002). The reliability of this test ranges between $r = 0.85$ and 0.96 (Hertel, Miller, and Deneger 2000). Although height and leg length were significantly related to excursion distance, foot type (pes planus, cavus, or rectus) and range of motion at the hip and ankle were not. Given that leg length accounted for

Table 12.3 Age–Gender Norms for 8 ft Timed Up and Go Test*

Percentile rank	TIME (SEC)													
	60-64 YR		65-69 YR		70-74 YR		75-79 YR		80-84 YR		85-89 YR		90-94 YR	
	F	M	F	M	F	M	F	M	F	M	F	M	F	M
95	3.2	3.0	3.6	3.1	3.8	3.2	4.0	3.3	4.0	4.0	4.5	4.0	5.0	4.3
90	3.7	3,0	4.1	3.6	4.0	3.6	4.3	3.5	4.4	4.1	4.7	4.3	5.3	4.5
85	4.0	3.3	4.4	3.9	4.3	3.9	4.6	3.9	4.9	4.5	5.3	4.5	6.1	5.1
80	4.2	3.6	4.6	4.1	4.7	4.2	5.0	4.3	5.4	4.9	5.8	5.0	6.7	5.7
75	4.4	3.8	4.8	4.3	4.9	4.4	5.2	4.6	5.7	5.2	6.2	5.5	7.3	6.2
70	4.6	4.0	5.0	4.5	5.2	4.6	5.5	4.9	6.1	5.5	6.6	5.8	7.7	6.6
65	4.7	4.2	5.1	4.6	5.4	4.8	5.7	5.2	6.3	5.7	6.9	6.2	8.2	7.0
60	4.9	4.4	5.3	4.8	5.6	5.0	5.9	5.4	6.7	6.0	7.3	6.5	8.6	7.4
55	5.0	4.5	5.4	4.9	5.8	5.1	6.1	5.7	6.9	6.2	7.6	6.9	9.0	7.7
50	5.2	4.7	5.6	5.1	6.0	5.3	6.3	5.9	7.2	6.4	7.9	7.2	9.4	8.1
45	5.4	4.9	5.8	5.3	6.2	5.5	6.5	6.1	7.5	6.6	8.2	7.5	9.8	8.5
40	5.5	5.0	5.9	5.4	6.4	5.6	6.7	6.4	7.8	6.9	8.5	7.9	10.2	8.8
35	5.7	5.2	6.1	5.6	6.6	5.8	6.9	6.6	8.1	7.1	8.9	8.2	10.6	9.2
30	5.8	5.4	6.2	5.7	6.8	6.0	7.1	6.9	8.3	7.3	9.2	8.6	11.1	9.6
25	6.0	5.6	6.4	5.9	7.1	6.2	7.4	7.2	8.7	7.6	9.6	8.9	11.5	10.0
20	6.2	5.8	6.6	6.1	7.3	6.4	7.6	7.5	9.0	7.9	10.0	9.4	12.1	10.5
15	6.4	6.1	6.8	6.3	7.7	6.7	8.0	7.9	9.5	8.3	10.5	9.9	12.7	11.1
10	6.7	6.4	7.1	6.6	8.0	7.0	8.3	8.3	10.0	8.7	11.1	10.5	13.5	11.8
5	7.2	6.8	7.6	7.1	8.6	7.4	8.9	9.0	10.8	9.4	12.0	11.5	14.6	12.9

*Score is measured in seconds.

F = females; M = males.

Based on R. Rikli and C. Jones, 2001, *Senior fitness test manual* (Champaign, IL: Human Kinetics).

23% of variance in excursion distance, Gribble and Hertel (2003) recommended normalizing the test scores for leg length. To accomplish this, divide the excursion distance by the client's leg length and multiply by 100. Leg length is measured as the distance from the anterior superior iliac spine to the center of medial malleolus with the client lying supine.

The star excursion balance test is performed with the client standing (preferably barefoot) in the middle of a grid formed by eight lines extending from the center at 45° from each other (see figure 12.3). The client is allowed six practice trials in each of the eight directions on each leg. Clients begin reaching in the anterior direction and progress clockwise around the grid. Three trials are administered in the eight directions for each limb. During the trials, the client reaches to the farthest point possible on the line with the most distal part of the reach foot, and the tester marks this point on the grid line. Between individual trials in each direction, the client is given a 10 sec rest. For each direction, the distance from the point of maximum excursion to the center of the grid is measured in centimeters using a standard tape measure. The average of the three trials is used to quantify reach distance in each direction. When both the dominant and nondominant limbs are tested, a 5 min rest is provided.

One limitation of the star excursion balance test is the amount of time needed to administer 48 practice trials and 24 test trials for each leg. Hertel and colleagues (2006) simplified this test using factor analysis. Results from the analysis showed that the posteromedial reach score is highly representative of all eight directions of the test. They recommended using just the anteromedial, medial, and posteromedial reach tasks to test for functional deficits caused by chronic ankle instability for young adults. Also, Robinson and Gribble (2008) recently reported that the number of practice trials may be reduced from six to four for each direction. Table 12.4 presents the average reach distances in the eight directions for young women and men (Gribble and Hertel 2003).

Assessing Dynamic Balance Using Test Batteries

As mentioned earlier, balance is a complex construct. Most balance test batteries are comprehensive and include multiple test items to assess both static and dynamic balance. These test batteries require the client to perform a variety of functional tasks that mimic ADL. The tasks usually include maintaining a fixed sitting or standing posture, walking, rising from a seated position, and transferring between chairs. This section presents commonly used balance test batteries.

Tinetti Performance-Oriented Mobility Assessment

The Performance-Oriented Mobility Assessment (POMA) is a test battery that was developed to assess balance and gait of older adults (Tinetti 1986). It contains 14 performance-based items that evaluate gait maneuvers and position changes encountered in normal daily activities such as standing from sitting position and stepping over an obstacle on an uneven surface. Each item is scored on a scale ranging from

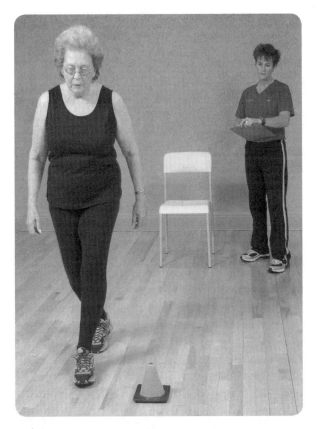

Figure 12.2 The 8 ft timed up and go test.

Reprinted, by permission, from M. Kettles, 2006, *Women's health and fitness guide* (Champaign, IL: Human Kinetics), 106.

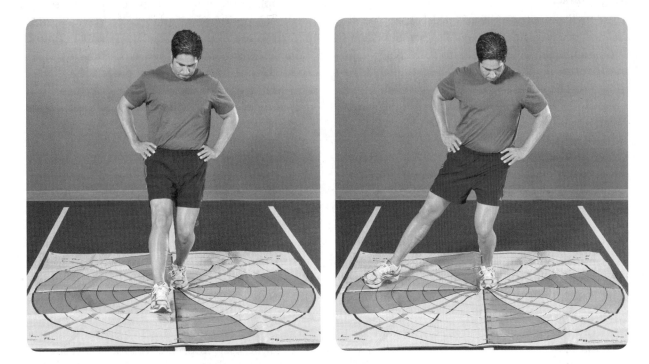

Figure 12.3 Star excursion balance test.

Reprinted, by permission, from M.P. Reiman, 2009, *Functional testing in human performance* (Champaign, IL: Human Kinetics), 108.

Table 12.4 Average Normalized Distances (%) for Star Excursion Balance Test*

Reach direction	Male	Female
Anterior	79.2	76.9
Anterolateral	73.8	74.7
Lateral	80.0	79.8
Posterolateral	90.4	85.5
Posterior	93.9	85.3
Posteromedial	95.6	89.1
Medial	97.7	90.7
Anteromedial	85.2	83.1

*Normalized score (%) = excursion distance / leg length × 100.

Distance and leg length in cm.

0 (cannot perform) to 2 (normal performance); the maximum score is 28. This test battery provides a reliable and valid assessment of balance in elderly, community-dwelling populations, and scores are associated with risk of falling (Berg et al. 1992; Tinetti, Speechley, and Ginter 1988). Scores greater than 25 are indicative of good balance and lower fall risk (Mayson et al. 2008). For detailed instructions about the POMA, see Tinetti 1986 and Tinetti and colleagues 1988.

Berg Balance Scale

The Berg Balance Scale (BBS) is widely used to evaluate balance performance of nursing home residents and community-dwelling older adults. Inter- and intrarater reliability for this scale is extremely high ($R = .98$). The BBS has good concurrent validity: $r = 0.91$ with POMA test scores and $r = -0.76$ with timed up and go scores (Podsiadlo and Richardson 1991; Tinetti 1986).

The BBS evaluates performance on 14 functional mobility tasks and takes about 15 min to administer. Participants are scored on a 5-point scale, with a score of 0 indicating that the task could not be completed and a score of 4 indicating that the task was performed independently (Berg et al. 1992). The maximum score is 56; a score of 45 or less used to identify individuals with greater risk for falls (Hawk et al. 2006). However, Muir and colleagues (2008) reported that the cutoff value of 45 has poor sensitivity (25% to 42%) for predicting one or more falls in a community-dwelling older population. They concluded that multiple factors contribute to risk of falls in older people and that balance impairment alone does not adequately predict future risk. For complete instructions about scoring each item of the BBS, see Berg and colleagues 1992.

Dynamic Gait Index

The Dynamic Gait Index (DGI) provides a valid and reliable composite measure of one's ability to adapt gait during movement-related tasks. This test battery consists of eight items that are scored on a scale of 0 (cannot perform) to 3 (normal performance), with a maximum score of 24. For some of the items, the task is supposed to be completed as quickly as possible. Also, some items require performing two tasks simultaneously, such as walking while turning the head and looking up on command. Mayson and colleagues (2008) reported a positive association between DGI scores and a measure of cognition. Performance on this test is dependent on balance, mobility, and cognitive function (Mayson et al. 2008). Scores >20 are associated with a lower incidence of falling (Riddle and Stratford 1999; Shumway-Cook et al. 1997). For detailed instructions and information about the DGI, see Shumway-Cook and Woollacott 1995.

Assessing Static and Dynamic Balance With Direct Measures

The application of technology to balance assessment has produced a number of excellent computerized systems to assess static and dynamic balance. The relatively high cost (ranging from $6000 to $90,000) of these computerized systems, however, precludes their usefulness in most field and clinical settings. These systems consist of a computerized force plate with three or more force transducers that quantify vertical pressures applied to the support platform. These vertical pressures are used to derive the anteroposterior and mediolateral coordinates of the **center of pressure**. The systems provide data about postural sway and steadiness while the client remains motionless, weight distribution between the feet, the ability to move the center of vertical force (center of pressure) to maintain balance, and automatic motor responses to platform disturbances (Guskiewicz and Perrin 1996). Force platform balance tests provide valid information about postural control that can be used to predict risk of falling among older people with and without a history of balance problems or falling (Pajala et al. 2008).

Computerized dynamic posturography is designed to assess the individual and composite functioning of sensory, motor, and biomechanical components of balance (e.g., NeuroCom Equitest). The motor control tests provide data about the client's responses to sudden movements of the force plate that threaten balance. The sensory organization tests examine the client's ability to maintain an upright posture when visual and proprioceptive sensory information is modified mechanically (Nashner 1997). The NeuroCom Balance Master can be used to assess functional tasks such as walking, turning, and changing posture (e.g., sitting to standing). It measures weight symmetry, weight shifts, and limits of stability.

The **limits of stability** test, a measure of the maximum excursion of the center of gravity, assesses the degree to which the individual is able to lean in several directions while maintaining balance over a fixed supporting base (Clark et al. 2005). Research shows that this test provides reliable scores and is predictive of risk of falling (Clark, Rose, and Fujimoto 1997; Wallman 2001). The limits of stability in normal adults is 12° in the anterior-posterior plane and 16° in the mediolateral direction.

The Biodex Stability System may be used to evaluate and train neuromuscular control by quantifying the ability to maintain dynamic postural stability on both stable and unstable surfaces. This system provides ongoing visual feedback to the individual while attempting to reproduce specified movement patterns of the center of gravity. Using the Biodex Stability System, one calculates the stability index by dividing the client's anterior-posterior score (measured in degrees) by the normal value (12°) and multiplying by 100. Similarly, to calculate the mediolateral stability index, one divides the client's score by the normal value (16°) and multiplies by 100. Combined values less than 100% are indicative of balance problems (de Bruin et al. 2009).

In fitness, athletic, and rehabilitation settings, less expensive balance systems can be used to assess neuromuscular control, proprioception, and mechanoreceptor input (e.g., Biodex Stability System and Kinesthetic Ability Trainer). These systems, however, do not have the ability to quantify the vestibular and visual components of balance. Typically they consist of a multiaxial platform positioned on a U-joint with eight movable springs and are used for balance training.

DESIGNING BALANCE TRAINING PROGRAMS

Balance training has been identified as one of the top 10 worldwide trends in the fitness industry. The 2008 "Physical Activity Guidelines for Americans" suggests balance training at least 3 days a week for inactive and active older adults (≥65 yr). Although the ACSM (2010) makes no specific recommendations for exercises to include in a balance training program, the guidelines state that neuromuscular training (i.e., balance, agility, and proprioceptive training) is effective for preventing falls. Also, a review of balance training studies concluded that balance exercises are effective for reducing the risk of ankle sprains in athletes; 6 wk of balance training after an acute ankle sprain substantially reduces the risk of a recurrent sprain (McKeon and Hertel 2008). General recommendations for designing balance training programs are presented in the following:

RECOMMENDATIONS FOR BALANCE TRAINING PROGRAMS (ACSM 2009b)

- Have clients engage in balance activities 2 or 3 days per week.
- Progressively increase the difficulty of the balance exercises by using a narrower base of support such as two-leg stance, semitandem stance, tandem stance, and one-leg stance.
- Include dynamic movements that challenge the center of gravity such as tandem walking and circle turns.
- Use exercises that stress postural muscles, such as heel stands and toe stands, and exercises that reduce sensory input such as standing with eyes closed.
- Prescribe tai chi.

Balance Training Exercise Prescription

Compared to the other physical fitness components, there is a lack of research dealing with balance training for athletes, children, and older adults. It is difficult to compare studies examining the effects of exercise on balance because of diversity in the populations (e.g., young athletes to frail older adults), as well as the lack of standardization in balance outcome measures and training regimens. Also, there is no gold standard measure of balance. The following questions address issues you should consider when prescribing balance training for your clients.

■ *What types of physical activities may be used to improve balance?*

Given that balance performance is affected by muscle strength and flexibility, resistance training and stretching programs may be useful for maintaining and improving balance. In addition to increasing strength and range of motion, Pilates, yoga, tai chi, dance, walking, and combinations of exercise modes may be suitable activities for improving balance. Balance discs, foam pads and rollers, balance boards, stability balls, and computerized balance training systems are tools that may add variety and challenge to balance training programs.

In a review of exercise interventions to improve balance, Howe and colleagues (2007) analyzed results from 34 studies having a total of 2883 participants. The researchers categorized the training interventions as follows: gait, balance, coordination, and functional tasks training; strength training; tai chi; general physical activity (walking); and

multimodal physical activity programs that used a combination of exercise modes. Table 12.5 summarizes the positive effects of these interventions on direct and indirect measures of balance.

■ *What types of balance training activities can be used with older adults?*

In addition to flexibility and resistance training, exercise programs specifically designed to improve the functional ability of the lower extremities may be effective for improving balance and preventing falls in older adults. Shigematsu and colleagues (2008) compared the effects of regular walking and square-stepping exercise on balance, leg power, agility, and reaction time of adults 65 to 74 yr. The participants exercised for 70 min, two times per week, for 12 wk. The square-stepping exercise program included forward, backward, lateral, and oblique stepping patterns performed on a felt mat (100 × 250 cm) that was partitioned into 40 squares, 25 cm each. Each stepping pattern was repeated 4 to 10 times, and the patterns became progressively more complex, ranging from elementary forward–backward stepping to advanced lateral, oblique, and anterior-posterior patterns of stepping. Compared to the walking program, square-stepping exercise produced significantly greater improvements in leg extension power, forward–backward tandem walking, stepping with both feet, walking around

Table 12.5 Positive Effects of Various Physical Activity Interventions on Balance*

Type of training	Direct measures	Indirect measures
Gait, balance, coordination, functional tasks training	Static and dynamic stability with force platform Limits of stability	One-leg stance with eyes open Berg Balance Test
Resistance training	Omni-directional tilt	Functional reach One-leg stance with eyes open Tandem stance Gait speed
Tai chi training		Walking on balance beam One-leg stance with eyes open
General physical activity (walking)		Tandem walking Tandem stance Functional reach Walking on balance beam Timed up and go
Multimodal training	Body sway Limits of stability	Functional reach Tandem stance Tandem walking

*Training significantly improved performance on the direct and indirect balance tests listed.

two cones, and reaction time. Preliminary results suggest that square-stepping exercise is more effective than regular walking in reducing risk factors associated with falling.

In another study, proprioceptive balance training involved bilateral dorsiflexion/plantar flexion and supination/pronation of the ankle and bilateral squats during standing on semicompressible foam roller devices (Bellew et al. 2005). These devices are approximately 13 × 6 in. (33 × 15 cm) and resemble a football cut lengthwise. During each exercise session, subjects performed two 2 min bouts of bilateral supination/pronation and two 2 min bouts of bilateral plantar flexion/dorsiflexion. Each 2 min set of bilateral movements of the ankle was followed by partial squats (one set of 10 reps). This balance training protocol was performed 2 days/wk for 5 wk. Compared to a sedentary control group, the training group showed significant improvements in functional reach test (25%) and a lower extremity reach test (16%).

Takeshima and associates (2007) compared the effects of aerobic, resistance, balance, flexibility, and tai chi training on the functional fitness of older adults. Exercise programs were performed for 12 wk, 2 days/wk, for each exercise training mode except for the aerobic training (3 days/wk for 90 min). While resistance training elicited the greatest improvement (31%) in upper body strength, balance training produced the greatest increase in lower body strength (40%). Resistance training, tai chi, and balance training each produced similar gains in balance and agility (10%).

Hill and colleagues (2007) examined the effects of physical activity that combined yoga, tai chi, and resistance training. At the end of this 6 mo program, strength, balance, and gait endurance of older adults were significantly improved. Those who attended classes 2 days per week improved more than those averaging only once per week.

■ *Does resistance training improve balance?*

Improved balance is often mentioned as one of the benefits of resistance training. Orr and colleagues (2008) recently published the first systematic review of studies that assessed the effect of progressive resistance exercise training on balance of older adults. They noted that only a small percentage of balance outcome measures were significantly improved due to resistance training: static balance (26%), dynamic balance (14%), func-

tional balance (57%), and computerized dynamic posturography (8%). Thus, resistance training as an isolated intervention does not consistently improve balance of older adults. Part of the discrepancy in results may be a function of the fact that in many of these studies, the researchers selected universal whole-body and lower body strength exercises for the resistance training programs instead of identifying key muscles used for balance.

These results also suggest that strength alone is not the major underlying mechanism for poor balance. Muscle power (force × velocity) may also be a limiting factor in balance control. Age-related decreases in neural processing may diminish the ability to develop force rapidly in response to postural challenges (Orr et al. 2008). Mayson and colleagues (2008) reported that leg press velocity was positively related to dynamic balance performance (i.e., Berg Balance Scale, POMA, and dynamic gait index), whereas greater leg strength was associated with better performance on static balance tests (e.g., unipedal stance test).

In future studies addressing the use of progressive resistance training, it may be prudent to focus on the type of balance to be developed (i.e., static, dynamic, or functional), as well as specific muscle groups critical for balance such as the ankle dorsiflexors and plantar flexors, the knee extensors and flexors, and the hip abductors and adductors. Hess and Woollacott (2005) reported that a high-intensity strength training program targeting key lower extremity muscle groups (i.e., knee flexors and extensors and ankle plantar flexors and dorsiflexors) significantly improved the postural control in balance-impaired older adults.

■ *Does balance training reduce the risk of ankle sprains?*

Research demonstrates that balance training using balance boards, elastic tubing, ankle discs, and foam pads may reduce the risk of ankle injury and reinjury in physically active individuals (Han et al. 2009; Hoffman and Payne 1995; Verhagen et al. 2004). These programs use a combination of strengthening and coordination exercises to rehabilitate injured ankles and to improve balance. Han and colleagues (2009) reported that dynamic balance of healthy young adults with and without a history of ankle sprains was improved following a 4 wk elastic tubing exercise program with lower body resistance exercises performed in four directions (i.e., front pull, back pull, crossover, and reverse crossover). For this program, participants performed three sets of 15 repetitions, three times per week. Improvement in balance performance was retained up to 4 wk posttraining, suggesting that this form of balance training may improve ankle stability.

■ *How effective is tai chi for improving balance and preventing falls in older adults?*

Over the past few decades, tai chi has increased in popularity. Between 1992 and 2001, there were 11 published randomized clinical trials in the tai chi literature compared to 31 published from 2002 to 2007 (Li et al. 2009). The National Institute on Aging sponsored two studies on tai chi for older adults (Wolf et al. 1996; Wolfson et al. 1996). In the first study, the effects of tai chi on strength, flexibility, cardiovascular endurance, body composition, functional ability, and occurrence of falls were examined. Tai chi reduced falls and had a favorable impact on components of fitness and functional ability. The second study demonstrated that improvements in balance (measured by one-leg stance, limits of stability, sensory organization tests) and lower body strength resulting from a 3 mo balance training intervention could be sustained by participation in a low-intensity maintenance program of tai chi for 6 mo after the intervention (Wolfson et al. 1996).

Li and colleagues (2005) studied the effects of a 6 mo tai chi program (three times per week) on balance and number of falls in older men and women 70 to 92 yr. Compared to results for a control group that participated in a stretching program, the risk of multiple falls was 55% lower for the tai chi intervention. Tai chi participants showed significant improvements in all measures of balance including the Berg Balance Scale, Dynamic Gait Index, functional reach, and one-leg stance. Studies suggest that tai chi is an effective form of exercise for reducing falls and improving dynamic and functional balance performance of older adults (Kuramoto 2006; Maciaszek et al. 2007; Rogers, Larkey, and Keller 2009).

Wu (2002) reported that tai chi interventions improved one-leg stance with eyes open and Romberg test scores in 20 to 60 yr and older (>75 yr) adults. Tai chi training had only a limited effect on walking and timed get up and go scores.

■ *What is the optimal style of tai chi for improving balance?*

Tai chi is practiced in a variety of styles, for example Yang, Wu, and Tai Chi Chih. Each style has its own movements and traditional length of practice. The Yang style uses a wide stance and steady, slow speed of movement with constant knee flexion. Shifting body weight in this stance demands strength and flexibility. In contrast, the Wu style uses higher stances with a narrower stance width and slower movements, requiring more balance than strength compared to other styles. Therefore, the Wu style of tai chi may be more appropriate for balance training programs and interventions (Wu 2002).

■ *How many tai chi sessions are needed to show improvement in balance?*

The research clearly shows that the number of tai chi sessions makes a difference in terms of training effects on balance. Generally, 40 or more sessions are needed to show significant improvements in balance performance. To reduce risk of falls, tai chi training programs should be a minimum of 15 wk. Due to age-related declines in physical abilities, the duration and frequency of tai chi programs for older adults may need to be increased to derive the degree of improvement seen in younger adults.

■ *Is yoga an effective exercise mode for improving balance?*

Despite the popularity of yoga, there are a limited number of randomized control studies assessing the effects of yoga on physical fitness and motor performance. Oken and colleagues (2006) reported that a 26 wk Hatha yoga intervention produced significant improvements in the timed one-leg stand with eyes open and chair sit-and-reach test scores of healthy older men and women 65 to 85 yr. The yoga training consisted of one 90 min session per week with unsupervised home practice during the week. During the training, participants were taught 18 poses; during the exercise sessions, seven or eight poses were held for 20 to 30 sec each.

Balance Training Programs

In light of the complex nature of balance and the paucity of research studies dealing with balance assessment and training, it is not possible at this time to make firm recommendations for prescribing

Sample Multimodal Balance Training Program

Client data

Age	65 yr	Method	Tai chi, Pilates, lunges, boxing, agility training
Gender	Female		
Body weight	145 lb	Frequency	3 or more days/wk
Program goal	Improve static and dynamic balance; prevent falls	Duration	45 to 60 min per session

Exercise mode	Principles	Actions	Progressions
Tai chi	■ Increase limits of stability ■ Improve rhythmic movements ■ Increase ROM ■ Control of center of gravity	■ Prayer wheel: slow, rhythmical weight shifts coordinated with large arm circles ■ Cat walk: slow and purposeful steps, with diagonal weight shifts ■ Cloud hands: slow lateral steps with trunk vertical ■ Part the horse's mane: coordination of arms and legs while walking forward ■ Repulsing the monkey: slow, backward walking with diagonal weight shifts	Learn one movement per week starting with weight shift and leg placement, progressing to coordinated arm and torso movements.
Agility	■ Improve coordination ■ Quick change in direction ■ Increase mobility in tight spaces	■ High knee stepping with hand slapping knees ■ Lateral shuffle ■ Tire course: wide-based quick high steps and turns	Begin exercises at self-paced tempo and gradually increase speed. Progress to quick changes in direction and pace. Add dual tasks like counting aloud while moving.
Lunges	■ Stepping for postural correction ■ Increase limits of stability ■ Quick change in direction	■ Postural correction: lean until center of mass is outside base of support, requiring a step; in all directions ■ Multidirectional stepping in clockwise direction ■ Dynamic lunge walking	Start with firm surface and progress to one foot on foam pad and then both feet on foam pad. Perform exercises in well-lit room and progress to wearing sunglasses and then blindfolded. Use arms reciprocally while lunging and then progress to lifting arms overhead while holding a ball.
Boxing	■ Anticipatory postural adjustments ■ Postural corrections ■ Backward walking ■ Fast arm and foot motions	■ Jab: short, straight punch from shoulder ■ Cross: power punch with trunk rotation ■ Hook: short, lateral punch ■ Combination: two or more punches delivered quickly	Start with lateral stance to punching bag; progress to pivoting on back foot and walking backward around bag. Start at a self-paced tempo and gradually increase bursts of speed for 15 to 30 sec.
Pilates	■ Improve postural control, functional transitions, and sequencing actions	■ Sit-to-stand maneuvers ■ Floor transfers and bridging ■ Rolling prone lying ■ Bird dog, cat-camel ■ Half-kneeling to stand	Gradually improve form and speed during the movements.

a balance training program for your clients. You can use the general guidelines presented in this section as a starting point. You should individualize programs to take into account your client's needs, goals, age, and physical activity status. Keep in mind that balance training is task specific. Task-specific exercises, targeting a single, specific balance or gait impairment, are more effective than generalized exercise for improving balance. Techniques from a variety of exercise modalities can be combined to form a comprehensive balance program that challenges your client. In the sample multimodal program, exercises from tai chi, Pilates, agility training, boxing, and lunges are used to improve balance and mobility of an older adult (see p. 311).

There are many excellent resources available for designing an individualized balance training program for your clients. *ABLE Bodies Balance Training* (see Scott 2008) presents a 16 wk exercise program that safely takes older adults through the exercise progressions for improving balance and mobility, flexibility, posture and core stability, strength, and cardiorespiratory endurance. Resources for

---

GUIDELINES FOR DESIGNING BALANCE TRAINING PROGRAMS

- **Mode:** Tai chi, Pilates, yoga, static and dynamic balance training exercises, resistance training, or a combination of modes
- **Equipment:** Balance discs, foam pads and rollers, balance boards, stability balls, computerized balance systems, and force platforms to add variety and challenge to the program
- **Frequency:** Minimum of 2 or 3 days/wk
- **Time:** 45 to 60 min per session
- **Duration:** 4 to 6 mo depending on exercise mode

---

developing safe exercise programs for improving balance and functional fitness of older adults are available (see Rose 2003; Scott 2008). For ideas about incorporating Pilates and yoga workouts into balance training programs, see Isacowitz (2006) and Shaw (2009).

Sources for Equipment

Product	Supplier's contact information
Balance discs, foam pads, balance boards, stability balls	Perform Better (888) 556-7462 www.performbetter.com
NeuroCom Pro Balance Master, Equitest, Smart Balance Master	NeuroCom International, Inc. (800) 767-6744 www.resourcesonbalance.com
Biodex stability systems	Biodex Medical Systems, Inc. (800) 224-6339 www.biodex.com
Kinesthetic ability trainers	Med-Fit Systems, Inc. (800) 831-7665 www.medfitsystems.com
Pilates equipment	Balanced Body, Inc. (800) 745-2837 www.pilates.com

KEY POINTS

- Balance training is one of the top 10 trends in the fitness industry.
- Balance is an important component of the functional fitness of older adults.
- To reduce risk of falling, older adults are encouraged to engage in balance activities 3 or more days per week.
- Static balance is the ability to maintain the center of gravity within the supporting base during standing or sitting.
- Dynamic balance is the ability to maintain an upright position while the center of gravity and supporting base are moving.
- Functional balance is the ability to perform daily movement tasks requiring balance.

- The dynamic systems model of balance describes balance control as adaptive and functional.
- Visual, somatosensory, and vestibular systems interact to maintain balance.
- Body size, foot size, gender, aging, and physical activity affect balance and risk of falling.
- Indirect measures of balance are valid and reliable and useful in field and clinical settings.
- Direct measures of balance can be used to assess static and dynamic balance but are costly and therefore may be more suitable for research settings.
- Pilates, yoga, tai chi, dancing, walking, and resistance training are effective training modes for improving balance.

KEY TERMS

Learn the definition for each of the following key terms. Definitions of terms can be found in the glossary on page 411.

balance
center of pressure
computerized dynamic posturography
dynamic balance

functional balance
limits of stability
line of gravity
static balance

REVIEW QUESTIONS

In addition to being able to define each of the key terms, test your knowledge and understanding of material by answering the following review questions.

1. Why is balance testing included in functional fitness test batteries?
2. Balance is a complex construct. Identify the biomechanical, neurological, and environmental systems that influence and control balance performance.
3. Define static and dynamic balance and give examples of tests that may be used to assess these types of balance.
4. Explain how the visual, proprioceptive, and vestibular systems interact to maintain and control balance.
5. Describe how aging affects balance.
6. Identify modes of exercise that can be used to improve balance.
7. What are the center of pressure and limits of stability, and how are these measures used to assess dynamic balance?
8. Briefly describe the generic exercise prescription for improving balance of older adults.

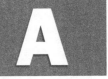
Health and Fitness Appraisal

This appendix includes questionnaires and forms that you can duplicate and use for the pretest health screening of your clients. The PAR-Q (appendix A.1) is used to identify individuals who need medical clearance from their physicians before taking any physical fitness tests or starting an exercise program. The Medical History Questionnaire (appendix A.2) is used to obtain a personal and family health history for your client. As part of the pretest health screening, ask your clients if they have any of the conditions or symptoms listed in the Checklist for Signs and Symptoms of Disease (appendix A.3). The

PARmed-X (appendix A.4) may be used by physicians to assess and convey medical clearance for physical activity participation of your clients.

You can obtain a lifestyle profile for your clients by using either the Lifestyle Evaluation form or the Fantastic Lifestyle Checklist provided in appendix A.5. Be sure that each participant signs the Informed Consent (appendix A.6) before conducting any physical fitness tests or allowing your client to engage in an exercise program. Appendix A.7 includes Web sites for selected professional organizations and institutes.

Physical Activity Readiness
Questionnaire - PAR-Q
(revised 2002)

PAR-Q & YOU
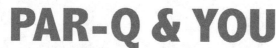

(A Questionnaire for People Aged 15 to 69)

Regular physical activity is fun and healthy, and increasingly more people are starting to become more active every day. Being more active is very safe for most people. However, some people should check with their doctor before they start becoming much more physically active.

If you are planning to become much more physically active than you are now, start by answering the seven questions in the box below. If you are between the ages of 15 and 69, the PAR-Q will tell you if you should check with your doctor before you start. If you are over 69 years of age, and you are not used to being very active, check with your doctor.

Common sense is your best guide when you answer these questions. Please read the questions carefully and answer each one honestly: check YES or NO.

YES	NO		
☐	☐	1.	Has your doctor ever said that you have a heart condition <u>and</u> that you should only do physical activity recommended by a doctor?
☐	☐	2.	Do you feel pain in your chest when you do physical activity?
☐	☐	3.	In the past month, have you had chest pain when you were not doing physical activity?
☐	☐	4.	Do you lose your balance because of dizziness or do you ever lose consciousness?
☐	☐	5.	Do you have a bone or joint problem (for example, back, knee or hip) that could be made worse by a change in your physical activity?
☐	☐	6.	Is your doctor currently prescribing drugs (for example, water pills) for your blood pressure or heart condition?
☐	☐	7.	Do you know of <u>any other reason</u> why you should not do physical activity?

If

you

answered

YES to one or more questions

Talk with your doctor by phone or in person BEFORE you start becoming much more physically active or BEFORE you have a fitness appraisal. Tell your doctor about the PAR-Q and which questions you answered YES.

- You may be able to do any activity you want — as long as you start slowly and build up gradually. Or, you may need to restrict your activities to those which are safe for you. Talk with your doctor about the kinds of activities you wish to participate in and follow his/her advice.
- Find out which community programs are safe and helpful for you.

NO to all questions

If you answered NO honestly to <u>all</u> PAR-Q questions, you can be reasonably sure that you can:
- start becoming much more physically active — begin slowly and build up gradually. This is the safest and easiest way to go.
- take part in a fitness appraisal — this is an excellent way to determine your basic fitness so that you can plan the best way for you to live actively. It is also highly recommended that you have your blood pressure evaluated. If your reading is over 144/94, talk with your doctor before you start becoming much more physically active.

DELAY BECOMING MUCH MORE ACTIVE:
- if you are not feeling well because of a temporary illness such as a cold or a fever — wait until you feel better; or
- if you are or may be pregnant — talk to your doctor before you start becoming more active.

PLEASE NOTE: If your health changes so that you then answer YES to any of the above questions, tell your fitness or health professional. Ask whether you should change your physical activity plan.

<u>Informed Use of the PAR-Q</u>: The Canadian Society for Exercise Physiology, Health Canada, and their agents assume no liability for persons who undertake physical activity, and if in doubt after completing this questionnaire, consult your doctor prior to physical activity.

No changes permitted. You are encouraged to photocopy the PAR-Q but only if you use the entire form.

NOTE: If the PAR-Q is being given to a person before he or she participates in a physical activity program or a fitness appraisal, this section may be used for legal or administrative purposes.

"I have read, understood and completed this questionnaire. Any questions I had were answered to my full satisfaction."

NAME _____

SIGNATURE _____ DATE _____

SIGNATURE OF PARENT _____ WITNESS _____
or GUARDIAN (for participants under the age of majority)

> **Note: This physical activity clearance is valid for a maximum of 12 months from the date it is completed and becomes invalid if your condition changes so that you would answer YES to any of the seven questions.**

CSEP
SCPE © Canadian Society for Exercise Physiology   Supported by: ▮✦ Health   Santé
                                                                    Canada   Canada

continued on other side...

...continued from other side

PAR-Q & YOU

Physical Activity Readiness
Questionnaire - PAR-Q
(revised 2002)

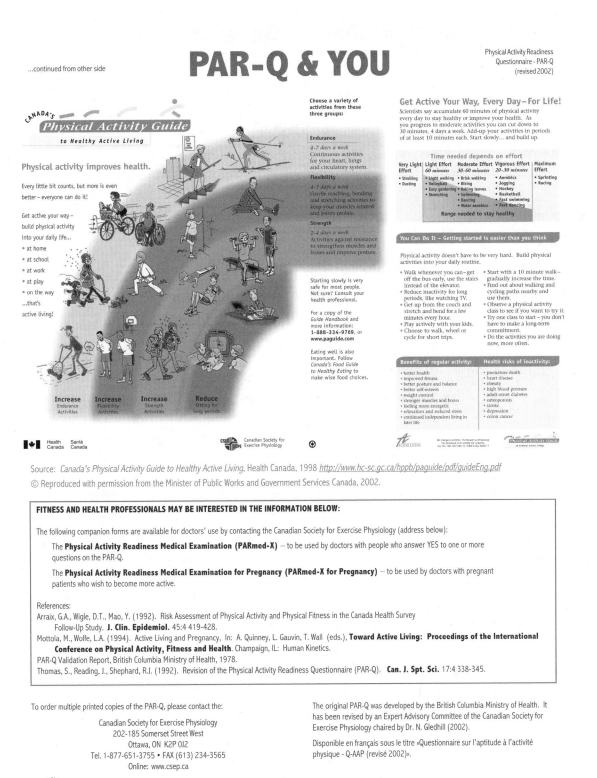

Source: *Canada's Physical Activity Guide to Healthy Active Living*, Health Canada, 1998 http://www.hc-sc.gc.ca/hppb/paguide/pdf/guideEng.pdf
© Reproduced with permission from the Minister of Public Works and Government Services Canada, 2002.

FITNESS AND HEALTH PROFESSIONALS MAY BE INTERESTED IN THE INFORMATION BELOW:

The following companion forms are available for doctors' use by contacting the Canadian Society for Exercise Physiology (address below):

The **Physical Activity Readiness Medical Examination (PARmed-X)** — to be used by doctors with people who answer YES to one or more questions on the PAR-Q.

The **Physical Activity Readiness Medical Examination for Pregnancy (PARmed-X for Pregnancy)** — to be used by doctors with pregnant patients who wish to become more active.

References:
Arraix, G.A., Wigle, D.T., Mao, Y. (1992). Risk Assessment of Physical Activity and Physical Fitness in the Canada Health Survey
    Follow-Up Study. **J. Clin. Epidemiol.** 45:4 419-428.
Mottola, M., Wolfe, L.A. (1994). Active Living and Pregnancy, In: A. Quinney, L. Gauvin, T. Wall (eds.), **Toward Active Living: Proceedings of the International**
    Conference on Physical Activity, Fitness and Health. Champaign, IL: Human Kinetics.
PAR-Q Validation Report, British Columbia Ministry of Health, 1978.
Thomas, S., Reading, J., Shephard, R.J. (1992). Revision of the Physical Activity Readiness Questionnaire (PAR-Q). **Can. J. Spt. Sci.** 17:4 338-345.

To order multiple printed copies of the PAR-Q, please contact the:

Canadian Society for Exercise Physiology
202-185 Somerset Street West
Ottawa, ON K2P 0J2
Tel. 1-877-651-3755 • FAX (613) 234-3565
Online: www.csep.ca

The original PAR-Q was developed by the British Columbia Ministry of Health. It has been revised by an Expert Advisory Committee of the Canadian Society for Exercise Physiology chaired by Dr. N. Gledhill (2002).

Disponible en français sous le titre «Questionnaire sur l'aptitude à l'activité physique - Q-AAP (revisé 2002)».

CSEP SCPE © Canadian Society for Exercise Physiology   Supported by: Health Canada Santé Canada

Source: Physical Activity Readiness Questionnaire (PAR-Q) © 2002. Reprinted with permission from the Canadian Society for Exercise Physiology. http://www.csep.ca/forms.asp

Medical History Questionnaire

Demographic Information

Last name	First name	Middle initial

Date of birth	Sex	Home phone

Address	City, State	Zip code

Work phone	Family physician	

Section A

1. When was the last time you had a physical examination?

2. If you are allergic to any medications, foods, or other substances, please name them.

3. If you have been told that you have any chronic or serious illnesses, please list them.

4. Give the following information pertaining to the last 3 times you have been hospitalized. *Note:* Women, do not list normal pregnancies.

	Hospitalization 1	Hospitalization 2	Hospitalization 3
Reason for hospitalization	_____	_____	_____
Month and year of hospitalization	_____	_____	_____
Hospital	_____	_____	_____
City and state	_____	_____	_____

Section B

During the past 12 months

1. Has a physician prescribed any form of medication for you?	❏ Yes	❏ No
2. Has your weight fluctuated more than a few pounds?	❏ Yes	❏ No
3. Did you attempt to bring about this weight change through diet or exercise?	❏ Yes	❏ No
4. Have you experienced any faintness, light-headedness, or blackouts?	❏ Yes	❏ No
5. Have you occasionally had trouble sleeping?	❏ Yes	❏ No
6. Have you experienced any blurred vision?	❏ Yes	❏ No
7. Have you had any severe headaches?	❏ Yes	❏ No
8. Have you experienced chronic morning cough?	❏ Yes	❏ No
9. Have you experienced any temporary change in your speech pattern, such as slurring or loss of speech?	❏ Yes	❏ No
10. Have you felt unusually nervous or anxious for no apparent reason?	❏ Yes	❏ No
11. Have you experienced unusual heartbeats such as skipped beats or palpitations?	❏ Yes	❏ No
12. Have you experienced periods in which your heart felt as though it were racing for no apparent reason?	❏ Yes	❏ No

From Vivian H. Heyward, 2010, *Advanced Fitness Assessment and Exercise Prescription*, 6th ed. (Champaign, IL: Human Kinetics).

At present

1. Do you experience shortness or loss of breath while walking with others your own age?　☐ Yes ☐ No

2. Do you experience sudden tingling, numbness, or loss of feeling in your arms, hands, legs, feet, or face?　☐ Yes ☐ No

3. Have you ever noticed that your hands or feet sometimes feel cooler than other parts of your body?　☐ Yes ☐ No

4. Do you experience swelling of your feet and ankles?　☐ Yes ☐ No

5. Do you get pains or cramps in your legs?　☐ Yes ☐ No

6. Do you experience any pain or discomfort in your chest?　☐ Yes ☐ No

7. Do you experience any pressure or heaviness in your chest?　☐ Yes ☐ No

8. Have you ever been told that your blood pressure was abnormal?　☐ Yes ☐ No

9. Have you ever been told that your serum cholesterol or triglyceride level was high?　☐ Yes ☐ No

10. Do you have diabetes?　☐ Yes ☐ No

    If yes, how is it controlled?

    ☐ Dietary means　　☐ Insulin injection

    ☐ Oral medication　　☐ Uncontrolled

11. How often would you characterize your stress level as being high?

    ☐ Occasionally　☐ Frequently　☐ Constantly

12. Have you ever been told that you have any of the following illnesses?　☐ Yes ☐ No

    ☐ Myocardial infarction　☐ Arteriosclerosis　☐ Heart disease　☐ Thyroid disease

    ☐ Coronary thrombosis　☐ Rheumatic heart　☐ Heart attack　☐ Heart valve disease

    ☐ Coronary occlusion　☐ Heart failure　☐ Heart murmer

    ☐ Heart block　☐ Aneurysm　☐ Angina

13. Have you ever had any of the following medical procedures?　☐ Yes ☐ No

    ☐ Heart surgery　　☐ Pacemaker implant

    ☐ Cardiac catheterization　☐ Defibrilator

    ☐ Coronary angioplasty　☐ Heart transplantation

Section C

Has any member of your immediate family been treated for or suspected to have had any of these conditions? Please identify their relationship to you (father, mother, sister, brother, etc.).

A. Diabetes

B. Heart disease

C. Stroke

D. High blood pressure

From Vivian H. Heyward, 2010, *Advanced Fitness Assessment and Exercise Prescription*, 6th ed. (Champaign, IL: Human Kinetics).

Checklist for Signs and Symptoms of Disease

Instructions: Ask your clients if they have any of the following conditions and risk factors. If so, refer them to their physicians to obtain a signed medical clearance prior to any exercise testing or participation. See the glossary on p. 411 for definitions of terms.

Client's name _____ Date _____

Condition	Yes	No	Comments
Cardiovascular			
Hypertension			
Hypercholesterolemia			
Heart murmurs			
Myocardial infarction (heart attack)			
Fainting/dizziness			
Claudication			
Chest pain			
Palpitations			
Ischemia			
Tachycardia (rhythm disturbances)			
Ankle edema			
Stroke			
Pulmonary			
Asthma			
Bronchitis			
Emphysema			
Nocturnal dyspnea			
Coughing up blood			
Exercise-induced asthma			
Breathlessness during or after mild exertion			
Metabolic			
Diabetes			
Obesity			

From Vivian H. Heyward, 2010, *Advanced Fitness Assessment and Exercise Prescription*, 6th ed. (Champaign, IL: Human Kinetics).

Condition	Yes	No	Comments
Metabolic (*continued*)			
Glucose intolerance			
McArdle's syndrome			
Hypoglycemia			
Thyroid disease			
Cirrhosis			
Musculoskeletal			
Osteoporosis			
Osteoarthritis			
Low back pain			
Prosthesis			
Muscular atrophy			
Swollen joints			
Orthopedic pain			
Artificial joints			
Risk factors*			
Male older than 45 yr			
Female older than 55 yr, or had hysterectomy, or are postmenopausal			
Smoking or quit smoking within previous 6 mo			
Blood pressure > 140/90 mmHg			
Don't know blood pressure			
Taking blood pressure medication			
Blood cholesterol > 200 mg · dl^{-1}			
Do not know cholesterol level			
Have close relative who had heart attack or heart surgery before age 55 (father or brother) or age 65 (mother or sister)			
Physically inactive (<30 min of physical activity more than 4 days/wk)			
Overweight by more than 20 lb (9 kg)			

*If you have two or more risk factors, you should consult your physician before engaging in exercise.

From Vivian H. Heyward, 2010, *Advanced Fitness Assessment and Exercise Prescription,* 6th ed. (Champaign, IL: Human Kinetics).

PARmed-X PHYSICAL ACTIVITY READINESS MEDICAL EXAMINATION

The PARmed-X is a physical activity-specific checklist to be used by a physician with patients who have had positive responses to the Physical Activity Readiness Questionnaire (PAR-Q). In addition, the Conveyance/Referral Form in the PARmed-X can be used to convey clearance for physical activity participation, or to make a referral to a medically-supervised exercise program.

Regular physical activity is fun and healthy, and increasingly more people are starting to become more active every day. Being more active is very safe for most people. The PAR-Q by itself provides adequate screening for the majority of people. However, some individuals may require a medical evaluation and specific advice (exercise prescription) due to one or more positive responses to the PAR-Q.

Following the participant's evaluation by a physician, a physical activity plan should be devised in consultation with a physical activity professional (CSEP-Professional Fitness & Lifestyle Consultant or CSEP-Exercise Therapist™). To assist in this, the following instructions are provided:

PAGE 1: • Sections A, B, C, and D should be completed by the participant BEFORE the examination by the physician. The bottom section is to be completed by the examining physician.

PAGES 2 & 3: • A checklist of medical conditions requiring special consideration and management.

PAGE 4: • Physical Activity & Lifestyle Advice for people who do not require specific instructions or prescribed exercise.

• Physical Activity Readiness Conveyance/Referral Form - an optional tear-off tab for the physician to convey clearance for physical activity participation, or to make a referral to a medically-supervised exercise program.

This section to be completed by the participant

A PERSONAL INFORMATION:

NAME _____

ADDRESS _____

_____

TELEPHONE _____

BIRTHDATE _____ GENDER _____

MEDICAL No. _____

B PAR-Q: Please indicate the PAR-Q questions to which you answered YES

❑	Q 1	Heart condition
❑	Q 2	Chest pain during activity
❑	Q 3	Chest pain at rest
❑	Q 4	Loss of balance, dizziness
❑	Q 5	Bone or joint problem
❑	Q 6	Blood pressure or heart drugs
❑	Q 7	Other reason:

_____

C RISK FACTORS FOR CARDIOVASCULAR DISEASE:
Check all that apply

❑ Less than 30 minutes of moderate physical activity most days of the week.

❑ Currently smoker (tobacco smoking 1 or more times per week).

❑ High blood pressure reported by physician after repeated measurements.

❑ High cholesterol level reported by physician.

❑ Excessive accumulation of fat around waist.

❑ Family history of heart disease.

Please note: *Many of these risk factors are modifiable. Please refer to page 4 and discuss with your physician.*

D PHYSICAL ACTIVITY INTENTIONS:

What physical activity do you intend to do?

_____

_____

_____

This section to be completed by the examining physician

Physical Exam:

Ht	Wt	BP	i)	/
		BP	ii)	/

Conditions limiting physical activity:

❑ Cardiovascular   ❑ Respiratory   ❑ Other

❑ Musculoskeletal   ❑ Abdominal

Tests required:

❑ ECG   ❑ Exercise Test   ❑ X-Ray

❑ Blood   ❑ Urinalysis   ❑ Other

Physical Activity Readiness Conveyance/Referral:

Based upon a current review of health status, I recommend:

Further Information:
❑ Attached
❑ To be forwarded
❑ Available on request

❑ No physical activity

❑ Only a medically-supervised exercise program until further medical clearance

❑ Progressive physical activity:

❑ with avoidance of: _____

❑ with inclusion of: _____

❑ under the supervision of a CSEP-Professional Fitness & Lifestyle Consultant or CSEP-Exercise Therapist™

❑ Unrestricted physical activity–start slowly and build up gradually

CSEP/SCPE © Canadian Society for Exercise Physiology

Supported by: Health Canada / Santé Canada

1

PARmed-X

PHYSICAL ACTIVITY READINESS MEDICAL EXAMINATION

Following is a checklist of medical conditions for which a degree of precaution and/or special advice should be considered for those who answered "YES" to one or more questions on the PAR-Q, and people over the age of 69. Conditions are grouped by system. Three categories of precautions are provided. Comments under Advice are general, since details and alternatives require clinical judgement in each individual instance.

	Absolute Contraindications	Relative Contraindications	Special Prescriptive Conditions	ADVICE
	Permanent restriction or temporary restriction until condition is treated, stable, and/or past acute phase.	Highly variable. Value of exercise testing and/or program may exceed risk. Activity may be restricted. Desirable to maximize control of condition. Direct or indirect medical supervision of exercise program may be desirable.	Individualized prescriptive advice generally appropriate: • limitations imposed; and/or • special exercises prescribed. May require medical monitoring and/or initial supervision in exercise program.	
Cardiovascular	❏ aortic aneurysm (dissecting) ❏ aortic stenosis (severe) ❏ congestive heart failure ❏ crescendo angina ❏ myocardial infarction (acute) ❏ myocarditis (active or recent) ❏ pulmonary or systemic embolism—acute ❏ thrombophlebitis ❏ ventricular tachycardia and other dangerous dysrhythmias (e.g., multi-focal ventricular activity)	❏ aortic stenosis (moderate) ❏ subaortic stenosis (severe) ❏ marked cardiac enlargement ❏ supraventricular dysrhythmias (uncontrolled or high rate) ❏ ventricular ectopic activity (repetitive or frequent) ❏ ventricular aneurysm ❏ hypertension—untreated or uncontrolled severe (systemic or pulmonary) ❏ hypertrophic cardiomyopathy ❏ compensated congestive heart failure	❏ aortic (or pulmonary) stenosis—mild angina pectoris and other manifestations of coronary insufficiency (e.g., post-acute infarct) ❏ cyanotic heart disease ❏ shunts (intermittent or fixed) ❏ conduction disturbances • complete AV block • left BBB • Wolff-Parkinson-White syndrome ❏ dysrhythmias—controlled ❏ fixed rate pacemakers	• clinical exercise test may be warranted in selected cases, for specific determination of functional capacity and limitations and precautions (if any). • slow progression of exercise to levels based on test performance and individual tolerance. • consider individual need for initial conditioning program under medical supervision (indirect or direct).
			❏ intermittent claudication	progressive exercise to tolerance
			❏ hypertension: systolic 160-180; diastolic 105+	progressive exercise; care with medications (serum electrolytes; post-exercise syncope; etc.)
Infections	❏ acute infectious disease (regardless of etiology)	❏ subacute/chronic/recurrent infectious diseases (e.g., malaria, others)	❏ chronic infections ❏ HIV	variable as to condition
Metabolic		❏ uncontrolled metabolic disorders (diabetes mellitus, thyrotoxicosis, myxedema)	❏ renal, hepatic & other metabolic insufficiency	variable as to status
			❏ obesity ❏ single kidney	dietary moderation, and initial light exercises with slow progression (walking, swimming, cycling)
Pregnancy		❏ complicated pregnancy (e.g., toxemia, hemorrhage, incompetent cervix, etc.)	❏ advanced pregnancy (late 3rd trimester)	refer to the "PARmed-X for PREGNANCY"

References:

Arraix, G.A., Wigle, D.T., Mao, Y. (1992). Risk Assessment of Physical Activity and Physical Fitness in the Canada Health Survey Follow-Up Study. **J. Clin. Epidemiol.** 45:4 419-428.

Mottola, M., Wolfe, L.A. (1994). Active Living and Pregnancy, In: A. Quinney, L. Gauvin, T. Wall (eds.), **Toward Active Living: Proceedings of the International Conference on Physical Activity, Fitness and Health**. Champaign, IL: Human Kinetics.

PAR-Q Validation Report, British Columbia Ministry of Health, 1978.

Thomas, S., Reading, J., Shephard, R.J. (1992). Revision of the Physical Activity Readiness Questionnaire (PAR-Q). **Can. J. Spt. Sci.** 17: 4 338-345.

The PAR-Q and PARmed-X were developed by the British Columbia Ministry of Health. They have been revised by an Expert Advisory Committee of the Canadian Society for Exercise Physiology chaired by Dr. N. Gledhill (2002).

No changes permitted. You are encouraged to photocopy the PARmed-X, but only if you use the entire form.

Disponible en français sous le titre
«Évaluation médicale de l'aptitude à l'activité physique (X-AAP)»

Continued on page 3...

2

	Special Prescriptive Conditions	**ADVICE**
Lung	❑ chronic pulmonary disorders	special relaxation and breathing exercises
	❑ obstructive lung disease	breath control during endurance exercises to tolerance; avoid polluted air
	❑ asthma	
	❑ exercise-induced bronchospasm	avoid hyperventilation during exercise; avoid extremely cold conditions; warm up adequately; utilize appropriate medication.
Musculoskeletal	❑ low back conditions (pathological, functional)	avoid or minimize exercise that precipitates or exasperates e.g., forced extreme flexion, extension, and violent twisting; correct posture, proper back exercises
	❑ arthritis—acute (infective, rheumatoid; gout)	treatment, plus judicious blend of rest, splinting and gentle movement
	❑ arthritis—subacute	progressive increase of active exercise therapy
	❑ arthritis—chronic (osteoarthritis and above conditions)	maintenance of mobility and strength; non-weightbearing exercises to minimize joint trauma (e.g., cycling, aquatic activity, etc.)
	❑ orthopaedic	highly variable and individualized
	❑ hernia	minimize straining and isometrics; stregthen abdominal muscles
	❑ osteoporosis or low bone density	avoid exercise with high risk for fracture such as push-ups, curl-ups, vertical jump and trunk forward flexion; engage in low-impact weight-bearing activities and resistance training
CNS	❑ convulsive disorder not completely controlled by medication	minimize or avoid exercise in hazardous environments and/or exercising alone (e.g.. swimming, mountainclimbing, etc.)
	❑ recent concussion	thorough examination if history of two concussions; review for discontinuation of contact sport if three concussions, depending on duration of unconsciousness, retrograde amnesia, persistent headaches, and other objective evidence of cerebral damage
Blood	❑ anemia—severe (< 10 Gm/dl)	control preferred; exercise as tolerated
	❑ electrolyte disturbances	
Medications	❑ antianginal ❑ antiarrhythmic ❑ antihypertensive ❑ anticonvulsant ❑ beta-blockers ❑ digitalis preparations ❑ diuretics ❑ ganglionic blockers ❑ others	NOTE: consider underlying condition. Potential for: exertional syncope, electrolyte imbalance, bradycardia, dysrhythmias, impaired coordination and reaction time, heat intolerance. May alter resting and exercise ECG's and exercise test performance.
Other	❑ post-exercise syncope	moderate program
	❑ heat intolerance	prolong cool-down with light activities; avoid exercise in extreme heat
	❑ temporary minor illness	postpone until recovered
	❑ cancer	if potential metastases, test by cycle ergometry, consider non-weight bearing exercises; exercise at lower end of prescriptive range (40-65% of heart rate reserve), depending on condition and recent treatment (radiation, chemotherapy); monitor hemoglobin and lymphocyte counts; add dynamic lifting exercise to strengthen muscles, using machines rather than weights.

*Refer to special publications for elaboration as required

The following companion forms are available online: http://www.csep.ca/forms.asp

The **Physical Activity Readiness Questionnaire (PAR-Q)** - a questionnaire for people aged 15-69 to complete before becoming much more physically active.

The **Physical Activity Readiness Medical Examination for Pregnancy (PARmed-X for PREGNANCY)** - to be used by physicians with pregnant patients who wish to become more physically active.

For more information, please contact the:

Canadian Society for Exercise Physiology
202 - 185 Somerset St. West
Ottawa, ON K2P 0J2
Tel. 1-877-651-3755 • FAX (613) 234-3565 • Online: www.csep.ca

---

Note to physical activity professionals...

It is a prudent practice to retain the completed Physical Activity Readiness Conveyance/Referral Form in the participant's file.

CSEP SCPE © Canadian Society for Exercise Physiology

Supported by: Health Canada Santé Canada

Continued on page 4...

3

PARmed-X PHYSICAL ACTIVITY READINESS MEDICAL EXAMINATION

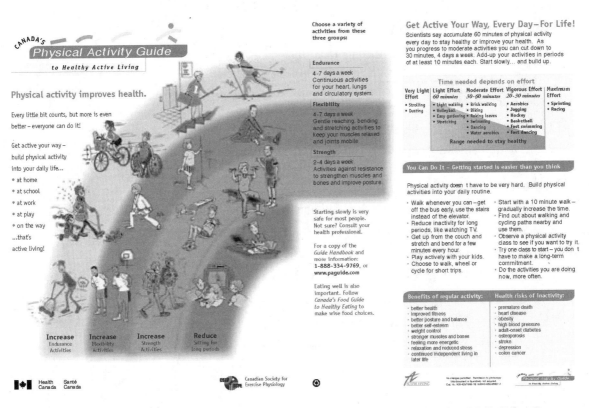

Source: Canada's Physical Activity Guide to Healthy Active Living, Health Canada, 1998 http://www.hc-sc.gc.ca/hppb/paguide/pdf/guideEng.pdf

© Reproduced with permission from the Minister of Public Works and Government Services Canada, 2002.

PARmed-X Physical Activity Readiness Conveyance/Referral Form

Based upon a current review of the health status of _____, I recommend:

❏ No physical activity

❏ Only a medically-supervised exercise program until further medical clearance

❏ Progressive physical activity

    ❏ with avoidance of: _____

    ❏ with inclusion of: _____

    ❏ under the supervision of a CSEP-Professional Fitness &

    Lifestyle Consultant or CSEP-Exercise Therapist™

❏ Unrestricted physical activity — start slowly and build up gradually

Further Information:
    ❏ Attached
    ❏ To be forwarded.
    ❏ Available on request

Physician/clinic stamp:

_____ M.D.

_____ 20_____
            (date)

4

NOTE: This physical activity clearance is valid for a maximum of six months from the date it is completed and becomes invalid if your medical condition becomes worse.

Source: Physical Activity Readiness Medical Examination (PARmed-X) © 2002. Reprinted with permission from the Canadian Society for Exercise Physiology. http://www.csep.ca/forms.asp.

Lifestyle Evaluation

Smoking habits

1. Have you ever smoked cigarettes, cigars, or a pipe?   ❏ Yes   ❏ No

2. Do you smoke presently?   ❏ Yes   ❏ No

   Cigarettes _____ a day

   Cigars _____ a day

   Pipefuls _____ a day

3. At what age did you start smoking? _____ years

4. If you have quit smoking, when did you quit? _____

Drinking habits

1. During the past month, how many days did you drink alcoholic beverages? _____

2. During the past month, how many times did you have 5 or more drinks per occasion?
   _____

3. On average, how many glasses of beer, wine, or highballs do you consume a week?

   Beer _____ glasses or cans

   Wine _____ glasses

   Highballs _____ glasses

   Other _____ glasses

Exercise habits

1. Do you exercise vigorously on a regular basis?   ❏ Yes   ❏ No

2. What activities do you engage in on a regular basis?

3. If you walk, run, or jog, what is the average number of miles you cover each workout?
   _____ miles

4. How many minutes on the average is each of your exercise workouts? _____ minutes

5. How many workouts a week do you participate in on average? _____ workouts

6. Is your occupation?

   _____ Inactive (e.g., desk job)

   _____ Light work (e.g., housework, light carpentry)

   _____ Heavy work (e.g., heavy carpentry, lifting)

From Vivian H. Heyward, 2010, *Advanced Fitness Assessment and Exercise Prescription*, 6th ed. (Champaign, IL: Human Kinetics).

APPENDIX A.5

7. Check those activities that you would prefer in a regular exercise program for yourself:

_____ Walking, running, or jogging _____ Handball, racquetball, or squash

_____ Stationary running _____ Basketball

_____ Jumping rope _____ Swimming

_____ Bicycling _____ Tennis

_____ Stationary cycling _____ Aerobic dance

_____ Step aerobics _____ Stair-climbing

  _____ Other (specify)

Dietary habits

1. What is your current weight? _____ lb _____ kg height? _____ in. _____ cm

2. What would you like to weigh? _____ lb _____ kg

3. What is the most you ever weighed as an adult? _____ lb _____ kg

4. What is the least you ever weighed as an adult? _____ lb _____ kg

5. What weight-loss methods have you tried? _____

_____

6. Which do you eat regularly?

❏ Breakfast ❏ Midafternoon snack

❏ Midmorning snack ❏ Dinner

❏ Lunch ❏ After-dinner snack

7. How often do you eat out each week? _____ times

8. What size portions do you normally have?

❏ Small ❏ Moderate ❏ Large ❏ Extra large ❏ Uncertain

9. How often do you eat more than one serving?

❏ Always ❏ Usually ❏ Sometimes ❏ Never

10. How long does it usually take you to eat a meal? _____ minutes

11. Do you eat while doing other activities (e.g., watching TV, reading, working)? _____

12. When you snack, how many times a week do you eat the following?

Cookies, cake, pie _____ Candy _____ Diet soda _____

Soft drinks _____ Doughnuts _____ Fruit _____

Milk or milk beverage _____ Potato chips, pretzels, etc. _____

Peanuts or other nuts _____ Ice cream _____

Cheese and crackers _____ Other _____

13. How often do you eat dessert? _____ times a day _____ times a week

14. What dessert do you eat most often? _____

15. How often do you eat fried foods? _____ times a week

16. Do you salt your food at the table? ❏ Yes ❏ No

❏ Before tasting it ❏ After tasting it

From Vivian H. Heyward, 2010, *Advanced Fitness Assessment and Exercise Prescription*, 6th ed. (Champaign, IL: Human Kinetics).

Fantastic Lifestyle Checklist

INSTRUCTIONS: Unless otherwise specified, place an 'X' beside the box which best describes your behaviour or situation in the past month. Explanations of questions and scoring are provided on the next page.

FAMILY FRIENDS	I have someone to talk to about things that are important to me	almost never	seldom	some of the time	fairly often	almost always
	I give and receive affection	almost never	seldom	some of the time	fairly often	almost always
ACTIVITY	I am vigorously active for at least 30 minutes per day e.g., running, cycling, etc.	less than once/week	1-2 times/week	3 times/week	4 times/week	5 or more times/week
	I am moderately active (gardening, climbing stairs, walking, housework)	less than once/week	1-2 times/week	3 times/week	4 times/week	5 or more times/week
NUTRITION	I eat a balanced diet (see explanation)	almost never	seldom	some of the time	fairly often	almost always
	I often eat excess 1) sugar, or 2) salt, or 3) animal fats, or 4) junk foods.	four of these	three of these	two of these	one of these	none of these
	I am within ____ kg of my healthy weight	not within 8 kg	8 kg (20 lbs)	6 kg (15 lbs)	4 kg (10 lbs)	2 kg (5 lbs)
TOBACCO TOXICS	I smoke tobacco	more than 10 times/week	1 - 10 times/week	none in the past 6 months	none in the past year	none in the past 5 years
	I use drugs such as marijuana, cocaine	sometimes				never
	I overuse prescribed or 'over the counter' drugs	almost daily	fairly often	only occasionally	almost never	never
	I drink caffeine-containing coffee, tea, or cola	more than 10/day	7-10/day	3-6/day	1-2/day	never
ALCOHOL	My average alcohol intake per week is____ (see explanation)	more than 20 drinks	13-20 drinks	11-12 drinks	8-10 drinks	0-7 drinks
	I drink more than four drinks on an occasion	almost daily	fairly often	only occasionally	almost never	never
	I drive after drinking	sometimes				never
SLEEP SEATBELTS STRESS SAFE SEX	I sleep well and feel rested	almost never	seldom	some of the time	fairly often	almost always
	I use seatbelts	never	seldom	some of the time	most of the time	always
	I am able to cope with the stresses in my life	almost never	seldom	some of the time	fairly often	almost always
	I relax and enjoy leisure time	almost never	seldom	some of the time	fairly often	almost always
	I practice safe sex (see explanation)	almost never	seldom	some of the time	fairly often	always
TYPE of behaviour	I seem to be in a hurry	almost always	fairly often	some of the time	seldom	almost never
	I feel angry or hostile	almost always	fairly often	some of the time	seldom	almost never
INSIGHT	I am a postive or optimistic thinker	almost never	seldom	some of the time	fairly often	almost always
	I feel tense or uptight	almost always	fairly often	some of the time	seldom	almost never
	I feel sad or depressed	almost always	fairly often	some of the time	seldom	almost never
CAREER	I am satisfied with my job or role	almost never	seldom	some of the time	fairly often	almost always

STEP 1 Total the X's in each column → ☐ ☐ ☐ ☐ ☐

STEP 2 Multiply the totals by the numbers indicated (write your answer in the box below) → 0 x 1 x 2 x 3 x 4

STEP 3 Add your scores across the bottom for your grand total → ☐ + ☐ + ☐ + ☐ = ☐

Grand total
(see explantion)

From Vivian H. Heyward, 2010, *Advanced Fitness Assessment and Exercise Prescription,* 6th ed. (Champaign, IL: Human Kinetics). Adapted, by permission, from D. Wilson, 1998, *Fantastic lifestyle assessment.*

A BALANCED DIET:

According to Canada's Food Guide to Healthy Eating (for people four years and over):

Different People Need Different Amounts of Food

The amount of food you need every day from the 4 food groups and other foods depends on your age, body size, activity level, whether you are male or female and if your are pregnant or breast feeding. That's why the Food Guide gives a lower and higher number of servings for each food group. For example, young children can choose the lower number of servings, while male teenagers can select the higher number. Most other people can choose servings somewhere in between.

Grain Products	Vegetables & Fruit	Milk Products	Meat & Alternatives	Other Foods
Choose whole grain and enriched products more often.	Choose dark green and orange vegetables more often.	Choose lower fat milk products more often.	Choose leaner meats, poultry and fish, as well as dried peas, beans and lentils more often.	Taste and enjoyment can also come from other foods and beverages that are not part of the 4 food groups. Some of these are higher in fat or calories, so use these foods in moderation.

recommended number of servings per day:

5-12	5-10	Children 4-9 years: 2-3 Youth 10-16 years: 3-4 Adults: 2-4 Pregnant and breast-feeding women: 3-4	2-3	

▼ ALCOHOL INTAKE:

1 drink equals:

		Canadian	Metric	U.S.
1 bottle of beer	5% alcohol	12 oz.	340.8 ml	10 oz.
1 glass wine	12% alcohol	5 oz.	142 ml	4.5 oz
1 shot spirits	40% alcohol	1.5 oz	42.6 ml	1.25 oz.

▼ SAFE SEX:

Refers to the use of methods of preventing infection or conception.

WHAT DOES THE SCORE MEAN?

➡	85-100	70-84	55-69	35-54	0-34
	EXCELLENT	VERY GOOD	GOOD	FAIR	NEEDS IMPROVEMENT

NOTE: A low total score does not mean that you have failed. There is always the chance to change your lifestyle — starting now. Look at the areas where you scored a 0 or 1 and decide which areas you want to work on first.

TIPS:

1. Don't try to change all the areas at once. This will be too overwhelming for you.

2. Writing down your proposed changes and your overall goal will help you to succeed.

3. Make changes in small steps towards the overall goal.

4. Enlist the help of a friend to make similar changes and/or to support you in your attempts.

5. Congratulate yourself for achieving each step. Give yourself appropriate rewards.

6. Ask your physical activity professional (CSEP-Professional Fitness and Lifestyle Consultant), family physician, nurse or health department for more information on any of these areas.

Adapted, by permission, from D. Wilson, 1998, *Fantastic lifestyle assessment*.

Informed Consent

In order to assess cardiovascular function, body composition, and other physical fitness components, the undersigned hereby voluntarily consents to engage in one or more of the following tests (check the appropriate boxes):

- ❏ Graded exercise stress test
- ❏ Body composition tests
- ❏ Muscle fitness tests
- ❏ Flexibility tests
- ❏ Balance tests

Explanation of the tests

The graded exercise test is performed on a cycle ergometer or motor-driven treadmill. The workload is increased every few minutes until exhaustion or until other symptoms dictate that we terminate the test. You may stop the test at any time because of fatigue or discomfort.

The underwater weighing procedure involves being completely submerged in a tank or tub after fully exhaling the air from your lungs. You will be submerged for 3 to 5 seconds while we measure your underwater weight. This test provides an accurate assessment of your body composition.

For muscle fitness testing, you lift weights for a number of repetitions using barbells or exercise machines. These tests assess the strength and endurance of the major muscle groups in the body.

For evaluation of flexibility, you perform a number of tests. During these tests, we measure the range of motion in your joints.

For balance tests, we will be measuring the amount of time you can maintain certain stances or the distance you are able to reach without losing balance.

Risks and discomforts

During the graded exercise test, certain changes may occur. These changes include abnormal blood pressure responses, fainting, irregularities in heartbeat, and heart attack. Every effort is made to minimize these occurrences. Emergency equipment and trained personnel are available to deal with these situations if they occur.

You may experience some discomfort during the underwater weighing, especially after you expire all the air from your lungs. However, this discomfort is momentary, lasting only 3 to 5 seconds. If this test causes you too much discomfort, an alternative procedure (e.g., skinfold or bioelectrical impedance test) can be used to estimate your body composition.

There is a slight possibility of pulling a muscle or spraining a ligament during the muscle fitness and flexibility testing. In addition, you may experience muscle soreness 24 or 48 hours after testing. These risks can be minimized by performing warm-up exercises prior to taking the tests. If muscle soreness occurs, appropriate stretching exercises to relieve this soreness will be demonstrated.

Expected benefits from testing

These tests allow us to assess your physical working capacity and to appraise your physical fitness status. The results are used to prescribe a safe, sound exercise program for you. Records are kept strictly confidential unless you consent to release this information.

From Vivian H. Heyward, 2010, *Advanced Fitness Assessment and Exercise Prescription*, 6th ed. (Champaign, IL: Human Kinetics).

APPENDIX A.6

Inquiries

Questions about the procedures used in the physical fitness tests are encouraged. If you have any questions or need additional information, please ask us to explain further.

Freedom of Consent

Your permission to perform these physical fitness tests is strictly voluntary. You are free to stop the tests at any point, if you so desire.

I have read this form carefully and I fully understand the test procedures that I will perform and the risks and discomforts. Knowing these risks and having had the opportunity to ask questions that have been answered to my satisfaction, I consent to participate in these tests.

_____	_____
Date	Signature of patient
_____	_____
Date	Signature of witness
_____	_____
Date	Signature of supervisor

From Vivian H. Heyward, 2010, *Advanced Fitness Assessment and Exercise Prescription*, 6th ed. (Champaign, IL: Human Kinetics).

Web Sites for Selected Professional Organizations and Institutes[a]

Name	Web site address
Aerobics and Fitness Association of America (AFAA)	www.afaa.com
American Association for Health, Physical Education, Recreation and Dance (AAHPERD)	www.aapherd.org
American Association of Cardiovascular and Pulmonary Rehabilitation (AACPR)	www.aacvpr.org
American College of Sports Medicine (ACSM)	www.acsm.org
American Council on Exercise (ACE)	www.acefitness.org
American Fitness Professionals and Associates (AFPA)	www.afpafitness.org
American Society of Exercise Physiologists (ASEP)	www.asep.org
Australian Association for Exercise and Sport Sciences (AAESS)	www.aaess.com.au
Canadian Academy of Sports Medicine (CASM)	www.casm-acms.org
Canadian Society for Exercise Physiology (CSEP)	www.csep.ca
Cooper Institute for Aerobics Research	www.cooperinst.org
Ethics and Safety Compliance Standards	www.escs.info
Gatorade Sport Science Institute (GSSI)	www.gssiweb.com
IDEA Health and Fitness Association	www.ideafit.com
International Association of Fitness Certifying Agencies	www.iafca.org
International Federation of Sports Medicine (FIMS)	www.fims.org
International Fitness Professionals Association (IFPA)	www.ifpa-fitness.com
International Health, Racquet, & Sportsclub Association	www.ihrsa.org
International Society for Aging and Physical Activity (ISAPA)	www.isapa.org
National Athletic Trainers Association (NATA)	www.nata.org
National Board of Fitness Examiners	www.nbfe.org
National Commission for Certifying Agencies (NCCA)	www.NOCA.org/
National Organization for Competency Assurance (NOCA)	www.NOCA.org
National Strength and Conditioning Association (NSCA)	www.nsca-lift.org
North American Society for Pediatric Exercise Medicine (NASPEM)	www.naspem.org
Sports Medicine Australia	www.sma.org.au
Sports Medicine New Zealand	www.sportsmedicine.co.nz

[a]Organizations and institutes dealing with exercise physiology, sports medicine, or physical fitness.

From Vivian H. Heyward, 2010, *Advanced Fitness Assessment and Exercise Prescription*, 6th ed. (Champaign, IL: Human Kinetics).

Cardiorespiratory Assessments

Appendix B.1 includes a Summary of GXT and Cardiorespiratory Field Test Protocols that are presented in more detail in chapter 4. This appendix summarizes popular maximal and submaximal protocols for treadmill, cycle ergometer, bench stepping, stair-climbing, rowing ergometer, and distance run/walk tests, as well as methods that you can use to obtain an estimate of your client's $\dot{V}O_2$max for each protocol.

Appendix B.2, the Rockport Fitness Charts, provides age-gender norms for the Rockport Walking Test. These charts may be used to classify your client's aerobic capacity.

Appendix B.3 presents a variety of step test protocols. Testing and scoring procedures are included for each protocol. For some protocols, prediction equations are available to estimate your client's $\dot{V}O_2$max.

Appendix B.4 presents OMNI RPE scales for children and adults engaging in running/walking, stepping, and resistance exercise. Instructions for administering these scales are provided.

Appendix B.5 provides the answers to questions posed in the sample case study presented in chapter 5 (see p. 122).

Summary of Graded Exercise Test and Cardiorespiratory Field Test Protocols

Test mode/Protocol	Population	Type	Method to estimate $\dot{V}O_2max$	Description (page)
Treadmill				
Balke	Active/sedentary men and women	Max or submax	Prediction equation Multistage equation/graphing	74
Modified Balke	Children	Max or submax	ACSM equations (walk/run) Multistage equations/graphing	96
Bruce	Active/sedentary men and women	Max or submax	Prediction equation Multistage equation/graphing	77
	Elderly	Max or submax	Prediction equation Multistage equation/graphing	
	Cardiac patients	Max or submax	Prediction equation Multistage equation/graphing	
Modified Bruce	High-risk and elderly	Max or submax	ACSM walking equation Multistage equation/graphing	77
Ebbeling (single-stage walking)	Healthy adults (20-59 years)	Submax	Prediction equation	86
George (single-stage jogging)	Healthy adults (18-28 years)	Submax	Prediction equation	86
Naughton	Male cardiac patients	Max or submax	Prediction equation Multistage equation/graphing	75
Cycle ergometer				
Åstrand	Healthy adults	Max	ACSM leg ergometry equation	82
Åstrand-Ryhming	Healthy adults	Submax	Nomogram	87
Fox	Healthy adults	Max or submax	ACSM leg ergometry equation Prediction equation	89
YMCA	Healthy adults	Submax	Multistage equation/graphing	88
McMaster	Children	Max or submax	ACSM leg ergometry equation Multistage equation/graphing	96
Swain	Healthy adults	Submax	ACSM leg ergometry equation	89
Bench stepping				
Åstrand-Ryhming	Healthy adults	Submax	Nomogram	89
Nagle	Healthy adults	Max	ACSM stepping equation	83
Queens College	Healthy adults (college age)	Submax	Prediction equation	90

From Vivian H. Heyward, 2010, *Advanced Fitness Assessment and Exercise Prescription,* 6th ed. (Champaign, IL: Human Kinetics).

APPENDIX B.1

Test mode/Protocol	Population	Type	Method to estimate $\dot{V}O_2max$	Description (page)
Stair-climbing				
Howley	Healthy adults	Submax	Multistage equation/graphing	91
Recumbent stepper				
Billinger	Healthy adults	Max	Multistage equation	84
Rowing ergometer				
Hagerman	Noncompetitive and unskilled rowers	Submax	Nomogram	92
Distance run/walk				
1.0-mile run/walk	Children (8-17 years)	Submax	Prediction equation	96
1.0-mile steady-state jog	Healthy adults (college age)	Submax	Prediction equation	94
1.5-mile run/walk	Healthy adults	Submax	Prediction equation	94
1.5-mile steady-state run	Healthy adults	Submax	Prediction equation	94
1.0-mile walk	Healthy adults	Submax	Prediction equation	94
9-min run	Healthy adults	Submax	Prediction equation	94
12-min run	Healthy adults	Submax	Prediction equation	92
20-meter shuttle run	Children (8-19 years)	Submax	Prediction equation	96

From Vivian H. Heyward, 2010, *Advanced Fitness Assessment and Exercise Prescription,* 6th ed. (Champaign, IL: Human Kinetics).

Rockport Fitness Charts

Age-Gender Norms for the Rockport Walking Test

Relative Fitness Level

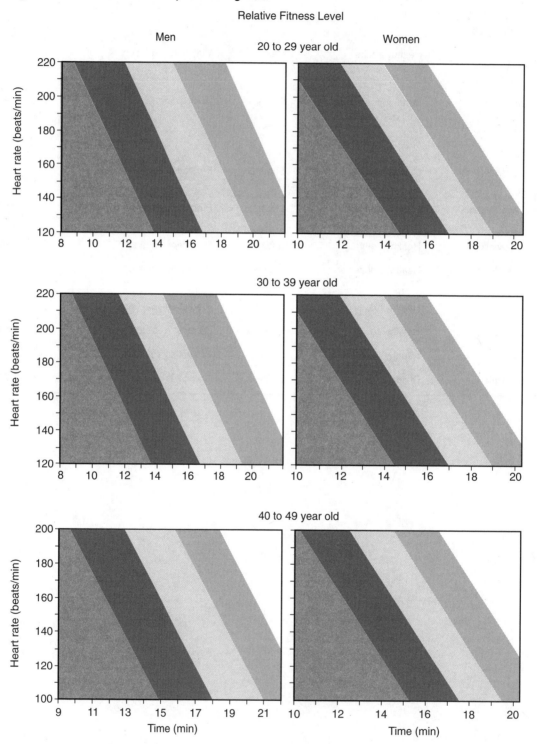

Reprinted with permission of The Rockport Company, Inc.

Age-Gender Norms for the Rockport Walking Test

Relative Fitness Level

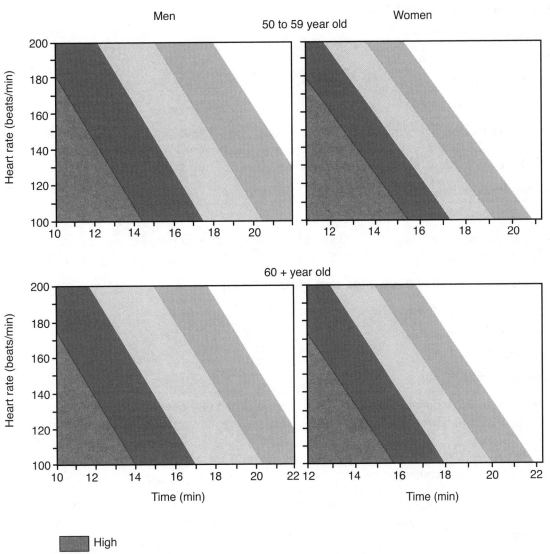

Men   50 to 59 year old   Women

60 + year old

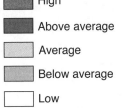

High

Above average

Average

Below average

Low

Step Test Protocols

Harvard Step Test (Brouha 1943)

Age and sex: Young men

Stepping rate: 30 steps·min^{-1}

Bench height: 20 in.

Duration of exercise: 5 min

Scoring procedures: Sit down immediately after exercise. The pulse rate is counted in 1/2-min counts, from 1 to 1 1/2, 2 to 2 1/2, and 3 to 3 1/2 min after exercise. The three 1/2-min pulse counts are summed and used in the following equation to determine physical efficiency index (PEI):

$$PEI = \frac{\text{duration of exercise (sec)} \times 100}{2 \times \text{sum of recovery HRs}}$$

You can evaluate the performance of college-age males using the following PEI classifications: <55 = poor, 55-64 = low average, 65-79 = average, 80-89 = good, and ≥90 = excellent.

Three-Minute Step Test (Hodgkins and Skubic 1963)

Age and sex: High school- and college-age women

Stepping rate: 24 steps·min^{-1}

Bench height: 18 in.

Duration of exercise: 3 min

Scoring procedures: Sit down immediately after exercise. The pulse rate is counted for 30 sec after 1 min of rest (1 to 1 1/2 min after exercise). Use the recovery pulse count in the following equation:

$$CV\text{ efficiency} = \frac{\text{duration of exercise (sec)} \times 100}{\text{recovery pulse} \times 5.6}$$

You can evaluate the performance of college-age women using the following classifications for cardio-vascular (CV) efficiency: 0-27 = very poor, 28-38 = poor, 39-48 = fair, 49-59 = good, 60-70 = very good, and 71-100 = excellent.

OSU Step Test (Kurucz, Fox, and Mathews 1969)

Age and sex: Men 19-56 years

Stepping rate: 24 to 30 steps·min^{-1}

Bench height: Split-level bench 15 and 20 in. high with an adjustable hand bar

Duration of exercise: 18 innings, 50 sec each

Phase I: 6 innings, 24 steps·min^{-1}, 15-in. bench

Phase II: 6 innings, 30 steps·min^{-1}, 15-in. bench

Phase III: 6 innings, 30 steps·min^{-1}, 20-in. bench

(Each inning consists of 30 sec of stepping and 20 sec of rest.)

Scoring procedures: Exactly 5 sec into each rest period, take a 10-sec pulse count. Terminate the test when the heart rate reaches 150 bpm (25 counts × 6). The score is the inning during which the heart rate reaches 150 bpm.

Eastern Michigan University Step Test (Witten 1973)

Age and sex: College-age women

Stepping rate: 24 to 30 steps·min^{-1}

Bench height: Tri-level bench 14 to 20 in.

Duration of exercise: 20 innings, 50 sec each

Phase I: 5 innings, 24 steps·min^{-1}, 14-in. bench

Phase II: 5 innings, 30 steps·min^{-1}, 14-in. bench

Phase III: 5 innings, 30 steps·min^{-1}, 17-in. bench

Phase IV: 5 innings, 30 steps·min^{-1}, 20-in. bench

(Each inning consists of 30 sec of stepping and 20 sec of rest.)

Scoring procedures: Exactly 5 sec into each rest period, take a 10-sec pulse count. Terminate the test when the heart rate reaches 168 bpm (28 counts × 6). The score is the inning during which the heart rate reaches 168 bpm.

Cotten Revision of OSU Step Test (Cotten 1971)

Age and sex: High school- and college-age men

Stepping rate: 24 to 36 steps·min^{-1}

Bench height: 17 in.

Duration of exercise: 18 innings, 50 sec each

Phase I: 6 innings, 24 steps·min^{-1}, 17-in. bench

Phase II: 6 innings, 30 steps·min^{-1}, 17-in. bench

Phase III: 6 innings, 36 steps·min^{-1}, 17-in. bench

(Each inning consists of 30 sec of stepping and 20 sec of rest.)

Scoring procedures: As with the OSU Step Test, the score is the inning during which the heart rate reaches 150 bpm (25 counts in 10 sec). $\dot{V}O_2$max in ml·kg^{-1}·min^{-1} can be estimated using the following equation:

$$\dot{V}O_2\text{max} = (1.69978 \times \text{step test score}) - (0.06252 \times \text{body weight in lb}) + 47.12525$$

Queens College Step Test (McArdle et al. 1972)

Age and sex: College-age women and men

Stepping rate: 22 steps·min^{-1} for women; 24 steps·min^{-1} for men

Bench height: 16 1/4 in.

Duration of exercise: 3 min

Scoring procedures: Remain standing after exercise. Beginning 5 sec after the cessation of exercise, take a 15-sec pulse count. Multiply the 15-sec count by 4 to express the score in beats per minute (bpm). $\dot{V}O_2$max in ml·kg^{-1}·min^{-1} can be estimated using the following equations:

Women: $\dot{V}O_2\text{max} = 65.81 - (0.1847 \times \text{HR})$

Men: $\dot{V}O_2\text{max} = 111.33 - (0.42 \times \text{HR})$

References

Brouha, L. 1943. The step test: A simple method of measuring physical fitness for muscular work in young men. Research Quarterly 14: 31–36.

Cotten, D.J. 1971. A modified step test for group cardiovascular testing. Research Quarterly 42: 91–95.

Hodgkins, J. and Skubic, V. 1963. Cardiovascular efficiency test scores for college women in the United States. Research Quarterly 34: 454–461.

Kurucz, R., Fox, E.L., and Mathews, D.K. 1969. Construction of a submaximal cardiovascular step test. Research Quarterly 40: 115–122.

McArdle, W.D., Katch, F.I., Pechar, G.S., Jacobson, L., and Ruck, S. 1972. Reliability and interrelationships between maximal oxygen intake, physical working capacity and step-test scores in college women. Medicine and Science in Sports 4: 182–186.

Witten, C. 1973. Construction of a submaximal cardiovascular step test for college females. Research Quarterly 44: 46–50.

OMNI RPE Scales

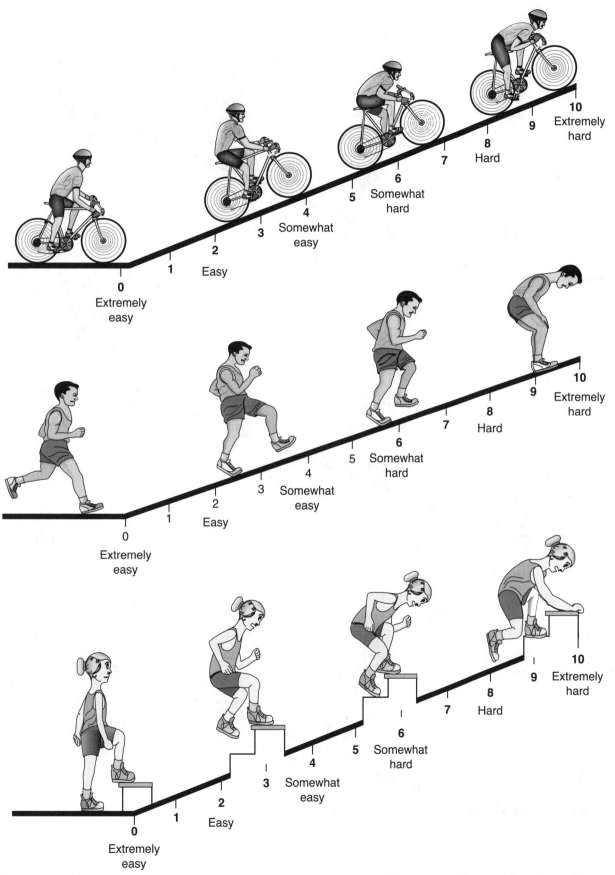

Reprinted, by permission, from R.J. Robertson, 2004, Perceived exertion for practitioners: Rating effort with the OMNI picture system (Champaign, IL: Human Kinetics), 141-150.

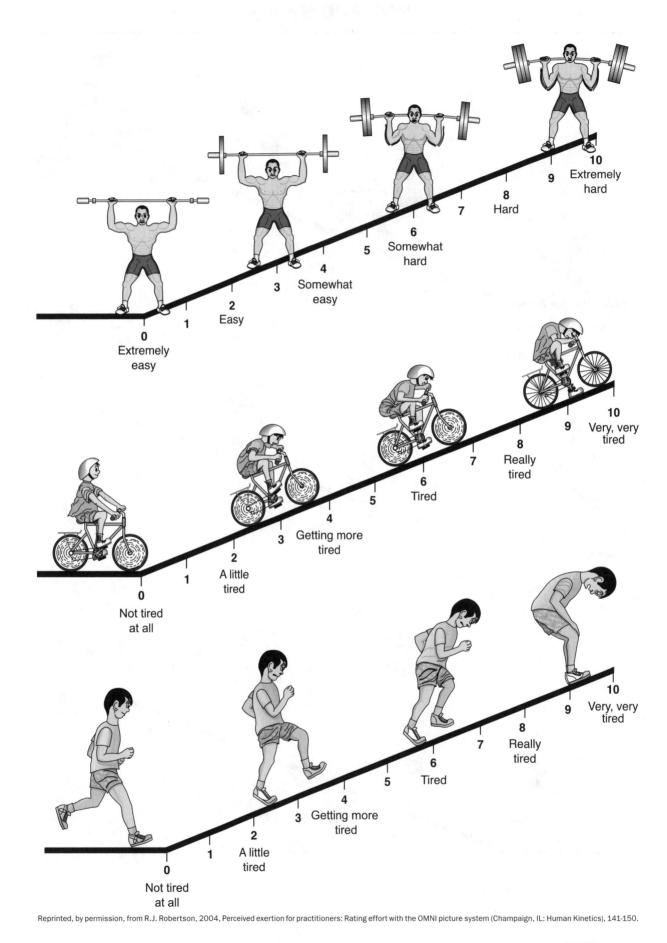

Reprinted, by permission, from R.J. Robertson, 2004, Perceived exertion for practitioners: Rating effort with the OMNI picture system (Champaign, IL: Human Kinetics), 141-150.

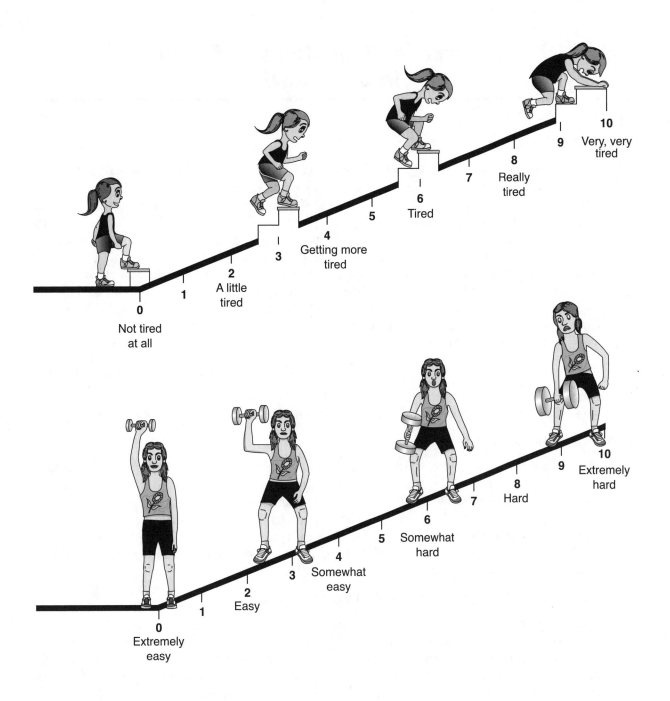

10
Very, very
tired

9

8
Really
tired

7

6
Tired

5

4
Getting more
tired

3

2
A little
tired

1

0
Not tired
at all

10
Extremely
hard

9

8
Hard

7

6
Somewhat
hard

5

4
Somewhat
easy

3

2
Easy

1

0
Extremely
easy

Reprinted, by permission, from R.J. Robertson, 2004, Perceived exertion for practitioners: Rating effort with the OMNI picture system (Champaign, IL: Human Kinetics), 141-150.

Analysis of Sample Case Study in Chapter 5

1. CHD Risk Profile

This client has risk factors for CHD. Her total cholesterol (TC; 220 mg·dl^{-1}) is borderline high (200 to 230 mg·dl^{-1}), and her blood pressure (140/82 mmHg) is categorized as Stage I hypertension (140 to 159 mm Hg). Also, her HDL-C (37 mg·dl^{-1}) and TC/HDL ratio (5.9) place her at higher risk (<40 mg·dl^{-1} and >5.0, respectively). She quit smoking cigarettes (one pack a day) three years ago, which is a step in the right direction. Following the National Cholesterol Education Program's recommendation, you should encourage this client to have her LDL-C assessed to determine if she needs a cholesterol treatment program. Engaging in an aerobic exercise program should lower her systolic blood pressure. Her triglycerides and blood glucose levels are normal. She should be encouraged to dine out less frequently and to eat three well-balanced meals a day. When dining out, she should select foods that are low in saturated fat, cholesterol, and sodium. This may help to lower her blood cholesterol and blood pressure.

The client is also at greater risk because of

- the high stress associated with her job (police officer) and lifestyle (divorced parent raising two children),
- family history of cardiovascular disease, and
- physical inactivity (she does not exercise regularly outside of work-related physical activity).

2. Special Considerations

The client has not exercised aerobically for the past six years, and she has gained 15 lb during that time. It is likely that she will experience some discomfort when she starts her aerobic exercise program. Thus, it is important to initially prescribe low-intensity exercise to minimize her physical discomfort.

You also need to consider her busy schedule to find a convenient time for her to exercise. She reports feeling dizzy after eating. The likely reason is that she is eating only one meal a day, and the insulin surge after eating is lowering her blood glucose level. It is important to convince this client to start eating at least three meals a day to avoid this problem.

3. HR, BP, and RPE Responses to Graded Exercise Test

The client's HR response to the graded exercise test was normal. The exercise HR increased during each stage of the exercise test. The maximal heart rate (190 bpm) was very close to her age-predicted maximal HR (220 – 28 = 192 bpm). The client's BP response to the graded exercise test was normal. The diastolic BP remained fairly constant (78 to 82 mmHg), and the systolic BP increased with each stage of the exercise test. The RPEs were normal. The ratings increased linearly with exercise intensity.

4. Functional Aerobic Capacity

The graded exercise test was voluntarily terminated by the client due to fatigue. This was most likely a maximal-effort exercise test as indicated by the RPE (18) and the exercise heart rate (190 bpm) during the last stage of the graded exercise test. The treadmill speed and grade during the last stage of the protocol was 2.5 mph and 12%, respectively. This corresponds to a functional aerobic capacity of 7.0 METs or 24.5 ml·kg^{-1}·min^{-1}. According to the norms, this client's cardiorespiratory fitness level is *poor* for her age.

5. & 6. Training HRs

The graph of the client's HR and RPE responses to the graded exercise test is presented in figure B.5 (see p. 346).

Given the client's poor cardiorespiratory fitness level and her lack of regular aerobic exercise, the initial minimal training intensity will be 50% $\dot{V}O_2R$ (4.0 METs), gradually increasing to a maximum intensity of 75% $\dot{V}O_2R$ (5.5 METs). The corresponding training HRs, extrapolated from figure B.4, are 152 bpm (50% $\dot{V}O_2R$ or 4.0 METs) and 174 bpm (75% $\dot{V}O_2R$ or 5.5 METs). The HRs and RPEs corresponding to the relative exercise intensities in the following chart were extrapolated from the graph.

%$\dot{V}O_2R$	METs	HR (bpm)	RPE
50%	4.0	152	12
60%	4.6	165	14
70%	5.2	170	15
75%	5.5	174	16

7. Speed Calculations (ACSM Formula for Walking on Level Course)

To calculate walking speed corresponding to 60% of client's $\dot{V}O_2R$ [.60 × (7 − 1) + 1] = 4.6 METs):

   a. Convert METs into $ml \cdot kg^{-1} \cdot min^{-1}$.

$$4.6 \text{ METs} \times 3.5 \text{ ml} \cdot kg^{-1} \cdot min^{-1} = 16.1 \text{ ml} \cdot kg^{-1} \cdot min^{-1}$$

   b. Substitute into ACSM walking equation and solve for speed ($m \cdot min^{-1}$).

$$\dot{V}O_2 = [\text{speed} \times 0.1] + [1.8 \times \text{speed} \times \text{grade}] + \text{resting } \dot{V}O_2$$

$$16.1 \text{ ml} \cdot kg^{-1} \cdot min^{-1} = [\text{speed} \times 0.1] + [1.8 \times \text{speed} \times 0\% \text{ grade}] + 3.5 \text{ ml} \cdot kg^{-1} \cdot min^{-1}$$

$$12.6 \text{ ml} \cdot kg^{-1} \cdot min^{-1} = m \cdot min^{-1} \times 0.1$$

$$126 \text{ m} \cdot min^{-1} = \text{speed}$$

   c. Convert speed ($m \cdot min^{-1}$) into miles per hour ($26.8 \text{ m} \cdot min^{-1}$ = 1 mph).

$$126 \text{ m} \cdot min^{-1}/26.8 \text{ m} \cdot min^{-1} = 4.7 \text{ mph}$$

   d. Convert miles per hour into minutes per mile walking pace.

$$60 \text{ min} \cdot hr^{-1}/4.7 \text{ mph} = 12.8 \text{ min} \cdot mile^{-1}, \text{ or } 12:48 \text{ (12 min, 48 sec per mile)}$$

Follow these same steps to calculate the walking speed corresponding to 70% $\dot{V}O_2R$ and 75% $\dot{V}O_2R$.

(Answers: 70% $\dot{V}O_2R$ = 5.5 mph; 75% $\dot{V}O_2R$ = 5.9 mph.)

8. Lifestyle Modifications

   ■ Eat three well-balanced meals a day.
   ■ Avoid fried foods high in saturated fats, cholesterol, and sodium.
   ■ Dine out less frequently and select restaurants offering healthy food choices (e.g., salad bar, grilled skinless chicken, or fish).
   ■ Exercise aerobically at least three days a week.
   ■ Try using relaxation techniques (e.g., stretching, progressive relaxation, mental imagery) to relax in the evening instead of drinking wine.

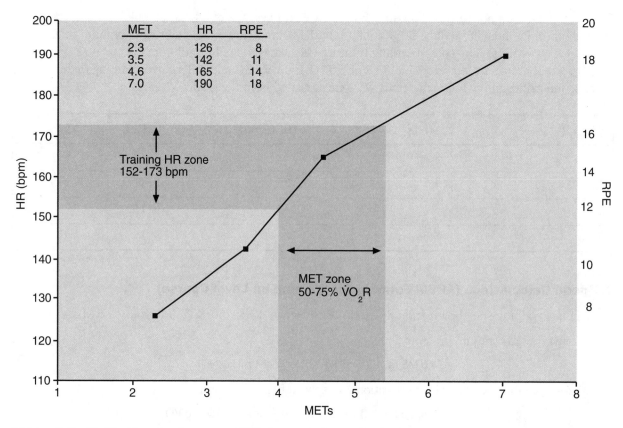

Figure B.5 Plotting heart rate versus METs for graded exercise test.

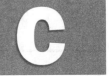

Muscular Fitness Exercises and Norms

Appendix C.1 describes standardized testing protocols for 11 muscle groups using digital, handheld dynamometry.

Appendix C.2 includes norms for isokinetic (Omni-Tron) muscular fitness tests. Average strength, endurance, and power values are presented for young adults, older adults, and resistance-trained individuals.

Appendix C.3 describes and illustrates some sample basic isometric exercises for a variety of muscle groups.

Appendix C.4 provides an extensive list of dynamic resistance training exercises. Exercises for the upper and lower extremities are organized by body region (e.g., chest, upper arm, thigh). For each exercise, equipment, body positions, joint actions, prime movers, and exercise variations are presented.

Standardized Testing Protocols
for Digital, Handheld Dynamometry

Muscle group	Position	Limb/joint position	Dynamometer placement
1. Elbow flexors	Supine	Shoulder 30° abducted, elbow 90° flexed, forearm supinated	Proximal to wrist on flexor surface of forearm
2. Elbow extensors	Supine	Same as for elbow flexors	Proximal to wrist on extensor surface of forearm
3. Shoulder extensors	Supine	Shoulder 90° anteflexed, elbow extended	Proximal to elbow on extensor surface of arm
4. Shoulder abductors	Supine	Shoulder 45° abducted, elbow extended	Proximal to lateral epicondyle of humerus
5. Wrist extensors	Sitting	Elbow 90° flexed, forearm supported and pronated, wrist in neutral position, finger flexed	Proximal to 3rd metacarpal head
6. Hip flexors	Supine	Hip 90° flexed, knee relaxed, ankle supported by tester	Proximal to knee on anterior surface of thigh
7. Hip extensors	Supine	Hip 90° flexed, knee relaxed	Proximal to knee on posterior surface of thigh
8. Hip abductors	Supine	Hips 45° flexed, knees 90° flexed, contralateral knee supported by chest of tester	Lateral epicondyle of knee
9. Knee flexors	Sitting	Knee 90° flexed	Proximal to ankle on posterior surface of leg
10. Knee extensors	Sitting	Knee 90° flexed	Proximal to ankle on anterior surface of leg
11. Ankle dorsiflexors	Sitting	Knee 90° flexed, foot in neutral position	Proximal to metatarsophalangeal joints on dorsal surface of foot

Data from van den Beld et al. 2000.

Average Strength, Endurance, and Power Values for Isokinetic (Omni-Tron) Tests

Strength[a]	Young adult[b]	Older adult[c]	Weight trained[d]
Females			
Chest press	88.1	76.7	131.8
Lateral row	82.6	77.4	111.4
Shoulder press	32.9	30.4	60.1
Lateral pull-down	70.8	66.3	101.2
Knee extension	67.7	59.3	82.7
Knee flexion	51.5	43.3	64.3
Males			
Chest press	173.8	154.9	218.6
Lateral row	153.5	143.2	178.6
Shoulder press	69.2	62.4	102.6
Lateral pull-down	134.8	115.3	176.0
Knee extension	110.9	95.5	127.2
Knee flexion	75.9	67.3	89.9

Note: Data courtesy of Hydra-Fitnesss, Belton, TX: 1988.
[a]Values of strength measured in foot-pounds at dial setting 10.
[b]Average age for females = 15.1 ± 2.6 years; for males = 15.8 ± 2.7 years.
[c]Average age for females = 38.2 ± 9.7 years; for males = 37.6 ± 9.6 years.
[d]Average age for females = 21.2 ± 2.0 years; for males = 20.6 ± 2.1 years.

Endurance[a]	Young adult[b]	Older adult[c]	Weight trained[d]
Females			
Chest press	64.3	53.4	125.7
Lateral row	102.4	85.7	143.7
Shoulder press	28.1	25.1	56.3
Lateral pull-down	109.1	91.5	216.3
Knee extension	88.7	86.6	111.6
Knee flexion	114.3	89.2	148.2
Males			
Chest press	211.8	167.3	321.1
Lateral row	266.9	221.2	312.5
Shoulder press	112.4	94.2	170.9
Lateral pull-down	352.2	296.3	501.5
Knee extension	72.9	80.8	98.9
Knee flexion	83.5	84.2	130.9

[a]Values of endurance measured in foot-pounds at dial setting 3.
[b]Average age for females = 15.1 ± 2.6 years; for males = 15.8 ± 2.7 years.
[c]Average age for females = 38.2 ± 9.7 years; for males = 37.6 ± 9.6 years.
[d]Average age for females = 21.2 ± 2.0 years; for males = 20.6 ± 2.1 years.

(continued)

Average Strength, Endurance, and Power Values for Isokinetic (Omni-Tron) Tests (continued)

Power[a]	Young adult[b]	Older adult[c]	Weight trained[d]
Females			
Chest press	86.3	73.7	163.0
Lateral row	121.3	113.6	156.3
Shoulder press	39.5	32.9	81.9
Lateral pull-down	165.4	128.4	254.1
Knee extension	101.9	73.4	122.5
Knee flexion	103.5	74.6	142.1
Males			
Chest press	264.9	228.4	392.3
Lateral row	302.4	268.4	345.0
Shoulder press	130.7	122.0	224.5
Lateral pull-down	430.9	354.7	550.9
Knee extension	198.4	159.4	233.5
Knee flexion	182.0	155.5	259.5

[a]Values of power measured in foot-pounds at dial setting 6.
[b]Average age for females = 15.1 ± 2.6 years; for males = 15.8 ± 2.7 years.
[c]Average age for females = 38.2 ± 9.7 years; for males = 37.6 ± 9.6 years.
[d]Average age for females = 21.2 ± 2.0 years; for males = 20.6 ± 2.1 years.

Isometric Exercises

Exercise 1: Chest Push

Muscle groups: Shoulder and elbow flexors

Equipment: None

Description:

1. Lock hands together.
2. Keep forearms parallel to ground and hands close to chest.
3. Push hands together.

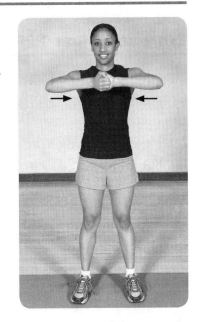

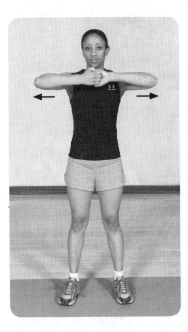

Exercise 2: Shoulder Pull

Muscle groups: Shoulder and elbow flexors

Equipment: None

Description:

    1. Using same position as in chest push, attempt to pull hands apart

Exercise 3: Triceps Extension

Muscle groups: Elbow extensors

Equipment: Towel or rope

Description:

1. Placing right hand over shoulder and left hand at small of back, grasp rope or towel behind back.
2. Attempt to pull towel or rope upward with right hand.
3. Change position of hands.

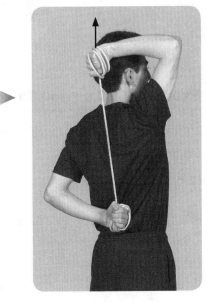

From Vivian H. Heyward, 2010, *Advanced Fitness Assessment and Exercise Prescription*, 6th ed. (Champaign, IL: Human Kinetics).

Exercise 4: Arm Curls

Muscle groups: Elbow flexors

Equipment: Towel or rope

Description:

1. Stand with knees flexed about 45°.
2. Place rope or towel behind thighs and grasp each end with hands shoulder-width apart.
3. Attempt to flex elbows.

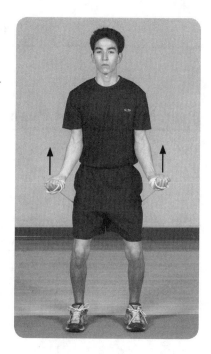

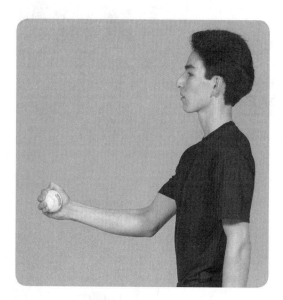

Exercise 5: Ball Squeeze

Muscle groups: Wrist and finger flexors

Equipment: Tennis ball

Description:

1. Hold tennis ball firmly in hand and squeeze maximally.

Exercise 6: Leg and Thigh Extensions

Muscle groups: Hip and knee extensors

Equipment: Rope

Description:

1. Stand on rope with knees flexed.
2. Grasp rope firmly with hands at sides, elbows fully extended.
3. Keeping trunk erect, attempt to extend legs by lifting upward.

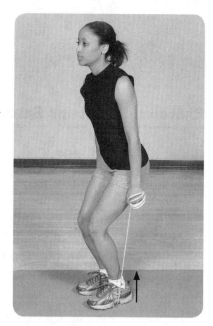

From Vivian H. Heyward, 2010, *Advanced Fitness Assessment and Exercise Prescription,* 6th ed. (Champaign, IL: Human Kinetics).

Exercise 7: Leg Press

Muscle groups: Hip and knee extensors

Equipment: Doorway

Description:

1. Sit in doorway facing side of door frame.
2. Grasp door frame behind head.
3. Attempt to extend legs by pushing feet against door frame.

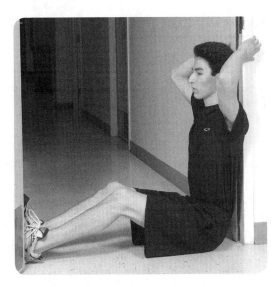

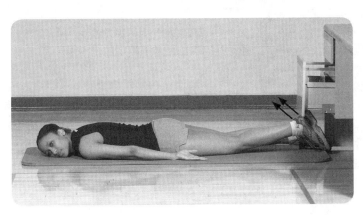

Exercise 8: Leg Curl

Muscle groups: Knee flexors

Equipment: Dresser or desk

Description:

1. Pull out lower dresser drawer slightly.
2. Lying prone, with knees flexed, hook heels under bottom of drawer.
3. Attempt to pull heels toward head.

Exercise 9: Knee Squeeze or Pull

Muscle groups: Hip adductors or abductors

Equipment: Chair

Description:

1. Sitting on chair with forearms crossed and hands on inside of knees, attempt to squeeze knees together (adductors).
2. Same position but place hands on outside of knees; attempt to pull knees apart (abductors).

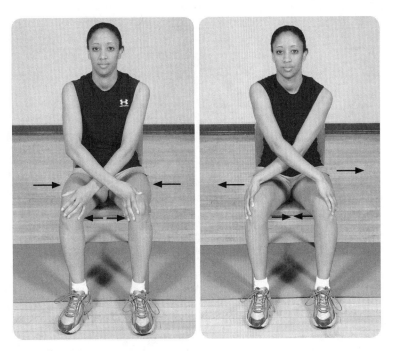

From Vivian H. Heyward, 2010, *Advanced Fitness Assessment and Exercise Prescription*, 6th ed. (Champaign, IL: Human Kinetics).

Exercise 10: Pelvic Tilt ▶

Muscle groups: Abdominals

Equipment: None

Description:

1. Supine with knees flexed and arms overhead.
2. Tighten abdominal muscles while pressing lower back into floor.

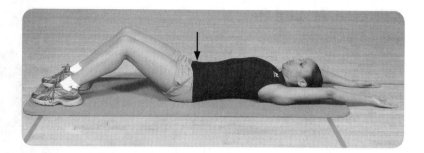

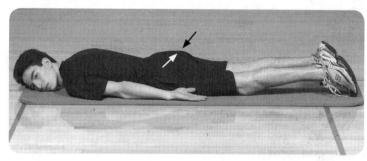

◀ Exercise 11: Gluteal Squeeze

Muscle groups: Hip extensors and abductors

Equipment: None

Description:

1. Lie prone with legs together and fully extended.
2. Tighten and squeeze the buttocks together.

From Vivian H. Heyward, 2010, *Advanced Fitness Assessment and Exercise Prescription*, 6th ed. (Champaign, IL: Human Kinetics).

APPENDIX C.3

Dynamic Resistance Training Exercises

Exercise	Type[a]	Variations	Equipment[b]	Body position	Joint actions	Prime movers
Upper extremity						
Chest						
Bench press	M-J	Flat	B, D, M	Supine lying on flat bench	Shoulder horizontal adduction, elbow extension	Pectoralis major (midsternal), triceps brachii
		Incline	B, D, M	Sitting on incline bench	Shoulder flexion, elbow extension	Pectoralis major (clavicular), triceps brachii
		Decline	B, D	Supine lying on decline bench	Shoulder flexion, elbow extension	Pectoralis major (lower sternal), triceps brachii
Push-up	M-J	Hands wider than shoulders	None	Prone; BW supported by hands and feet	Shoulder horizontal adduction, elbow extension	Pectoralis major (midsternal), triceps brachii
		Hands narrower than shoulders	None	Same as above	Shoulder flexion, elbow extension	Pectoralis major (clavicular, ant deltoid, triceps brachii
Bar dip	M-J	Neutral grip	Parallel bars	Vertically supported by bars	Shoulder flexion, elbow extension	Pectoralis major (clavicular, ant deltoid, triceps brachii
		Pronated grip		Same as above	Shoulder adduction, elbow extension	Pectoralis major (midsternal), triceps brachii
Fly	S	Flat	D	Supine lying on flat bench	Shoulder adduction	Pectoralis major (midsternal)
Pullover (bent arm)	S	Flat	B, D	Supine lying on flat bench	Shoulder extension	Pectoralis major (lower sternal), post deltoid, latissimus dorsi

(continued)

From Vivian H. Heyward, 2010, *Advanced Fitness Assessment and Exercise Prescription*, 6th ed. (Champaign, IL: Human Kinetics).

Dynamic Resistance Training Exercises (continued)

Exercise	Type[a]	Variations	Equipment[b]	Body position	Joint actions	Prime movers
Upper extremity (cont.)						
Shoulders						
Overhead press	M-J	Military	B, D, M	Sitting or standing	Shoulder flexion, elbow extension	Pectoralis major (clavicular), ant deltoid, triceps brachii
		Behind the head	B	Sitting	Shoulder abduction, elbow extension	Ant/mid deltoid, supraspinatus
Upright row	M-J		B, D	Standing	Shoulder abduction, scapula upward rotation, elbow flexion	Mid deltoid, supraspinatus, trapezius (upper), brachialis
Front arm raise	S		B, C, D	Standing	Shoulder flexion	Pectoralis major (clavicular), ant deltoid
Lateral arm raise	S		C, D, M	Sitting or standing	Shoulder abduction	Mid deltoid, supraspinatus, pectoralis major (clavicular)
Reverse fly	S		C, D	Standing	Shoulder horizontal extension	Post deltoid, infraspinatus, teres minor
Upper arm						
Arm curl	S	Supinated grip	B, D, M	Standing or sitting on incline bench or preacher bench	Elbow flexion	Biceps brachii, brachialis
	S	Neutral grip	Same as above		Elbow flexion	Brachioradialis, brachialis, biceps brachii
	S	Pronated grip	Same as above		Elbow flexion	Brachialis
Triceps press-down	M-J		M	Seated	Shoulder flexion, elbow extension	Ant deltoid, pectoralis major (clavicular), triceps brachii

Exercise	Type[a]	Variations	Equipment[b]	Body position	Joint actions	Prime movers
Upper extremity (cont.)						
Upper arm (cont.)						
Triceps extension	S		B	Supine lying on flat bench	Elbow extension	Triceps brachii
Triceps push-down	S	V-bar or strength bar	C	Standing	Elbow extension	Triceps brachii
French press	S		D	Standing or sitting	Elbow extension	Triceps brachii (medial head)
Overhead press	S		C, R	Standing with trunk flexed 45°	Elbow extension	Triceps brachii
Triceps kickback	S		D	Standing with one knee/hand on flat bench and trunk horizontal to floor	Elbow extension	Triceps brachii (long head)
Forearm						
Radioulnar rotation	S		D	Forearm/elbow supported on bench; hand free	Supination and pronation	Supinator, pronator teres, biceps brachii, brachioradialis
Wrist curl	S		D	Same as above	Wrist flexion	FCU, FCR
Reverse wrist curl	S		D	Same as above	Wrist extension	ECU, ECR (longus, brevis)
Radioulnar flexion	S		D	Standing with arm at side	Radial flexion, ulna flexion	FCR, ECR, FCU, ECU
Upper-mid back						
Lat pull-down	M-J	Pronated, wide grip	M	Sitting	Shoulder adduction, scapula adduction	Latissimus dorsi (upper), teres major, pectoralis major (upper), trapezius, rhomboids
	M-J	Narrow, neutral grip	M	Sitting	Shoulder extension, elbow flexion	Latissimus dorsi (lower), pectoralis major (lower sternal), biceps brachii

(continued)

From Vivian H. Heyward, 2010, *Advanced Fitness Assessment and Exercise Prescription*, 6th ed. (Champaign, IL: Human Kinetics).

Dynamic Resistance Training Exercises (continued)

Exercise	Type[a]	Variations	Equipment[b]	Body position	Joint actions	Prime movers
Upper mid-back (cont.)						
Seated row	M-J	Neutral grip	M	Sitting	Shoulder extension, elbow flexion	Latissimus dorsi (lower), biceps brachii
	M-J	Pronated grip	M	Sitting with elbows horizontal to floor	Shoulder horizontal extension, elbow flexion	Post deltoid, latissimus dorsi (upper), infraspinatus, brachialis
Bent-over row	M-J	Neutral grip	D	Standing with trunk flexed 90°	Shoulder extension, elbow flexion	Latissimus dorsi, biceps brachii
	M-J	Pronated grip	D	Standing with trunk flexed 90° and elbows out	Shoulder horizontal extension, elbow flexion	Post deltoid, infraspinatus, latissimus dorsi, brachialis
Pull-up	M-J	Pronated grip	Pull-up bar	Vertically hanging from bar	Shoulder adduction, elbow flexion	Latissimus dorsi (upper), pectoralis major (sternal), brachialis
Chin-up	M-J	Supinated or neutral grip	Pull-up bar	Vertically hanging from bar	Shoulder extension, elbow flexion	Latissimus dorsi (lower), pectoralis major (sternal), biceps brachii
Shoulder shrug	S	Regular	B, D, M	Standing	Shoulder girdle (scapula and clavicle) elevation	Trapezius (upper), levator scapulae, rhomboids
	S	Elevation with shoulder roll		Standing	Shoulder girdle elevation, scapula adduction	Trapezius (mid), rhomboids
Lower back						
Trunk extension	M-J		M	Sitting with pelvis/thighs stabilized	Spinal extension	Erector spinae
Back raise	M-J		Glut-ham developer	Prone with pelvis supported; trunk flexed	Spinal extension	Erector spinae
Side bends	M-J		D	Standing	Spinal lateral flexion	Quadratus lumborum

From Vivian H. Heyward, 2010, *Advanced Fitness Assessment and Exercise Prescription*, 6th ed. (Champaign, IL: Human Kinetics).

Exercise	Type[a]	Variations	Equipment[b]	Body position	Joint actions	Prime movers
Lower back (cont.)						
Isometric side support (side bridge)	M-J		None	Side-lying with BW supported by forearm and feet	None	Quadratus lumborum, abdominal obliques
Single-leg extension	M-J		None	Hands and knees	Spinal extension, hip extension	Erector spinae, gluteus maximus, hamstrings (upper)
Abdomen						
Curl-up	M-J	Bent knee	None	Supine lying with knees bent	Spinal flexion	Rectus abdominis
	M-J	With twist	None	Same as above	Spinal flexion	Abdominal obliques
Abdominal crunch	M-J		M	Sitting	Spinal flexion	Rectus abdominis
Reverse sit-up	M-J		None	Supine lying on floor on bench	Spinal flexion	Rectus abdominis (lower)
Lower extremity						
Hip						
Half squat	M-J		B, M	Standing	Hip extension, knee extension	Gluteus maximus, hamstrings (upper), quadriceps femoris
Leg press	M-J		M	Sitting	Hip extension, knee extension	Gluteus maximus, hamstrings (upper), quadriceps femoris
Lunge	M-J		B, D	Standing	Hip extension, knee extension	Gluteus maximus hamstrings (upper), quadriceps femoris
Glut-ham raise	M-J		Glut-ham developer	Prone with thighs supported and trunk flexed	Hip extension and knee flexion	Gluteus maximus, hamstrings

(continued)

From Vivian H. Heyward, 2010, *Advanced Fitness Assessment and Exercise Prescription*, 6th ed. (Champaign, IL: Human Kinetics).

Dynamic Resistance Training Exercises (continued)

Exercise	Type[a]	Variations	Equipment[b]	Body position	Joint actions	Prime movers
Lower extremity (cont.)						
Hip (cont.)						
Hip flexion	S		C, M	Standing	Hip flexion	Iliopsoas, rectus femoris (upper)
Hip extension	S		C, M	Standing	Hip extension	Gluteus maximus, hamstrings (upper)
Hip adduction	S		M	Sitting or supine lying	Hip adduction	Adductor longus, brevis, and magnus; gracilis
Hip abduction	S		M	Sitting or supine lying	Hip abduction	Gluteus medius
Side leg raise	S		None	Lying on side	Hip abduction	Gluteus medius, hamstrings (upper)
Good morning exercise	S		B, D	Standing	Hip extension	Gluteus maximus, hamstrings (upper)
Thigh						
Leg extension	S		M	Seated	Knee extension	Quadriceps femoris
Leg curl	S	Straight	M	Prone lying, seated, or standing	Knee flexion	Hamstrings (lower)
	S	Knee externally rotated	M	Same as above	Knee flexion	Biceps femoris
	S	Knees internally rotated	M	Same as above	Knee flexion	Semitendinosus, semimembranosus
Lower leg						
Heel raise	S	Standing	D, M	Standing	Ankle plantar flexion	Gastrocnemius
	S	Seated	M	Sitting	Ankle plantar flexion	Soleus
Toe raise	S		Strength bar	Sitting	Ankle dorsiflexion	Tibialis anterior, peroneus tertius, extensor digitorum longus

Note: FCU = flexor carpi ulnaris; ECU = extensor carpi ulnaris; FCR = flexor carpi radialis; ECR = extensor carpi radialis.

[a]Type of exercise: M-J = multijoint exercise; S = single-joint exercise; [b]Equipment codes: B = barbell; C = cables; D = dumbbells; M = exercise machine; R = rope.

From Vivian H. Heyward, 2010, *Advanced Fitness Assessment and Exercise Prescription*, 6th ed. (Champaign, IL: Human Kinetics).

Body Composition Assessments

Appendix D.1 presents prediction equations for estimating residual lung volume. Use these equations only when it is not possible to directly measure your client's residual lung volume.

Appendix D.2 describes and illustrates the standardized sites for skinfold measurements, and appendix D.3 describes the skinfold sites and measurement procedures for Jackson's generalized skinfold prediction equations for men and women.

Standardized sites for circumference (appendix D.4) and bony breadth (appendix D.5) measurements are also provided. Follow these procedures to identify and measure various sites.

Appendix D.6 contains the Ashwell Body Shape Chart. Use this chart to compare your client's waist circumference to standing height.

Prediction Equations
for Residual Volume

Population	Smoking history[a]	n	Equation[b]
MEN			
Boren, Kory, and Syner (1966)	Mixed	422	RV = 0.0115 (Age) + 0.019 (HT) − 2.24 r = 0.57, *SEE* = 0.53 L
Goldman and Becklake (1959)			RV = 0.017 (Age) + 0.027 (HT) − 3.477
Berglund et al. (1963)			RV = 0.022 (Age) + 0.0198 (HT) − 0.015 (WT) − 1.54
WOMEN			
O'Brien and Drizd (1983)	Nonsmokers	926	RV = 0.03 (Age) + 0.0387 (HT) − 0.73 (BSA) − 4.78 r = 0.66, *SEE* = 0.49 L
Black, Offord, and Hyatt (1974)	Mixed	110	RV = 0.021 (Age) + 0.023 (HT) − 2.978 r = 0.70, *SEE* = 0.46 L
Goldman and Becklake (1959)			RV = 0.009 (Age) + 0.032 (HT) − 3.9
Berglund et al. (1963)			RV = 0.007 (Age) + 0.0268 (HT) − 3.42

[a]Mixed indicates that sample included both smokers and nonsmokers.
[b]Age (in yr); HT = height (in cm); BSA = body surface area (in m²); WT = body mass (in kg).

References

Berglund, E., Birath, G., Bjure, J., Grimby, G., Kjellmar, I., Sandvist, L., and Soderholm, B. 1963. Spirometric studies in normal subjects. I. Forced expirograms in subjects between 7 and 70 years of age. *Acta Medica Scandinavica* 173: 185-192.

Black, L.F., Offord, K., and Hyatt, R.E. 1974. Variability in the maximum expiratory flow volume curve in asymptomatic smokers and nonsmokers. *American Review of Respiratory Diseases* 110: 282–292.

Boren, H.G., Kory, R.C., and Syner, J.C. 1966. The Veteran's Administration-Army cooperative study of pulmonary function: II. The lung volume and its subdivisions in normal men. *American Journal of Medicine* 41: 96–114.

Goldman, H.I., and Becklake, M.R. 1959. Respiratory function tests: Normal values at medium altitudes and the prediction of normal results. *American Review of Tuberculosis and Respiratory Diseases* 79: 457-467.

O'Brien, R.J., and Drizd, T.A. 1983. Roentgenographic determination of total lung capacity: Normal values from a national population survey. *American Review of Respiratory Diseases* 128: 949–952.

Standardized Sites
for Skinfold Measurements

Site	Direction of fold	Anatomical reference	Measurement
Chest	Diagonal	Axilla and nipple	Fold is taken between axilla and nipple as high as possible on anterior axillary fold, with measurement taken 1 cm below fingers.
Subscapular	Diagonal	Inferior angle of scapula	Fold is along natural cleavage line of skin just inferior to inferior angle of scapula, with caliper applied 1 cm below fingers.
Midaxillary	Horizontal	Xiphisternal junction (point where costal cartilage of ribs 5-6 articulates with sternum, slightly above inferior tip of xiphoid process)	Fold is taken on midaxillary line at level of xiphisternal junction.
Suprailiac	Oblique	Iliac crest	Fold is grasped posteriorly to midaxillary line and superiorly to iliac crest along natural cleavage of skin with caliper applied 1 cm below fingers.
Abdominal	Horizontal	Umbilicus	Fold is taken 3 cm lateral and 1 cm inferior to center of the umbilicus.
Triceps	Vertical (midline)	Acromial process of scapula and olecranon process of ulna	Using a tape measure, distance between lateral projection of acromial process and inferior margin of olecranon process is measured on lateral aspect of arm with elbow flexed 90°. Midpoint is marked on lateral side of arm. Fold is lifted 1 cm above marked line on posterior aspect of arm. Caliper is applied at marked level.
Biceps	Vertical (midline)	Biceps brachii	Fold is lifted over belly of the biceps brachii at the level marked for the triceps and on line with anterior border of the acromial process and the antecubital fossa. Caliper is applied 1 cm below fingers.
Thigh	Vertical (midline)	Inguinal crease and patella	Fold is lifted on anterior aspect of thigh midway between inguinal crease and proximal border of patella. Body weight is shifted to left foot and caliper is applied 1 cm below fingers.
Calf	Vertical (medial aspect)	Maximal calf circumference	Fold is lifted at level of maximal calf circumference on medial aspect of calf with knee and hip flexed to 90°.

Adapted from Harrison et al. 1988.

From Vivian H. Heyward, 2010, *Advanced Fitness Assessment and Exercise Prescription,* 6th ed. (Champaign, IL: Human Kinetics).

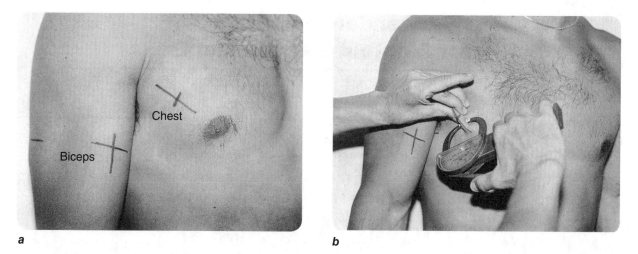

Figure D.2.1 *(a)* Site and *(b)* measurement of the chest skinfold. Photos courtesy of Linda K. Gilkey.

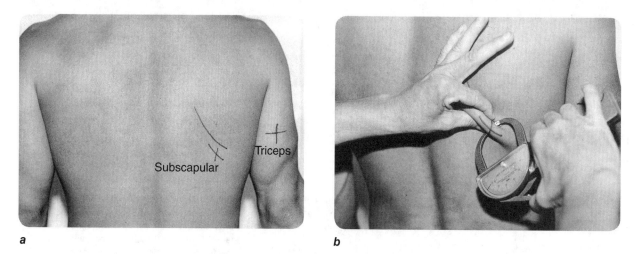

Figure D.2.2 *(a)* Site and *(b)* measurement of the subscapular skinfold. Photos courtesy of Linda K. Gilkey.

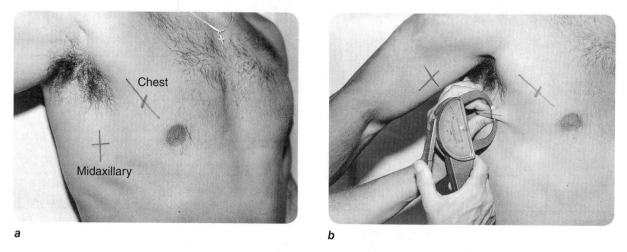

Figure D.2.3 *(a)* Site and *(b)* measurement of the midaxillary skinfold. Photos courtesy of Linda K. Gilkey.

From Vivian H. Heyward, 2010, *Advanced Fitness Assessment and Exercise Prescription*, 6th ed. (Champaign, IL: Human Kinetics).

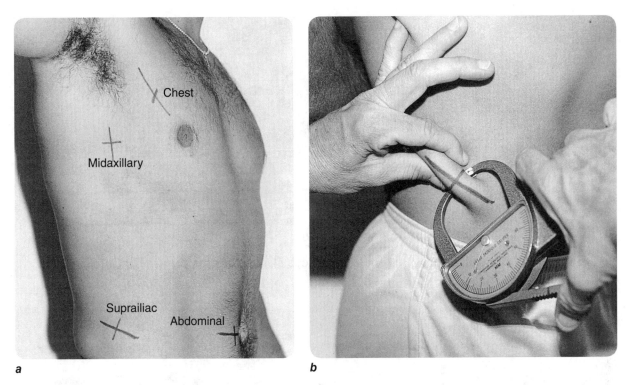

a

b

Figure D.2.4 *(a)* Site and *(b)* measurement of the suprailiac skinfold. Photos courtesy of Linda K. Gilkey.

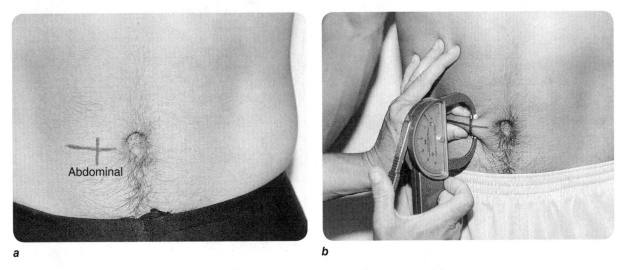

a

b

Figure D.2.5 *(a)* Site and *(b)* measurement of the abdominal skinfold. Photos courtesy of Linda K. Gilkey.

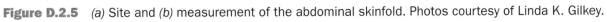

From Vivian H. Heyward, 2010, *Advanced Fitness Assessment and Exercise Prescription,* 6th ed. (Champaign, IL: Human Kinetics).

APPENDIX D.2

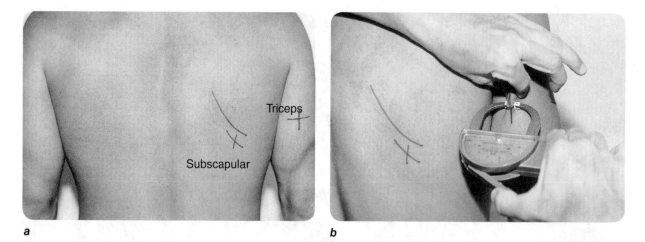

a   b

Figure D.2.6 *(a)* Site and *(b)* measurement of the triceps skinfold. Photos courtesy of Linda K. Gilkey.

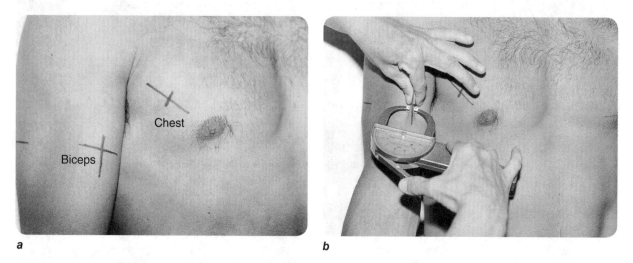

a   b

Figure D.2.7 *(a)* Site and *(b)* measurement of the biceps skinfold. Photos courtesy of Linda K. Gilkey.

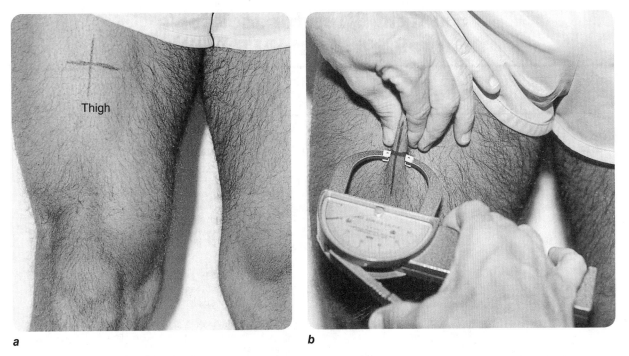

a *b*

Figure D.2.8 *(a)* Site and *(b)* measurement of the thigh skinfold. Photos courtesy of Linda K. Gilkey.

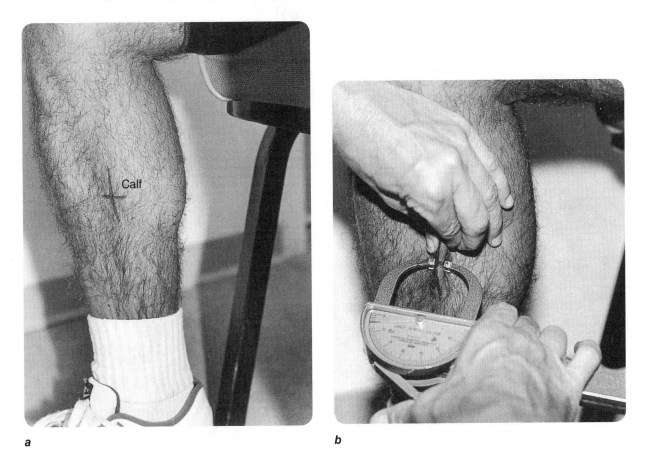

a *b*

Figure D.2.9 *(a)* Site and *(b)* measurement of the calf skinfold. Photos courtesy of Linda K. Gilkey.

From Vivian H. Heyward, 2010, *Advanced Fitness Assessment and Exercise Prescription*, 6th ed. (Champaign, IL: Human Kinetics).

Skinfold Sites for Jackson's Generalized Skinfold Equations

Site	Direction of fold	Anatomical reference	Measurement
Chest	Diagonal	Axilla and nipple	Fold is taken 1/2 the distance between the anterior axillary line and nipple for men and 1/3 of this distance for women.
Subscapular	Oblique	Vertebral border and inferior angle of scapula	Fold is taken on diagonal line coming from the vertebral border, 1-2 cm below the inferior angle.
Midaxillary	Vertical	Xiphoid process of sternum	Fold is taken at level of xiphoid process along the midaxillary line.
Suprailiac	Diagonal	Iliac crest	Fold is taken diagonally above the iliac crest along the anterior axillary line.
Abdominal	Vertical	Umbilicus	Fold is taken vertically 2 cm lateral to the umbilicus.

Adapted from Jackson and Pollock 1978 and Jackson, Pollock, and Ward 1980.

From Vivian H. Heyward, 2010, *Advanced Fitness Assessment and Exercise Prescription*, 6th ed. (Champaign, IL: Human Kinetics).

APPENDIX D.3

Standardized Sites
for Circumference Measurements

Site	Anatomical reference	Position	Measurement
Neck	Laryngeal prominence ("Adam's apple")	Perpendicular to long axis of neck	Apply tape with minimal pressure just inferior to the Adam's apple.
Shoulder	Deltoid muscles and acromion processes of scapula	Horizontal	Apply tape snugly over maximum bulges of the deltoid muscles, inferior to acromion processes. Record measurement at end of normal expiration.
Chest	Fourth costosternal joints	Horizontal	Apply tape snugly around the torso at level of fourth costosternal joints. Record at end of normal expiration.
Waist	Narrowest part of torso, level of the "natural" waist between ribs and iliac crest	Horizontal	Apply tape snugly around the waist at level of narrowest part of torso. An assistant is needed to position tape behind the client. Take measurement at end of normal expiration.
Abdominal	Maximum anterior protuberance of abdomen, usually at umbilicus	Horizontal	Apply tape snugly around the abdomen at level of greatest anterior protuberance. An assistant is needed to position tape behind the client. Take measurement at end of normal expiration.
Hip (buttocks)	Maximum posterior extension of buttocks	Horizontal	Apply tape snugly around the buttocks. An assistant is needed to position tape on opposite side of body.
Thigh (proximal)	Gluteal fold	Horizontal	Apply tape snugly around thigh, just distal to the gluteal fold.
Thigh (mid)	Inguinal crease and proximal border of patella	Horizontal	With client's knee flexed 90° (right foot on bench), apply tape at level midway between inguinal crease and proximal border of patella.
Thigh (distal)	Femoral epicondyles	Horizontal	Apply tape just proximal to the femoral epicondyles.
Knee	Patella	Horizontal	Apply tape around the knee at midpatellar level with knee relaxed in slight flexion.
Calf	Maximum girth of calf muscle	Perpendicular to long axis of leg	With client sitting on end of table and legs hanging freely, apply tape horizontally around the maximum girth of calf.
Ankle	Malleoli of tibia and fibula	Perpendicular to long axis of leg	Apply tape snugly around minimum circumference of leg, just proximal to the malleoli.
Arm (biceps)	Acromion process of scapula and olecranon process of ulna	Perpendicular to long axis of arm	With client's arms hanging freely at sides and palms facing thighs, apply tape snugly around the arm at level midway between the acromion process of scapula and olecranon process of ulna (as marked for triceps and biceps skinfolds).
Forearm	Maximum girth of forearm	Perpendicular to long axis of forearm	With client's arms hanging down and away from trunk and forearm supinated, apply tape snugly around the maximum girth of the proximal part of the forearm.
Wrist	Styloid processes of radius and ulna	Perpendicular to long axis of forearm	With client's elbow flexed and forearm supinated, apply tape snugly around wrist, just distal to the styloid processes of the radius and ulna.

Adapted from Callaway et al. 1988.

From Vivian H. Heyward, 2010, *Advanced Fitness Assessment and Exercise Prescription*, 6th ed. (Champaign, IL: Human Kinetics).

Standardized Sites for
Bony Breadth Measurements

Site	Anatomical reference	Position	Measurement
Biacromial (shoulder)	Lateral borders of acromion processes of scapula	Horizontal	With client standing, arms hanging vertically and shoulders relaxed, downward and slightly forward, apply blades of anthropometer to lateral borders of acromion processes. Measurement is taken from the rear.
Chest	Sixth rib on midaxillary line or fourth costosternal joints anteriorly	Horizontal	With client standing, arms slightly abducted, apply the large spreading caliper tips lightly on the sixth ribs on the midaxillary line. Take measurement at end of normal expiration.
Bi-iliac (bicristal)	Iliac crests	45° downward angle	With client standing, arms folded across the chest, apply anthropometer blades firmly at a 45° downward angle, at maximum breadth of iliac crest. Measurement is taken from rear.
Bitrochanteric	Greater trochanter of femur	Horizontal	With client standing, arms folded across the chest, apply anthropometer blade with considerable pressure to compress soft tissues. Measure maximum distance between the trochanters from the rear.
Knee	Femoral epicondyles	Diagonal or horizontal	With client sitting and knee flexed to 90°, apply caliper blades firmly on lateral and medial femoral epicondyles.
Ankle (bimalleolar)	Malleoli of tibia and fibula	Oblique	With client standing and weight evenly distributed, place the caliper blades on the most lateral part of lateral malleolus and most medial part of medial malleolus. Measurement is taken on an oblique plane from the rear.
Elbow	Epicondyles of humerus	Oblique	With client's elbow flexed 90°, arm raised to the horizontal, and forearm supinated, apply the caliper blades firmly to the medial and lateral humeral epicondyles at an angle that bisects the right angle at the elbow.
Wrist	Styloid process of radius and ulna, anatomical "snuff box"	Oblique	With client's elbow flexed 90°, upper arm vertical and close to torso, and forearm pronated, apply caliper tips firmly at an oblique angle to the styloid processes of the radius (at proximal part of anatomical snuff box) and ulna.

Adapted from Wilmore et al. 1988.

From Vivian H. Heyward, 2010, *Advanced Fitness Assessment and Exercise Prescription,* 6th ed. (Champaign, IL: Human Kinetics).

Ashwell Body Shape Chart

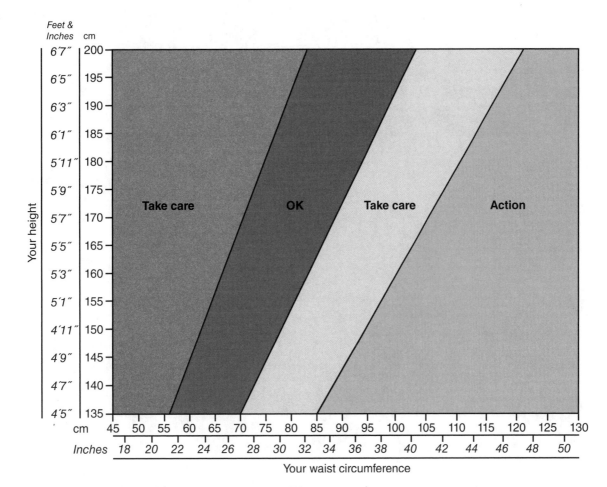

Adapted, by permission, from Ashwell Associates. © Dr. Margaret Ashwell OBE.

From Vivian H. Heyward, 2010, *Advanced Fitness Assessment and Exercise Prescription,* 6th ed. (Champaign, IL: Human Kinetics).

Energy Intake and Expenditure

You can use the Food Record and RDA Profile (appendix E.1) to obtain information about your client's energy intake and daily energy needs. Appendix E.2 shows a sample computerized analysis of food intake that summarizes your client's recommended daily nutrients, compares the daily intake to caloric needs, and provides a detailed nutrient analysis for each food item ingested.

Your clients may use the Physical Activity Log (appendix E.3) to record the type and duration of physical activities they engage in on a daily basis. This provides an estimate of the client's daily caloric expenditure due to activity. Appendix E.4 presents MET estimates of gross expenditure for conditioning exercises, sports, and recreational activities. You can use these estimates to calculate your client's energy expenditure ($kcal \cdot min^{-1}$) for a variety of activities. Appendix E.5 includes illustrations of healthy eating pyramids for Asian, Latin American, Mediterranean, and Vegetarian diets.

Food Record and RDA Profile

Food code	Amount	Description

Food code: This is generally for office use. If you have the food code list, however, use this space to more precisely describe your food item.

Amount: You can use common measures (cup, slice, etc.) or weight for your foods.

Food description: Be specific. For example, bread choices include soft and firm textures; vegetables may be raw or cooked fresh, frozen, or canned; meats should be lean only or lean with some fat; fruit juices are fresh, frozen, or canned; and cheese might be cream or skim, soft, hard, or cottage.

From Vivian H. Heyward, 2010, *Advanced Fitness Assessment and Exercise Prescription,* 6th ed. (Champaign, IL: Human Kinetics).

RDA Profile Information

Name: _____

Age: _____   Height: _____

Sex: Male _____   Weight: _____

    Female _____   Activity level: _____
                                                 (enter number from choices below)

        Pregnant _____

        Nursing _____

Most people engage in a variety of activities in a 24-hr period, and each activity can use a different amount of energy. Thus, any table of activity levels must depend on averages. Choose the level that represents your *normal daily average*.

1. Sedentary

   Inactive, sometimes under someone else's care. Energy level is for basal metabolism plus about 15% for minimal activities.

2. Lightly active

   Most professionals (lawyers, doctors, accountants, architects, etc.), office workers, shop workers, teachers, homemakers with mechanical appliances, unemployed persons.

3. Moderately active

   Most persons in light industry, building workers (excluding heavy laborers), many farm workers, active students, department store workers, soldiers not in active service, people engaged in commercial fishing, homemakers without mechanical household appliances.

4. Very active

   Full-time athletes, dancers, unskilled laborers, some agricultural workers (especially in peasant farming), forestry workers, army recruits, soldiers in active service, mine workers, steel workers.

5. Exceptionally active

   Lumberjacks, blacksmiths, women construction workers, rickshaw pullers.

From ESHA Research, 606 Juntura Way SE, Salem, OR 97302; phone: (503) 585-6242.

From Vivian H. Heyward, 2010, *Advanced Fitness Assessment and Exercise Prescription,* 6th ed. (Champaign, IL: Human Kinetics).

Sample Computerized Analysis of Food Intake

Jane Doe Personal Profile Report

Gender:	Female
Activity Level:	Lightly Active
Height:	5 ft 3 in
Weight:	132 lbs
Age:	25 yrs
BMI:	23.38

Recommended Daily Nutrients

Basic Components			
Calories	2044		*
Protein	47.9	g	
Carbohydrates	296	g	**
Dietary Fiber	20	g	#
Fat - Total	68	g	**
Saturated Fat	20	g	**
Mono Fat	25	g	**
Poly Fat	23	g	**
Cholesterol	300	mg	

Vitamins			
Vitamin A IU	4000	IU	
Vitamin A RE	800	RE	
Thiamin-B_1	1.02	mg	
Riboflavin-B_2	1.23	mg	
Niacin	13.49	NE	
Vitamin-B_6	1.60	mg	
Vitamin-B_{12}	2.00	mcg	
Biotin	65.00	mcg **	
Vitamin C	60.00	mg	

Vitamin D mcg	5.00	mcg	
Vit E-Alpha Equiv.	8.00	mg	
Folate	180.00	mcg	
Vitamin K	6.00	mcg	
Pantothenic	7.00	mg **	

Minerals			
Calcium	800.00	mg	
Chromium	125.00	mcg **	
Copper	2.50	mg **	
Fluoride	2.75	mg **	
Iodine	150	mcg	
Iron	15	mg	
Magnesium	280	mg	
Manganese	3.50	mg **	
Molybdenum	163	mcg **	
Phosphorus	800	mg	
Potassium	3750	mg	
Selenium	55	mcg	
Sodium	2400	mg	
Zinc	12	mg	

* Suggested values within recommended ranges
** Dietary goals   \# Fiber = 1 gram/100 kcal

The Food Processor® Nutrition Analysis program from ESHA Research, Salem, Oregon.

From Vivian H. Heyward, 2010, *Advanced Fitness Assessment and Exercise Prescription,* 6th ed. (Champaign, IL: Human Kinetics).

Source of Calories

Ratios and Percents

		0	25	50	75	100
Protein	19%					
Carbohydrates	58%					
Fat - Total	22%					
Alcohol	0%					

Source of Fat

		0	6	11	17	22
Saturated (7-10%)	10%					
Mono Unsat (10-15%)	6%					
Poly Unsat (up to 10%)	4%					
Other/Missing	2%					

Exchanges

Bread / Starch:	8.0	Fruit:	4.6
Other Carbs / Sugar:	2.6	Vegetables:	3.8
Very Lean Meat / Protein:	4.5	Milk - Skim:	0.5
Lean Meat:	2.9	Fat:	5.4

Ratios

P : S (Poly / Saturated Fat)	0.39 : 1
Potassium : Sodium	1.61 : 1
Calcium : Phosphorus	0.53 : 1
CSI (Cholesterol / Saturated Fat Index)	28.21

Daily Intake

June 23, 1997

% comparison to: Jane Doe

Bar Graph

Nutrient	Value	Goal%	0	25	50	75	100
Basic Components							
Calories	1691.39	83%					
Protein	84.04 g	175%					
Carbohydrates	251.82 g	85%					
Dietary fiber	20.71 g	101%					
Fat - Total	42.41 g	62%					
Saturated fat	19.24 g	94%					
Mono fat	11.86 g	47%					
Poly fat	7.47 g	33%					
Cholesterol	175.49 mg	58%					
Vitamins							
Vitamin A RE	1326.90 RE	166%					
Thiamin B_1	1.79 mg	176%					
Riboflavin B_2	2.11 mg	171%					
Niacin B_3	37.54 mg	278%					
Vitamin B_6	3.37 mg	211%					
Vitamin B_{12}	2.55 mcg	127%					
Vitamin C	266.19 mg	444%					
Vitamin D mcg	7.07 mcg	141%					
Vit E-Alpha Equiv.	3.79 mg	47%					
Folate	440.36 mcg	245%					
Pantothenic Acid	4.87 mg	70%					
Minerals							
Calcium	665.59 mg	83%					
Copper	1.24 mg	49%					
Iron	12.83 mg	86%					
Magnesium	267.18 mg	95%					
Manganese	2.25 mg	64%					
Phosphorus	1254.53 mg	157%					
Potassium	3187.63 mg	85%					
Selenium	144.48 mcg	263%					
Sodium	1974.93 mg	82%					
Zinc	5.78 mg	48%					

From Vivian H. Heyward, 2010, *Advanced Fitness Assessment and Exercise Prescription*, 6th ed. (Champaign, IL: Human Kinetics).

Spreadsheet

Amount	Food Item	Weight (g)	Cals	Prot (g)	Carb (g)	Fiber (g)	Fat-T (g)
1/2 cup	Orange Juice prepared from frozen	124.50	56.03	0.85	13.45	0.25	0.07
2 oz-wt	Kelloggs Corn Flakes Cereal	56.70	220.56	4.59	48.82	1.47	0.17
1 each	Banana--Medium size	118.00	108.56	1.22	27.61	2.83	0.57
1/2 cup	Skim Milk-Vitamin A Added	122.50	42.75	4.18	5.94	0	0.22
1 piece	Whole Wheat Bread-Toasted	25.00	69.25	2.73	12.93	1.85	1.20
2 tsp	Jelly	12.67	34.33	0.05	8.97	0.13	0.01
1 each	White Pita Pocket Bread 6 1/2"diameter	60.00	165.00	5.46	33.42	1.32	0.72
1/2 cup	Tuna Salad	102.50	191.67	16.40	9.65	0	9.49
1/4 cup	Alfalfa Sprouts-Raw	8.25	2.39	0.33	0.31	0.21	0.06
2 piece	Fresh Tomato Wedge(1/4 of Medium Tomato)	62.00	13.02	0.53	2.88	0.68	0.20
8 oz-wt	Diet soda pop - average assorted	226.80	0	0	0	0	0
1 each	Medium Apple w/Peel	138.00	81.42	0.26	21.11	3.73	0.50
4 oz-wt	Chicken light meat - roasted	113.40	173.50	30.73	0	0	4.62
1 each	Baked Potato w/skin - medium	122.00	132.98	2.82	30.74	2.93	0.12
1 oz-wt	Cheddar Cheese-Shredded	28.35	114.25	7.06	0.36	0	9.38
4 oz-wt	Broccoli Pieces-Steamed	113.40	31.75	3.39	5.95	3.40	0.40
1/2 cup	Rich Vanilla Ice Cream	74.00	178.34	2.59	16.58	0	11.99
1/2 cup	Fresh Strawberries-Slices-Cup	83.00	24.90	0.51	5.83	1.91	0.31
2 tbs	Frozen Dessert Topping-Semi Solid	9.38	29.81	0.12	2.17	0	2.37
1 cup	Brewed Coffee	237.00	4.74	0.24	0.95	0	0.01
1 tsp	White Granulated Sugar	4.17	16.13	0	4.16	0	0
	Totals	1841.61	1691.39	84.04	251.82	20.71	42.41

Amount	Food Item	Fat-S (g)	Fat-M (g)	Fat-P (g)	Chol (mg)	A-RE (RE)	B_1 (mg)
1/2 cup	Orange Juice prepared from frozen	0.01	0.01	0.01	0	9.96	0.10
2 oz-wt	Kelloggs Corn Flakes Cereal	0.02	0.09	0.03	0	750.71	0.74
1 each	Banana--Medium size	0.22	0.05	0.11	0	9.44	0.05
1/2 cup	Skim Milk-Vitamin A Added	0.14	0.06	0.01	2.21	74.73	0.04
1 piece	Whole Wheat Bread-Toasted	0.26	0.47	0.28	0	0	0.08
2 tsp	Jelly	0.00	0.00	0.01	0	0.25	0.00
1 each	White Pita Pocket Bread 6 1/2"diameter	0.10	0.06	0.32	0	0	0.36
1/2 cup	Tuna Salad	1.58	2.96	4.22	13.32	27.67	0.03
1/4 cup	Alfalfa Sprouts-Raw	0.01	0.00	0.03	0	1.32	0.01
2 piece	Fresh Tomato Wedge(1/4 of Medium Tomato)	0.03	0.03	0.08	0	38.44	0.04
8 oz-wt	Diet soda pop - average assorted	0	0	0	0	0	0
1 each	Medium Apple w/Peel	0.08	0.02	0.14	0	6.90	0.02
4 oz-wt	Chicken light meat - roasted	1.24	1.75	1.05	85.05	9.07	0.07
1 each	Baked Potato w/skin - medium	0.03	0.00	0.05	0	0	0.13
1 oz-wt	Cheddar Cheese-Shredded	6.01	2.66	0.27	29.77	85.90	0.01
4 oz-wt	Broccoli Pieces-Steamed	0.06	0.03	0.19	0	165.79	0.07
1/2 cup	Rich Vanilla Ice Cream	7.39	3.45	0.45	45.14	136.16	0.03
1/2 cup	Fresh Strawberries-Slices-Cup	0.02	0.04	0.15	0	2.49	0.02
2 tbs	Frozen Dessert Topping-Semi Solid	2.05	0.15	0.05	0	8.06	0
1 cup	Brewed Coffee	0.00	0	0.00	0	0	0
1 tsp	White Granulated Sugar	0	0	0	0	0	0
	Totals	19.24	11.86	7.47	175.49	1326.90	1.79

The Food Processor Nutrition Analysis program from ESHA Research, Salem, Oregon.

Spreadsheet

Amount	Food Item	B₂ (mg)	B₃ (mg)	B₆ (mg)	B₁₂ (mcg)	Vit C (mg)	D-mcg (mcg)
1/2 cup	Orange Juice prepared from frozen	0.02	0.25	0.05	0	48.43	0
2 oz-wt	Kelloggs Corn Flakes Cereal	0.86	9.98	1.02	0	30.05	1.98
1 each	Banana--Medium size	0.12	0.64	0.68	0	10.74	0
1/2 cup	Skim Milk-Vitamin A Added	0.17	0.11	0.05	0.46	1.20	1.23
1 piece	Whole Wheat Bread-Toasted	0.05	0.97	0.05	0.00	0	0.05
2 tsp	Jelly	0.00	0.00	0.00	0	0.11	0
1 each	White Pita Pocket Bread 6 1/2"diameter	0.20	2.78	0.02	0	0	0
1/2 cup	Tuna Salad	0.07	6.87	0.08	1.23	2.25	3.31
1/4 cup	Alfalfa Sprouts-Raw	0.01	0.04	0.00	0	0.68	0
2 piece	Fresh Tomato Wedge(1/4 of Medium Tomato)	0.03	0.39	0.05	0	11.84	0
8 oz-wt	Diet soda pop - average assorted	0	0	0	0	0	0
1 each	Medium Apple w/Peel	0.02	0.11	0.07	0	7.87	0
4 oz-wt	Chicken light meat - roasted	0.11	11.91	0.61	0.35	0	0.34
1 each	Baked Potato w/skin - medium	0.04	2.01	0.42	0	15.74	0
1 oz-wt	Cheddar Cheese-Shredded	0.11	0.02	0.02	0.23	0	0.09
4 oz-wt	Broccoli Pieces-Steamed	0.13	0.69	0.16	0	89.70	0
1/2 cup	Rich Vanilla Ice Cream	0.12	0.06	0.03	0.27	0.52	0.07
1/2 cup	Fresh Strawberries-Slices-Cup	0.05	0.19	0.05	0	47.06	0
2 tbs	Frozen Dessert Topping-Semi Solid	0	0	0	0	0	0
1 cup	Brewed Coffee	0	0.53	0	0	0	0
1 tsp	White Granulated Sugar	0.00	0	0	0	0	0
	Totals	2.11	37.54	3.37	2.55	266.19	7.07

Amount	Food Item	E-aTE (mg)	Fola (mcg)	Panto (mg)	Calc (mg)	Copp (mg)	Iron (mg)
1/2 cup	Orange Juice prepared from frozen	0.24	54.53	0.20	11.21	0.05	0.12
2 oz-wt	Kelloggs Corn Flakes Cereal	0.14	200.15	0.10	1.70	0.04	3.58
1 each	Banana--Medium size	0.32	22.54	0.31	7.08	0.12	0.37
1/2 cup	Skim Milk-Vitamin A Added	0.05	6.37	0.40	150.68	0.01	0.05
1 piece	Whole Wheat Bread-Toasted	0.23	9.75	0.10	20.25	0.08	0.93
2 tsp	Jelly	0	0.13	0.02	1.01	0.00	0.03
1 each	White Pita Pocket Bread 6 1/2"diameter	0.02	14.40	0.24	51.60	0.10	1.57
1/2 cup	Tuna Salad	0.97	7.48	0.27	17.42	0.15	1.02
1/4 cup	Alfalfa Sprouts-Raw	0.00	2.97	0.05	2.64	0.01	0.08
2 piece	Fresh Tomato Wedge(1/4 of Medium Tomato)	0.24	9.30	0.15	3.10	0.05	0.28
8 oz-wt	Diet soda pop - average assorted	0	0	0	0	0	0
1 each	Medium Apple w/Peel	0.44	3.86	0.08	9.66	0.06	0.25
4 oz-wt	Chicken light meat - roasted	0.30	3.40	1.03	14.74	0.05	1.22
1 each	Baked Potato w/skin - medium	0.06	13.42	0.68	12.20	0.37	1.66
1 oz-wt	Cheddar Cheese-Shredded	0.10	5.16	0.12	204.40	0.01	0.19
4 oz-wt	Broccoli Pieces-Steamed	0.54	68.27	0.58	54.32	0.05	1.00
1/2 cup	Rich Vanilla Ice Cream	0	3.70	0.27	86.58	0.02	0.04
1/2 cup	Fresh Strawberries-Slices-Cup	0.12	14.69	0.28	11.62	0.04	0.32
2 tbs	Frozen Dessert Topping-Semi Solid	0.02	0	0	0.59	0.00	0.01
1 cup	Brewed Coffee	0	0.24	0.00	4.74	0.02	0.12
1 tsp	White Granulated Sugar	0	0	0	0.04	0.00	0.00
	Totals	3.79	440.36	4.87	665.59	1.24	12.83

From Vivian H. Heyward, 2010, *Advanced Fitness Assessment and Exercise Prescription*, 6th ed. (Champaign, IL: Human Kinetics).

Spreadsheet

Amount	Food Item	Magn (mg)	Mang (mg)	Phos (mg)	Potas (mg)	Sel (mcg)	Sod (mg)
1/2 cup	Orange Juice prepared from frozen	12.45	0.02	19.92	236.55	0.25	1.25
2 oz-wt	Kelloggs Corn Flakes Cereal	6.80	0.05	35.72	52.16	2.89	580.04
1 each	Banana--Medium size	34.22	0.18	23.60	467.28	1.18	1.18
1/2 cup	Skim Milk-Vitamin A Added	13.97	0.00	123.73	203.35	1.23	63.09
1 piece	Whole Wheat Bread-Toasted	24.25	0.65	64.50	70.75	10.25	148.00
2 tsp	Jelly	0.76	0.02	0.63	8.11	0.25	4.56
1 each	White Pita Pocket Bread 6 1/2"diameter	15.60	0.29	58.20	72.00	18.00	321.60
1/2 cup	Tuna Salad	19.47	0.04	182.45	182.45	70.01	412.05
1/4 cup	Alfalfa Sprouts-Raw	2.23	0.02	5.78	6.52	--	0.50
2 piece	Fresh Tomato Wedge(1/4 of Medium Tomato)	6.82	0.07	14.88	137.64	0.25	5.58
8 oz-wt	Diet soda pop - average assorted	0	0	90.72	34.02	0	113.40
1 each	Medium Apple w/Peel	6.90	0.06	9.66	158.70	0.41	0
4 oz-wt	Chicken light meat - roasted	26.08	0.02	246.08	267.62	28.92	57.83
1 each	Baked Potato w/skin - medium	32.94	0.28	69.54	509.96	1.95	9.76
1 oz-wt	Cheddar Cheese-Shredded	7.88	0.00	145.15	27.90	4.03	176.05
4 oz-wt	Broccoli Pieces-Steamed	28.35	0.25	74.73	367.42	--	30.62
1/2 cup	Rich Vanilla Ice Cream	8.14	0.01	70.30	117.66	4.00	41.44
1/2 cup	Fresh Strawberries-Slices-Cup	8.30	0.24	15.77	137.78	0.75	0.83
2 tbs	Frozen Dessert Topping-Semi Solid	0.17	0.01	0.72	1.71	--	2.37
1 cup	Brewed Coffee	11.85	0.06	2.37	127.98	0.11	4.74
1 tsp	White Granulated Sugar	0	0.00	0.08	0.08	0.01	0.04
	Totals	267.18	2.25	1254.53	3187.63	144.48	1974.93

Amount	Food Item	Zinc (mg)
1/2 cup	Orange Juice prepared from frozen	0.06
2 oz-wt	Kelloggs Corn Flakes Cereal	0.16
1 each	Banana--Medium size	0.19
1/2 cup	Skim Milk-Vitamin A Added	0.49
1 piece	Whole Wheat Bread-Toasted	0.55
2 tsp	Jelly	0.01
1 each	White Pita Pocket Bread 6 1/2"diameter	0.50
1/2 cup	Tuna Salad	0.57
1/4 cup	Alfalfa Sprouts-Raw	0.08
2 piece	Fresh Tomato Wedge(1/4 of Medium Tomato)	0.06
8 oz-wt	Diet soda pop - average assorted	0
1 each	Medium Apple w/Peel	0.06
4 oz-wt	Chicken light meat - roasted	0.88
1 each	Baked Potato w/skin - medium	0.39
1 oz-wt	Cheddar Cheese-Shredded	0.88
4 oz-wt	Broccoli Pieces-Steamed	0.45
1/2 cup	Rich Vanilla Ice Cream	0.30
1/2 cup	Fresh Strawberries-Slices-Cup	0.11
2 tbs	Frozen Dessert Topping-Semi Solid	0.00
1 cup	Brewed Coffee	0.05
1 tsp	White Granulated Sugar	0.00
	Totals	5.78

The Food Processor Nutrition Analysis program from ESHA Research, Salem, Oregon.

From Vivian H. Heyward, 2010, *Advanced Fitness Assessment and Exercise Prescription,* 6th ed. (Champaign, IL: Human Kinetics).

Physical Activity Log

Name: _____ Date: _____

Day and date	Activity	Duration (min)	X	kcal·min^{-1}	= Total (kcal)

From Vivian H. Heyward, 2010, *Advanced Fitness Assessment and Exercise Prescription,* 6th ed. (Champaign, IL: Human Kinetics).

Gross Energy Expenditure for Conditioning Exercises, Sports, and Recreational Activities

METs	Description	METs	Description
Conditioning Exercises			
5.0	Aerobic dancing, low impact	12.5	Rollerblading, in-line skating, vigorous effort
8.5	Aerobics, step, with 6-8 in. step	8.0	Rope skipping, slow
10.0	Aerobics, step, with 10-12 in. step	10.0	Rope skipping, moderate
3.0	Bicycling, stationary, 50 W, very light effort	12.0	Rope skipping, fast
5.5	Bicycling, stationary, 100 W, light effort	9.5	Skiing, Nordic (machine)
7.0	Bicycling, stationary, 150 W, moderate effort	6.0	Slimnastics, Jazzercize
10.5	Bicycling, stationary, 200 W, vigorous effort	9.0	Stair-climbing (machine), step ergometer
12.5	Bicycling, stationary, 250 W, very vigorous effort	2.5	Stretching, hatha yoga
8.0	Calisthenics (e.g., push-ups, pull-ups, jumping jacks, sit-ups), vigorous	10.0	Swimming, laps, freestyle, fast, vigorous effort
3.5	Calisthenics, light or moderate effort	7.0	Swimming, laps, freestyle, slow, moderate or light effort
8.0	Circuit resistance training, including some aerobic activity and minimal rest (e.g., super circuit resistance training)	7.0	Swimming, backstroke
8.0	Elliptical training, machine, 125 strides·min^{-1} with resistance	10.0	Swimming, breaststroke
3.5	Rowing (machine), 50 W, light effort	11.0	Swimming, butterfly
7.0	Rowing (machine), 100 W, moderate effort	11.0	Swimming, crawl, fast, vigorous effort
8.5	Rowing (machine), 150 W, vigorous effort	8.0	Swimming, crawl, slow, moderate or light effort
12.0	Rowing (machine), 200 W, very vigorous effort	8.0	Swimming, sidestroke
8.0	Running, 5 mph (12 min·mile^{-1})	4.0	Swimming, treading water, moderate effort
9.0	Running, 5.2 mph (11.5 min·mile^{-1})	4.0	Tai chi
10.0	Running, 6.0 mph (10 min·mile^{-1})	5.0	Treading, walking, variable speed 2.5-4.0 mph and grade 0-10%
11.0	Running, 6.7 mph (9 min·mile^{-1})	11.0	Treading, running, variable speed 5.8-7.5 mph and grade 0-10%
11.5	Running, 7.0 mph (8.5 min·mile^{-1})	2.5	Walking, 2.0 mph
12.5	Running, 7.5 mph (8 min·mile^{-1})	3.0	Walking, 2.5 mph
13.5	Running, 8 mph (7.5 min·mile^{-1})	3.3	Walking, 3.0 mph
14.0	Running, 8.6 mph (7 min·mile^{-1})	3.8	Walking, 3.5 mph
15.0	Running, 9 mph (6.5 min·mile^{-1})	5.0	Walking, 4.0 mph
16.0	Running, 10 mph (6 min·mile^{-1})	6.3	Walking, 4.5 mph
18.0	Running, 10.9 mph (5.5 min·mile^{-1})	4.0	Water aerobics, water calisthenics
9.0	Running, cross country	8.0	Water jogging
7.0	Jogging, general	3.0	Weightlifting (free weights/machines), light to moderate effort
6.0	Jogging/walking combination (jogging component less than 10 min)	6.0	Weightlifting (free weights/machines), powerlifting, bodybuilding, vigorous effort
4.5	Jogging on a mini-trampoline		

From Vivian H. Heyward, 2010, *Advanced Fitness Assessment and Exercise Prescription,* 6th ed. (Champaign, IL: Human Kinetics).

METs	Description	METs	Description
	Sports and recreational activities		
3.5	Archery (non-hunting)	3.0	Diving, springboard or platform
7.0	Badminton, competitive	6.0	Fencing
4.5	Badminton, social singles or doubles	4.0	Fishing and hunting from riverbank and walking
5.0	Baseball, general	2.5	Fishing and hunting from boat, sitting
8.0	Basketball, game	6.0	Fishing in stream, in waders
4.5	Basketball, shooting baskets	2.0	Fishing, ice, sitting
6.5	Basketball, wheelchair	2.5	Fishing and hunting, bow and arrow, crossbow
8.5	Bicycling, BMX or mountain	2.5	Fishing and hunting, pistol shooting, trap shooting, standing
4.0	Bicycling, <10 mph, leisure, pleasure	9.0	Football, competitive
6.0	Bicycling, 10-11.9 mph	2.5	Football or baseball, playing catch
8.0	Bicycling, 12-13.9 mph	8.0	Football, touch, flag
10.0	Bicycling, 14-15.9 mph	3.0	Frisbee, playing, general
12.0	Bicycling, 16-19 mph	8.0	Frisbee, ultimate
16.0	Bicycling, ≥ 20 mph	3.0	Gardening, lawn work, general
5.0	Bicycling, unicycle	4.5	Golfing, walking and carrying clubs
2.5	Billiards, pool	3.0	Golfing, miniature, driving range
2.5	Bird watching	4.3	Golfing, walking and pulling clubs
3.0	Bowling	3.5	Golfing, power cart
3.0	Bowling, lawn	4.0	Gymnastics, general
12.0	Boxing, in ring	4.0	Hacky sack
6.0	Boxing, punching bag	12.0	Handball, general
9.0	Boxing, sparring	8.0	Handball, team
7.0	Broomball	3.5	Hang gliding
12.0	Boxing, in run	6.0	Hiking, cross country
6.0	Boxing, punching bag	8.0	Hockey, field
9.0	Boxing, sparring	8.0	Hockey, ice
7.0	Broomball	4.0	Horseback riding, general
3.0	Canoeing, 2.0-3.9 mph, light effort	3.0	Horseshoe pitching, quoits
7.0	Canoeing, 4.0-5.9 mph, moderate effort	12.0	Jai alai
12.0	Canoeing, ≥ 6.0 mph, vigorous effort	10.0	Judo, jujitsu, kick boxing, tae kwon do
5.0	Children's games, hopscotch, dodgeball, T-ball, tetherball, playground	4.0	Juggling
5.0	Cricket (batting and bowling)	5.0	Kayaking and whitewater rafting
2.5	Croquet	7.0	Kickball
4.0	Curling	8.0	Lacrosse
4.8	Dancing, ballet or modern, twist, jazz, tap, jitterbug	4.0	Motor-cross
4.5	Dancing, Greek, Middle Eastern, belly, hula, flamenco, swing	9.0	Orienteering
4.5	Dancing, ballroom, fast, disco, folk, square, line dancing, Irish step dancing, polka, contra, country	10.0	Paddleball, competitive
3.0	Dancing, slow, waltz, foxtrot, samba, tango, mamgo, cha-cha	6.0	Paddleball, casual, general
5.5	Dancing, traditional American Indian dancing	4.0	Paddle boating
2.5	Darts, wall or lawn	8.0	Polo

(continued)

From Vivian H. Heyward, 2010, *Advanced Fitness Assessment and Exercise Prescription,* 6th ed. (Champaign, IL: Human Kinetics).

Gross Energy Expenditure *(continued)*

METs	Description	METs	Description
	Sports and recreational activities *(continued)*		
6.5	Race walking	8.0	Snow shoeing
10.0	Racquetball, competitive	10.0	Soccer, competitive
7.0	Racquetball, casual, general	7.0	Soccer, casual, general
11.0	Rock climbing, ascending	5.0	Softball, fast or slow pitch
8.0	Rock climbing, rappelling	6.0	Softball, pitching
10.0	Rugby	12.0	Squash
3.0	Sailing, boat and board sailing, wind surfing, ice surfing	3.0	Surfing, body or board
7.0	Scuba diving, skin diving	6.0	Swimming, leisurely, not laps
3.0	Shuffleboard	8.0	Swimming, synchronized
5.0	Skateboarding	4.0	Table tennis, Ping-Pong
7.0	Skating, roller or ice	7.0	Tennis, general
15.0	Skating, speed skating	5.0	Tennis, doubles
7.0	Skiing, cross-country, 2.5 mph, light effort	8.0	Tennis, singles
8.0	Skiing, cross-country, 4.0-4.9 mph, moderate effort	4.0	Track and field, shot, discus, hammer throw
9.0	Skiing, cross-country, 5.0-7.9 mph, vigorous effort	6.0	Track and field, high jump, long jump, triple jump, javelin, pole vault
14.0	Skiing, cross-country, >8.0 mph, racing	10.0	Track and field, steeplechase, hurdles
5.0	Skiing, downhill, light effort	3.5	Trampoline
6.0	Skiing, downhill, moderate effort	8.0	Volleyball, competitive
8.0	Skiing, downhill, vigorous effort, racing	8.0	Volleyball, beach
6.0	Skiing, water	3.0	Volleyball, noncompetitive
7.0	Skimobiling	10.0	Water polo
3.5	Skydiving	3.0	Water volleyball
7.0	Sledding, tobogganing, bobsledding, luge	7.0	Wallyball
5.0	Snorkeling	6.0	Wrestling

From Vivian H. Heyward, 2010, *Advanced Fitness Assessment and Exercise Prescription*, 6th ed. (Champaign, IL: Human Kinetics).

Healthy Eating Pyramids

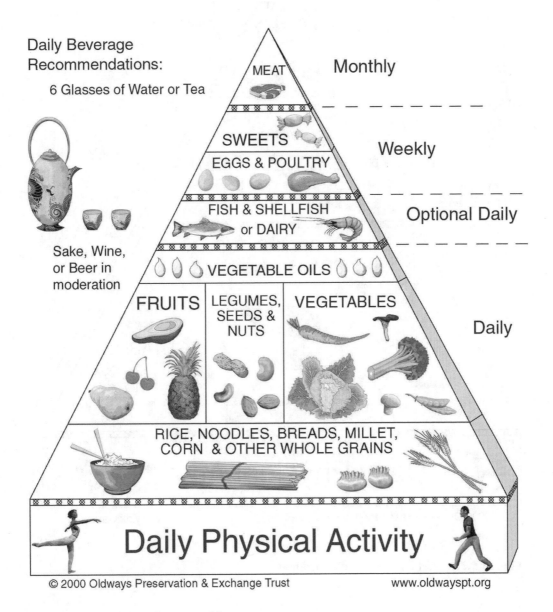

Daily Beverage
Recommendations:

6 Glasses of Water or Tea

Sake, Wine,
or Beer in
moderation

MEAT — Monthly

SWEETS
EGGS & POULTRY — Weekly

FISH & SHELLFISH
or DAIRY — Optional Daily

VEGETABLE OILS

FRUITS | LEGUMES, SEEDS & NUTS | VEGETABLES — Daily

RICE, NOODLES, BREADS, MILLET, CORN & OTHER WHOLE GRAINS

Daily Physical Activity

www.oldwayspt.org

Figure E.5.1   Asian diet pyramid.

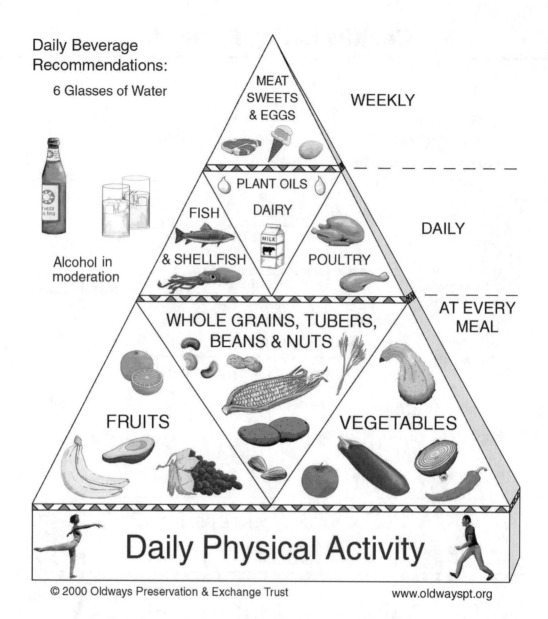

Figure E.5.2 Latin American diet pyramid.

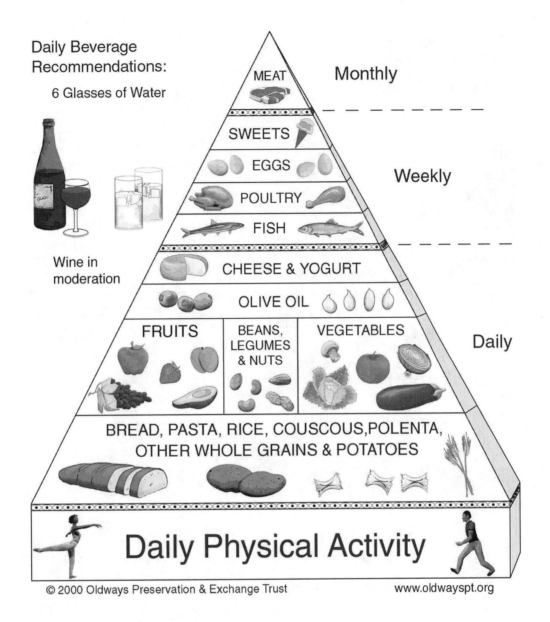

Daily Beverage Recommendations:

6 Glasses of Water

Wine in moderation

Monthly

MEAT

Weekly

SWEETS
EGGS
POULTRY
FISH

Daily

CHEESE & YOGURT
OLIVE OIL
FRUITS | BEANS, LEGUMES & NUTS | VEGETABLES
BREAD, PASTA, RICE, COUSCOUS, POLENTA, OTHER WHOLE GRAINS & POTATOES

Daily Physical Activity

© 2000 Oldways Preservation & Exchange Trust   www.oldwayspt.org

Figure E.5.3   Mediterranean diet pyramid.

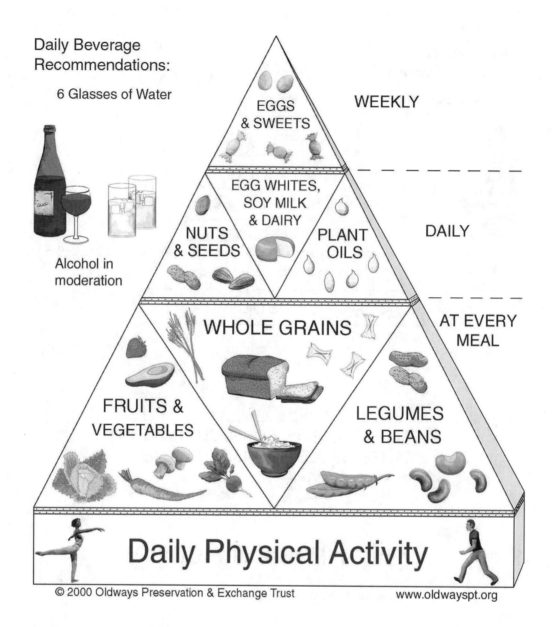

Daily Beverage Recommendations:

6 Glasses of Water

Alcohol in moderation

WEEKLY

EGGS & SWEETS

DAILY

EGG WHITES, SOY MILK & DAIRY

NUTS & SEEDS

PLANT OILS

AT EVERY MEAL

WHOLE GRAINS

FRUITS & VEGETABLES

LEGUMES & BEANS

Daily Physical Activity

© 2000 Oldways Preservation & Exchange Trust

www.oldwayspt.org

Figure E.5.4 Vegetarian diet pyramid.

Flexibility and Low Back Care Exercises

Appendix F.1 describes and illustrates selected static stretching exercises for flexibility. This information is organized by body region and muscle groups. Appendix F.2 summarizes Exercise Do's and Don'ts. For each contraindicated exercise, a safe alternative exercise is presented.

Recommended exercises for low back care programs are illustrated in appendix F.3. This appendix provides a description and identifies muscle groups involved for each exercise.

Selected Flexibility Exercises

ANTERIOR THIGH REGION

Muscle Groups: Quadriceps and Hip Flexors

Exercise 1

Description: From a standing position, raise one foot toward hips and grasp ankle. Pull leg upward toward buttocks.

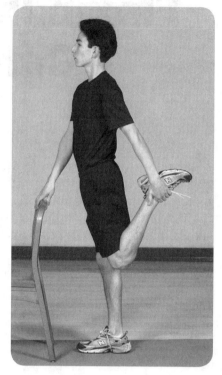

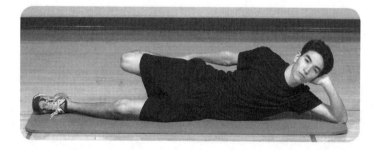

Exercise 2

Description: Lying on your side, flex the knee and grasp the ankle. Press the foot into the hand and squeeze pelvis forward. Do not pull the foot.

Exercise 3

Description: In a prone position, flex the knee and grasp ankle or foot with both hands. Do not pull on the foot. Keep knees on the floor and do not arch the back.

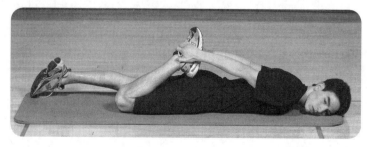

From Vivian H. Heyward, 2010, *Advanced Fitness Assessment and Exercise Prescription*, 6th ed. (Champaign, IL: Human Kinetics).

Muscle Groups:
Hamstrings and Hip Extensors

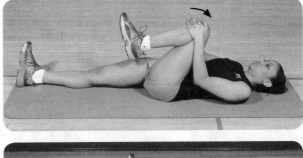

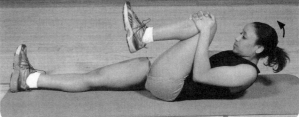

Exercise 1

Description: In a supine position, grasp knee and pull knee toward chest, then flex head to knee.

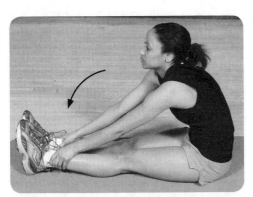

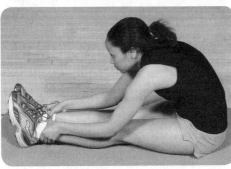

Exercise 2

Description: From a long-sitting position, grasp ankles and flex trunk to legs.

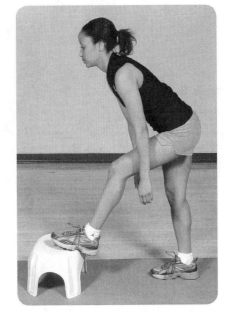

Exercise 3

Description: From a standing position, place your foot on a low step, keep the knee flexed slightly, and bend from the hips until you feel the stretch.

(continued)

From Vivian H. Heyward, 2010, *Advanced Fitness Assessment and Exercise Prescription,* 6th ed. (Champaign, IL: Human Kinetics).

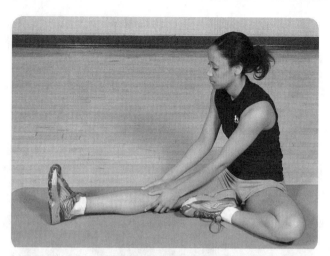

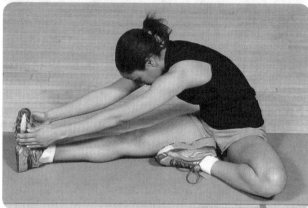

Exercise 4

Description: From a sitting position, with one knee flexed, flex the trunk keeping the spine extended until you feel tension.

Exercise 5

Description: From a lying position, with one leg extended and the other leg flexed, grasp leg with both hands and flex thigh to trunk.

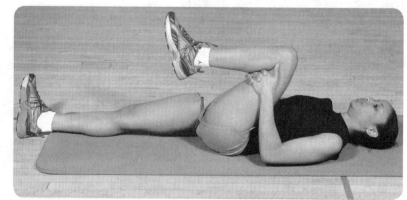

From Vivian H. Heyward, 2010, *Advanced Fitness Assessment and Exercise Prescription,* 6th ed. (Champaign, IL: Human Kinetics).

Muscle Groups: Hip Adductors

Exercise 1

Description: From a tailor-sitting position, with soles of feet together, place hands on inside of knees and push downward slowly.

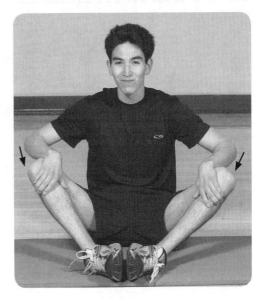

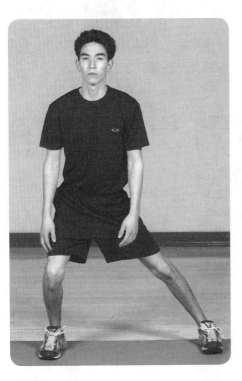

Exercise 2

Description: From a straddle-standing position, flex one knee and hip, lowering body closer to floor.

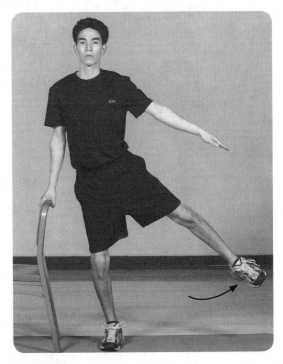

Exercise 3

Description: Standing on one leg while supporting yourself against wall or chair abduct hip, keeping leg straight. Have partner grasp ankle and passively stretch the muscle further.

From Vivian H. Heyward, 2010, *Advanced Fitness Assessment and Exercise Prescription,* 6th ed. (Champaign, IL: Human Kinetics).

Muscle Groups: Hip Abductors and Trunk Lateral Flexors

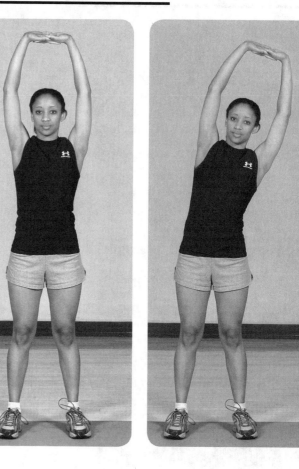

Exercise 1

Description: From standing position, with arms overhead, clasp hands together and laterally flex trunk to side no more than 20°.

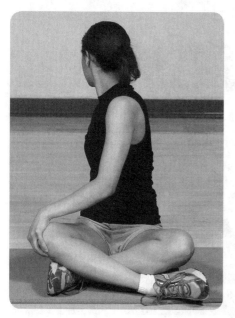

Exercise 2

Description: From a crossed-leg sitting position, rotate trunk to the right. Place hands on right side of thigh and pull. Repeat to opposite side.

From Vivian H. Heyward, 2010, *Advanced Fitness Assessment and Exercise Prescription*, 6th ed. (Champaign, IL: Human Kinetics).

Muscle Group: Plantar Flexors

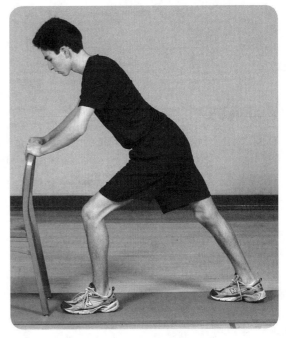

Exercise 1

Description: Assume front-leaning position against wall or chair with one foot ahead of the other. Flex hip, knee, and ankle to lower your body closer to the ground, keeping feet flat on floor.

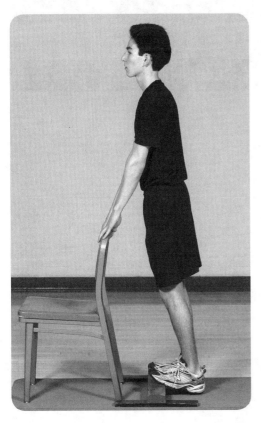

Exercise 2

Description: Standing with balls of feet on stairs, curb, or wood block, lower heels to floor.

From Vivian H. Heyward, 2010, *Advanced Fitness Assessment and Exercise Prescription,* 6th ed. (Champaign, IL: Human Kinetics).

ANTERIOR LEG REGION

Muscle Group: Dorsiflexors

Exercise 1

Description: Standing with ankle of the nonsupporting leg fully extended, stretch the dorsiflexors by slowly flexing the knee of the supporting leg.

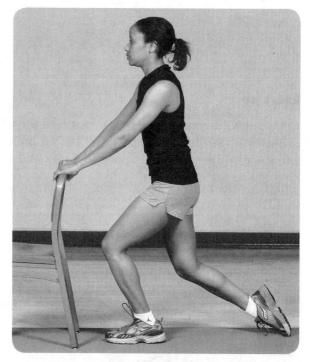

UPPER AND LOWER BACK REGIONS

Muscle Group: Trunk Extensors

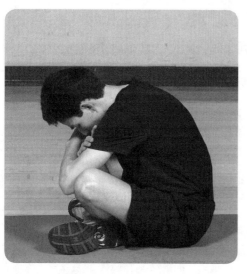

Exercise 1

Description: Sit with legs crossed and arms relaxed. Tuck chin and curl forward attempting to touch forehead to knees.

From Vivian H. Heyward, 2010, *Advanced Fitness Assessment and Exercise Prescription,* 6th ed. (Champaign, IL: Human Kinetics).

Exercise 2

Description: In a supine position, with knees flexed, grasp thighs below the knee caps and bring knees to chest. Flatten lower back to floor.

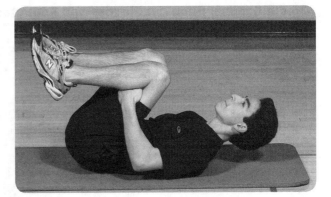

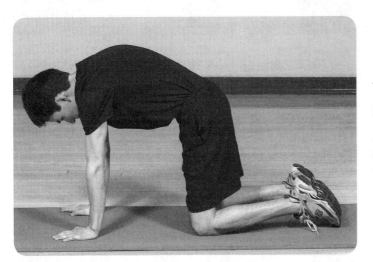

Exercise 3

Description: From a kneeling position, bring chin to chest. Contract abdomen and buttocks muscles while rounding lower back.

ANTERIOR CHEST, SHOULDER, AND ABDOMINAL REGIONS

Muscle Groups: Shoulder Flexors and Adductors, Trunk Flexors

Exercise 1

Description: In a prone position, push up until elbows are fully extended. Keep pelvis and hips on floor.

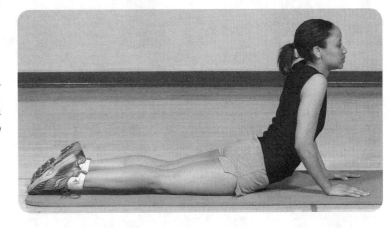

(continued)

From Vivian H. Heyward, 2010, *Advanced Fitness Assessment and Exercise Prescription,* 6th ed. (Champaign, IL: Human Kinetics).

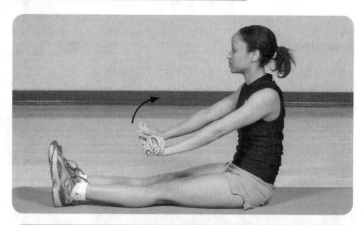

Exercise 2

Description: Grasp towel or rope with both hands. Rotate arms overhead behind trunk.

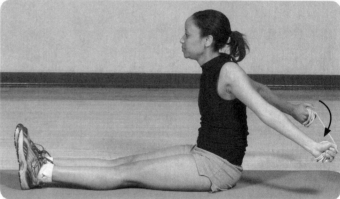

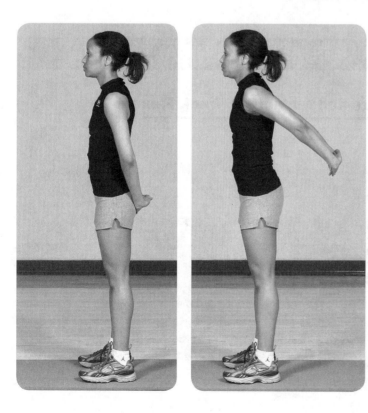

Exercise 3

Description: Clasp hands together behind trunk with elbows extended. Slowly raise arms upward.

From Vivian H. Heyward, 2010, *Advanced Fitness Assessment and Exercise Prescription,* 6th ed. (Champaign, IL: Human Kinetics).

Exercise Do's and Don'ts

DON'T: Neck Hyperextension

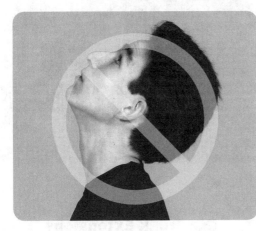

DO: Neck Lateral Flexion

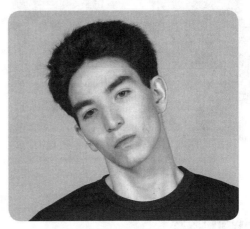

DON'T: Head Throws in a Crunch

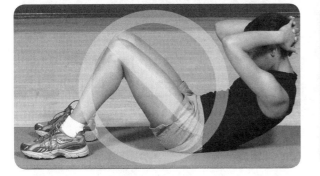

DO: Partial Sit-Up

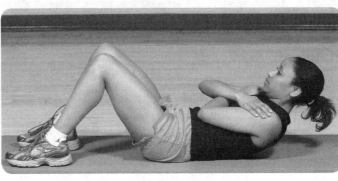

DON'T: Unsupported Hip/Trunk Flexion

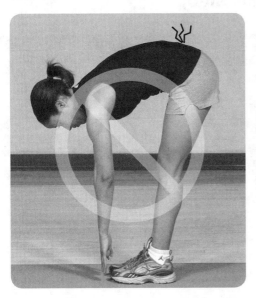

DO: Seated Hip/Trunk Flexion

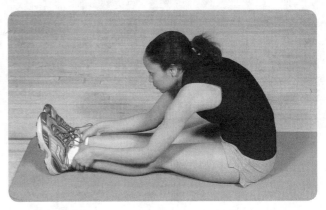

From Vivian H. Heyward, 2010, *Advanced Fitness Assessment and Exercise Prescription,* 6th ed. (Champaign, IL: Human Kinetics).

DON'T: The Plow

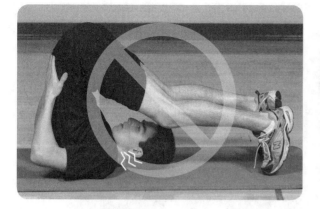

DO: Camel

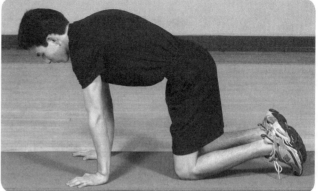

DON'T: Swan Lifts

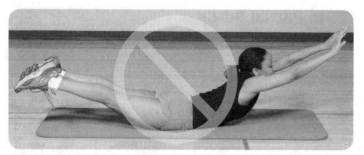

DO: Trunk Extensions

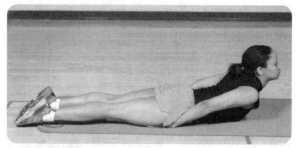

DON'T: V-Sits

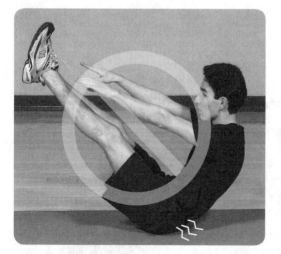

DO: Partial Sit-Up

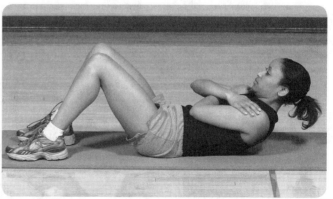

From Vivian H. Heyward, 2010, *Advanced Fitness Assessment and Exercise Prescription*, 6th ed. (Champaign, IL: Human Kinetics).

400

DON'T: Leg Lifts With Trunk Hyperextended

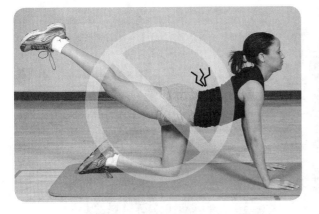

DO: Leg Lifts With Trunk and Leg in Straight Line

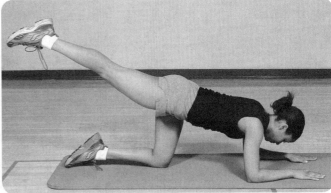

DON'T: Hamstring Stretch— Leg on Bar

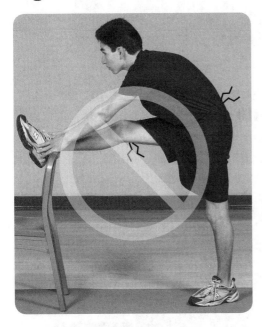

DO: Hamstring Stretch—Knee to Chest

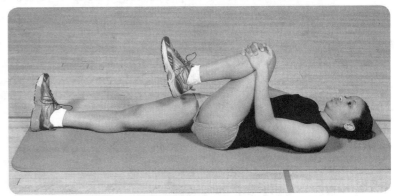

DON'T: Hurdler's Stretch

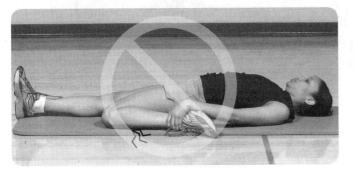

DO: Quad Stretch

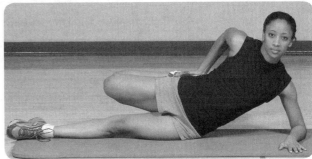

From Vivian H. Heyward, 2010, *Advanced Fitness Assessment and Exercise Prescription*, 6th ed. (Champaign, IL: Human Kinetics).

DON'T: Squats & Deep Knee Bends

DO: Half-Squats

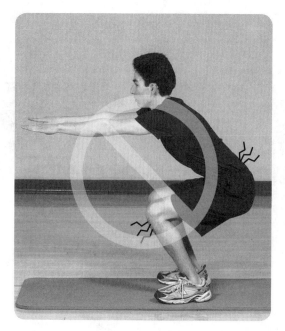

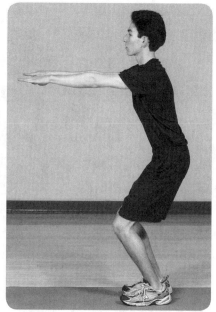

DON'T: Lunges (with knee forward of supporting foot)

DO: Lunges (with knee in line with supporting heel)

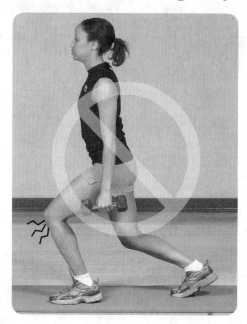

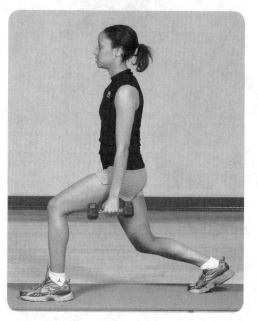

From Vivian H. Heyward, 2010, *Advanced Fitness Assessment and Exercise Prescription*, 6th ed. (Champaign, IL: Human Kinetics).

DON'T: Fast Twists & Jump Twists

DO: Jump Without Twist

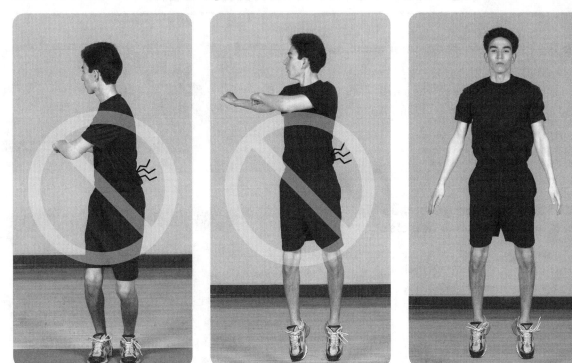

From Vivian H. Heyward, 2010, *Advanced Fitness Assessment and Exercise Prescription,* 6th ed. (Champaign, IL: Human Kinetics).

Exercises for Low Back Care

Pelvic Tilt (stretches abdominal muscles)

Lie on your back with knees bent, feet flat on the floor, and arms at your sides. Flatten the small of your back against the floor. (Your hips will tilt upward.) Hold.

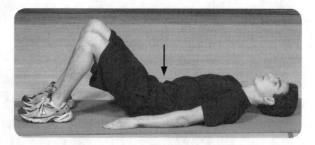

Double Knee to Chest (stretches hip, buttock, and lower back muscles)

Lie on your back with knees bent, feet flat on the floor, and arms at your sides. Raise both knees, one at a time, to your chest and hold with your hands. Lower your legs, one at a time, to the floor and rest briefly.

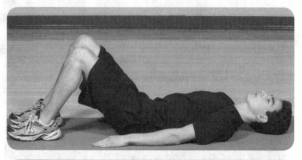

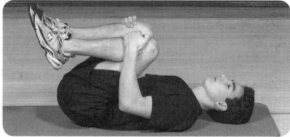

Trunk Flex (stretches back, abdominal, and leg muscles)

On your hands and knees, tuck in your chin and arch your back. Slowly sit back on your heels, letting your shoulders drop toward the floor. Hold.

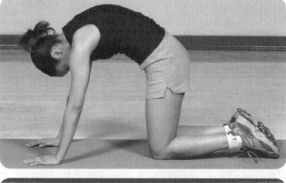

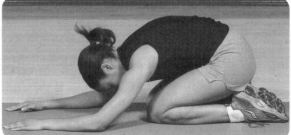

From Vivian H. Heyward, 2010, *Advanced Fitness Assessment and Exercise Prescription,* 6th ed. (Champaign, IL: Human Kinetics).

Cat and Camel (strengthens back and abdominal muscles)

On your hands and knees with your head parallel to the floor, arch your back and then let it slowly sag toward the floor. Try to keep your arms straight.

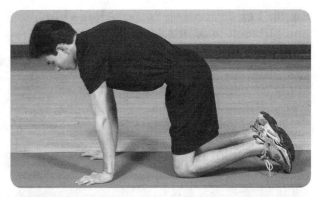

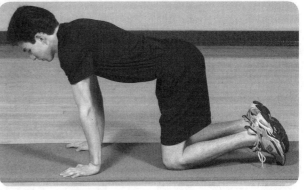

Partial Sit-Up (strengthens abdominal muscles)

Lie on your back with knees bent, feet flat on the floors, and arms crossed over your chest. Keeping your middle and lower back flat on the floor, raise your head and shoulders off the floor, and hold. Gradually increase your holding time.

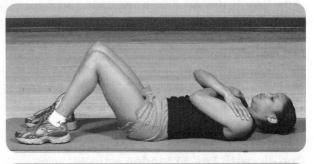

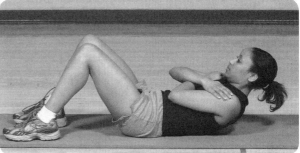

From Vivian H. Heyward, 2010, *Advanced Fitness Assessment and Exercise Prescription,* 6th ed. (Champaign, IL: Human Kinetics).

Single-Leg Extension (strengthens hip and buttock muscles, and stretches abdominal and leg muscles)

Lie on your stomach with your arms folded under your chin. Slowly lift one leg—not too high—without bending it, while keeping your pelvis flat on the floor. Slowly lower your leg and repeat with the other leg.

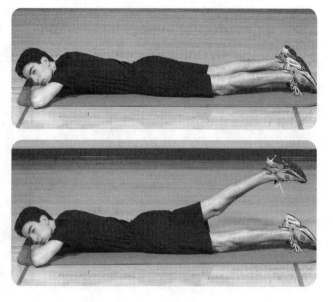

Single-Leg Extension Hold (strengthens the trunk extensors)

On your hands and knees with your head parallel to the floor, extend your thigh and leg and hold this position. Raising the contralateral arm simultaneously is more difficult and increases the extensor muscle activity and spinal compression.

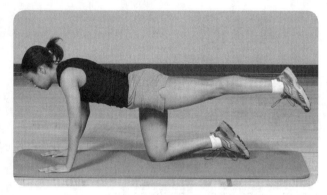

Curl-Up with Leg Extended (strengthens abdominal muscles)

Lie on your back with one knee flexed (foot flat on floor) and the other knee extended. Place your hands under the lumbar spine to preserve the neutral spine position. Slowly raise your head and shoulders off the floor.

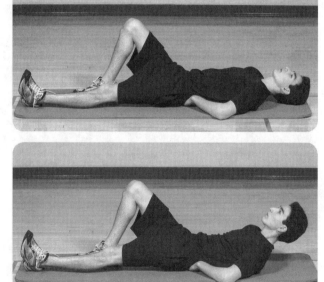

From Vivian H. Heyward, 2010, *Advanced Fitness Assessment and Exercise Prescription*, 6th ed. (Champaign, IL: Human Kinetics).

Isometric Side Support or Side Bridge (strengthens the lateral muscles of trunk and abdomen)

Assume a side support position with body supported by the knee, thigh, and forearm (flexed to 90°), and hold this position. Supporting the body with the feet, instead of the knee and the thigh, increases the muscle activity and spinal load.

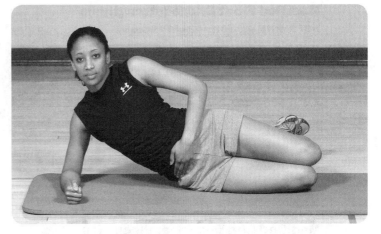

Standing Cat and Camel (strengthens back and abdominal muscles)

Stand with feet shoulder-width apart and with hands on knees. Straighten back and hold this position. Perform 10 to 20 repetitions.

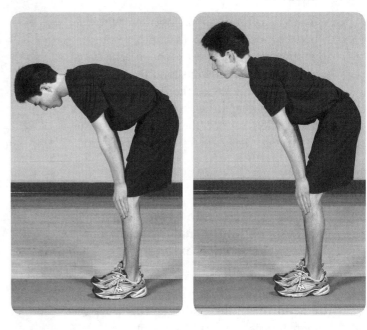

Bent-Knee Curl-Up (strengthens abdominal muscles)

Lie on your back with one knee bent and with foot flat on the floor. Place arms across chest. Lift shoulders off ground and hold this position momentarily. Perform 10 to 20 repetitions.

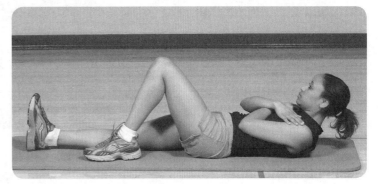

From Vivian H. Heyward, 2010, *Advanced Fitness Assessment and Exercise Prescription,* 6th ed. (Champaign, IL: Human Kinetics).

Modified Front Bridge (strengthens back and abdominal muscles)

Assume a front support position with the body supported by the forearms (elbows flexed to 90°), knees, and toes. Hold this position for 10 to 20 counts.

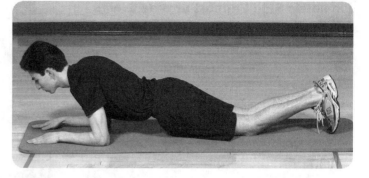

Modified Bird Dog (strengthens hip extensors)

Assume a front support position with the body supported by both hands (shoulder-width apart and elbows extended), one knee, and one foot. Extend unsupported leg so that thigh is parallel with the trunk. Hold this position momentarily. Perform 10 repetitions for each leg. Support the body with one arm to increase the difficulty of this exercise.

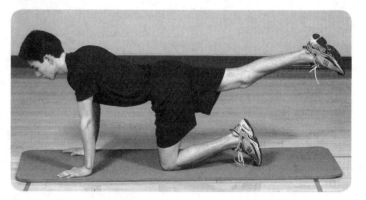

Standing McKenzie Exercise (stretches abdominal muscles and strengthens back extensors)

Assume a standing position with feet shoulder-width apart and with hands placed on hips. Extend the trunk and hold this position momentarily. Perform 10 repetitions.

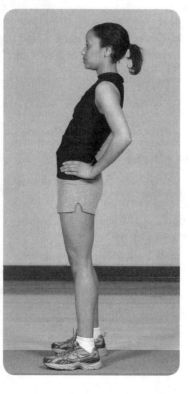

From Vivian H. Heyward, 2010, *Advanced Fitness Assessment and Exercise Prescription,* 6th ed. (Champaign, IL: Human Kinetics).

List of Abbreviations

Terms	
%BF	Relative body fat
AAHPERD	American Alliance for Health, Physical Education, Recreation and Dance
ACSM	American College of Sports Medicine
ADL	Activities of daily living
AI	Adequate intake
ATP	Adenosine triphosphate
AV	Atrioventricular
BIA	Bioelectrical impedance analysis
BM	Body mass
BMI	Body mass index
BMR	Basal metabolic rate
BP	Blood pressure
BSA	Body surface area
BV	Body volume
BW	Body weight
C	Circumference
CDC	Centers for Disease Control and Prevention
CE	Constant error
CHD	Coronary heart disease
CP	Creatine phosphate
CRAC	Contract-relax with agonist contraction
CSA	Cross-sectional area
CSEP	Canadian Society for Exercise Physiology
CV	Cardiovascular
CVD	Cardiovascular disease
D	Skeletal diameter
Db	Body density
DOMS	Delayed-onset muscle soreness
DXA	Dual-energy X-ray absorptiometry
ECG	Electrocardiogram
EIMD	Exercise-induced muscle damage
EMG	Electromyography
F	Force
FFB	Fat-free body
FFM	Fat-free mass

Terms	
FITT	Frequency, intensity, time, and type of exercise
FM	Fat mass
FRC	Functional residual lung capacity
GH	Growth hormone
GI	Glycemic index
GIS	Geographical information system
GPS	Global positioning system
GV	Volume of air in gastrointestinal tract
GXT	Graded exercise test
HDL	High-density lipoprotein
HDL-C	High-density lipoprotein cholesterol
HMB	β-Hydroxy-β-methylbutyrate
HR	Heart rate
HRmax	Maximal heart rate
HRrest	Resting heart rate
HRA	Health risk appraisal
HRR	Heart rate reserve
HT	Standing height
HT^2/R	Resistance index
HW	Hydrostatic weighing
LDL	Low-density lipoprotein
LDL-C	Low-density lipoprotein cholesterol
LP	Linear periodization
MET	Metabolic equivalent
MRI	Magnetic resonance imaging
MVIC	Maximal voluntary isometric contraction
N	Sample size
NCEP	National Cholesterol Education Program
NIDDM	Non-insulin-dependent diabetes mellitus
NIH	National Institutes of Health
NIR	Near-infrared interactance
P	Power output
p	Specific resistivity
PAL	Physical activity level
PAR-Q	Physical Activity Readiness Questionnaire

Terms

PARmed-X	Physical Activity Readiness Medical Examination Questionnaire
PEI	Physical efficiency index
$\dot{Q}$	Cardiac output
R	Resistance for bioimpedance analysis
r	Pearson product–moment correlation
RDA	Recommended dietary allowance
rep	Repetition
RER	Respiratory exchange ratio
RLP	Reverse linear periodization
RM	Repetition maximum
R_{mc}	Multiple correlation coefficient
RMR	Resting metabolic rate
ROM	Range of motion
RPE	Rating of perceived exertion
RV	Residual lung volume
SAD	Sagittal abdominal diameter
SEE	Standard error of estimate
SKF	Skinfold
ΣSKF	Sum of skinfolds
SV	Stroke volume
TBW	Total body water
TC	Total cholesterol
TC/HDL-C	Ratio of total cholesterol to HDL-cholesterol
TE	Total error
TEE	Total energy expenditure
TGV	Thoracic gas volume
TLC	Total lung capacity
TLCNS	Total lung capacity, head not submerged
UWW	Underwater weight
UP	Undulating periodization
VLDL	Very low-density lipoprotein
$\dot{V}O_2$	Volume of oxygen consumed per minute
$\dot{V}O_2$max	Maximal oxygen uptake
$\dot{V}O_2$R	Oxygen uptake reserve
WHTR	Waist-to-height ratio
WHR	Waist-to-hip ratio
X_c	Reactance
YMCA	Young Men's Christian Association
Z	Impedance

Units of Measure

bpm	beats per minute
C	Celsius
cc	cubic centimeter
cm	centimeter
dl	deciliter
F	Fahrenheit
ft-lb	foot-pound
g	gram
hr	hour
in.	inch
kcal	kilocalorie
kg	kilogram
kgm	kilogram-meter
km	kilometer
L	liter
lb	pound
m	meter
meq	milli-equivalent
mg	milligram
min	minute
ml	milliliter
mm	millimeter
mmHg	millimeters of mercury
mph	miles per hour
N	newton
Nm	newton-meter
rpm	revolutions per minute
sec	second
W	watt
wk	week
yr	year
μg	microgram
μg RE	retinol equivalent
Ω	ohm

Glossary

absolute $\dot{V}O_2$—Measure of rate of oxygen consumption and energy cost of non-weight-bearing activities; measured in $L \cdot min^{-1}$ or $ml \cdot min^{-1}$.

accelerometer—Device used to record body acceleration minute to minute, providing detailed information about frequency, duration, intensity, and patterns of movement.

accommodating-resistance exercise—Type of exercise in which fluctuations in muscle force throughout the range of motion are matched by an equal counterforce as the speed of limb movement is kept at a constant velocity; isokinetic exercise.

acquired immune deficiency syndrome (AIDS)—Disease characterized as a deficiency in the body's immune system, caused by human immunodeficiency virus (HIV).

active-assisted stretching—Stretching technique that involves voluntarily moving a body part to the end of its active range of motion followed by an assistant's moving the body part beyond its active range of motion.

active stretching—Stretching technique that involves moving a body part without external assistance; voluntary muscle contraction.

activities of daily living (ADL)—Normal everyday activities such as getting out of a chair or car, climbing stairs, shopping, dressing, and bathing.

acute-onset muscle soreness—Soreness or pain occurring during or immediately after exercise; caused by ischemia and accumulation of metabolic waste products in the muscle.

air displacement plethysmography (ADP)—Densitometric method to estimate body volume using air displacement and pressure–volume relationships.

android obesity—Type of obesity in which excess body fat is localized in the upper body; upper body obesity; apple-shaped body.

aneurysm—Dilation of a blood vessel wall causing a weakness in the vessel's wall; usually caused by atherosclerosis and hypertension.

angina pectoris—Chest pain.

ankylosis—Limited range of motion at a joint.

anorexia nervosa—Eating disorder characterized by excessive weight loss.

anthropometry—Measurement of body size and proportions including skinfold thicknesses, circumferences, bony widths and lengths, stature, and body weight.

aortic stenosis—Narrowing of the aortic valve, obstructing blood flow from the left ventricle into the aorta.

Archimedes' principle—Principle stating that weight loss underwater is directly proportional to the volume of water displaced by the body's volume.

arrhythmia—Abnormal heart rhythm.

arteriosclerosis—Hardening of the arteries, or thickening and loss of elasticity in the artery walls that obstruct blood flow; caused by deposits of fat, cholesterol, and other substances.

asthma—Respiratory disorder characterized by difficulty in breathing and wheezing due to constricted bronchi.

at risk for overweight—Characterizing children with a body mass index between the 85th and 94th percentiles for age and sex.

ataxia—Impaired ability to coordinate movement characterized by staggering gait or postural imbalance.

atherosclerosis—Buildup and deposition of fat and fibrous plaque in the inner walls of the coronary arteries.

atrial fibrillation—Cardiac dysrhythmia in which the atria quiver instead of pumping in an organized fashion.

atrial flutter—Type of atrial tachycardia in which the atria contract at rates of 230 to 380 bpm.

atrophy—A wasting or decrease in size of a body part.

attenuation—Weakening of X-ray energy as it passes through fat, lean tissue, and bone.

augmented unipolar leads—Three ECG leads (aVF, aVL, aVR) that compare voltage across each limb

411

lead to the average voltage across the two opposite electrodes.

auscultation—Method used to measure heart rate or blood pressure by listening to heart and blood sounds.

balance—Complex construct involving multiple biomechanical, neurological, and environmental systems.

ballistic stretching—Type of stretching exercise that uses a fast bouncing motion to produce stretch and increase range of motion.

basal metabolic rate (BMR)—Measure of minimal amount of energy needed to maintain basic and essential physiological functions.

behavior modification model—Psychological theory of change; clients become actively involved with the change process by setting short- and long-term goals.

β-hydroxy-β-methyl butyrate (HMB)—Dietary supplement known to increase lean body mass and strength of individuals engaging in resistance training.

bias—In regression analysis, a systematic over- or underestimation of actual scores caused by technical error or biological variability between validation and cross-validation samples; constant error.

biaxial joint—Joint allowing movement in two planes; condyloid and saddle joints.

bioelectrical impedance analysis (BIA)—Field method for estimating the total body water or fat-free mass using measures of impedance to current flowing through the body.

bioimpedance spectroscopy (BIS) – Type of bioimpedance analysis that combines upper body, lower body, and whole-body bioimpedance to estimate FFM and %BF.

Bland and Altman method—Statistical approach used to assess the degree of agreement between methods by calculating the 95% limits of agreement and confidence intervals; used to judge the accuracy of a prediction equation or method for estimating measured values of individuals in a group.

body composition—A component of physical fitness; absolute and relative amounts of muscle, bone, and fat tissues composing body mass.

body density (Db)—Overall density of fat, water, mineral, and protein components of the human body; total body mass expressed relative to total body volume.

body mass (BM)—Measure of the size of the body; body weight.

body mass index (BMI)—Crude index of obesity; body mass (kg) divided by height squared (m^2).

body surface area—Amount of surface area of the body estimated from the client's height and body weight.

body volume (BV)—Measure of body size estimated by water or air displacement.

body weight (BW)—Mass or size of the body; body mass.

bone strength—Function of mineral content and density of bone tissue; related to risk of bone fracture.

Boyle's law—Isothermal gas law stating that volume and pressure are inversely related.

bradycardia—Resting heart rate <60 bpm.

bronchitis—Acute or chronic inflammation of the bronchi of the lungs.

caloric threshold—Method to estimate duration of exercise based on the caloric cost of the exercise and to estimate the total amount of exercise needed per week for health benefits.

cardiac arrest—Sudden loss of heart function usually caused by ventricular fibrillation.

cardiomyopathy—Any disease that affects the structure and function of the heart.

cardiorespiratory endurance—Ability of heart, lungs, and circulatory system to supply oxygen to working muscles efficiently.

cardiovascular disease (CVD)—Disease of the heart, blood vessels, or both; types of cardiovascular disease include atherosclerosis, hypertension, coronary heart disease, congestive heart failure, and stroke.

center of pressure—Vertical force applied to the supporting base or a force platform during sitting or standing.

chest leads—Six ECG leads (V_1 to V_6) used to measure voltage across specific areas of the chest.

cholesterol—Waxy, fatlike substance found in all animal products (e.g., meats, dairy products, and eggs).

chylomicron—Type of lipoprotein derived from intestinal absorption of triglycerides.

circumference (C)—Measure of the girth of body segments.

cirrhosis—Chronic, degenerative disease of the liver in which the lobes are covered with fibrous tissue; associated with chronic alcohol abuse.

claudication—Cramp-like pain in the calves due to poor circulation to leg muscle.

complex carbohydrates—Macronutrients found in plant-based foods, whole grains, and low-fat dairy products, for example starch and cellulose.

compound sets—Advanced resistance training system in which two sets of exercises for the same muscle group are performed consecutively, with little or no rest between sets.

computerized dynamic posturography—Computer system designed to assess the individual and composite functioning of sensory, motor, and biomechanical components of balance.

concentric contraction—Type of dynamic muscle contraction in which muscle shortens as it exerts tension.

congestive heart failure—Impaired cardiac pumping caused by myocardial infarction, ischemic heart disease, or cardiomyopathy.

constant error (CE)—Average difference between measured and predicted values for cross-validation group; bias.

constant-resistance exercise—Type of exercise in which the external resistance remains the same throughout the range of motion (e.g., lifting free weights or dumbbells).

continuous exercise test—Type of graded exercise test that is performed with no rest between workload increments.

continuous training—One continuous, aerobic exercise bout performed at low-to-moderate intensity.

contract-relax agonist contract (CRAC) technique—Type of proprioceptive neuromuscular facilitation technique in which the target muscle is isometrically contracted and then stretched; stretching is assisted by a submaximal contraction of the agonistic muscle group.

contract–relax (CR) technique—Type of proprioceptive neuromuscular facilitation technique in which the target muscle is isometrically contracted and then stretched.

contracture—Shortening of resting muscle length caused by disuse or immobilization.

core stability—Ability to maintain ideal alignment of neck, spine, scapulae, and pelvis while exercising.

core strengthening—Strengthening core muscle groups (erector spinae and abdominal movers and stabilizers) used for core stability.

coronary heart disease (CHD)—Disease of the heart caused by a lack of blood flow to heart muscle, resulting from atherosclerosis.

criterion method—Gold standard or reference method; typically a direct measure of a component used to validate other tests.

cross training—Type of training in which the client participates in a variety of exercise modes to develop one or more components of physical fitness.

cuff hypertension—Overestimation of blood pressure caused by use of a bladder that is too small for the arm circumference.

cyanosis—Bluish discoloration of skin caused by lack of oxygenated hemoglobin in the blood.

decision-making theory—Theory stating that individuals decide whether or not to engage in a behavior by weighing the perceived benefits and costs of that behavior.

delayed-onset muscle soreness (DOMS)—Soreness in the muscle occurring 24 to 48 hr after exercise.

densitometry—Measurement of total body density; hydrodensitometry and air displacement plethysmography are densitometry methods.

diabetes—Complex disorder of carbohydrate, fat, and protein metabolism resulting from a lack of insulin secretion (type 1) or defective insulin receptors (type 2).

diastolic blood pressure (DBP)—Lowest pressure in the artery during the cardiac cycle.

dietary thermogenesis—Energy needed for digesting, absorbing, transporting, and metabolizing foods.

digital activity log—A hand computer used to record the type and duration of physical activities performed during the day.

diminishing return principle—Training principle; as genetic ceiling is approached, rate of improvement slows or evens off.

discontinuous exercise test—Type of graded exercise test that is performed with 5 to 10 min of rest between increments in workload.

discontinuous training—Several intermittent, low- to high-intensity aerobic exercise bouts interspersed with rest or relief intervals.

dose–response relationship—The volume of physical activity is directly related to health benefits from that activity

dual-energy X-ray absorptiometry (DXA)—Method used to measure total body bone mineral density, bone mineral content, fat, and lean soft tissue mass.

dynamic balance—Ability to maintain an upright position while the center of gravity and base of support are moving.

dynamic contraction—Type of muscle contraction producing visible joint movement; concentric, eccentric, or isokinetic contraction.

dynamic flexibility—Measure of the rate of torque or resistance developed during stretching throughout the range of joint motion.

dynapenia—Age-related loss in muscle strength.

dyslipidemia—Abnormal blood lipid profile.

dyspnea—Shortness of breath or difficulty breathing

caused by certain heart conditions, anxiety, or strenuous exercise.

eccentric contraction—Type of muscle contraction in which the muscle lengthens as it produces tension to resist gravity or decelerate a moving body segment.

edema—Accumulation of interstitial fluid in tissues such as pericardial sac and joint capsules.

elastic deformation—Deformation of the muscle–tendon unit that is proportional to the load or force applied during stretching.

electrocardiogram (ECG)—A composite record of the electrical events in the heart during the cardiac cycle.

embolism—Piece of tissue or thrombus that circulates in the blood until it lodges in a vessel.

emphysema—Pulmonary disease causing damage in alveoli and loss of lung elasticity.

exercise-induced hypertrophy—Increase in size of muscle as a result of resistance training.

exercise-induced muscle damage (EIMD)—Skeletal muscle damage induced through exercise.

factorial method—Method used to assess energy needs; the sum of the resting metabolic rate and the additional calories expended during work, household chores, personal daily activities, and exercise.

false negative—An error in which individuals are incorrectly identified as having no risk factors when in fact they do have risk factors

false positive—An error in which individuals are incorrectly identified as having risk factors when they do not have risk factors.

fat-free body (FFB)—All residual, lipid-free chemicals and tissues in the body, including muscle, water, bone, connective tissue, and internal organs.

fat-free mass (FFM)—*See* fat-free body; weight or mass of the fat-free body.

fat mass (FM)—All extractable lipids from adipose and other tissues in the body.

FITT principle (FITT)—Describes four components of an exercise prescription: frequency, intensity, time, and type of activity.

flexibility—Ability to move joints fluidly through complete range of motion without injury.

flexibility training—Systematic program of stretching exercises designed to progressively increase the range of motion of joints over time.

flexometer—Device for measuring range of joint motion using a weighted 360° dial and pointer.

free-motion machines—Resistance exercise machines that have adjustable seats, lever arms, and cable pulleys for exercising muscle groups in multiple planes.

functional balance—Ability to perform daily activities requiring balance, for example picking up an object from the floor.

functional fitness—Ability to perform everyday activities safely and independently without fatigue; requires aerobic endurance, flexibility, balance, agility, and muscular strength.

functional training—System of exercise progressions for specific muscle groups using a stepwise approach that increases the difficulty level (strength) and skill (balance and coordination) required for each exercise in the progression.

generalized prediction equations—Prediction equations that are applicable to a diverse, heterogeneous group of individuals.

geographical information system (GIS)—Computer system that stores information about location and the surrounding environment.

global positioning system (GPS)—System that uses 24 satellites and ground stations to calculate geographic locations and accurately track a specific activity.

glucose intolerance—Inability of body to metabolize glucose.

glycemic index (GI)—Rating of the body's glycemic response to a food compared to the reference value (GI = 100 for white bread or glucose).

goniometer—Protractor-like device used to measure joint angle at the extremes of the range of motion.

graded exercise test (GXT)—A multistage submaximal or maximal exercise test requiring the client to exercise at gradually increasing workloads; may be continuous or discontinuous; used to estimate $\dot{V}O_2$max.

Graves disease—Disease associated with an overactive thyroid gland that secretes greater than normal amounts of thyroid hormones; also known as hyperthyroidism or thyrotoxicosis.

gross $\dot{V}O_2$—Total rate of oxygen consumption, reflecting the caloric cost of both rest and exercise.

gynoid obesity—Type of obesity in which excess fat is localized in the lower body; lower body obesity; pear-shaped body.

HDL-cholesterol (HDL-C)—Cholesterol transported in the blood by high-density lipoproteins.

health belief model—Model suggesting that individuals will change a behavior because they perceive a threat of disease if they do not change.

healthy body weight—Body mass index from 18.5 to 25 kg/m².

heart block—Interference in the conduction of electrical impulses that control normal contraction of the heart muscle; may occur at sinoatrial node, atrioventricular node, bundle of HIS, or a combination of these sites.

heart rate monitor—Device used to assess heart rate and to monitor exercise intensity.

heart rate reserve (HRR)—Maximal heart rate minus the resting heart rate.

hepatitis—Inflammation of the liver characterized by jaundice and gastrointestinal discomfort.

high blood pressure—Hypertension; chronic elevation of blood pressure.

high CHD risk—One or more signs or symptoms of cardiovascular and pulmonary disease; or characterizing individuals with known cardiovascular, pulmonary, or metabolic disease.

high-density lipoprotein (HDL)—Type of lipoprotein involved in the reverse transport of cholesterol to the liver.

high intensity–low repetitions—Optimal training stimulus for strength development; 85% to 100% 1-RM or 1- to 6-RM.

hybrid sphygmomanometer—Device used to measure blood pressure that combines features of electronic and auscultatory devices.

hydrodensitometry—Method used to estimate body volume by measuring weight loss when the body is fully submerged; underwater weighing.

hydrostatic weighing (HW)—*See* hydrodensitometry.

hypercholesterolemia—Excess of total cholesterol, LDL-cholesterol, or both in blood.

hyperlipidemia—Excess lipids in blood.

hypermobility—Excessive range of motion at a joint.

hyperplasia—Increase in number of cells.

hypertension—High blood pressure; chronic elevation of blood pressure.

hyperthyroidism—Overactive thyroid gland that secretes greater than normal amounts of thyroid hormones; also known as thyrotoxicosis or Graves disease.

hypertrophy—Increase in size of cells.

hypoglycemia—Low blood glucose level.

hypokalemia—Inadequate amount of potassium in the blood characterized by an abnormal ECG, weakness, and flaccid paralysis.

hypomagnesemia—Inadequate amount of magnesium in the blood resulting in nausea, vomiting, muscle weakness, and tremors.

hypothyroidism—Underactive thyroid gland that secretes lower than normal amounts of thyroid hormones; also known as myxedema.

hypoxia—Inadequate oxygen at the cellular level.

impedance (Z)—Measure of total amount of opposition to electrical current flowing through the body; function of resistance and reactance.

improvement stage—Stage of exercise program in which client improves most rapidly; frequency, intensity, duration are systematically increased; usually lasting 16 to 20 wk.

inclinometer—Gravity-dependent goniometer used to measure the angle between the long axis of the moving segment and the line of gravity.

initial conditioning stage—Stage of exercise program used as a primer to familiarize client with exercise training, usually lasting 4 wk.

initial values principle—Training principle; the lower the initial value of a component, the greater the relative gain and the faster the rate of improvement in that component; the higher the initial value, the slower the improvement rate.

insulin-dependent diabetes mellitus (IDDM)—Type 1 diabetes, caused by lack of insulin production by the pancreas.

interindividual variability principle—Training principle; individual responses to training stimulus are variable and depend on age, initial fitness level, and health status.

interval training—A repeated series of exercise work bouts interspersed with rest or relief periods.

ischemia—Decreased supply of oxygenated blood to body part or organ.

ischemic heart disease—Pathologic condition of the myocardium caused by lack of oxygen to the heart muscle.

isokinetic contraction—Maximal contraction of a muscle group at a constant velocity throughout entire range of motion.

isometric contraction—Type of muscle contraction in which there is no visible joint movement; static contraction.

isotonic contraction—Type of muscle contraction producing visible joint movement; dynamic contraction.

joint laxity—Looseness or instability of a joint, increasing risk of musculoskeletal injury.

Karvonen method—Method to prescribe exercise intensity as a percentage of the heart rate reserve added to the resting heart rate; percent heart rate reserve method.

kilocalorie (kcal)—Amount of heat needed to raise the temperature of 1 kg of water 1° C; measure of energy need and expenditure.

LDL-cholesterol (LDL-C)—Cholesterol transported in the blood by low-density lipoproteins.

limb leads—Three ECG leads (I, II, III) measuring the voltage differential between left and right arms

(I) and between the left leg and right (II) and left (III) arms.

limits of agreement—Statistical method used to assess the extent of agreement between methods; also known as the Bland and Altman method.

limits of stability—Measure of the maximum excursion of the center of gravity during maintenance of balance over a fixed supporting base.

linear periodization (LP)—Strength training method that progressively increases training intensity as training volume decreases between microcycles.

line of best fit—Regression line depicting relationship between reference measure and predictor variables in an equation.

line of gravity—Vertical projection of the center of gravity of the body to the supporting base.

line of identity—Straight line with a slope equal to 1 and an intercept equal to 0; used in a scatter plot to illustrate the differences in the measured and predicted scores of a cross-validation sample.

lipoprotein—Molecule used to transport and exchange lipids among the liver, intestine, and peripheral tissues.

low back pain—Pain produced by muscular weakness or imbalance resulting from lack of physical activity.

low CHD risk—Characterizing younger individuals (men <45 yr and women <55 yr) who are asymptomatic and have no more than one risk factor.

low-density lipoprotein (LDL)—Primary transporter of cholesterol in the blood; product of very low-density lipoprotein metabolism.

lower body obesity—Type of obesity in which excess body fat is localized in the lower body; gynoid obesity; pear-shaped body.

low intensity–high repetitions—Optimal training stimulus for development of muscular endurance; ≤60% 1-RM or 15- to 20-RM.

lumbar stabilization—Maintaining a static position of the lumbar spine by isometrically cocontracting the abdominal wall and low back muscles during exercise.

macrocycle—Phase of periodized resistance training program usually lasting 9 to 12 mo.

maintenance stage—Stage of exercise program designed to maintain level of fitness achieved by end of improvement stage; should be continued on a regular, long-term basis.

maximal exercise test—Graded exercise test in which exercise intensity increases gradually until the $\dot{V}O_2$ plateaus or fails to rise with a further increase in workload.

maximum oxygen consumption—Maximum rate of oxygen utilization by muscles during exercise; $\dot{V}O_2$ max.

maximum oxygen uptake ($\dot{V}O_2$max)—Maximum rate of oxygen utilization of muscles during aerobic exercise.

maximum voluntary isometric contraction (MVIC)—Measure of the maximum force exerted in a single contraction against an immovable resistance.

McArdle's syndrome—Inherited metabolic disease characterized by inability to metabolize muscle glycogen, resulting in excessive amounts of glycogen stored in skeletal muscles.

mesocycle—Phase of a periodized resistance training program usually lasting 3 to 4 mo.

metabolic equivalents (METs)–the ratio of the person's working (exercising) metabolic rate to the resting metabolic rate.

metabolic syndrome—A combination of cardiovascular disease risk factors associated with hypertension, dyslipidemia, insulin resistance, and abdominal obesity.

microcycle—Phase of a periodized resistance training program usually lasting 1 to 4 wk.

miscuffing—Source of blood pressure measurement error caused by use of a blood pressure cuff that is not appropriately scaled for the client's arm circumference.

moderate CHD risk—Characterizing older individuals (men ≥45 yr and women ≥55 yr), or individuals of any age having two or more risk factors.

multicomponent model—Body composition model that takes into account interindividual variations in water, protein, and mineral content of the fat-free body.

multimodal exercise program—Type of exercise program that uses a variety of aerobic exercise modalities.

multiple correlation coefficient (R_{mc})—Correlation between reference measure and predictor variables in a prediction equation.

murmur—Low-pitched fluttering or humming sound.

muscle balance—Ratio of strength between opposing muscle groups, contralateral muscle groups, and upper and lower body muscle groups.

muscular endurance—Ability of muscle to maintain submaximal force levels for extended periods.

muscular strength—Maximal force or tension level produced by a muscle or muscle group.

musculoskeletal fitness—Ability of skeletal and muscular systems to perform work.

myocardial infarction—Heart attack.

myocardial ischemia—Lack of blood flow to the heart muscles.

myocarditis—Inflammation of the heart muscle caused by viral, bacterial, or fungal infection.

myxedema—Disease associated with an underactive thyroid gland that secretes lower than normal amounts of thyroid hormones; also known as hypothyroidism.

near-infrared interactance (NIR)—Field method that estimates %BF based on optical density of tissues at the measurement site; presently, validity of this method is questionable.

negative energy balance—Excess of energy expenditure in relation to energy intake.

net $\dot{V}O_2$—Rate of oxygen consumption in excess of the resting $\dot{V}O_2$; used to describe the caloric cost of exercise.

nonaxial joint—Type of joint allowing only gliding, sliding, or twisting rather than movement about an axis of rotation; gliding joint.

non-insulin-dependent diabetes mellitus (NIDDM)—Type 2 diabetes, caused by decreased insulin receptor sensitivity.

normotensive—Referring to normal blood pressure, defined as values less than 120/80 mmHg.

obesity—Excessive amount of body fat relative to body mass; BMI of 30 kg/m^2 or more.

objectivity—Intertester reliability; ability of test to yield similar scores for a given individual when the same test is administered by different technicians.

objectivity coefficient—Correlation between pairs of test scores measured on the same individuals by two different technicians.

occlusion—Blockage of blood flow to body part or organ.

omnikinetic exercise—Type of accommodating-resistance exercise that adjusts for fluctuations in both muscle force and speed of joint rotation throughout range of motion.

one-repetition maximum (1-RM)—Maximal weight that can be lifted for one complete repetition of a movement.

optical density—Measure of the amount of near-infrared light reflected by the body's tissues at specific wavelengths.

oscillometry—Method for measuring blood pressure that uses an automated electronic manometer to measure oscillations in pressure when the cuff is deflated.

osteoarthritis—Degenerative disease of the joints characterized by excessive amounts of bone and cartilage in the joint

osteopenia—Low bone mineral mass; precursor to osteoporosis.

osteoporosis—Disorder characterized by low bone mineral and bone density; occurring most frequently in postmenopausal women and sedentary individuals.

overcuffing—Using a blood pressure cuff with a bladder too large for the arm circumference, leading to an underestimation of blood pressure.

overload principle—Training principle; physiological systems must be taxed beyond normal to stimulate improvement.

overweight—BMI between 25 and 29.9 kg/m^2 in adults; BMI greater than or equal to 95th percentile for age and sex in children.

pallor—Unnatural paleness or absence of skin color.

palpation—Method used to measure heart rate by feeling the pulse at specific anatomical sites.

palpitations—Racing or pounding of the heart.

passive stretching—Stretching technique that involves a body part being moved by an assistant as the client relaxes the target muscle group.

pedometer—A device used to count the number of steps taken throughout the day.

pelvic stabilization—Maintenance of a static position of the pelvis during performance of exercises for the low back extensor muscles.

percent body fat (%BF)—Fat mass expressed relative to body mass; relative body fat.

percent heart rate maximum (%HRmax)—Method used to prescribe exercise intensity as a percentage of the measured or age-predicted maximum heart rate.

percent heart rate reserve (%HRR)—Method used to prescribe exercise intensity as a percentage of the heart rate reserve (HRR = HRmax − HRrest) added to the resting heart rate; Karvonen method.

percent $\dot{V}O_2$ reserve (%$\dot{V}O_2$R)—Method used to prescribe exercise intensity as a percentage of $\dot{V}O_2$ reserve ($\dot{V}O_2$R = $\dot{V}O_2$max − $\dot{V}O_2$rest) added to the resting $\dot{V}O_2$.

pericarditis—Inflammation of the pericardium caused by trauma, infection, uremia, or heart attack.

periodization—Advanced form of training that systematically varies the volume and intensity of the training exercises.

persuasive technology—A computer system, device, or application that is intentionally designed to change a person's attitude or behavior.

physical activity level (PAL)—The ratio of total energy expenditure to basal metabolic rate; PAL = TEE / BMR.

physical fitness—Ability to perform occupational, recreational, and daily activities without undue fatigue.

population-specific equations—Prediction equations intended only for use with individuals from a specific homogeneous group.

positive energy balance—Excess of energy intake in relation to energy expenditure.

prehypertension—Systolic blood pressure of 120 to 139 mmHg or diastolic pressure of 80 to 89 mmHg.

PR interval—Part of ECG tracing that indicates delay in the impulse at the atrioventricular node.

progression principle—Training principle; training volume must be progressively increased to impose overload and stimulate further improvements.

proprioceptive neuromuscular facilitation (PNF)—Mode of stretching designed to increase range of joint motion through spinal reflex mechanisms such as reciprocal inhibition.

prosthesis—An artificial replacement of a missing body part, such as an artificial limb or joint.

pulmonary ventilation—Movement of air into and out of the lungs.

pulse pressure—Difference between the systolic and diastolic blood pressures.

P wave—Part of ECG tracing that reflects depolarization of the atria.

pyramiding—Advanced resistance training system in which a relatively light weight is lifted in the first set and progressively heavier weights are lifted in subsequent sets; light-to-heavy system.

QRS complex—Part of ECG tracing reflecting ventricular depolarization and contraction.

ramp protocols—Graded exercise tests that are individualized and that provide for continuous, frequent (every 10-20 sec) increments in work rate so that $\dot{V}O_2$ increases linearly.

range of motion (ROM)—Degree of movement at a joint; measure of static flexibility.

rating of perceived exertion (RPE)—A scale used to measure a client's subjective rating of exercise intensity.

reactance (X_c)—Measure of opposition to electrical current flowing through body due to the capacitance of cell membranes; a vector of impedance.

reciprocal inhibition—Reflex that inhibits the contraction of antagonistic muscles when the prime mover is voluntarily contracted.

reference method—Gold standard or criterion method; typically a direct measure of a component used to validate other tests.

regression line—Line of best fit depicting relationship between reference measure and predictor variables.

relative body fat (%BF)—Fat mass expressed as a percentage of total body mass; percent body fat.

relative strength—Muscular strength expressed relative to the body mass or lean body mass; 1-RM/BM.

relative $\dot{V}O_2$max—Rate of oxygen consumption expressed relative to the body mass or lean body mass; measured in $ml \cdot kg^{-1} \cdot min^{-1}$.

reliability—Ability of a test to yield consistent and stable scores across trials and over time.

reliability coefficient—Correlation depicting relationship between trial 1 and trial 2 scores or day 1 and day 2 scores of a test.

repetition maximum (RM)—Measure of intensity for resistance exercise expressed as maximum weight that can be lifted for a given number of repetitions.

repetitions—Number of times a specific exercise movement is performed in a set.

residual score—Difference between the actual and predicted scores (Y – Y').

residual volume (RV)—Volume of air remaining in lungs following a maximal expiration.

resistance (R)—Measure of pure opposition to electrical current flowing through body; a vector of impedance.

resistance index (ht^2/R)—Predictor variable in some BIA regression equations that is calculated by dividing standing height squared by resistance.

respiratory exchange ratio (RER)—Ratio of expired CO_2 to inspired O_2.

resting energy expenditure (REE)—Energy required to maintain essential physiological processes at rest; resting metabolic rate.

resting metabolic rate (RMR)—Energy required to maintain essential physiological processes in a relaxed, awake, and reclined state; resting energy expenditure.

reverse linear periodization (RLP)—Strength training method that progressively decreases training intensity as training volume increases between microcycles.

reversibility principle—Training principle; physiological gains from training are lost when individual stops training (detraining).

rheumatic heart disease—Condition in which the heart valves are damaged by rheumatic fever, contracted from a streptococcal infection (strep throat).

rheumatoid arthritis—Chronic, destructive disease of the joints characterized by inflammation and thickening of the synovial membranes and swelling of the joints.

sagittal abdominal diameter (SAD)—Measure of the anteroposterior thickness of the abdomen at the umbilical level.

sarcopenia—Age-related loss in muscle mass.

self-determination theory—Theory describing how the presence or absence of specific psychological needs affects behavior.

self-efficacy—Individuals' perception of their ability to perform a task and their confidence in making a specific behavioral change.

sensitivity—Probability of a test correctly identifying individuals with risk factors for a specific disease.

set—Defines the number of times a specific number of repetitions of a given exercise is repeated; single or multiple sets.

simple carbohydrates—Simple sugars (e.g., glucose and fructose) found in fruits, berries, table sugar, honey, and some vegetables.

skeletal diameter (D)—Measure of the width of bones.

skinfold (SKF)—Measure of the thickness of two layers of skin and the underlying subcutaneous fat.

social cognitive model—Psychological theory of behavior change; based on concepts of self-efficacy and outcome expectation.

specificity—Measure of a test's ability to correctly identify individuals with no risk factors for a specific disease.

specificity principle—Training principle; physiological and metabolic responses and adaptations to exercise training are specific to type of exercise and muscle groups involved.

sphygmomanometer—Device used to measure blood pressure manually, consisting of a blood pressure cuff and a manometer.

spinning—Group-led exercise that involves stationary cycling at various cadences and resistances.

split routine—Advanced resistance training system in which different muscle groups are targeted on consecutive days to avoid overtraining.

stages of motivational readiness for change model—Psychological theory of behavior change; ability to make long-term behavioral change is based on client's emotional and intellectual readiness; stages of readiness are precontemplation, contemplation, preparation, action, and maintenance.

standard error of estimate (SEE)—Measure of error for prediction equation; quantifies the average deviation of individual data points around the line of best fit.

static balance—Ability to maintain the center of gravity within the supporting base during standing or sitting.

static contraction—Type of muscle contraction in which there is no visible joint movement; isometric contraction.

static flexibility—Measure of the total range of motion at a joint.

static stretching—Mode of exercise used to increase range of motion by placing the joint at the end of its range of motion and slowly applying torque to the muscle to stretch it further.

stress relaxation—Decreased tension within musculotendinous unit when it is held at a fixed length during static stretching.

stretch tolerance—Measure of the amount of resistive force to stretch within target muscles that can be tolerated before experiencing pain.

stroke—Rupture or blockage of blood flow to the brain caused by a blood clot or some other particle.

ST segment—Part of ECG tracing reflecting ventricular repolarization; used to detect coronary occlusion and myocardial infarct.

submaximal exercise test—Graded exercise test in which exercise is terminated at some predetermined submaximal heart rate or workload; used to estimate $\dot{V}O_2max$.

super circuit resistance training—Type of circuit resistance training that intersperses a short, aerobic exercise bout between each resistance training exercise station.

supersetting—Advanced resistance training system in which exercises for agonist and antagonistic muscle groups are done consecutively without rest.

syncope—Brief lapse in consciousness caused by lack of oxygen to the brain.

systolic blood pressure (SBP)—Highest pressure in the arteries during systole of the heart.

tachycardia—Resting heart rate >100 bpm.

talk test—Method to monitor exercise intensity; measure of the client's ability to converse comfortably while exercising; based on the relationship between exercise intensity and pulmonary ventilation.

tare weight—Weight of chair or platform and its supporting equipment used in hydrostatic weighing.

telomeres—Repeated DNA sequences that determine structure and function of chromosomes.

theory of planned behavior—An extension of the theory of reasoned action that takes into consideration the individual's perception of behavioral control.

theory of reasoned action—Theory that proposes a way to understand and predict an individual's behavior; intention is the most important determinant of behavior.

thoracic gas volume (TGV)—Volume of air in the lungs and thorax.

thrombophlebitis—Inflammation of a vein often accompanied by formation of a blood clot.

thrombus—Lump of cellular elements of the blood attached to inner walls of an artery or vein, sometimes blocking blood flow through the vessel.

thyrotoxicosis—Overactive thyroid gland that secretes greater than normal amounts of thyroid hormones; also known as Graves disease or hyperthyroidism.

tonic vibration reflex—Reflex that activates muscle spindles and alpha motor neurons of muscles stimulated by vibration loading.

total cholesterol (TC)—Absolute amount of cholesterol in the blood.

total energy expenditure (TEE)—Sum of energy expenditures for resting metabolic rate, dietary thermogenesis, and physical activity.

total energy expenditure (TEE) method—Method for determining energy expenditure measured by doubly labeled water or predicted from equations.

total error (TE)—Average deviation of individual scores of the cross-validation sample from the line of identity.

training volume—Total amount of training as determined by the number of sets and exercises for a muscle group, intensity, and frequency of training.

transtheoretical model—Model describing the process a client goes through when adopting a change in health behavior.

treading—Type of group-led interval training that involves walking, jogging, and running at various speeds and grades on a treadmill with relief intervals interspersed.

triaxial joint—Type of joint allowing movement in three planes; ball-and-socket joint.

tri-sets—Advanced resistance training system in which three different exercises for the same muscle group are performed consecutively with little or no rest between the exercises.

T wave—Part of ECG tracing corresponding to ventricular repolarization.

two-component model—Body composition model that divides the body into fat and fat-free body components.

type A activity—Endurance activity requiring minimal skill or fitness, for example walking.

type B activity—Endurance activity requiring minimal skill but average fitness, for example jogging.

type C activity—Physical activity requiring both skill and physical fitness, for example swimming.

type D activity—Recreational sports that may improve physical fitness, for example basketball.

type 1 diabetes—Insulin-dependent diabetes, caused by lack of insulin production by the pancreas.

type 2 diabetes—Non-insulin-dependent diabetes, caused by decreased insulin receptor sensitivity.

undercuffing—Using a blood pressure cuff with a bladder too small for the arm circumference, leading to an overestimation of blood pressure.

underwater weight (UWW)—Method used to estimate body volume by measuring weight loss when the body is fully submerged; hydrostatic weighing.

underweight—BMI <18.5 kg/m^2.

undulating periodization (UP)—Strength training method that varies training intensity and volume weekly or even daily.

uniaxial joint—Type of joint allowing movement in one plane; hinge or pivot joint.

upper body obesity—Type of obesity in which excess fat is localized to the upper body; android obesity; apple-shaped body.

uremia—Excessive amounts of urea and other nitrogen waste products in the blood associated with kidney failure.

validity—Ability of a test to accurately measure, with minimal error, a specific component.

validity coefficient—Correlation between reference measure and predicted scores.

valvular heart disease—Congenital disorder of a heart valve characterized by obstructed blood flow, valvular degeneration, and regurgitation of blood.

variable-resistance exercise—Type of exercise in which resistance changes during the range of motion due to levers, pulleys, and cams.

ventilatory threshold—Point at which there is an exponential increase in pulmonary ventilation relative to exercise intensity and rate of oxygen consumption.

ventricular ectopy—Premature (out of sequence) contraction of the ventricles.

ventricular fibrillation—Cardiac dysrhythmia marked by rapid, uncoordinated, and unsynchronized contractions of the ventricles, so that no blood is pumped by the heart.

vertigo—Dizziness or inability to maintain normal balance in a standing or seated position.

very low-density lipoprotein (VLDL)—Lipoprotein made in the liver for transporting triglycerides.

vibration training—Training method that uses whole-body mechanical vibration to increase strength, balance, and bone integrity.

viscoelastic properties—Tension within the muscle–tendon unit caused by the elastic and viscous deformation of the unit when force is applied during stretching.

viscous deformation—Deformation of the muscle–tendon unit that is proportional to the speed at which tension is applied during stretching.

$\dot{V}O_2max$—Maximum rate of oxygen utilization of muscles during exercise.

$\dot{V}O_2peak$—Measure of highest rate of oxygen consumption during an exercise test regardless of whether or not a $\dot{V}O_2$ plateau is reached.

$\dot{V}O_2reserve$—The $\dot{V}O_2max$ minus the $\dot{V}O_2rest$.

waist-to-height ratio (WHTR)—Waist circumference divided by standing height; used as a measure of abdominal obesity.

waist-to-hip ratio (WHR)—Waist circumference divided by hip circumference; used as a measure of upper body or abdominal obesity.

white coat hypertension—Condition in which individuals have normal blood pressure but become hypertensive when blood pressure is measured by a health professional.

References

Abercromby, A.F.J., Amonette, W.E., Layne, C.S., McFarlin, B.K., Hinman, M.R., and Paloski, W.H. 2007. Vibration exposure and biodynamic responses during whole-body vibration training. *Medicine & Science in Sports & Exercise* 39: 1794-1800.

Abraham, W.M. 1977. Factors in delayed muscle soreness. *Medicine and Science in Sports* 9: 11–20.

Adams, J., Mottola, M., Bagnall, K.M., and McFadden, K.D. 1982. Total body fat content in a group of professional football players. *Canadian Journal of Applied Sport Sciences* 7: 36-44.

Ahlback, S.O., and Lindahl, O. 1964. Sagittal mobility of the hip-joint. *Acta Orthopaedica Scandinavica* 34: 310–313.

Ainsworth, B.E., Haskell, W.L., Whitt, M.C., Irwin, M.L., Swartz, A.M., Strath, S.J., O'Brien, W.L., Bassett, D.R. Jr., Schmitz, K.H., Emplaincourt, P.O., Jacobs, D.R., and Leon, A.S. 2000. Compendium of physical activities: An update of activity codes and MET intensities. *Medicine & Science in Sports & Exercise* 32(Suppl.): S498–S516.

Albert, W.J., Bonneau, J., Stevenson, J.M., and Gledhill, N. 2001. Back fitness and back health assessment considerations for the Canadian Physical Activity, Fitness and Lifestyle Appraisal. *Canadian Journal of Applied Physiology* 26: 291–317.

Alter, M.J. 2004. *Science of flexibility.* 3rd ed. Champaign, IL: Human Kinetics.

Altunkan, S., and Altunkan, E. 2006. Validation of the Omron 637IT wrist blood pressure device with a position sensor according to the International Protocol in the elderly. *Blood Pressure Monitoring* 11: 97-102.

Altunkan, S., Ilman, N., Kayaturk, N., and Altunkan, E. 2007. Validation of the Omron M6 (HEM-7001-E) upper-arm blood pressure measuring device according to the International Protocol in adults and obese adults. *Blood Pressure Monitoring* 12(4): 219-225.

Altunkan, S., Oztas, K., and Altunkan, E. 2006. Validation of the Omron 637IT wrist blood pressure measuring device with a position sensor according to the International Protocol in adults and obese adults. *Blood Pressure Monitoring* 11: 79-85.

Alway, S.E., Grumbt, W.H., Gonyea, W.J., and Stray-Gundersen, J. 1989. Contrasts in muscle and myofibers of elite male and female bodybuilders. *Journal of Applied Physiology* 67: 24–31.

American Cancer Society. 2006. At-a-glance—nutrition and physical activity. www.cancer.org/docroot/PED/content/PED_3_2X_Recommendations.asp?sitearea=PED.

American Alliance for Health, Physical Education, Recreation and Dance. 1988. *The AAHPERD physical best program.* Reston, VA: Author.

American College of Sports Medicine. 1996. Position stand on exercise and fluid replacement. *Medicine & Science in Sports & Exercise* 28(1): i-vii.

American College of Sports Medicine. 2004. NCCA accreditation. *ACSM's Certified News* 14(3): 1.

American College of Sports Medicine. 2006. *ACSM's guidelines for exercise testing and prescription,* 7th ed. Philadelphia: Lippincott Williams & Wilkins.

American College of Sports Medicine. 2009a. Appropriate physical activity intervention strategies for weight loss and prevention of weight regain for adults. *Medicine & Science in Sports & Exercise* 41: 459-471.

American College of Sports Medicine. 2009b. *Balance training tools for older adults.* www.acsm.org.

American College of Sports Medicine. 2010. *ACSM's guidelines for exercise testing and prescription,* 8th ed. Philadelphia: Lippincott Williams & Wilkins.

American College of Sports Medicine. 2010. *ACSM's resource manual for guidelines for exercise testing and prescription,* 6th ed. Philadelphia: Wolters Kluwer/Lippincott Williams & Wilkins.

American College of Sports Medicine and American Diabetes Association. 1997. Joint position statement on diabetes mellitus and exercise. *Medicine & Science in Sports & Exercise* 27(12): i-vi.

American College of Sports Medicine, American Dietetic Association, and Dietitians of Canada. 2009. Nutrition and athletic performance: Joint position statement. *Medicine & Science in Sports & Exercise* 41: 709-731.

American Council on Exercise. 1997. Absolute certainty: Do abdominal trainers work any better than the average crunch? *ACE Fitness Matters* 3(2): 1-2.

American Dietetic Association. 2000. Position of the American Dietetic Association, Dietitians of Canada, and the American College of Sports Medicine: Nutrition and athletic performance. *Journal of American Dietetic Association* 100: 1543-1556.

American Dietetic Association. 2003. *Let the evidence speak: Indirect calorimetry and weight management guides.* Chicago: Author.

American Fitness Professionals and Associates. 2004. AFPA news flash: What is the National Board of Fitness Examiners (NBFE) and how does it work? www.afpafitness.com.

American Heart Association. 1999. *2000 heart and stroke statistical update.* Dallas: Author.

American Heart Association. 2001. *International cardiovascular disease statistics.* Dallas: Author.

American Heart Association. 2004. *Heart disease and stroke statistics—2004 update.* Dallas: Author.

American Heart Association. 2008a. Diabetes mellitus—statistics. Statistical fact sheet—risk factors 2008 update. www.Americanheart.org.

American Heart Association. 2008b. High blood cholesterol and other lipids—statistics. Statistical fact sheet—risk factors 2008 update. www.Americanheart.org.

American Heart Association. 2008c. High blood pressure—statistics. Statistical fact sheet—risk factors 2008 update. www.Americanheart.org.

American Heart Association. 2008d. International cardiovascular disease statistics. Statistical fact sheet—populations 2008 update. www.Americanheart.org.

American Heart Association. 2008e. Metabolic syndrome—statistics. Statistical fact sheet—risk factors 2008 update. www.Americanheart.org.

American Heart Association. 2008f. Overweight and obesity—statistics. Statistical fact sheet—risk factors 2008 update. www.Americanheart.org.

American Heart Association. 2008g. Physical inactivity. Statistical fact sheet—risk factors 2008 update. www.Americanheart.org.

American Heart Association. 2008h. Tobacco—statistics. Statistical fact sheet—risk factors 2008 update. www.Americanheart.org.

American Heart Association. 2009. Heart disease and stroke statistics 2009 update. A report from the American Heart Association Statistics Committee and Stroke Statistics Subcommittee. *Circulation* 119: e21-e181.

American Medical Association. 1988. *Guides to the evaluation of permanent impairment,* 3rd ed. Chicago, IL: Author.

American Society of Exercise Physiologists. 2004. Standards of professional practice. www.css.edu/ASEP/Standardsof-ProfessionalPractice.

Anderson, B., and Burke, E.R. 1991. Scientific, medical, and practical aspects of stretching. *Clinics in Sports Medicine* 10: 63-86.

Anderson, G.S. 1992. The 1600-m and multistage 20-m shuttle run as predictive tests of aerobic capacity in children. *Pediatric Exercise Science* 4: 312–318.

Anderson, R. 1980. *Stretching.* Fullerton, CA: Shelter.

Andrews, A.W., Thomas, M.W., and Bohannon, R.W. 1996. Normative values for isometric muscle force measurements obtained with hand-held dynamometers. *Physical Therapy* 76: 248-259.

Antonio, J., and Gonyea, W.J. 1993. Skeletal muscle fiber hyperplasia. *Medicine & Science in Sports & Exercise* 25: 1333–1345.

Ardern, C.I., Katzmarzyk, P.T., and Ross, R. 2003. Discrimination of health risk by combined body mass index and waist circumference. *Obesity Research* 11: 135-142.

Armsey, T.D., and Grime, T.E. 2002. Protein and amino acid supplementation in athletes. *Current Sports Medicine Reports* 4: 253-256.

Armstrong, R.B. 1984. Mechanisms of exercise-induced delayed onset muscular soreness: A brief review. *Medicine & Science in Sports & Exercise* 16: 529–538.

Ashwell, M., and Hsieh, S.D. 2005. Six reasons why the waist-to-height ratio is a rapid and effective global indicator for health risks of obesity and how its use could simplify the international public health message on obesity. *International Journal of Food Sciences and Nutrition* 56: 303-307.

Ashwell, M., McCall, S.A., Cole, T.J., and Dixon, A.K. 1985. Fat distribution and its metabolic complications: Interpretations. In *Human body composition and fat distribution,* ed. N.G. Norgan, 227–242. Wageningen, Netherlands: Euronut.

Åstrand, I. 1960. Aerobic capacity in men and women with special reference to age. *Acta Physiologica Scandinavica* 49(Suppl. 169): 1–92.

Åstrand, P.O. 1956. Human physical fitness with special reference to age and sex. *Physiological Reviews* 36: 307–335.

Åstrand, P.O. 1965. *Work tests with the bicycle ergometer.* Varberg, Sweden: AB Cykelfabriken Monark.

Åstrand, P.O., and Rodahl, K. 1977. *Textbook of work physiology.* New York: McGraw-Hill.

Åstrand, P.O., and Ryhming, I. 1954. A nomogram for calculation of aerobic capacity (physical fitness) from pulse rate during submaximal work. *Journal of Applied Physiology* 7: 218–221.

Atterhog, J.H., Jonsson, B., and Samuelsson, R. 1979. Exercise testing: A prospective study of complication rates. *American Heart Journal* 98: 572-580.

Australian Bureau of Statistics. 2008. Australian statistics on overweight and obesity in adults 2004-05. www.ausstats.abs.gov.au/ausstats.

Axler, C.T., and McGill, S.M. 1997. Low back loads over a variety of abdominal exercises: Searching for the safest abdominal challenge. *Medicine & Science in Sports & Exercise* 29: 804-810.

Baechle, T.R. 1994. *Essentials of strength training and conditioning.* Champaign, IL: Human Kinetics.

Baechle, T.R., Earle, R.W., and Wathen, D. 2000. Resistance training. In *Essentials of strength training and conditioning,* eds. T.R. Baechle and R.W. Earle. Champaign, IL: Human Kinetics.

Bahr, R., Ingnes, I., Vaage, O., Sjersted, O.M., and Newsholme, E.A. 1987. Effect of duration of exercise on excess postexercise O_2 consumption. *Journal of Applied Physiology* 62: 485–490.

Baker, D., Wilson, G., and Carlyon, R. 1994. Periodization: The effect on strength of manipulating volume and intensity. *Journal of Strength and Conditioning Research* 8: 235–242.

Bakhtiary, A.H., Safavi-Farokhi, Z., and Aminian-Far, A. 2007. Influence of vibration on delayed onset of muscle soreness following eccentric exercise. *British Journal of Sports Medicine* 41: 145-148.

Balke, B. 1963. A simple field test for the assessment of physical fitness. *Civil Aeromedical Research Institute Report, 63–18.* Oklahoma City: Federal Aviation Agency.

Balke, B., and Ware, R. 1959. An experimental study of physical fitness of Air Force personnel. *US Armed Forces Medical Journal* 10: 675–688.

Ball, T.E., and Rose, K.S. 1991. A field test for predicting maximum bench press lift of college women. *Journal of Applied Sport Science Research* 5: 169–170.

Ballor, D.L., and Keesey, R.E. 1991. A meta-analysis of the factors affecting exercise-induced changes in body mass, fat mass, and fat-free mass in males and females. *International Journal of Obesity* 15: 717-726.

Bandura, A. 1982. Self-efficacy mechanism in human agency. *American Psychologist* 37: 122–147.

Bandy, W.D., and Irion, J.M. 1994. The effect of time on static stretch on the flexibility of the hamstring muscles. *Physical Therapy* 74: 845-851.

Barreira, T., Kang, M., Caputo, J., Farley, S., and Renfrow, M. 2009. Validation of the Actiheart monitor for the measurement of physical activity. *International Journal of Exercise Science* 2(1): article 7. http://digitalcommons.wku.edu/ijes/vol2/iss1/7.

Baumgartner, R.N., Heymsfield, S.B., and Roche, A.F. 1995. Human body composition and the epidemiology of chronic disease. *Obesity Research* 3: 73–95.

Baumgartner, R.N., Heymsfield, S.B., Lichtman, S., Wang, J., and Pierson, R.N. 1991. Body composition in elderly people: Effect of criterion estimates on predictive equations. *American Journal of Clinical Nutrition* 53: 1–9.

Baumgartner, T.A. 1978. Modified pull-up test. *Research Quarterly* 49: 80–84.

Baumgartner, T.A., and Jackson, A.S. 1975. *Measurement for evaluation in physical education.* Boston: Houghton Mifflin.

Baumgartner, T.A., East, W.B., Frye, P.A., Hensley, L.D., Knox, D.F., and Norton, C.J. 1984. Equipment improvements and additional norms for the modified pull-up test. *Research Quarterly for Exercise and Sport* 55: 64–68.

Baun, W.B., and Baun, M.R. 1981. A nomogram for the estimate of percent body fat from generalized equations. *Research Quarterly for Exercise and Sport* 52: 380–384.

Beaulieu, J.E. 1980. *Stretching for all sports.* Pasadena, CA: Athletic Press.

Beenakker, E.A.C., van der Hoeven, J.H., Fock, J.M., and Maurits, N.M. 2001. Reference values of maximum iso-

metric muscle force obtained in 270 children aged 4-16 years by hand-held dynamometry. *Neuromuscular Disorders* 11: 441-446.

Beevers, G., Lip, G.Y.H., and O'Brien, E. 2001a. ABC of hypertension. Blood pressure measurement. Part I—Sphygmomanometry: Factors common to all techniques. *British Medical Journal* 322: 981-985.

Beevers, G., Lip, G.Y.H., and O'Brien, E. 2001b. ABC of hypertension. Blood pressure measurement. Part II—Conventional sphygmomanometry: Technique of auscultatory blood pressure measurement. *British Medical Journal* 322: 1043-1047.

Behm, D.G., Faigenbaum, A.D., Falk, B., and Klentrou, P. 2008. Canadian Society for Exercise Physiology position paper: Resistance training in children and adolescents. *Applied Physiology, Nutrition, and Metabolism* 33: 547-561.

Behnke, A.R. 1961. Quantitative assessment of body build. *Journal of Applied Physiology* 16: 960–968.

Behnke, A.R., and Wilmore, J.H. 1974. *Evaluation and regulation of body build and composition.* Englewood Cliffs, NJ: Prentice Hall.

Bellew, J.W., Fenter, P.C., Chelette, B., Moore, R., and Loreno, D. 2005. Effects of a short-term dynamic balance training program in healthy older women. *Journal of Geriatric Physical Therapy* 28: 4-8, 27.

Benardot, D., Clarkson, P., Coleman, E., and Manore, M. 2001. Can vitamin supplements improve sport performance? *Gatorade Sports Science Exchange Roundtable* 12(3): 1-4.

Bentzur, K.M., Kravitz, L., and Lockner, D.W. 2008. Evaluation of the Bod Pod for estimating percent body fat in collegiate track and field female athletes: A comparison of four methods. *Journal of Strength and Conditioning Research* 22: 1985-1991.

Berg, K.O., Wood-Dauphinee, S.L., Williams, J.I., and Maki, B. 1992. Measuring balance in the elderly: Validation of an instrument. *Canadian Journal of Public Health* 83(2): S7-S11.

Bergsma-Kadijk, J.A., Baumeister, B., and Deurenberg, P. 1996. Measurement of body fat in young and elderly women: Comparison between a four-compartment model and widely used reference methods. *British Journal of Nutrition* 75: 649-657.

Berlin, J.A., and Colditz, G.A. 1990. A meta-analysis of physical activity in the prevention of coronary heart disease. *American Journal of Epidemiology* 132: 612–628.

Berry, M.J., Cline, C.C., Berry, C.B., and Davis, M. 1992. A comparison between two forms of aerobic dance and treadmill running. *Medicine & Science in Sports & Exercise* 24: 946–951.

Bielinski, R., Schultz, Y., and Jequier, E. 1985. Energy metabolism during the postexercise recovery in man. *American Journal of Clinical Nutrition* 42: 69–82.

Billinger, S.A., Loudon, J.K., and Gajewski, B.J. 2008. Validity of a total body recumbent stepper exercise test to assess cardiorespiratory fitness. *Journal of Strength and Conditioning Research* 22: 1556-1562.

Birk, T.J., and Birk, C.A. 1987. Use of ratings of perceived exertion for exercise prescription. *Sports Medicine* 4: 1–8.

Bjorntorp, P. 1988. Abdominal obesity and the development of non-insulin diabetes mellitus. *Diabetes and Metabolism Reviews* 4: 615–622.

Blair, D., Habricht, J.P., Sims, E.A., Sylwester, D., and Abraham, S. 1984. Evidence of an increased risk for hypertension with centrally located body fat, and the effect of race and sex on this risk. *American Journal of Epidemiology* 119: 526–540.

Blair, S.N. 2009. Physical inactivity: The biggest public health problem of the 21st century. *British Journal of Sports Medicine* 43: 1-2.

Blair, S.N., LaMonte, M.J., and Nichaman, M.Z. 2004. The evolution of physical activity recommendations: How much is enough? *American Journal of Clinical Nutrition* 79 (Suppl.): 913S-920S.

Bland, J.M., and Altman, D.G. 1986. Statistical methods for assessing agreement between two methods of clinical measurement. *The Lancet* 12: 307-310.

Blessing, D.L., Wilson, D.G., Puckett, J.R., and Ford, H.T. 1987. The physiological effects of 8 weeks of aerobic dance with and without hand-held weights. *American Journal of Sports Medicine* 15: 508–510.

Blum, V., Carriere, E.G.J., Kolsters, W., Mosterd, W.L., Schiereck, P., and Wesseling, K.H. 1997. Aortic and peripheral blood pressure during isometric and dynamic exercise. *International Journal of Sports Medicine* 18: 30-34.

Bohannon, R.W. 1997. Reference values for extremity muscle strength obtained by hand-held dynamometry from adults aged 20 to 79 years. *Archives of Physical Medicine and Rehabilitation* 78: 26-32.

Bohannon, R.W. 2006a. Reference values for the timed up and go test: A descriptive meta-analysis. *Journal of Geriatric Physical Therapy* 29(2): 64-68.

Bohannon, R.W. 2006b. Single leg stance times. A descriptive meta-analysis of data from individuals at least 60 years of age. *Topics in Geriatric Rehabilitation* 22: 70-77.

Bohe, J., Low, A., Wolfe, R.R., and Rennie, M.J. 2003. Human muscle protein synthesis is modulated by extracellular, not intramuscular amino acid availability: A dose-response study. *Journal of Physiology* 552: 315-324.

Bompa, T.O., DiPasquale, M.D., and Cornacchia, L.J. 2003. *Serious strength training.* 2nd ed. Champaign, IL: Human Kinetics.

Bonci, L. 2009. *Sport nutrition for coaches.* Champaign, IL: Human Kinetics.

Bonge, D., and Donnelly, J.E. 1989. Trials to criteria for hydrostatic weighing at residual volume. *Research Quarterly for Exercise and Sport* 60: 176-179.

Borg, G. 1998. *Borg's perceived exertion and pain scales.* Champaign, IL: Human Kinetics.

Borg, G.V., and Linderholm, H. 1967. Perceived exertion and pulse rate during graded exercise in various age groups. *Acta Medica Scandinavica* 472(Suppl.): 194–206.

Borms, J., Van Roy, P., Santens, J.P., and Haentjens, A. 1987. Optimal duration of static stretching exercises for improvement of coxo-femoral flexibility. *Journal of Sports Science* 5: 39-47.

Bosco, C.M., Colli, R., Introini, E., Cardinale, M., Tsarpela, O., Madella, A., Tihanyi, J., and Viru, A. 1999. Adaptive responses of human skeletal muscle to vibration exposure. *Clinical Physiology* 19: 183-187.

Bouchard, C. 2001. Physical activity and health: Introduction to the dose-response symposium. *Medicine & Science in Sports & Exercise* 33 (Suppl.): S347–S350.

Bouchard, C., Perusse, L., Leblanc, C., Tremblay, A., and Theriault, G. 1988. Inheritance of the amount and distribution of human body fat. *International Journal of Obesity* 12: 205–215.

Bouchard, C., Shephard, R.J., and Stephens, T., eds. 1994. *Physical activity, fitness, and health. International proceedings and conference statement.* Champaign, IL: Human Kinetics.

Bouchard, C., Tremblay, A., Despres, J.P., Nadeau, A., Lupien, P.J., Theriault, G., Dussault, J., Moorjani, S., Pinault, S., and Fournier, G. 1990. The response of long-term overfeeding in identical twins. *New England Journal of Medicine* 322: 1477–1482.

Bracko, M.R. 2002. Can stretching prior to exercise and sports improve performance and prevent injury. *ACSM's Health & Fitness Journal* 6(5): 17-22.

Bracko, M.R. 2004. Can we prevent back injuries? *ACSM's Health & Fitness Journal* 8(4): 5–11.

Brahler, C.J., and Blank, S.E. 1995. VersaClimbing elicits higher V.O$_2$max than does treadmill running or rowing ergometry. *Medicine & Science in Sports & Exercise* 27: 249–254.

Braith, R.W., Graves, J.E., Leggett, S.H., and Pollock, M.L. 1993. Effect of training on the relationship between maximal and submaximal strength. *Medicine & Science in Sports & Exercise* 25: 132–138.

Branch, J.D. 2003. Effect of creatine supplementation on body composition and performance: A meta-analysis. *International Journal of Sport Nutrition and Exercise Metabolism* 13: 198–226.

Brandenburg, J.P. 2006. Duration of stretch does not influence the degree of force loss following static stretching. *Journal of Sports Medicine and Physical Fitness* 46: 526-534.

Bravata, D.M., Sanders, L., Huang, J., Krumholz, H.M., Olkin, I., Gardner, C.D., Bravata, D.M. 2003. Efficacy and safety of low-carbohydrate diets: A systematic review. *Journal of the American Medical Association* 289: 1837-1850.

Bravata, D.M., Smith-Spangler, C., Sundaram, V., Gienger, A.L., Lin, N., Lewis, R., Stave, C.D., Olkin, I., and Sirard, J.R. 2007. Using pedometers to increase physical activity and improve health: A systematic review. *Journal of the American Medical Association* 298: 2296-2304.

Bray, G.A. 1978. Definitions, measurements and classifications of the syndromes of obesity. *International Journal of Obesity* 2: 99–113.

Bray, G.A., and Gray, D.S. 1988a. Anthropometric measurements in the obese. In *Anthropometric standardization reference manual,* ed. T.G. Lohman, A.F. Roche, and R. Martorell, 131–136. Champaign, IL: Human Kinetics.

Bray, G.A., and Gray, D.S. 1988b. Obesity. Part I—Pathogenesis. *Western Journal of Medicine* 149: 429–441.

Brehm, B.A. 1988. Elevation of metabolic rate following exercise—implications for weight loss. *Sports Medicine* 6: 72–78.

British Heart Foundation. 2004. Statistics database. www.heartstats.org/temp/bloodsppressures2004.pdf.

British Heart Foundation. 2006. Diet, physical activity, and obesity statistics, 2006 edition. www.bhf.org.

British Heart Foundation. 2008. Coronary heart disease statistics, 2007 edition. www.bhf.org.

British Heart Foundation Health Promotion Research Group. 2005. European cardiovascular disease statistics, 2005 edition. www.bhf.org.

Brooks, G.A., Butte, N.F., Rand, W.M., Flatt, J.P., and Caballero, B. 2004. Chronicle of the Institute of Medicine physical activity recommendation: How a physical activity recommendation came to be among dietary recommendations. *American Journal of Clinical Nutrition* 79 (Suppl.): 921S-930S.

Brose, A., Parise, G., and Tarnopolsky, M.A. 2003. Creatine supplementation enhances isometric strength and body composition improvements following strength exercise training in older adults. *Journals of Gerontology Series A: Biological Sciences and Medical Sciences* 58: 11-19.

Brown, D.A., and Miller, W.C. 1998. Normative data for strength and flexibility of women throughout life. *European Journal of Applied Physiology* 78: 77–82.

Brozek, J., Grande, F., Anderson, J.T., and Keys, A. 1963. Densiometric analysis of body composition: Revision of some quantitative assumptions. *Annals of the New York Academy of Sciences* 110: 113–140.

Bruce, R.A., Kusumi, F., and Hosmer, D. 1973. Maximal oxygen intake and nomographic assessment of functional aerobic impairment in cardiovascular disease. *American Heart Journal* 85: 546–562.

Bryner, R.W., Ullrich, I.H., Sauers, J., Donley, D., Hornsby, G., Kolar, M., and Yeater, R. 1999. Effects of resistance vs. aerobic training combined with an 800 calorie liquid diet on lean body mass and resting metabolic rate. *Journal of the American College of Nutrition* 18(2): 115–121.

Brzycki, M. 1993. Strength testing—predicting a one-rep max from reps-to-fatigue. *Journal of Physical Education, Recreation and Dance* 64 (1): 88–90.

Brzycki, M. 2000. Assessing strength. *Fitness Management* 16(7): 34–37.

Buchholz, A.C., and Schoeller, D.A. 2004. Is a calorie a calorie? *American Journal of Clinical Nutrition* 79 (Suppl.): 899S-906S.

Bunt, J.C., Lohman, T.G., and Boileau, R.A. 1989. Impact of total body water fluctuations on estimation of body fat from body density. *Medicine & Science in Sports & Exercise* 21: 96–100.

Buresh, R., and Berg, K. 2002. Scaling oxygen uptake to body size and several practical applications. *Journal of Strength and Conditioning Research* 16: 461-465.

Burke, D.G., Culligan, C.J., and Holt, L.E. 2000. The theoretical basis of proprioceptive neuromuscular facilitation. *Journal of Strength and Conditioning Research* 14: 496-500.

Burke, L.M., Kiens, B., and Ivy, J.L. 2004. Carbohydrates and fat for training and recovery. *Journal of Sports Science* 22: 15-30.

Byrnes, W.C., Clarkson, P.M., and Katch, F.I. 1985. Muscle soreness following resistive exercise with and without eccentric contraction. *Research Quarterly for Exercise and Sport* 56: 283–285.

Cable, A., Nieman, D.C., Austin, M., Hogen, E., and Utter, A.C. 2001. Validity of leg-to-leg bioelectrical impedance measurement in males. *Journal of Sports Medicine and Physical Fitness* 41: 411-414.

Callaway, C.W., Chumlea, W.C., Bouchard, C., Himes, J.H., Lohman, T.G., Martin, A.D., Mitchell, C.D., Mueller, W.H., Roche, A.F., and Seefeldt, V.D. 1988. Circumferences. In *Anthropometric standardization reference manual,* ed. T.G. Lohman, A.F. Roche, and R. Martorell, 39–54. Champaign, IL: Human Kinetics.

Campbell, W.W., and Geik, R.A. 2004. Nutritional considerations for the older athlete. *Nutrition* 20: 603-608.

Campbell, W.W., Johnson, C.A., McCabe, G.P., and Carnell, N.S. 2008. Dietary protein requirements of younger and older adults. *American Journal of Clinical Nutrition* 88: 1322-1329.

Canadian Society for Exercise Physiology. 2003. *The Canadian physical activity, fitness and lifestyle approach: CSEP-Health & Fitness Program's Health-Related Appraisal and Counselling Strategy.* 3rd ed. Ottawa, ON: Author.

Canning, P.M., Courage, M.L., and Frizzell, L.M. 2004. Prevalence of overweight and obesity in a provincial population of Canadian preschool children. *Canadian Medical Association Journal* 171: 240-242.

Carns, M.L., Schade, M.L., Liba, M.R., Hellebrandt, F.A., and Harris, C.W. 1960. Segmental volume reduction by localized and generalized exercise. *Human Biology* 32: 370–376.

Carpenter, D.M., and Nelson, B.W. 1999. Low back strengthening for the prevention and treatment of low back pain. *Medicine & Science in Sports & Exercise* 31: 18-24.

Carter, N.D., Kannus, P., and Khan, K.M. 2001. Exercise in the prevention of falls in older people. A systematic literature review examining the rationale and the evidence. *Sports Medicine* 31: 427-438.

Casa, D.L., Armstrong, L.E., Hillman, S.K., Montain, S.J., Reiff, R.V., Rich, B.S.E., Roberts, W.O., and Stone, J.A. 2002. National Athletic Trainers' Association position statement: Fluid replacement for athletes. *Journal of Athletic Training* 35(2): 21-224.

Cassady, S.L., Nielsen, D.H., Janz, K.F., Wu, Y., Cook, J.S., and Hansen, J.R. 1993. Validity of near infrared body composition analysis in children and adolescents. *Medicine & Science in Sports & Exercise* 25: 1185-1191.

Cataldo, D., and Heyward, V. 2000. Pinch an inch: A comparison of several high-quality and plastic skinfold calipers. *ACSM's Health & Fitness Journal* 4(3): 12–16.

Caton, J.R., Mole, P.A., Adams, W.C., and Heustis, D.S. 1988. Body composition analysis by bioelectrical impedance: Effect of skin temperature. *Medicine & Science in Sports & Exercise* 20: 489–491.

Cavill, N., Kahlmeier, S., and Racioppi, F., eds. 2006. Physical activity and health in Europe: Evidence for action. World Health Organization. www.who.int/moveforhealth.

Centers for Disease Control. 2003. Prevalence of physical activity, including lifestyle activities among adults—United States, 2000-2001. *Morbidity and Mortality Weekly* 52(32): 764-769.

Centers for Disease Control and Prevention. 2005. Adult participation in recommended levels of physical activity: United States, 2001 and 2003. *Morbidity and Mortality Weekly Report* 54: 1208-1212.

Centers for Disease Control and Prevention. 2005. NHANES 2001-2002 data documentation MEC examination. Balance examination (BAX_B). http://www.cdc.gov/nchs/data/nhanes/nhanes_01_02/bax_b_doc.pdf.

Centers for Disease Control and Prevention. 2007. Cigarette smoking among adults—United States, 2006. *Morbidity and Mortality Weekly Report* [serial online] 56(44): 1157-1161.

Centers for Disease Control and Prevention. 2009. Falls among older adults: An overview. http://www.cdc.gov/HomeandRecreationalSafety/Falls/adultfalls.html.

Chalmers, G. 2004. Re-examination of the possible role of Golgi tendon organ and muscle spindle reflexes in proprioceptive neuromuscular facilitation muscle stretching. *Sports Biomechanics* 3: 159-183.

Chamberlin, B., and Gallagher, R. (May 7, 2008). Exergames: Using video games to promote physical activity. Paper presented at Children, Youth and Families at Risk (CYFAR) Conference, San Antonio, TX.

Chapman, E.A., deVries, H.A., and Swezey, R. 1972. Joint stiffness: Effects of exercise on young and old men. *Journal of Gerontology* 27: 218–221.

Charette, S.L., McEvoy, L., Pyka, G., Snow-Harter, C., Guido, D., Wiswell, R.A., and Marcus, R. 1991. Muscle hypertrophy response to resistance training in older women. *Journal of Applied Physiology* 70: 1912–1916.

Cherkas, L.F., Hunkin, J.L., Kato, B.S., Richards, J.B., Gardner, J.P., Surdulescu, G.L., Kimura, M., Lu, X., Spector, T.D., and Aviv, A. 2008. The association between physical activity in leisure time and leukocyte telomere length. *Archives of Internal Medicine* 168(2): 154-158.

Chewning, B., Yu, T., and Johnson, J. 2000. T'ai chi (part 2): Effects on health. *ACSM's Health & Fitness Journal* 4(3): 17–19, 28, 30.

Chobanian, A.V., Bakris, G.L., Black, H.R., Cushman, W.C., Green, L.A., Izzo, J.L., Jones, D.W., Materson, B.J., Oparil, S., Wright, J.T. Jr., Roccella, E.J., and the National High Blood Pressure Education Coordinating Committee. 2003.

The seventh report of the Joint National Committee on prevention, detection, evaluation, and treatment of high blood pressure. *Hypertension* 42: 1206-1252. Also available in *Journal of the American Medical Association* 289 (2003): 2560-2572.

Chung, I., and Lip, G.Y.H. 2003. White coat hypertension: Not so benign after all? *Journal of Human Hypertension* 17: 807-809.

Cipriani, D., Abel, B., and Pirrwitz, D. 2003. A comparison of two stretching protocols on hip range of motion: Implications for total daily stretch duration. *Journal of Strength and Conditioning Research* 17: 274-278.

Clark, B.C., and Manini, T.M. 2008. Sarcopenia ≠ dynapenia. *Journal of Gerontology* 63A: 829-834.

Clark, N. 2008. *Nancy Clark's sport nutrition guidebook,* 4th ed. Champaign, IL: Human Kinetics.

Clark, S., Iltis, P.W., Anthony, C.J., and Toews, A. 2005. Comparison of older adult performance during the functional-reach and limits-of-stability tests. *Journal of Aging and Physical Activity* 13: 266-275.

Clark, S., Rose, D.J., and Fujimoto, K. 1997. Generalizability of the limits of stability test in the evaluation of dynamic balance among older adults. *Archives of Physical Medicine and Rehabilitation* 78: 1078-1084.

Clarke, D.H. 1975. *Exercise physiology.* Englewood Cliffs, NJ: Prentice Hall.

Clarke, H.H. 1966. *Muscular strength and endurance in man.* Englewood Cliffs, NJ: Prentice Hall.

Clarke, H.H., and Monroe, R.A. 1970. *Test manual: Oregon cable-tension strength test batteries for boys and girls from fourth grade through college.* Eugene, OR: University of Oregon.

Clarkson, P.M. 1990. Tired blood: Iron deficiency in athletes and effects of iron supplementation. *Sports Science Exchange* 3(28). Gatorade Sports Science Institute, Quaker Oats Co.

Clarkson, P.M., and Haymes, E.M. 1994. Trace mineral requirements for athletes. *International Journal of Sport Nutrition* 4: 104–119.

Clarkson, P.M., Byrnes, W.C., McCormick, K.M., Turcotte, L.P., and White, J.S. 1986. Muscle soreness and serum creatine kinase activity following isometric, eccentric and concentric exercise. *International Journal of Sports Medicine* 7: 152–155.

Clarys, J.P., Martin, A.D., Drinkwater, D.T., and Marfell-Jones, M.J. 1987. The skinfold: Myth and reality. *Journal of Sports Sciences* 5: 3–33.

Clemons, J.M., Duncan, C.A., Blanchard, O.E., Gatch, W.H., Hollander, D.B., and Doucer, J.L. 2004. Relationships between the flexed-arm hang and select measures of muscular fitness. *Journal of Strength and Conditioning Research* 18: 630-636.

Cohen, A. 2004. It's getting personal. *Athletic Business,* July, 52-54, 56, 58, 60.

Colberg, S.R. 2001. *The diabetic athlete.* Champaign, IL: Human Kinetics.

Cole, T.J., Bellizzi, M.C., Flegal, K.M., and Dietz, W.H. 2000. Establishing a standard definition for child overweight and obesity worldwide: International survey. *British Medical Journal* 320: 1240-1245.

Collins, M., Millard-Stafford, M., Sparling, P., Snow, T., Rosskopf, L., Webb, S., and Omer, J. 1999. Evaluation of the Bod Pod for assessing body fat in collegiate football players. *Medicine & Science in Sports & Exercise* 31: 1350–1356.

Conley, D., Cureton, K., Dengel, D., and Weyand, P. 1991. Validation of the 12-min swim as a field test of peak aerobic power in young men. *Medicine & Science in Sports & Exercise* 23: 766–773.

Conley, D., Cureton, K., Hinson, B., Higbie, E., and Weyand, P. 1992. Validation of the 12-minute swim as a field test of peak aerobic power in young women. *Research Quarterly for Exercise and Sport* 63: 153–161.

Cooper Institute for Aerobics Research. 1992. *The Prudential FITNESSGRAM test administration manual.* Dallas: Author.

Cooper Institute for Aerobics Research. 1994. *Fitnessgram user's manual.* Dallas: Author.

Cooper Institute for Aerobics Research. 2005. *The fitness specialist certification manual.* Dallas: Author.

Cooper, K.H. 1968. A means of assessing maximal oxygen intake. *Journal of the American Medical Association* 203: 201–204.

Cooper, K.H. 1977. *The aerobics way.* New York: Evans.

Corbin, C.B., Dowell, L.J., Lindsey, R., and Tolson, H. 1978. *Concepts in physical education.* Dubuque, IA: Brown.

Costill, D.L., Coyle, E.F., Fink, W.F., Lesmes, G.R., and Witzmann, F.A. 1979. Adaptations in skeletal muscle following strength training. *Journal of Applied Physiology* 46: 96–99.

Costill, D.L., and Fox, E.L. 1969. Energetics of marathon running. *Medicine and Science in Sports* 1: 81–86.

Costill, D.L., Thomason, H., and Roberts, E. 1973. Fractional utilization of the aerobic capacity during distance running. *Medicine and Science in Sports* 5: 248–252.

Cote, C., Simoneau, J.A., Lagasse, P., Bouley, M., Thibault, M.C., Marcotte, M., and Bouchard, C. 1988. Isokinetic strength training protocols: Do they induce skeletal muscle fiber hypertrophy? *Archives of Physical Medicine and Rehabilitation* 69: 281–285.

Cote, D.K., and Adams, W.C. 1993. Effect of bone density on body composition estimates in young adult black and white women. *Medicine & Science in Sports & Exercise* 25: 290–296.

Cotte, U.V., Faltenbacher, V.H., von Willich, W., and Bogner, J.R. 2008. Trial of validation of two devices for self-measurement of blood pressure according to the European Society of Hypertension International Protocol: The Citizen CH-432B and the Citizen CH-656C. *Blood Pressure Monitoring* 13: 55-62.

Cotten, D.J. 1972. A comparison of selected trunk flexibility tests. *American Corrective Therapy Journal* 26: 24.

Coyle, E.F. 1995. Fat metabolism during exercise. *Sports Science Exchange* 8(6). Gatorade Sports Science Institute, Quaker Oats Co.

Coyle, E.F., Feiring, D.C., Rotkis, T.C., Cote, R.W. III, Roby, F.B., Lee, W., and Wilmore, J.H. 1981. Specificity of power improvements through slow and fast isokinetic training. *Journal of Applied Physiology* 51: 1437–1442.

Cribb, P.J., Williams, A.D., and Hayes, A. 2007. A creatine-carbohydrate supplement enhances responses to resistance training. *Medicine & Science in Sports & Exercise* 39: 1960-1968.

Cribb, P.J., Williams, A.D., Hayes, A., and Carey, M.F. 2006. The effect of whey isolate on strength, body composition, and plasma glutamine. *International Journal of Sports Nutrition and Exercise Metabolism* 16: 494-509.

Cribb, P.J., Williams, A.D., Stathis, C.G., Carey, M.F., and Hayes, A. 2007. Effect of whey isolate, creatine, and resistance training on muscle hypertrophy. *Medicine & Science in Sports & Exercise* 39: 298-307.

Crommett, A., Kravitz, L., Wongsathikun, J., and Kemerly, T. 1999. Comparison of metabolic and subjective response of three modalities in college-age subjects. *Medicine & Science in Sports & Exercise* 31(Suppl.): S158 [abstract].

Crouter, S.E., Churilla, J.R., and Bassett, D.R. 2008. Accuracy of the Actiheart for the assessment of energy expenditure in adults. *European Journal of Clinical Nutrition* 62: 704-711.

Cullinen, K., and Caldwell, M. 1998. Weight training increases fat-free mass and strength in untrained young women. *Journal of the American Dietetic Association* 98(4): 414–418.

Curb, J.D., Ceria-Ulep, C.D., Rodriquez, B.L., Grove, J., Guralnik, J., Willcox, B.J., Donlon, T.A., Masaki, K.H., and Chen, R. 2006. Performance-based measures of physical function for high-function populations. *Journal of the American Geriatrics Society* 54: 737-742.

Cureton, K.J., Collins, M.A., Hill, D.W., and McElhannon, F.M. Jr. 1988. Muscle hypertrophy in men and women. *Medicine & Science in Sports & Exercise* 20: 338–344.

Cureton, K.J., Sloniger, M., O'Bannon, J., Black, D., and McCormack, W. 1995. A generalized equation for prediction of VO₂peak from 1-mile run/walk performance. *Medicine & Science in Sports & Exercise* 27: 445–451.

Cureton, K.J., Sparling, P.B., Evans, B.W., Johnson, S.M., Kong, U.D., and Purvis, J.W. 1978. Effect of experimental alterations in excess weight on aerobic capacity and distance running performance. *Medicine and Science in Sports* 10: 194–199.

Cureton, T.K., and Sterling, L.F. 1964. Interpretation of the cardiovascular component resulting from the factor analysis of 104 test variables measured in 100 normal young men. *Journal of Sports Medicine and Physical Fitness* 4: 1–24.

Curioni, C.C., and Lourenco, P.M. 2005. Long-term weight loss after diet and exercise: A systematic review. *International Journal of Obesity* 29: 1168-1174.

Davis, D.S., Quinn, R.O., Whiteman, C.T., Williams, J.D., and Young, C.R. 2008. Concurrent validity of four clinical tests to measure hamstring flexibility. *Journal of Strength and Conditioning Research* 22: 583-588.

Davis, J.A., Dorado, S., Keays, K.A., Reigel, R.A., Valencia, K.S., and Pham, P.H. 2007. Reliability and validity of the lung volume measurement made by the Bod Pod body composition system. *Clinical Physiology and Functional Imaging* 27: 42-46.

Day, J.R., Rossiter, H.B., Coats, E.M., Skasick, A., and Whipp, B.J. 2003. The maximally attainable V.O₂ during exercise in humans: The peak vs. maximum issue. *Journal of Applied Physiology* 95: 1901-1907.

de Bruin, E.D., Swanenburg, J., Betschon, E., and Murer, K. 2009. A randomized controlled trial investigating motor skill training as a function of attentional focus in old age. *BMC Geriatrics* 9: 15-24.

Deci, E.L., and Ryan, R.M. 2000. The "what" and "why" of goal pursuits: Human needs and the self-determination of behavior. *Psychological Inquiry* 11(4): 227-268.

del Rio-Navarro, B.E., Velazquez-Monroy, O., Sanchez-Castillo, C.P., Lara-Esqueda, A., Berber, A., Fanghanel, G., Violante, R., Tapia-Conyer, R., and James, W.P.T. 2004. The high prevalence of overweight and obesity in Mexican children. *Obesity Research* 12: 215-223.

Delecluse, C., Roelants, M., and Verschueren, S. 2003. Strength increase after whole-body vibration compared with resistance training. *Medicine & Science in Sports & Exercise* 35: 1033-1041.

Demerath, E.W., Guo, S.S., Chumlea, W.C., Towne, B., Roche, A.F., and Siervogel, R.M. 2002. Comparison of percent body fat estimates using air displacement plethysmography and hydrodensitometry in adults and children. *International Journal of Obesity and Related Metabolic Disorders* 26: 389-397.

Demont, R.G., Lephart, S.M., Giraldo, J.L., Giannantonio, F.P., Yuktanandana, P., and Fu, F.H. 1999. Comparison of two abdominal training devices with an abdominal crunch using strength and EMG measurements. *Journal of Sports Medicine and Physical Fitness* 39: 253-258.

Dempster, P., and Aitkens, S. 1995. A new air displacement method for the determination of human body composition. *Medicine & Science in Sports & Exercise* 27: 1692–1697.

Demura, S., Yamaji, S., Goshi, F., Kobayashi, H., Sato, S., and Nagasawa, Y. 2002. The validity and reliability of relative body fat estimates and the construction of new prediction equations for young Japanese adult males. *Journal of Sports Sciences* 20: 153-164.

Deschenes, M.R., and Kraemer, W.J. 2002. Performance and physiologic adaptations to resistance training. *American Journal of Physical Medicine and Rehabilitation* 8 (Suppl.): S3-S16.

de Souza, R.J., Swain, J.F., Appel, L.J., and Sacks, F.M. 2008. Alternatives for macronutrient intake and chronic disease: A comparison of the OmniHeart diets with popular diets and with dietary recommendations. *American Journal of Clinical Nutrition* 88: 1-11.

Despres, J.P., and Lamarche, B. 1994. Low-intensity endurance training, plasma lipoproteins, and the risk of coronary heart disease. *Journal of Internal Medicine* 236: 7–22.

Despres, J.P., Bouchard, C., Tremblay, A., Savard, R., and Marcotte, M. 1985. Effects of aerobic training on fat dis-tribution in male subjects. *Medicine & Science in Sports & Exercise* 17: 113–118.

Deurenberg, P. 2001. Universal cut-off BMI points for obesity are not appropriate. *British Journal of Nutrition* 85: 135-136.

Deurenberg, P., and Deurenberg-Yap, M. 2001. Differences in body-composition assumptions across ethnic groups: Practical consequences. *Current Opinion in Clinical Nutrition and Metabolic Care* 4: 377-383.

Deurenberg, P., and Deurenberg-Yap, M. 2002. Validation of skinfold thickness and hand-held impedance measurements for estimation of body fat percentage among Singaporean Chinese, Malay and Indian subjects. *Asia Pacific Journal of Clinical Nutrition* 11: 1-7.

Deurenberg, P., van der Kooy, K., Evers, P., and Hulshof, T. 1990. Assessment of body composition by bioelectrical impedance in a population aged >60 y. *American Journal of Clinical Nutrition* 51: 3–6.

Deurenberg, P., van der Kooy, K., and Leenan, R. 1989. Differences in body impedance when measured with different instruments. *European Journal of Clinical Nutrition* 43: 885-886.

Deurenberg, P., Weststrate, J.A., Paymans, I., and van der Kooy, K. 1988. Factors affecting bioelectrical impedance measurements in humans. *European Journal of Clinical Nutrition* 42: 1017–1022.

Deurenberg. P., Weststrate, J.A., and Seidell, J.C. 1991. Body mass index as a measure of body fatness: Age- and sex-specific prediction formulas. *British Journal of Nutrition* 65: 105–114.

Deurenberg, P., Yap, M., and van Staveren, W.A. 1998. Body mass index and percent body fat: A meta analysis among different ethnic groups. *International Journal of Obesity* 22: 1164-1171.

Deurenberg-Yap, M., Schmidt, G., van Staveren, W.A., Hautvast, J.G.A.J., and Deurenberg, P. 2001. Body fat measurement among Singaporean Chinese, Malays and Indians: A comparative study using a four-compartment model and different two-compartment models. *British Journal of Nutrition* 85: 491-498.

deVries, H.A. 1961. Prevention of muscular distress after exercise. *Research Quarterly* 32: 177–185.

deVries, H.A. 1962. Evaluation of static stretching procedures for improvement of flexibility. *Research Quarterly* 33: 222–229.

deVries, H.A., and Klafs, C.E. 1965. Prediction of maximal oxygen intake from submaximal tests. *Journal of Sports Medicine and Physical Fitness* 5: 207–214.

deWeijer, V.C., Gorniak, G.C., and Shamus, E. 2003. The effect of static stretch and warm-up exercise on hamstring length over the course of 24 hours. *Journal of Orthopaedic and Sports Physical Therapy* 33: 727-733.

Dewit, O., Fuller, N.J., Fewtrell, M.S., Elia, M., and Wells, J.C.K. 2000. Whole body air displacement plethysmography compared with hydrodensitometry for body composition analysis. *Archives of Disease in Childhood* 82: 159-164.

Dickinson, R.V. 1968. The specificity of flexibility. *Research Quarterly* 39: 792–793.

Disch, J., Frankiewicz, R., and Jackson, A. 1975. Construct validation of distance run tests. *Research Quarterly* 46: 169–176.

Dishman, R.K. 1994. Prescribing exercise intensity for healthy adults using perceived exertion. *Medicine & Science in Sports & Exercise* 26: 1087–1094.

Dolezal, B.A., and Potteiger, J.A. 1998. Concurrent resistance and endurance training influence basal metabolic rate in nondieting individuals. *Journal of Applied Physiology* 85: 695–700.

Donahue, B., Turner, D., and Worrell, T. 1994. The use of functional reach as a measurement of balance in boys and girls without disabilities ages 5 to 15 years. *Pediatric Physical Therapy* 6: 189-193.

Donahue, C.P., Lin, D.H., Kirschenbaum, D.S., and Keesey, R.E. 1984. Metabolic consequence of dieting and exercise in the treatment of obesity. *Journal of Counseling and Clinical Psychology* 52: 827–836.

Donnelly, J.R., Brown, T.E., Israel, R.G., Smith-Sintek, S., O'Brien, K.F., and Caslavka, B. 1988. Hydrostatic weighing without head submersion: Description of a method. *Medicine & Science in Sports & Exercise* 20: 66–69.

Dons, B., Bollerup, K., Bonde-Petersen, F., and Hancke, S. 1979. The effect of weight-lifting exercise related to muscle fiber composition and muscle cross-sectional area in humans. *European Journal of Applied Physiology* 40: 95–106.

Dorigatti, F., Bonzo, E., Zanier, A., and Palatini, P. 2007. Validation of Heine Gamma G7 (G5) and XXL-LF aneroid devices for blood pressure measurement. *Blood Pressure Monitoring* 12(1): 29-33.

Downs, D.S. 2006. Understanding exercise intention in an ethnically diverse sample of postpartum women. *Journal of Sport and Exercise Psychology* 28: 159-180.

Dubin, D. 2000. *Rapid interpretation of EKGs: An interactive course*, 6th ed. Tampa: Cover.

Ducimetier, P., Richard, J., and Cambien, F. 1989. The pattern of subcutaneous fat distribution in middle-aged men and the risk of coronary heart disease: The Paris prospective study. *International Journal of Obesity* 10: 229–240.

Dudley, G.A., and Fleck, S.J. 1987. Strength and endurance training: Are they mutually exclusive? *Sports Medicine* 4: 79–85.

Dunbar, C., and Saul, B. 2009. *ECG interpretation for the clinical exercise physiologist*. Philadelphia: Lippincott, Williams, and Wilkins.

Dunbar, C.C., Robertson, R.J., Baun, R., Blandin, M.F., Metz, K., Burdett, R., and Goss, F.L. 1992. The validity of regulating exercise intensity by ratings of perceived exertion. *Medicine & Science in Sports & Exercise* 24: 94–99.

Duncan, P.W., Studenski, S., Chandler, J., and Prescott, B. 1992. Functional reach: Predictive validity in a sample of elderly male veterans. *Journal of Gerontology* 47(3): M93-M98.

Duncan, P.W., Weiner, D.K., Chandler, J., and Studenski, S. 1990. Functional reach: A new clinical measure of balance. *Journal of Gerontology* 45: M192-M197.

Dunn, A.L., Marcus, B.H., Kampert, J.B., Garcia, M.E., Kohl, H.W. III, and Blair, S.N. 1999. Project Active—A 24-month randomized trial to compare lifestyle and structured physical activity interventions. *Journal of the American Medical Association* 281: 327-334.

Durstine J.L., Grandjean, P.W., Cox, C.A., and Thompson, P.D. 2002. Lipids, lipoproteins, and exercise. *Journal of Cardiopulmonary Rehabilitation* 22: 385-398.

Ebbeling, C., Ward, A., Puleo, E., Widrick, J., and Rippe, J. 1991. Development of a single-stage submaximal treadmill walking test. *Medicine & Science in Sports & Exercise* 23: 966–973.

Eckert, S., and Horstkotte, D. 2002. Comparison of Portapres non-invasive blood pressure measurement in the finger with intra-aortic pressure measurement during incremental bicycle exercise. *Blood Pressure Monitoring* 7: 179-183.

Edgerton, V.R. 1970. Morphology and histochemistry of the soleus muscle from normal and exercised rats. *American Journal of Anatomy* 127: 81–88.

Edgerton, V.R. 1973. Exercise and the growth and development of muscle tissue. In *Physical activity, human growth and development,* ed. G.L. Rarick, 1–31. New York: Academic Press.

Edwards, D.A., Hammond, W.H., Healy, M.J., Tanner, J.M., and Whitehouse, R.H. 1955. Design and accuracy of calipers for measuring subcutaneous tissue thickness. *British Journal of Nutrition* 9: 133–143.

Eickhoff-Shemek, J., and Herbert, D.L. 2007. Is licensure in your future?: Issues to consider—part 1. *ACSM's Health & Fitness Journal* 11(5): 35-37.

Eickhoff-Shemek, J., and Herbert, D.L. 2008a. Is licensure in your future?: Issues to consider—part 2. *ACSM's Health & Fitness Journal* 12 (1): 36-38.

Eickhoff-Shemek, J., and Herbert, D.L. 2008b. Is licensure in your future?: Issues to consider—part 3. *ACSM's Health & Fitness Journal* 12 (3): 36-38.

El Feghali, R.N., Topouchian, J.A., Pannier, B.M., El Assaad, H.A., and Asmar, R.G. 2007. Validation of the OMRON M7 (HEM-780-E) blood pressure measuring device in a population requiring large cuff use according to the International Protocol of the European Society of Hypertension. *Blood Pressure Monitoring* 12(3): 173-178.

Elia, M., Parkinson, S.A., and Diaz, E. 1990. Evaluation of near infra-red interactance as a method for predicting body composition. *European Journal of Clinical Nutrition* 44: 113–121.

Elliott, W.J., Young, P.E., DeVivo, L., Feldstein, J., and Black, H.R. 2007. A comparison of two sphymomanometers that may replace the traditional mercury column in the healthcare workplace. *Blood Pressure Monitoring* 12(1): 23-28.

Ellis, K.J., Bell, S.J., Chertow, G.M., Chumlea, W.C., Knox, T.A., Kotler, D.P., Lukaski, H.C., and Schoeller, D.A. 1999. Bioelectrical impedance methods in clinical research: A follow-up to the NIH technology assessment conference. *Nutrition* 15: 874-880.

Elsen, R., Siu, M.L., Pineda, O., and Solomons, N.W. 1987. Sources of variability in bioelectrical impedance determinations in adults. In *In vivo body composition studies,* ed. K.J. Ellis, S. Yasamura, and W.D. Morgan, 184–188. London: Institute of Physical Sciences in Medicine.

Emery, C.A. 2003. Is there a clinical standing balance measurement appropriate for use in sports medicine? A review of the literature. *Journal of Science and Medicine in Sport* 6: 492-504.

Emery, C.A., Cassidy, J.D., Klassen, T.P., Rosychuk, R.J., and Rowe, B.H. 2005. Development of a clinical static and dynamic standing balance measurement tool appropriate for use in adolescents. *Physical Therapy* 85(6): 502-514.

Enwemeka, C.S. 1986. Radiographic verification of knee goniometry. *Scandinavian Journal of Rehabilitation Medicine* 18: 47–49.

Epstein, L.H., Beecher, M.D., Graf, J.L., and Roemmich, J.L. 2007. Choice of interactive dance and bicycle games in overweight and non-overweight youth. *Annals of Behavioral Medicine* 33: 124-131.

Esmark, B., Andersen, J.L., Olsen, S., Richter, E.A., Mizuno, M., and Kjaer, M. 2001. Timing of postexercise protein intake is important for muscle hypertrophy with resistance training in elderly humans. *Journal of Physiology,* 535:301-311.

Etnyre, B.R., and Abraham, L.D. 1986. H-reflex changes during static stretching and two variations of proprioceptive neuromuscular facilitation techniques. *Electroencephalography and Clinical Neurophysiology* 63: 174-179.

Ettinger, B., Genault, H.K., and Cann, C.E. 1987. Postmenopausal bone loss is prevented by treatment with low-dosage estrogen with calcium. *Annals of Internal Medicine* 106: 40–45.

Evans, E.M., Rowe, D.A., Misic, M.M., Prior, B.M., and Arngrimsson, S.A. 2005. Skinfold prediction equation for athletes developed using a four-component model. *Medicine & Science in Sports & Exercise* 37: 2006-2011.

Evans, W., and Rosenberg, I. 1992. *Biomarkers.* New York: Simon & Schuster.

Fagard, R.H. 1999. Physical activity in the prevention and treatment of hypertension in the obese. *Medicine & Science in Sports & Exercise* 31(Suppl.): S624–S630.

Fahey, T.D., Rolph, R., Moungmee, P., Nagel, J., and Mortara, S. 1976. Serum testosterone, body composition, and strength of young adults. *Medicine and Science in Sports* 8: 31–34.

Faigenbaum, A.D. 2003. Youth resistance training. *President's Council on Physical Fitness and Sports Research Digest,* September: 1-8.

Faigenbaum, A.D., Milliken, L.A., and Westcott, W.L. 2003. Maximal strength testing in healthy children. *Journal of Strength and Conditioning Research* 17: 162-166.

Faigenbaum, A.D., Westcott, W.L., Loud, R.L., and Long, C. 1999. The effects of different resistance training protocols on muscular strength and endurance development in children. *Pediatrics* 104(1): e5.

Feigenbaum, M.S., and Pollock, M.L. 1999. Prescription of resistance training for health and disease. *Medicine & Science in Sports & Exercise* 31: 38–45.

Feland, J.B., Myrer, J.W., Schulthies, S.S., Fellingham, G.W., and Measom, G.W. 2001. The effect of duration of stretching of the hamstring muscle group for increasing range of motion in people aged 65 years or older. *Physical Therapy* 81: 1110-1117.

Fenstermaker, K., Plowman, S., and Looney, M. 1992. Validation of the Rockport walking test in females 65 years and older. *Research Quarterly for Exercise and Sport* 63: 322–327.

Ferber, R., Osternig, L., and Gravelle, D. 2002. Effect of PNF stretch techniques on knee flexor muscle EMG activity in older adults. *Journal of Electromyography and Kinesiology* 12: 391-397.

Ferland, M., Despres, J.P., Tremblay, A., Pinault, S., Nadeau, A., Moorjani, S., Lupien, P.J., Theriault, G., and Bouchard, C. 1989. Assessment of adipose distribution by computed axial tomography in obese women: Association with body density and anthropometric measurements. *British Journal of Nutrition* 61: 139-148.

Fess, E.E. 1992. Grip Strength. In *Clinical assessment recommendations,* American Society of Hand Therapists, 41–45, Chicago, IL: American Society of Hand Therapists.

Fiatarone, M.A., Marks, E.C., Ryan, N.D., Meredith, C.N., Lipsitz, L.A., and Evans, W.J. 1991. High-intensity strength training in nonagenarians. Effects on skeletal muscle. *Journal of the American Medical Association* 263: 3029–3034.

Fields, D.A., and Goran, M.I. 2000. Body composition techniques and the four-compartment model in children. *Journal of Applied Physiology* 89: 6113-620.

Fields, D.A., Goran, M.I., and McCrory, M.A. 2002. Body-composition assessment via air-displacement plethysmography in adults and children: A review. *American Journal of Clinical Nutrition* 75: 453-467.

Fields, D.A., Hunter, G.R., and Goran, M.I. 2000. Validation of the Bod Pod with hydrostatic weighing: Influence of body clothing. *International Journal of Obesity* 24: 200-205.

Fields, D.A., Wilson, G.D., Gladden, L.B., Hunter, G.R., Pascoe, D.D., and Goran, M.I. 2001. Comparison of the Bod Pod with the four-compartment model in adult females. *Medicine & Science in Sports & Exercise* 33: 1605-1610.

Fitness Canada. 1986. *Canadian standardized test of fitness (CSTF) operations manual,* 3rd ed., Ottawa, ON: Fitness and Amateur Sport Canada.

Fleck, S.J. 1999. Periodized strength training: A critical review. *Journal of Strength and Conditioning Research* 13(1): 82–89.

Fleck, S.J., and Falkel, J.E. 1986. Value of resistance training for the reduction of sports injuries. *Sports Medicine* 3: 61–68.

Fleck, S.J., and Kraemer, W.J. 2004. *Designing resistance training programs.* 3rd ed. Champaign, IL: Human Kinetics.

Flegal, K.M., Carroll, M.D., Ogden, C.L., and Johnson, C.L. 2002. Prevalence and trends in obesity among U.S. adults, 1999-2000. *Journal of the American Medical Association* 288(14): 1723-1727.

Flegal, K.M., Shepherd, J.A., Looker, A.C., Graubard, B.I., Borrud, L.G., Ogden, C.L., Harris, T.B., Everhart, J.E., and Schenker, N. 2009. Comparisons of percentage body fat, body mass index, waist circumference, and waist-stature ratio in adults. *American Journal of Clinical Nutrition* 89: 500-508.

FMpulse. 2004. Standards sought for personal trainers. *Fitness Management* 20(6): 16.

Fogelholm, G.M., Sievanan, H.T., Kukkonen-Harjula, K. Oja, P. and Vuori, I. 1993. Effects of a meal and its electrolytes on bioelectrical impedance. In *Human body composition: In vivo methods, models and assessment*, ed. K.J. Ellis and J.D. Eastman, 331-332. New York: Plenum Press.

Fogg, B.J. 2003. *Persuasive technology: Using computers to change what we think and do.* New York: Morgan Kaufmann.

Fogg, B.J., and Eckles, D., eds. 2007. *Mobile persuasion: 20 perspectives on the future of behavior change.* Palo Alto, CA: Stanford University.

Fohlin, L. 1977. Body composition, cardiovascular and renal function in adolescent patients with anorexia nervosa. *Acta Paediatrica Scandinavica* 268(Suppl.): 7–20.

Forbes, G.B. 1976. Adult decline in the lean body mass. *Human Biology* 48: 151–173.

Fornetti, W.C., Pivarnik, J.M., Foley, J.M., and Fiechtner, J.J. 1999. Reliability and validity of body composition measures in female athletes. *Journal of Applied Physiology* 87: 1114-1122.

Foster, C., Jackson, A.S., Pollock, M.L., Taylor, M.M., Hare, J., Sennett, S.M., Rod, J.L., Sarwar, M., and Schmidt, D.H. 1984. Generalized equations for predicting functional capacity from treadmill performance. *American Heart Journal* 107: 1229–1234.

Foster, C., Pollock, M.L., Rod, J.L., Dymond, D.S., Wible, G., and Schmidt, D.H. 1983. Evaluation of functional capacity during exercise radionuclide angiography. *Cardiology* 70: 85–93.

Foster, G.D., Wyatt, H.R., Hill, J.O., McGuckin, B.G., Brill, C., Selma Mohammed, B., Szapary, P.O., Rader, D.J., Edman, J.S., and Klien, S. 2003. A randomized trial of a low-carbohydrate diet for obesity. *New England Journal of Medicine* 348: 2082-2090.

Foster-Powell, K., and Miller, J. 1995. International tables of glycemic index. *American Journal of Clinical Nutrition* 62: 871S–893S.

Fowles, J.R., Sale, D.G., and MacDougall, J.D. 2000. Reduced strength after passive stretch of the human plantar flexors. *Journal of Applied Physiology* 89: 1179-1188.

Fox, E.L. 1973. A simple, accurate technique for predicting maximal aerobic power. *Journal of Applied Physiology* 35: 914–916.

Franchignoni, F., Tesio, L., Martino, M.T., and Ricupero, C. 1998. Reliability of four simple, quantitative tests of balance and mobility in healthy elderly females. *Aging* 10(1): 26-31.

Francis, P.R., Kolkhorst, F.W., Pennuci, M., Pozos, R.S., and Buono, M.J. 2001. An electromyographic approach to the evaluation of abdominal exercises. *ACSM's Health & Fitness Journal* 5(4): 8-14.

Friden, J. 2002. Delayed onset muscle soreness. *Scandinavian Journal of Medicine and Science in Sports* 12: 327-328.

Friden, J., Sjostrom, M., and Ekblom, B. 1983. Myofibrillar damage following intense eccentric exercise in man. *International Journal of Sports Medicine* 4: 170–176.

Friedl, K.E., DeLuca, J.P., Marchitelli, L.J., and Vogel, J.A. 1992. Reliability of body-fat estimations from a four-compartment model by using density, body water, and bone mineral measurements. *American Journal of Clinical Nutrition* 55: 764-770.

Frisancho, A.R. 1984. New standard of weight and body composition by frame size and height for assessment of nutritional status of adults and the elderly. *American Journal of Clinical Nutrition* 40: 808–819.

Frontera, W.R., Meredith, C.N., O'Reilly, K.P., Knuttgen, H.G., and Evans, W.J. 1988. Strength conditioning in older men: Skeletal muscle hypertrophy and improved function. *Journal of Applied Physiology* 64: 1038–1044.

Fuller, N.J., Sawyer, M.B., and Elia, M. 1994. Comparative evaluation of body composition methods and predictions, and calculation of density and hydration fraction of fat-free mass, in obese women. *International Journal of Obesity* 18: 503-512.

Gajdosik, R.L., Vander Linden, D.W., and Williams, A.K. 1999. Influence of age on length and passive elastic stiffness characteristics of the calf muscle-tendon unit of women. *Physical Therapy* 79: 827–838.

Gallagher, D., Visser, M., Sepulveda, D., Pierson, R.N., Harris, T., and Heymsfield, S.B. 1996. How useful is body mass index for comparison of body fatness across age, sex, and ethnic groups? *American Journal of Epidemiology* 143: 228-239.

Gallagher, M.R., Walker, K.Z., and O'Dea, K. 1998. The influence of a breakfast meal on the assessment of body composition using bioelectrical impedance. *European Journal of Clinical Nutrition* 52: 94-97.

Gellish, R.L., Goslin, B.R., Olson, R.E., McDonald, A., Russi, G.D., and Moudgil, V.K. 2007. Longitudinal modeling of the relationship between age and maximal heart rate. *Medicine & Science in Sports & Exercise* 39: 822-829.

Genton, L., Hans, D., Kyle, U.G., and Pichard, C. 2002. Dual-energy X-ray absorptiometry and body composition: Differences between devices and comparison with reference methods. *Nutrition* 18: 66-70.

Genton, L., Karsegard, V.L., Kyle, U.G., Hans, D.B., Michel, J.P., and Pichard, C. 2001. Comparison of four bioelectrical impedance analysis formulas in healthy elderly subjects. *Gerontology* 47: 315-323.

George, J., Vehrs, P., Allsen, P., Fellingham, G., and Fisher, G. 1993. VO_2max estimation from a submaximal 1-mile track jog for fit college-age individuals. *Medicine & Science in Sports & Exercise* 25: 401–406.

Gettman, L.R., Ayres, J.J., Pollock, M.L., and Jackson, A. 1978. The effect of circuit weight training on strength, cardio-respiratory function, and body composition of adult men. *Medicine and Science in Sports* 10: 171–176.

Gettman, L.R., and Pollock, M.L. 1981. Circuit weight training: A critical review of its physiological benefits. *The Physician and Sportsmedicine* 9: 44–60.

Gibbons, R.J., Balady, G.J., Bricker, J.T., Chaitman, B.R., Fletcher, G.F., Froelicher, V.F., Mark, D.B., McCallister, B.D., Mooss, A.N., O'Reilly, M.G., and Winters, W.L. Jr. 2002. ACC/AHA 2002 guideline update for exercise testing: A report of the American College of Cardiology/American Heart Association Task Force on Practice Guidelines (Committee on Exercise Testing). www.acc.org/clinical/guidelines/exercise/dirIndex.htm.

Gibson, A., Heyward, V., and Mermier, C. 2000. Predictive accuracy of Omron Body Logic Analyzer in estimating relative body fat of adults. *International Journal of Sport Nutrition and Exercise Metabolism* 10: 216–227.

Gibson, A.L., Holmes, J.C., Desautels, R.L., Edmonds, L.B., and Nuudi, L. 2008. Ability of new octapolar bioimpedance spectroscopy analyzers to predict 4-component-model percentage body fat in Hispanic, black, and white adults. *American Journal of Clinical Nutrition* 87: 332-338.

Gillman, M.W. 2008. The first months of life: A critical period for development of obesity. *American Journal of Clinical Nutrition* 87: 1587-1589.

Girouard, C.K., and Hurley, B.F. 1995. Does strength training inhibit gains in range of motion from flexibility training in older adults? *Medicine & Science in Sports & Exercise* 27: 1444–1449.

Gledhill, N., and Jamnik, R. 1995. Determining power outputs for cycle ergometers with different sized flywheels. *Medicine & Science in Sports & Exercise* 27: 134–135.

Gleichauf, C.N., and Rose, D.A. 1989. The menstrual cycle's effect on the reliability of bioimpedance measurements for assessing body composition. *American Journal of Clinical Nutrition* 50: 903–907.

Goldberg, A., Etlinger, J., Goldspink, D., and Jablecki, C. 1975. Mechanism of work-induced hypertrophy of skeletal muscle. *Medicine and Science in Sports* 7: 185–198.

Goldenberg, L., and Twist, P. 2007. *Strength ball training.* Champaign, IL: Human Kinetics.

Golding, L. 2000. *The Y's way to physical fitness.* Champaign, IL: Human Kinetics.

Gonyea, W.J., Ericson, G.C., and Bonde-Petersen, F. 1977. Skeletal muscle fiber splitting induced by weight-lifting exercise in cats. *Acta Physiologica Scandinavica* 99: 105–109.

Goran, M.I., Allison, D.B., and Poehlman, E.T. 1995. Issues relating to normalization of body fat content in men and women. *International Journal of Obesity* 19: 638-643.

Goran, M.I., Toth, M.J., and Poehlman, E.T. 1998. Assessment of research-based body composition techniques in healthy elderly men and women using the 4-component model as a criterion method. *International Journal of Obesity* 22: 135-142.

Gordon, D.J., Probstfield, J.L., Garrison, R.J., Neaton, J.D., Castelli, W.P., Knoke, J.D., Jacobs, D.R., Bangdiwala, S., and Tyroler, H.A. 1989. High-density lipoprotein cholesterol and cardiovascular disease: Four prospective American studies. *Circulation* 79: 8-15.

Gordon-Larsen, P., Hou, N., Sidney, S., Sternfeld, B., Lewis, C., Jacobs Jr., D., and Popkin, B. 2009. Fifteen-year longitudinal trends in walking patterns and their impact on weight change. *American Journal of Clinical Nutrition* 89: 19-26.

Gormley, S.E., Swain, D.P., High, R., Spina, R.J., Dowling, E.A., Kotipalli, U.S., and Gandrakota, R. 2008. Effect of intensity of aerobic training on VO$_2$max. *Medicine & Science in Sports & Exercise* 40: 1336-1343.

Goto, K., Ishii, N., Sugihara, S., Yoshioka, T., and Takamatsu, K. 2007. Effects of resistance exercise on lipolysis during subsequent submaximal exercise. *Medicine & Science in Sports & Exercise* 39: 308-315.

Graves, J.D., Webb, M., Pollock, M.L., Matkozich, J., Leggett, S.H., Carpenter, D.M., Foster, D.N., and Cirulli, J. 1994. Pelvic stabilization during resistance training: Its effect on the development of lumbar extension strength. *Archives of Physical Medicine and Rehabilitation* 75: 211-215.

Graves, J.E., Pollock, M.L., Colvin, A.B., Van Loan, M., and Lohman, T.G. 1989. Comparison of different bioelectrical impedance analyzers in the prediction of body composition. *American Journal of Human Biology* 1: 603–611.

Graves, L., Stratton, G., Ridgers, N.D., and Cable, N.T. 2007. Comparison of energy expenditure in adolescents when playing new generation and sedentary computer games: Cross-sectional study. *British Medical Journal* 335: 1282-1284.

Graves, L.E.F., Ridgers, N.D., and Stratton, G. 2008. The contribution of upper limb and total body movement to adolescents' energy expenditure whilst playing Nintendo Wii. *European Journal of Applied Physiology* 104: 617-623.

Gray, D.S., Bray, G.A., Gemayel, N., and Kaplan, K. 1989. Effect of obesity on bioelectrical impedance. *American Journal of Clinical Nutrition* 50: 255–260.

Greene, W.B., and Heckman, J.D. 1994. *The clinical measurement of joint motion.* Rosemont, IL: American Academy of Orthopaedic Surgeons.

Grembowski, D., Patrick, D., Diehr, P., Durham, M., Beresford, S., Kay, E., and Hecht, J. 1993. Self-efficacy and health behavior among older adults. *Journal of Health and Social Behavior* 34(6): 89–104.

Grenier, S.G., Russell, C., and McGill, S.M. 2003. Relationships between lumbar flexibility, sit-and-reach test, and a previous history of low back discomfort in industrial workers. *Canadian Journal of Applied Physiology* 28: 165-177.

Gribble, P.A., and Hertel, J. 2003. Considerations for normalizing measures of the star excursion balance test. *Measurement in Physical Education and Exercise Science* 7: 89-100.

Grier, T.D., Lloyd, L.K., Walker, J.L., and Murray, T.D. 2002. Metabolic cost of aerobic dance bench stepping at varying cadences and bench heights. *Journal of Strength and Conditioning Research* 16: 242-249.

Griffin, S., Robergs, R., and Heyward, V. 1997. Assessment

of exercise blood pressure: A review. *Medicine & Science in Sports & Exercise* 29: 149–159.

Gruber, J.J., Pollock, M.L., Graves, J.E., Colvin, A.B., and Braith, R.W. 1990. Comparison of Harpenden and Lange calipers in predicting body composition. *Research Quarterly for Exercise and Sport* 61: 184-190.

Gudivaka, R., Schoeller, D., and Kushner, R.F. 1996. Effect of skin temperature on multifrequency bioelectrical impedance analysis. *Journal of Applied Physiology* 81: 838-845.

Guskiewicz, K.M., and Perrin, D.H. 1996. Research and clinical applications of assessing balance. *Journal of Sport Rehabilitation* 5: 45-63.

Gustavsen, P.H., Hoegholm, A., Bang, L.E., and Kristensen, K.S. 2003. White coat hypertension is a cardiovascular risk factor. A 10-year follow-up study. *Journal of Human Hypertension* 17: 811-817.

Guy, J.A., and Micheli, L.J. 2001. Strength training for children and adolescents. *Journal of the American Academy of Orthopaedic Surgeons* 9: 29-36.

Habash, D. 2002. Tactile and interpersonal techniques for fatfold anthropometry. School of Medicine. Ohio State Unversity. Unpublished paper.

Habib, Z., and Westcott, S. 1998. Assessment of anthropometric factors on balance tests in children. *Pediatric Physical Therapy* 10: 101-109.

Hagerman, F. 1993. *Concept II rowing ergometer nomogram for prediction of maximal oxygen consumption* [abstract]. Morrisville, VT: Concept II.

Han, K., Ricard, M.D., and Fellingham, G.W. 2009. Effects of a 4-week exercise program on balance using elastic tubing as a perturbation force for individuals with a history of ankle sprains. *Journal of Orthopaedic & Sports Physical Therapy* 39: 246-255.

Harris, J.A., and Benedict, F.G. 1919. *A biometric study of basal metabolism in man* (publication no. 279). Washington, D.C.: Carnegie Institute.

Harris, M.L. 1969. A factor analytic study of flexibility. *Research Quarterly* 40: 62–70.

Harrison, G.G., Buskirk, E.R., Carter, L.J.E., Johnston, F.E., Lohman, T.G., Pollock, M.L., Roche, A.F., and Wilmore, J.H. 1988. Skinfold thicknesses and measurement technique. In *Anthropometric standardization reference manual,* ed. T.G. Lohman, A.F. Roche, and R. Martorell, 55–70. Champaign, IL: Human Kinetics.

Hartley, L.H. 1975. Growth hormone and catecholamine response to exercise in relation to physical training. *Medicine and Science in Sports* 7: 34–36.

Hartley, L.H., Mason, J.W., Hogan, R.P., Jones, L.G., Kotchen, T.A., Mougey, E.H., Wherry, R., Pennington, L., and Ricketts, P. 1972. Multiple hormonal responses to graded exercise in relation to physical conditioning. *Journal of Applied Physiology* 33: 602–606.

Hartley-O'Brien, S.J. 1980. Six mobilization exercises for active range of hip flexion. *Research Quarterly for Exercise and Sport* 51: 625–635.

Harvard School of Public Health. 2004. *Food Pyramids.* www.hsph.harvard.edu/nutritionsource/pyramids.html.

Haskell, W.L., Lee, I.M., Pate, R.R., Powell, K.E., Blair, S.N., Franklin, B.A., Macera, C.A., Heath, G.W., Thompson, P.D., and Bauman, A. 2007. Physical activity and public health: Updated recommendation for adults from the American College of Sports Medicine and the American Heart Association. *Medicine & Science in Sports & Exercise* 39(8): 1423-1434.

Hass, C.J., Garzarella, L., De Hoyas, D., and Pollock, M. 2000. Single versus multiple sets in long-term recreational weightlifters. *Medicine & Science in Sports & Exercise* 32: 235–242.

Hasson, R.E., Haller, J., Pober, D.M., Staudenmayer, J., and Freedson, P.S. 2009. Validity of the Omron HJ-112 pedometer during treadmill walking. *Medicine & Science in Sports & Exercise* 41: 805-809.

Hather, B.M., Tesch, P.A., Buchanan, P., and Dudley, G.A. 1991. Influence of eccentric actions on skeletal muscle adaptations to resistance training. *Acta Physiologica Scandinavica* 143: 177–185.

Hawk, C., Hyland, J.K., Rupert, R., Colonvega, M., and Hall, S. 2006. Assessment of balance and risk for falls in a sample of community-dwelling adults aged 65 and older. *Chiropractic & Osteology* 14: 3-10.

Hawkins, M.N., Raven, P.B., Snell, P.G., Stray-Gundersen, J., and Levine, B.D. 2007. Maximal oxygen uptake as a parametric measure of cardiorespiratory capacity. *Medicine & Science in Sports & Exercise* 39: 103-107.

Hayes, A., and Cribb, P.J. 2008. Effect of whey protein isolate on strength, body composition, and muscle hypertrophy during resistance training. *Current Opinion in Clinical Nutrition and Metabolic Care* 11: 40-44.

Hayes, P.A., Sowood, P.J., Belyavin, A., Cohen, J.B., and Smith, F.W. 1988. Sub-cutaneous fat thickness measured by magnetic resonance imaging, ultrasound, and calipers. *Medicine & Science in Sports & Exercise* 20: 303–309.

Health Canada. 2003. *Canada's physical activity guide to healthy active living.* Version 9. www.hc-sc.ca/english/lifestyles/index.html.

Hedley, A.A., Ogden, C.L., Johnson, C.L., Carroll, M.D., Curtin, L.R., and Flegal, K.M. 2004. Prevalence of overweight and obesity among U.S. children, adolescents, and adults, 1999-2002. *Journal of the American Medical Association* 291(23): 2847-2850.

Heil, D.P. 1997. Body mass scaling of peak oxygen uptake in 20- to 79-year-old adults. *Medicine & Science in Sports & Exercise* 29: 1602-1608.

Heitmann, B.L., Kondrup, J., Engelhart, M., Kristensen, J.H., Podenphant, J., Hoie, L.H., and Andersen, V. 1994. Changes in fat free mass in overweight patients with rheumatoid arthritis on a weight reducing regimen. A comparison of eight different body composition methods. *International Journal of Obesity* 18: 812-819.

Helgerud, J., Hoydal, K., Wang, E., Karlsen, T., Berg, P., Bjerkaas, M., Simonsen, T., Helgesen, C., Hjorth, N., Bach,

R., and Hoff, J. 2007. Aerobic high-intensity intervals improve VO$_2$ max more than moderate training. *Medicine & Science in Sports & Exercise* 39: 665-671.

Henwood, T.R., and Taaffe, D.R. 2003. Beneficial effects of high-velocity resistance training in older adults. *Medicine & Science in Sports & Exercise* 35 (Suppl.): S292 [abstract].

Herbert, D.L. 1995. First state licenses exercise physiologists. *Fitness Management,* October, 26–27.

Herbert, D.L. 2004. New law to regulate personal trainers proposed in Oregon. *The Exercise Standards and Malpractice Reporter* 18(2): 17, 20-24.

Herbert, R.D., and de Noronha, M. 2007. Stretching to prevent or reduce muscle soreness after exercise. *Cochrane Database of Systematic Reviews,* Issue 4, CD004577. DOI: 10.1002/14651858.CD004577.pub2.

Herbert, R.D., and Gabriel, M. 2002. Effects of stretching on muscle soreness and risk of injury: A meta-analysis. *British Medical Journal* 325: 468-471.

Hermansen, L., and Saltin, B. 1969. Oxygen uptake during maximal treadmill and bicycle exercise. *Journal of Applied Physiology* 26: 31–37.

Hertel, J., Braham, R.A., Hale, S.A., and Olmsted-Kramer, L.C. 2006. Simplifying the star excursion balance test: Analyses of subjects with and without chronic ankle instability. *Journal of Orthopaedic & Sports Physical Therapy* 36: 131-137.

Hertel, J., Miller, S.J., and Denegar, C.R. 2000. Intratester and intertester reliability during the star excursion balance tests. *Journal of Sport Rehabilitation* 9: 104-116.

Hess, J.A., and Woollacott, M. 2005. Effect of high-intensity strength-training on functional measures of balance ability in balance-impaired older adults. *Journal of Manipulative and Physiological Therapeutics* 28: 582-590.

Hettinger, T., and Muller, E.A. 1953. Muskelleistung und muskeltraining. *European Journal of Applied Physiology* 15: 111–126.

Heymsfield, S.B., Wang, J., Lichtman, S., Kamen, Y., Kehayias, J., and Pierson, R.N. 1989. Body composition in elderly subjects: A critical appraisal of clinical methodology. *American Journal of Clinical Nutrition* 50: 1167–1175.

Heyward, V.H., Cook, K.L., Hicks, V.L., Jenkins, K.A., Quatrochi, J.A., and Wilson, W. 1992. Predictive accuracy of three field methods for estimating relative body fatness of nonobese and obese women. *International Journal of Sport Nutrition* 2: 75–86.

Heyward, V.H., and Wagner, D.R. 2004. *Applied body composition assessment,* 2nd ed. Champaign, IL: Human Kinetics.

Hickson, R.C., and Rosenkoetter, M.A. 1981. Reduced training frequencies and maintenance of increased aerobic power. *Medicine & Science in Sports & Exercise* 13: 13–16.

Higgins, P.B., Fields, D.A., Hunter, G.R., and Gower, B.A. 2001. Effect of scalp and facial hair on air displacement plethysmography estimates of percentage of body fat. *Obesity Research* 9: 326-330.

Hill, J.O., and Melanson, E.L. 1999. Overview of the determinants of overweight and obesity: Current evidence and research issues. *Medicine & Science in Sports & Exercise* 31(Suppl.): S515–S521.

Hill, K., Smith, R., Fearn, M., Rydberg, M., and Oliphant, R. 2007. Physical and psychological outcomes of a supported physical activity program for older carers. *Journal of Aging and Physical Activity* 15: 257-271.

Himes, J.H., and Frisancho, R.A. 1988. Estimating frame size. In *Anthropometric standardization reference manual,* ed. T.G. Lohman, A.F. Roche, and R. Martorell, 121-124. Champaign, IL: Human Kinetics.

Hirsh, J. 1971. Adipose cellularity in relation to human obesity. *Advances in Internal Medicine* 17: 289–300.

Hoeger, W.W.K. 1989. *Lifetime physical fitness and wellness.* Englewood Cliffs, NJ: Morton.

Hoeger, W.W.K., and Hopkins, D.R. 1992. A comparison of the sit-and-reach and the modified sit-and-reach in the measurement of flexibility in women. *Research Quarterly for Exercise and Sport* 63: 191–195.

Hoeger, W.W.K., Hopkins, D.R., Button, S., and Palmer, T.A. 1990. Comparing the sit and reach with the modified sit and reach in measuring flexibility in adolescents. *Pediatric Exercise Science* 2: 156–162.

Hoffman, M., and Payne, V.G. 1995. The effects of proprioceptive ankle disk training on healthy subjects. *Journal of Orthopaedic & Sports Physical Therapy* 21: 90-93.

Holbrook, E.A., Barreira, T.V., and Kang, M. 2009. Validity and reliability of Omron pedometers for prescribed and self-paced walking. *Medicine & Science in Sports & Exercise* 41: 670-674.

Holt, L.E., Travis, T.M., and Okita, T. 1970. Comparative study of three stretching techniques. *Perceptual and Motor Skills* 31: 611-616.

Houtkooper, L.B., Going, S.G., Lohman, T.G., Roche, A.F., and VanLoan, M. 1992. Bioelectrical impedance estimation of fat-free body mass in children and youth: A cross-validation study. *Journal of Applied Physiology* 72: 366-373.

Houtkooper, L.B., Going, S.B., Westfall, C.H., Lohman, T.G. 1989. Prediction of fat-free body corrected for bone mass from impedance and anthropometry in adult females. *Medicine & Science in Sports & Exercise* 21: 539 [abstract].

Howatson, G., and van Someren, K.A. 2008. The prevention and treatment of exercise-induced muscle damage. *Sports Medicine* 38: 483-503.

Howe, T.E., Rochester, L., Jackson, A., and Blair, V.A. 2007. Exercise for improving balance in older people (review). *Cochrane Database Systematic Reviews,* Issue 4, CD004963.

Howley, E.T. 2007. VO$_2$max and the plateau—needed or not? *Medicine & Science in Sports & Exercise* 39: 101-102.

Howley, E. 2008. Physical activity guidelines for Americans. *President's Council on Physical Fitness and Sports Research Digest Series* 9(4), December.

Howley, E.T., Colacino, D.L., and Swensen, T.C. 1992. Factors affecting the oxygen cost of stepping on an electronic stepping ergometer. *Medicine & Science in Sports & Exercise* 24: 1055–1058.

Hsieh, S.D., Yoshinaga, H., and Muto, T. 2003. Waist-to-height ratio, a simple and practical index for assessing central fat distribution and metabolic risk in Japanese men and women. *International Journal of Obesity* 27: 610-616.

Hubley-Kozey, C.L. 1991. Testing flexibility. In *Physiological testing of the high-performance athlete*, ed. J.D. MacDougall, H.A. Wenger, and H.J. Green, 309–359. Champaign, IL: Human Kinetics.

Hudson, J., Hiripi, E., Pope, H., and Kessler, R. 2007. The prevalence and correlates of eating disorders in the National Comorbidity Survey Replication .*Biological Psychiatry* 61(3): 348-358.

Hui, S.C., and Yuen, P.Y. 2000. Validity of the modified back-saver sit-and-reach test: A comparison with other protocols. *Medicine & Science in Sports & Exercise* 32: 1655–1659.

Hui, S.C., Yuen, P.Y., Morrow, J.R., and Jackson, A.W. 1999. Comparison of the criterion-related validity of sit-and-reach tests with and without limb length adjustment in Asian adults. *Research Quarterly for Exercise and Sport* 70: 401–406.

Hultborn, H., Illert, M., and Santini, M. 1974. Disynaptic inhibition of the interneurons mediating the reciprocal Ia inhibition of motor neurones. *Acta Physiologica Scandinavica* 91: 14A-16A.

Human Kinetics. 1995. *Practical body composition kit*. Champaign, IL: Author.

Human Kinetics. 1999. *Assessing body composition*. Champaign, IL: Author.

Hunter, G.R., Wetzstein, C.J., McLafferty, C.L., Zuckerman, P.A., Landers, K.A., and Bamman, M.M. 2001. High-resistance versus variable-resistance training in older adults. *Medicine & Science in Sports & Exercise* 33: 1759-1764.

Idema, R.N., van den Meiracker, A.H., and Imholz, B.P.M. 1989. Comparison of Finapres non-invasive beat-to-beat finger blood pressure with intrabrachial artery pressure during and after bicycle ergometry. *Journal of Hypertension* 7 (Suppl. 6): S58-S59.

Ikai, M., and Fukunaga, T. 1968. Calculation of muscle strength per unit cross-sectional area of human muscle by means of ultrasonic measurement. *European Journal of Applied Physiology* 26: 26–32.

Institute of Medicine. 2002. *Dietary reference intakes for energy, carbohydrates, fiber, fat, fatty acids, cholesterol, protein, and amino acids*. Washington, D.C.: National Academies Press.

International Association for the Study of Obesity. 2007. Adult overweight and obesity in the European Union (EU25). www.iaso.org.

International Association for the Study of Obesity. 2007. Overweight in children in the European Union. www.iaso.org.

International Dance and Exercise Association. 2004. Personal fitness trainer certification. *IDEA Health & Fitness Source,* March: 15.

International Osteoporosis Foundation. 2009a. Epidemiology. www.iofbonehealth.org/health-professionals/about-osteoporosis/epidemiology.

International Osteoporosis Foundation. 2009b. FRAX® tool now available for use in 12 countries. www.iofbonehealth.org/news/news-detail.html?newsID=254.

Invergo, J.J., Ball, T.E., and Looney, M. 1991. Relationship of pushups and absolute muscular endurance to bench press strength. *Journal of Applied Sport Science Research* 5: 121–125.

Irving, B.A., Davis, C.K., Brock, D.W., Weltman, J.Y., Swift, D., Barrett, E.J., Gaesser, G.A., and Weltman, A. 2008. Effect of exercise training intensity on abdominal visceral fat and body composition. *Medicine & Science in Sports & Exercise* 40: 1863-1872.

Isacowitz, R. 2006. *Pilates*. Champaign, IL: Human Kinetics.

Jackson, A. 1984. Research design and analysis of data procedures for predicting body density. *Medicine & Science in Sports & Exercise* 16: 616–620.

Jackson, A.S., Ellis, K.J., McFarlin, B.K., Sailors, M.H., and Bray, M.S. 2009. Cross-validation of generalized body composition equations with diverse young men and women: The Training Intervention and Genetics of Exercise Response (TIGER) Study. *British Journal of Nutrition* 101: 871-878.

Jackson, A.S., and Pollock, M.L. 1976. Factor analysis and multivariate scaling of anthropometric variables for the assessment of body composition. *Medicine & Science in Sports & Exercise* 8: 196–203.

Jackson, A.S., and Pollock, M.L. 1978. Generalized equations for predicting body density of men. *British Journal of Nutrition* 40: 497–504.

Jackson, A.S., and Pollock, M.L. 1985. Practical assessment of body composition. *The Physician and Sportsmedicine* 13: 76–90.

Jackson, A.S., Pollock, M.L., Graves, J.E., and Mahar, M.T. 1988. Reliability and validity of bioelectrical impedance in determining body composition. *Journal of Applied Physiology* 64: 529–534.

Jackson, A.S., Pollock, M.L., and Ward, A. 1980. Generalized equations for predicting body density of women. *Medicine & Science in Sports & Exercise* 12: 175–182.

Jackson, A.W., and Langford, N.J. 1989. The criterion-related validity of the sit-and-reach test: Replication and extension of previous findings. *Research Quarterly for Exercise and Sport* 60: 384–387.

Jackson, A.W., Morrow, J.R., Brill, P.A., Kohl, H.W., Gordon, N.F., and Blair, S.N. 1998. Relations of sit-up and sit-and-reach tests to low back pain in adults. *Journal of Orthopaedic and Sports Physical Therapy* 27: 22–26.

Janssen, I., Heymsfield, S.B., Allison, D.B., Kotler, D.P., and Ross, R. 2002. Body mass index and waist circumference independently contribute to the prediction of nonabdominal, abdominal subcutaneous, and visceral fat. *American Journal of Clinical Nutrition* 75: 683-688.

Janssen, I., Katzmarzyk, P.T., and Ross, R. 2004. Waist circumference and not body mass index explain obesity-related health risk. *American Journal of Clinical Nutrition* 79: 379-384.

Jenkins, W.L., Thackaberry, M., and Killian, C. 1984. Speed-specific isokinetic training. *Journal of Orthopaedic and Sports Physical Therapy* 6: 181–183.

Johns, R.J., and Wright, V. 1962. Relative importance of various tissues in joint stiffness. *Journal of Applied Physiology* 17: 824–828.

Johnson, B.L., and Nelson, J.K., eds. 1986. *Practical measurements for evaluation in physical education*. Minneapolis: Burgess.

Jones, B.H., and Knapik, J.J. 1999. Physical training and exercise-related injuries. *Sports Medicine* 27: 111–125.

Jones, C.J., Rikli, R.E., Max, J., and Noffal, G. 1998. The reliability and validity of a chair sit-and-reach test as a measure of hamstring flexibility in older adults. *Research Quarterly for Exercise and Sport* 69: 338–343.

Jones, D.W., Frohlich, E.D., Grim, C.M., Grim, C.E., and Taubert, K.A. 2001. Mercury sphygmomanometers should not be abandoned: An advisory statement from the Council for High Blood Pressure Research, American Heart Association. *Hypertension* 37: 185-186.

Juker, D., McGill, S., Kropf, P., and Steffen, T. 1998. Quantitative intramuscular myoelectric activity of lumbar portions of psoas and the abdominal wall during a wide variety of tasks. *Medicine & Science in Sports & Exercise* 30: 301-310.

Kaminsky, L.A., and Whaley, M.H. 1998. Evaluation of a new standardized ramp protocol: The BSU/Bruce ramp protocol. *Journal of Cardiopulmonary Rehabilitation* 18: 438-444.

Kanis, J.A., Borgstrom, F., De Laet, C., Johansson, H., Johnell, O., Jonsson, B., Oden, A., Zethraeus, N., Pfleger, B., and Khaltaev, N. 2005. Assessment of fracture risk. *Osteoporosis International* 16: 581-589.

Katch F.I., Clarkson, P.M., Kroll, W., McBride, T., and Wilcox, A. 1984. Effects of sit-up exercise training on adipose cell size and adiposity. *Research Quarterly for Exercise and Sport* 55: 242–247.

Katch, F.I., McArdle, W.D., Czula, R., and Pechar, G.S. 1973. Maximal oxygen intake, endurance running performance, and body composition in college women. *Research Quarterly* 44: 301–312.

Kattus, A.A., Hanafee, W.N., Longmire, W.P., MacAlpin, R.N., and Rivin, A.U. 1968. Diagnosis, medical and surgical management of coronary insufficiency. *Annals of Internal Medicine* 69: 115–136.

Kay, A.D., and Blazevich, A.J. 2008. Reductions in active plantarflexor moment are significantly correlated with static stretch duration. *European Journal of Sport Science* 8: 41-46.

Keim, N.L., Blanton, C.A., and Kretsch, M.J. 2004. America's obesity epidemic: Measuring physical activity to promote an active lifestyle. *Journal of the American Dietetic Association* 104: 1398-1409.

Kelley, D.E., and Goodpaster, B.H. 1999. Effects of physical activity on insulin action and glucose tolerance in obesity. *Medicine & Science in Sports & Exercise* 31(Suppl.): S619–S623.

Kelley, G.A., and Kelley, K.S. 2006. Aerobic exercise and lipids and lipoproteins in men: A meta-analysis of randomized controlled trials. *Journal of Men's Health & Gender* 3(1): 61-70.

Kesaniemi, Y.K., Danforth, E., Jensen, M.D., Kopelman, P.G., Lefebvre, P., and Reeder, B.A. 2001. Dose-response issues concerning physical activity and health: An evidenced-based symposium. *Medicine & Science in Sports & Exercise* 33 (Suppl.): S351–S358.

Keys, A., and Brozek, J. 1953. Body fat in adult man. *Physiological Reviews* 33: 245–325.

Khaled, M.A., McCutcheon, M.J., Reddy, S., Pearman, P.L., Hunter, G.R., and Weinsier, R.L. 1988. Electrical impedance in assessing human body composition: The BIA method. *American Journal of Clinical Nutrition* 47: 789–792.

Kim, P.S., Mayhew, J.L., and Peterson, D.F. 2002. A modified bench press test as a predictor of 1 repetition maximum bench press strength. *Journal of Strength and Conditioning Research* 16: 440-445.

Kimball, S.R., and Jefferson, L.S. 2002. Control of protein synthesis by amino acid availability. *Current Opinions in Clinical Nutrition and Metabolic Care* 5: 63-67.

Kinser, A.M., Ramsey, M.W., O'Bryant, H.S., Ayres, C.A., Sands, W.A., and Stone, M.H. 2008. Vibration and stretching effects on flexibility and explosive strength in young gymnasts. *Medicine & Science in Sports & Exercise* 40: 133-140.

Kirby, R.L., Simms, F.C., Symington, V.J., and Garner, J.B. 1981. Flexibility and musculoskeletal symptomatology in female gymnasts and age-matched controls. *American Journal of Sports Medicine* 9: 160–164.

Klein, S., Allison, D.B., Heymsfield, S.B., Kelley, D.E., Leibel, R.L., Nonas, C., and Kahn, R. 2007. Waist circumference and cardiometabolic risk: A consensus statement from Shaping America's Health: Association for Weight Management and Obesity Prevention; NAASO, The Obesity Society; the American Society for Nutrition; and the American Diabetes Assocation. *American Journal of Clinical Nutrition* 85: 1197-1202.

Klein-Geltink, J.E., Choi, B.C.K., and Fry, R. 2006. Multiple exposures to smoking, alcohol, physical inactivity, and overweight: Prevalences according to the Canadian Community Health Survey Cycle 1.1. *Chronic Diseases in Canada* 27(1): 25-33.

Kline, G.M., Porcari, J.P., Hintermeister, R., Freedson, P.S., Ward, A., McCarron, R.F., Ross, J. and Rippe, J.M. 1987. Estimation of VO_2max from a one-mile track walk, gender, age, and body weight. *Medicine & Science in Sports & Exercise* 19: 253–259.

Knowler, W.C., Barrett-Conner, E., Fowler, S.E., Hamman, R.F., Lachin, J.M., Walker, E.A., and Nathan, D.M. 2002. Reduction in incidence of type 2 diabetes with lifestyle intervention or metformin. Diabetes Prevention Program Research Group. *New England Journal of Medicine* 346: 393-403.

Knudson, D. 2001. The validity of recent curl-up tests in young adults. *Journal of Strength and Conditioning Research* 15: 81-85.

Knudson, D., and Johnston, D. 1995. Validity and reliability of a bench trunk-curl test of abdominal endurance. *Journal of Strength and Conditioning Research* 9: 165-169.

Knudson, D., and Johnston, D. 1998. Analysis of three test durations of the bench trunk-curl. *Journal of Strength and Conditioning Research* 12: 150-151.

Knudson, D., and Noffal, G. 2005. Time course of stretch-induced isometric strength deficits. *European Journal of Applied Physiology* 94: 348-351.

Knudson, D.V. 1999. Issues in abdominal fitness: Testing and technique. *Journal of Physical Education, Recreation & Dance* 70(3): 49-55.

Knudson, D.V., Magnusson, P., and McHugh, M. 2000. Current issues in flexibility fitness. *President's Council on Physical Fitness and Sports Research Digest* 3(10): 1–8.

Knuttgen, H.G., and Kraemer, W.J. 1987. Terminology and measurement in exercise performance. *Journal of Applied Sport Science Research* 1: 1–10.

Knutzen, K.M., Brilla, L.R., and Caine, D. 1999. Validity of 1RM prediction equations for older adults. *Journal of Strength and Conditioning Research* 13: 242-246.

Kohrt, W.M. 1998. Preliminary evidence that DEXA provides an accurate assessment of body composition. *Journal of Applied Physiology* 84: 372-377.

Kohrt, W.M., Bloomfield, S.A., Little, K.D., Nelson, M.E., and Yingling, V.R. 2004. American College of Sports Medicine position stand: Physical activity and bone health. *Medicine & Science in Sports & Exercise* 36: 1985-1996.

Kohrt, W.M., Spina, R.J., Holloszy, J.O., and Ehsani, A.A. 1998. Prescribing exercise intensity for older women. *Journal of the American Geriatric Society* 46: 129–133.

Kokkinos, P.F., and Fernhall, B. 1999. Physical activity and high density lipoprotein cholesterol levels: What is the relationship? *Sports Medicine* 28: 307–314.

Kokkinos, P.F., Hurley, B.F., Smutok, M.A., Farmer, C., Reece, C., Shulman, R., Charabogos, C., Patterson, J., Will, S., Devane-Bell, J., and Goldberg, A.P. 1991. Strength training does not improve lipoprotein–lipid profiles in men at risk for CHD. *Medicine & Science in Sports & Exercise* 23: 1134–1139.

Komi, P.V., Viitasalo, J.T., Rauramaa, R., and Vihko, V. 1978. Effect of isometric strength training on mechanical, electrical, and metabolic aspects of muscle function. *European Journal of Applied Physiology* 40: 45–55.

Kostek, M.A., Pescatello, L.S., Seip, R.L., Angelopoulos, T.J., Clarkson, P.M., Gordon, P.M., Moyna, N.M., Visich, P.S., Zoeller, R.F., Thompson, P.D., Hoffman, R.P., and Price, T.B. 2007. Subcutaneous fat alterations resulting from an upper-body resistance training program. *Medicine & Science in Sports & Exercise* 39: 1177-1185.

Koulmann, N., Jimenez, C., Regal, D., Bolliet, P., Launay, J., Savourey, G., and Melin, B. 2000. Use of bioelectrical impedance analysis to estimate body fluid compartments after acute variations of the body hydration level. *Medicine & Science in Sports & Exercise* 32: 857-864.

Kraemer, W.J. 2003. Strength training basics. *The Physician and Sportsmedicine* 31(8): 39-45.

Kraemer, W.J., Adams, K., Cafarelli, E., Dudley, G.A., Dooly, C., Feigenbaum, M.S., Fleck, S.J., Franklin, B., Fry, A.C.,

Hoffman, J.R., Newton, R.U., Potteiger, J., Stone, M.H., Ratamess, N.A., and Triplett-McBride, T. 2002. ACSM Position Stand: Progression models in resistance training for healthy adults. *Medicine & Science in Sports & Exercise* 34: 364-380.

Kraemer, W.J., Deschenes, M.R., and Fleck, S.J. 1988. Physiological adaptations to resistance exercise: Implications for athletic conditioning. *Sports Medicine* 6: 246–256.

Kraemer, W.J., and Fleck, S.J. 2007. *Optimizing strength training.* Champaign, IL: Human Kinetics.

Kraemer, W.J., Fleck, S.J., and Evans, W.J. 1996. Strength and power training: Physiological mechanisms of adaptation. In *Exercise and Sport Sciences Reviews,* ed. J.O. Holloszy, 24: 363–397. Baltimore: Williams & Wilkins.

Kraemer, W.J., Gordon, S.J., Fleck, S.J., Marchitelli, L.J., Mello, R., Dziados, J.E., Friedl, K., Harman, E., Maresh, C., and Fry, A.C. 1991. Endogenous anabolic hormonal and growth factor responses to heavy resistance exercise in males and females. *International Journal of Sports Medicine* 12: 228–235.

Kraemer, W.J., Häkkinen, K., Newton, R.U., Nindl, B.C., Volek, J.S., McCormick, M., Gotshalk, L.A., Gordon, S.E., Fleck, S.J., Campbell, W.W., Putukian, M., and Evans, W.J. 1999. Effects of heavy-resistance training on hormonal response patterns in younger vs. older men. *Journal of Applied Physiology* 87: 982–992.

Kraemer, W.J., Nindl, B.C., Ratamess, N.A., Gotshalk, L.A., Volek, J.S., Fleck, S.J., Newton, R.U., and Hakkinen, K. 2004. Changes in muscle hypertrophy in women with periodized resistance training. *Medicine & Science in Sports & Exercise* 36: 697-708.

Kraemer, W.J., Noble, B.J., Clark, M.J., and Culver, B.W. 1987. Physiologic responses to heavy-resistance exercise with very short rest periods. *International Journal of Sports Medicine* 8: 247–252.

Kraemer, W.J., Patton, J., Gordon, S.E., Harman, E.A., Deschenes, M.R., Reynolds, K., Newton, R.U., Triplett, N.T., and Dziados, J.E. 1995. Compatibility of high intensity strength and endurance training on hormonal and skeletal muscle adaptations. *Journal of Applied Physiology* 78: 976–989.

Kraemer, W.J., and Ratamess, N.A. 2004. Fundamentals of resistance training: Progression and exercise prescription. *Medicine & Science in Sports & Exercise* 36: 674-688.

Kraemer, W.J., Volek, J.S., Clark, K.L., Gordon, S.E., Puhl, S.M., Koziris, L.P., McBride, J.M., Triplett-McBride, N.T., Putukian, M., Newton, R.U., Häkkinen, K., Bush, J.A., and Sabastianelli, W.J. 1999. Influence of exercise training on physiological and performance changes with weight loss in men. *Medicine & Science in Sports & Exercise* 31: 1320–1329.

Kravitz, L., and Heyward, V.H. 1995. Flexibility training. *Fitness Management* 11(2): 32-38.

Kravitz, L., Cizar, C., Christensen, C., and Setterlund, S. 1993. The physiological effects of step training with and without handweights. *Journal of Sports Medicine and Physical Fitness* 33: 348–358.

Kravitz, L., Heyward, V., Stolarczyk, L., and Wilmerding, V. 1997. Effects of step training with and without handweights on physiological profiles of women. *Journal of Strength and Conditioning Research* 11: 194–199.

Kravitz, L., Robergs, R., and Heyward, V. 1996. Are all aerobic exercise modes equal? *Idea Today* 14: 51–58.

Kravitz, L., Robergs, R.A., Heyward, V.H., Wagner, D.R., and Powers, K. 1997. Exercise mode and gender comparisons of energy expenditure at self-selected intensities. *Medicine & Science in Sports & Exercise* 29: 1028–1035.

Kravitz, L., Wax, B., Mayo, J.J., Daniels, R., and Charette, K. 1998. Metabolic response of elliptical exercise training. *Medicine & Science in Sports & Exercise* 30(Suppl.): S169 [abstract].

Kreider, R.B., Melton, C., Rasmussen, C.J., Greenwood, M., Lancaster, S., Cantler, E.C., Milnor, P., and Almada, A.L. 2003. Long-term creatine supplementation does not significantly affect clinical markers of health in athletes. *Molecular and Cellular Biochemistry* 244: 95-104.

Kretsch, M.J., Blanton, C.A., Baer, D., Staples, R., Horn, W.F., and Keim, N. 2004. Measuring energy expenditure with simple, low-cost tools. *Journal of the American Dietetic Association* 104: A-13.

Kriska, A.M., Blair, S.N., and Pereira, M.A. 1994. The potential role of physical activity in the prevention of non-insulin dependent diabetes mellitus: The epidemiological evidence. In *Exercise and Sport Sciences Reviews*, ed. J.O. Holloszy, 22: 121–143.

Krotkiewski, M., Gudmundsson, M., Backstrom, P., and Mandroukas, K. 1982. Zinc and muscle strength and endurance. *Acta Physiologica Scandinavica* 116: 309–311.

Kubo, K., Kaneshisa, H., Takeshita, D., Kawakami, Y., Fukashiro, S., and Fukunaga, T. 2000. In vivo dynamics of human medial gastrocnemius muscle-tendon complex curing stretch-shortening cycle exercise. *Acta Physiologica Scandinavica* 170: 127–135.

Kubo, K., Kawakami, Y., and Fukunaga, T. 1999. Influence of elastic properties of tendon structures on jump performance in humans. *Journal of Applied Physiology* 87: 2090–2096.

Kuntzelman, B.A. 1979. *The complete guide to aerobic dancing.* Skokie, IL: Publications International.

Kuramoto, A.K., and Payne, V.G. 1995. Predicting muscular strength in women: A preliminary study. *Research Quarterly for Exercise and Sport* 66: 168–172.

Kuramoto, A.M. 2006. Therapeutic benefits of tai chi exercise: Research review. *Wisconsin Medical Journal* 105(7): 42-46.

Kushner, R.F. 1992. Bioelectrical impedance analysis: A review of principles and applications. *Journal of the American College of Nutrition* 11: 199–209.

Kushner, R.F., Gudivaka, R., and Schoeller, D.A. 1996. Clinical characteristics influencing bioelectrical impedance analysis measurements. *American Journal of Clinical Nutrition* 64: 423S-427S.

Kushner, R.F., and Schoeller, D.A. 1986. Estimation of total body water in bioelectrical impedance analysis. *American Journal of Clinical Nutrition* 44: 417–424.

Kyle, U.G., Genton, L., Karsegard, L., Slosman, D.O., and Pichard, C. 2001. Single prediction equation for bioelectrical impedance analysis in adults aged 20-94 years. *Nutrition* 17: 248-253.

LaMonte, M.J., Ainsworth, B.E., and Reis, J.P. 2006. Measuring physical activity. In *Measurement theory and practice in kinesiology,* eds. T.M. Wood and W. Zhu, 237-272. Champaign, IL: Human Kinetics.

Lan, C., Lai, J., Chen, S., and Wong, M. 1998. 12-month tai chi training in the elderly: Its effects on health fitness. *Medicine & Science in Sports & Exercise* 30: 345–351.

Larsen, G.E., George, J.D., Alexander, J.L., Fellingham, G.W., Aldana, S.G., and Parcell, A.C. 2002. Prediction of maximum oxygen consumption from walking, jogging, or running. *Research Quarterly for Exercise and Sport* 73: 66-72.

Law, R.Y.W., and Herbert, R.D. 2007. Warm-up reduces delayed-onset muscle soreness but cool-down does not: A randomized controlled trial. *Australian Journal of Physiotherapy* 53: 91-95.

Layne, J.E., and Nelson, M.E. 1999. The effects of progressive resistance training on bone density: A review. *Medicine & Science in Sports & Exercise* 31:25–30.

Leger, L.A., Lambert, J., and Martin, P. 1982. Validity of plastic skinfold caliper measurements. *Human Biology* 54: 667–675.

Leger, L.A., Mercier, D., Gadoury, C., and Lambert, J. 1988. The multistage 20-metre shuttle run test for aerobic fitness. *Journal of Sports Sciences* 6: 93–101.

Leighton, J.R. 1955. An instrument and technique for measurement of range of joint motion. *Archives of Physical Medicine and Rehabilitation* 36: 571–578.

Lemieux, S., Prud'homme, D., Bouchard, C., Tremblay, A., and Despres, J-P. 1996. A single threshold value of waist girth identifies normal-weight and overweight subjects with excess visceral adipose tissue. *American Journal of Clinical Nutrition* 64: 685-693.

Lemon, P.W. 2000. Beyond the Zone: Protein needs of active individuals. *Journal of the American College of Nutrition* 19: 513S-521S.

Lermen, J., Bruce, R.A., Sivarajan, E., Pettet, G., and Trimble, S. 1976. Low-level dynamic exercises for earlier cardiac rehabilitation: Aerobic and hemodynamic responses. *Archives of Physical Medicine and Rehabilitation* 57: 355-360.

Lesmes, G.R., Costill, D.L., Coyle, E.F., and Fink, W.J. 1978. Muscle strength and power changes during maximal isokinetic training. *Medicine and Science in Sports* 10: 266–269.

Levine, B., Zuckerman, J., and Cole, C. 1998. Medical complications of exercise. In *ACSM's resource manual for guidelines for exercise testing and prescription*, ed. J.L. Roitman, 488–498. Philadelphia: Lippincott Williams & Wilkins.

Lewiecki, E.M., and Watts, N.B. 2009. New guidelines for the prevention and treatment of osteoporosis. *Southern Medical Journal* 102: 175-179.

Li, F., Harmer, P., Fisher, K.J., McAuley, E., Chaumeton, N., Eckstrom, E., and Wilson, N.L. 2005. Tai chi and fall reductions in older adults: A randomized controlled trial. *Journal of Gerontology* 60: 187-194.

Li, J.Y., Zhang, Y.F., Smith, G.S., Xue, C.J., Luo, Y.N., Chen, W.H., Skinner, C.J., and Finkelstein, J. 2009. Quality of reporting of randomized clinical trials in tai chi interventions—a systematic review. *eCam Advance Access.* doi: 10:1093/ecam/nep022.

Liang, M.T.C., Su, H., and Lee, N. 2000. Skin temperature and skin blood flow affect bioelectrical impedance study of female fat-free mass. *Medicine & Science in Sports & Exercise* 32: 221-227.

Liang, M.Y., and Norris, S. 1993. Effects of skin blood flow and temperature on bioelectrical impedance after exercise. *Medicine & Science in Sports & Exercise* 25: 1231-1239.

Litchell, H., and Boberg, J. 1978. The lipoprotein lipase activity of adipose tissue from different sites in obese women and relationship to cell size. *International Journal of Obesity* 2: 47–52.

Lockner, D., Heyward, V., Baumgartner, R., and Jenkins, K. 2000. Comparison of air-displacement plethysmography, hydrodensitometry, and dual X-ray absorptiometry for assessing body composition of children 10 to 18 years of age. *Annals of the New York Academy of Sciences* 904: 72–78.

Lohman, T.G. 1981. Skinfolds and body density and their relation to body fatness: A review. *Human Biology* 53: 181–115.

Lohman, T.G. 1987. *Measuring body fat using skinfolds* [videotape]. Champaign, IL: Human Kinetics.

Lohman, T.G. 1989. Bioelectrical impedance. In *Applying new technology to nutrition: Report of the ninth roundtable on medical issues,* 22–25. Columbus, OH: Ross Laboratories.

Lohman, T.G. 1992. *Advances in body composition assessment. Current issues in exercise science series.* Monograph no. 3. Champaign, IL: Human Kinetics.

Lohman, T.G. 1996. Dual energy X-ray absorptiometry. In *Human body composition,* ed. A.F. Roche, S.B. Heymsfield, and T.G. Lohman, 63-78. Champaign, IL: Human Kinetics.

Lohman, T.G., Boileau, R.A., and Slaughter, M.H. 1984. Body composition in children and youth. In *Advances in pediatric sport sciences,* ed. R.A. Boileau, 29–57. Champaign, IL: Human Kinetics.

Lohman, T.G., Going, S.B., and Metcalfe, L. 2004. Seeing ourselves through the obesity epidemic. *President's Council on Physical Fitness and Sports Research Digest Series* 5(3): 1-8.

Lohman, T.G., Going, S., Pamenter, R., Hall, M., Boyden, T., Houtkooper, L., Ritenbaugh, C., Bare, L., Hill, A., and Aickin, M. 1995. Effects of resistance training on regional and total bone mineral density in premenopausal women: A randomized prospective study. *Journal of Bone Mineral Research* 10: 1015–1024.

Lohman, T.G., Harris, M., Teixeira, P.J., and Weiss, L. 2000. Assessing body composition and changes in body composition: Another look at dual-energy X-ray absorptiometry. *Annals of the New York Academy of Sciences* 904: 45-54.

Lohman, T.G., Houtkooper, L., and Going, S. 1997. Body fat measurement goes high-tech: Not all are created equal. *ACSM's Health & Fitness Journal* 7: 30–35.

Lohman, T.G., Pollock, M.L., Slaughter, M.H., Brandon, L.J., and Boileau, R.A. 1984. Methodological factors and the prediction of body fat in female athletes. *Medicine & Science in Sports & Exercise* 16: 92–96.

Lohman, T.G., Roche, A.F., and Martorell, R., eds. 1988. *Anthropometric standardization reference manual.* Champaign, IL: Human Kinetics.

Londeree, B., and Moeschberger, M. 1984. Influence of age and other factors on maximal heart rate. *Journal of Cardiac Rehabilitation* 4: 44–49.

Loudon, J.K., Cagle, P.E., Figoni, S.F., Nau, K.L., and Klein, R.M. 1998. A submaximal all-extremity exercise test to predict maximal oxygen consumption. *Medicine & Science in Sports & Exercise* 30: 1299-1303.

Lounana, J., Campion, F., Noakes, T.D., and Medelli, J. 2007. Relationship between %HRmax, %HR reserve, %VO$_2$max, and %VO$_2$ reserve in elite cyclists. *Medicine & Science in Sports & Exercise* 39: 350-357.

Loy, S., Likes, E., Andrews, P., Vincent, W., Holland, G.J., Kawai, H., Cen, S., Swenberger, J., VanLoan, M., Tanaka, K., Heyward, V., Stolarczyk, L., Lohman, T.G., and Going, S.B. 1998. Easy grip on body composition measurements. *ACSM's Health & Fitness Journal* 2(5): 16–19.

Lozano, A., Rosell, J., and Pallas-Areny, R. 1995. Errors in prolonged electrical impedance measurements due to electrode repositioning and postural changes. *Physiological Measurement* 16: 121-130.

Ludwig, D.S., and Eckel, R.H. 2002. The glycemic index at 20 y. *American Journal of Clinical Nutrition* 76 (Suppl.): 264S-265S.

Lukaski, H.C. 1986. Use of the tetrapolar bioelectrical impedance method to assess human body composition. In *Human body composition and fat patterning,* ed. N.G. Norgan, 143–158. Wageningen, Netherlands: Euronut.

Lukaski, H.C. 1993. Soft tissue composition and bone mineral status: Evaluation by dual-energy X-ray absorptiometry. *Journal of Nutrition* 123: 438-443.

Lukaski, H.C., and Bolonchuk, W.W. 1988. Estimation of body fluid volumes using tetrapolar impedance measurements. *Aviation, Space, and Environmental Medicine* 59: 1163-l169.

Lukaski, H.C., Johnson, P.E., Bolonchuk, W.W., and Lykken, G.I. 1985. Assessment of fat-free mass using bioelectric impedance measurements of the human body. *American Journal of Clinical Nutrition* 41: 810-817.

Luthi, J.M., Howald, H., Claasen, H., Rosler, K., Vock, P., and Hoppeler, H. 1986. Structural changes in skeletal muscle tissue with heavy resistance exercise. *International Journal of Sports Medicine* 7: 123–127.

MacDougall, J.D., Sale, D.G., Moroz, J.R., Elder, G.C., Sutton, J.R., and Howalk, H. 1979. Mitochondrial volume density in human skeletal muscle following heavy resistance training. *Medicine and Science in Sports* 11: 164–166.

Macedonio, M.A., and Dunford, M. 2009. *The athlete's guide to making weight.* Champaign, IL: Human Kinetics.

Maciaszek, J., Osinski, W., Szeklicki, R., and Stemplewski, R. 2007. Effect of tai chi on body balance: Randomized controlled trial in men with osteopenia or osteoporosis. *American Journal of Chinese Medicine* 35: 1-9.

Mackey, A.L., Bojsen-Moller, J., Qvortrup, K., Langberg, H., Suetta, C., Kalliokoski, K.K., Kjaer, M., and Magnusson, S.P. 2008. Evidence of skeletal muscle damage following electrically stimulated isometric muscle contractions in humans. *Journal of Applied Physiology* 105: 1620-1627.

Magarey, A.M., Daniels, L.A., and Boulton, T.J. 2001. Prevalence of overweight and obesity in Australian children and adolescents: Reassessment of 1985 and 1995 data against new standard international definitions. *Medical Journal of Australia* 174: 561-564.

Magnusson, S.P. 1998. Passive properties of human skeletal muscle during stretch maneuvers. A review. *Scandinavian Journal of Medicine and Science in Sports* 8(2): 65–77.

Magnusson, S.P., Simonsen, E.B., Aagaard, P., Bueson, J., Johannson, F., and Kjaer, M. 1997. Determinants of musculoskeletal flexibility: Visoelastic properties, cross-sectional area, EMG and stretch tolerance. *Scandinavian Journal of Medicine and Science in Sports* 7: 195–202.

Mahieu, N.N., McNair, P., DeMuynck, M., Stevens, V., Blanckaert, I., Smits, N., and Witvrouw, E. 2007. Effect of static and ballistic stretching on the muscle—tendon tissue properties. *Medicine & Science in Sports & Exercise* 39: 494-501.

Maksud, M.G., and Coutts, K.D. 1971. Comparison of a continuous and discontinuous graded treadmill test for maximal oxygen uptake. *Medicine and Science in Sports* 3: 63–65.

Malek, M.H., Nalbone, D.P., Berger, D.E., and Coburn, J.W. 2002. Importance of health science education for personal fitness trainers. *Journal of Strength and Conditioning Research* 16: 19-24.

Manore, M.M. 2004. Nutrition and physical activity: Fueling the active individual. *President's Council on Physical Fitness and Sports Research Digest* 5(1): 1-8.

Manore, M.M., Meyer, N.L., and Thompson, J. 2009. *Sport nutrition for health and performance,* 2nd ed. Champaign, IL: Human Kinetics.

Manson, J.E., Nathan, D.M., Krolewski, A.S., Stampfer, M.J., Willett, W.C., and Hennekens, C.H. 1992. A prospective study of exercise and incidence of diabetes among US male physicians. *Journal of the American Medical Association* 268: 63–67.

Manson, J.E., Rimm, E.B., Stampfer, M.J., Rosner, B., Hennekens, C.H., Speizer, F.E., Colditz, G.A., Willett, W.C., and Krolewski, A.S. 1991. Physical activity incidence of non-insulin dependent diabetes mellitus in women. *Lancet* 338: 774–778.

Marcus, B.H., Bock, B.C., Pinto, B.M., Forsyth, L.H., Roberts, M.B., and Traficante, R.M. 1998. Efficacy of an individualized, motivationally tailored physical activity intervention. *Annals of Behavioral Medicine* 20: 174-180.

Marcus, B.H., Ciccolo, J.T., and Sciamanna, C.N. 2009. Using electronic/computer interventions to promote physical activity. *British Journal of Sports Medicine* 43: 102-105.

Marcus, B.H., and Forsyth, L.H. 2003. *Motivating people to be physically active.* Champaign, IL: Human Kinetics.

Marcus, B.H., and Lewis, B.A. 2003. Physical activity and the stages of motivational readiness for change model. *President's Council on Physical Fitness and Sports Research Digest* 4(1): 1-8.

Marcus, B.H., Rakowski, W., and Rossi, R.S. 1992. Assessing motivational readiness and decision-making for exercise. *Health Psychology* 11: 257-261.

Markandu, N.D., Whitcher, F., Arnold, A., and Carney, C. 2000. The mercury sphygmomanometer should be abandoned before it is proscribed. *Journal of Human Hypertension* 14: 31-36.

Markland, D., and Ingledew, L. 1997. The measurement of exercise motives: Factorial validity and invariance across gender of a revised exercise motivation inventory. *British Journal of Health Psychology* 2: 361-376.

Markland, D., and Tobin, V.J. 2004. A modification of the Behavioral Regulation in Exercise Questionnaire to include an assessment of amotivation. *Journal of Sport and Exercise Psychology* 26: 191-196.

Marks, B.L., Ward, A., Morris, D.H., Castellani, J., and Rippe, J.M. 1995. Fat-free mass is maintained in women following a moderate diet and exercise program. *Medicine & Science in Sports & Exercise* 27: 1243–1251.

Marley, W., and Linnerud, A. 1976. A three-year study of the Åstrand-Ryhming step test. *Research Quarterly* 47: 211–217.

Martin, A.D., Drinkwater, D.T., and Clarys, J.P. 1992. Effects of skin thickness and skinfold compressibility on skinfold thickness measurements. *American Journal of Human Biology* 4: 453–460.

Martin, A.D., Ross, W.D., Drinkwater, D.T., and Clarys, J.P. 1985. Prediction of body fat by skinfold caliper: Assumptions and cadaver evidence. *International Journal of Obesity* 9 (Suppl. 1): 31–39.

Martin, S.B., Jackson, A.W., Morrow, J.R., and Liemohn, W. 1998. The rationale for the sit and reach test revisited. *Measurement in Physical Education and Exercise Science* 2: 85–92.

Marx, J.O., Ratamess, N.A., Nindl, B.C., Gotshalk, L.A., Volek, J.S., Dohi, K., Bush, J.A., Gomez, A.L., Mazzetti, S.A., Fleck, S.J., Hakkinen, K., Newton, R.U., and Kraemer, W.J. 2001. Low-volume circuit versus high-volume periodized resistance training in women. *Medicine & Science in Sports & Exercise* 33: 635-643.

Mayer, J. 1968. *Overweight: Causes, costs and control.* Englewood Cliffs, NJ: Prentice Hall.

Mayer, T.G., Tencer, A.F., and Kristoferson, S. 1984. Use of noninvasive technique for quantification of spinal range-of-motion in normal subjects and chronic low back dysfunction patients. *Spine* 9: 588–595.

Mayhew, J.L., Ball, T.E., Arnold, M.D., and Bowen, J.C. 1992. Relative muscular endurance performance as a predictor of bench press strength in college men and women. *Journal of Applied Sport Science Research* 6: 200–206.

Mayson, D.J., Kiely, D.K., LaRose, S.I., and Bean, J.F. 2008. Leg strength or velocity of movement. Which is more influential on the balance of mobility limited elders? *American Journal of Physical Medicine and Rehabilitation* 87: 969-976.

Mazess, R.B., Barden, H.S., and Ohlrich, E.S. 1990. Skeletal and body-composition effects of anorexia nervosa. *American Journal of Clinical Nutrition* 52: 438–441.

McArdle, W.D., Katch, F.I., and Katch, V.L. 1996. *Exercise physiology: Energy, nutrition and human performance,* 4th ed. Baltimore: Williams & Wilkins.

McArdle, W.D., Katch, F.I., and Pechar, G.S. 1973. Comparison of continuous and discontinuous treadmill and bicycle tests for VO$_2$max. *Medicine and Science in Sports* 5: 156–160.

McArdle, W.D., Katch, F.I., Pechar, G.S., Jacobson, L., and Ruck, S. 1972. Reliability and interrelationships between maximal oxygen intake, physical working capacity and step-test scores in college women. *Medicine and Science in Sports* 4: 182–186.

McAtee, R., and Charland, J. 2007. *Facilitated stretching,* 3rd ed. Champaign, IL: Human Kinetics.

McConnell, T., and Clark, B. 1987. Prediction of maximal oxygen consumption during handrail-supported treadmill exercise. *Journal of Cardiopulmonary Rehabilitation* 7: 324–331.

McCrory, M.A., Gomez, T.D., Bernauer, E.M., and Mole, P.A. 1995. Evaluation of a new displacement plethysmograph for measuring human body composition. *Medicine & Science in Sports & Exercise* 27: 1686–1691.

McCrory, M.A., Mole, P.A., Gomez, T.D., Dewey, K.G., and Bernauer, E.M. 1998. Body composition by air displacement plethysmography using predicted and measured thoracic gas volumes. *Journal of Applied Physiology* 84: 1475-1479.

McCue, B.F. 1953. Flexibility of college women. *Research Quarterly* 24: 316–324.

McGill, S. 2007. *Low back disorders: Evidence based prevention and rehabilitation.* 2nd ed. Champaign, IL: Human Kinetics.

McGill, S.M. 1998. Low back exercises: Prescription for the healthy back and when recovering from injury. In *ACSM's resource manual for guidelines for exercise testing and prescription,* 3rd ed., Senior ed. J. Roitman.116-126. Philadelphia: Lippincott, Williams & Wilkins.

McGill, S.M. 2001. Low back stability: From formal description to issues for performance and rehabilitation. *Exercise and Sport Sciences Reviews* 29(1): 26–31.

McGill, S.M., Childs, A., and Liebenson, D.C. 1999. Endurance times for low back stabilization exercises: Clinical targets for testing and training from a normal database. *Archives of Physical Medicine and Rehabilitation* 80: 941-944.

McHugh, M.P. Kremenic, I.J., Fox, M.B., and Gleim, G.W. 1998. The role of mechanical and neural restraints to joint range of motion during passive stretch. *Medicine & Science in Sports & Exercise* 30: 928–932.

McHugh, M.P., Magnusson, S.P., Gleim, G.W., and Nicholas, J.A. 1992. Viscoelastic stress relaxation in human skeletal muscle. *Medicine & Science in Sports & Exercise* 24: 1375–1382.

McInnis, K., and Balady, G. 1994. Comparison of submaximal exercise responses using the Bruce vs modified Bruce protocols. *Medicine & Science in Sports & Exercise* 26: 103–107.

McKeon, P.O., and Hertel, J. 2008. Systematic review of postural control and lateral ankle instability. Part II: Is balance training clinically effective? *Journal of Athletic Training* 43(3): 305-315.

Mcrae, I.F., and Wright, V. 1969. Measurement of back movement. *Annals of Rheumatic Diseases* 28: 584–589.

McTiernan, A., Kooperberg, C., White, E., Wilcox, S., Coates, R., Adams-Campbell, L.L., Woods, N. and Okene, J. 2003. Recreational physical activity and the risk of breast cancer in postmenopausal women: The Women's Health Initiative Cohort Study. *Journal of the American Medical Association* 290(10): 1331-1336.

Mears, J., and Kilpatrick, M. 2008. Motivation for exercise: Applying theory to make a difference in adoption and adherence. *ACSM's Health & Fitness Journal* 12(1): 20-26.

Meldrum, D., Cahalane, E., Conroy, R., Fitzgerald, D., and Hardiman, O. 2007. Maximum voluntary isometric contraction: Reference values and clinical application. *Amyotrophic Lateral Sclerosis and Other Motor Neuron Disorders* 8: 47-55.

Meldrum, D., Cahalane, E., Keogan, F., and Hardiman, O. 2003. Maximum voluntary isometric contraction: Investigation of reliability and learning effect. *Amyotrophic Lateral Sclerosis and Other Motor Neuron Disorders* 4: 36-44.

Messier, S.P., Royer, T.D., Craven, T.E., O'Toole, M.L., Burns, R., and Ettinger W.H. Jr. 2000. Long-term exercise and its effect on balance in older, osteoarthritic adults: Results from the Fitness, Arthritis, and Seniors Trial (FAST). *Journal of the American Geriatrics Society* 48: 131-138.

Micozzi, M.S., Albanes, D., Jones, Y., and Chumlea, W.C. 1986. Correlations of body mass indices with weight, stature, and body composition in men and women in NHANES I and II. *American Journal of Clinical Nutrition* 44: 725–731.

Midgley, A.W., Bentley, D.J., Luttikholt, H., McNaughton, L.R., and Millet, G.P. 2008. Challenging a dogma of exercise physiology. Does an incremental exercise test for valid VO$_2$max determination really need to last between 8 and 12 minutes? *Sports Medicine* 38: 441-447.

Mifflin, M.D., St. Jeor, S.T., Hill, L.A., Scott, B.J., Daugherty, S.A., and Koh, Y.O. 1990. A new predictive equation for resting energy expenditure in healthy individuals. *American Journal of Clinical Nutrition* 51: 241-247.

Mikesky, A.E., Giddings, C.J., Matthews, W., and Gonyea, W.J. 1991. Changes in fiber size and composition in response to heavy-resistance exercise. *Medicine & Science in Sports & Exercise* 23: 1042–1049.

Milburn, S., and Butts, N.K. 1983. A comparison of the training responses to aerobic dance and jogging in college females. *Medicine & Science in Sports & Exercise* 15: 510–513.

Millard-Stafford, M.L., Collins, M.A., Evans, E.M., Snow, T.K., Cureton, K.J., and Rosskopf, L.B. 2001. Use of air displacement plethysmography for estimating body fat in a four-component model. *Medicine & Science in Sports & Exercise* 33: 1311-1317.

Miller, J.B. 2001. *GI research*. www.glycemicindex.com.

Minkler, S., and Patterson, P. 1994. The validity of the modified sit-and-reach test in college-age students. *Research Quarterly for Exercise and Sport* 65: 189–192.

Mischi, M., and Cardinale, M. 2009. The effects of a 28-Hz vibration on arm muscle activity during isometric exercise. *Medicine & Science in Sports & Exercise* 41: 645-653.

Moffatt, R.J., Stamford, B.A., and Neill, R.D. 1977. Placement of tri-weekly training sessions: Importance regarding enhancement of aerobic capacity. *Research Quarterly* 48: 583–591.

Moffroid, M.T., and Whipple, R.H. 1970. Specificity of speed of exercise. *Physical Therapy* 50: 1699–1704.

Mole, P.A., Oscai, L.B., and Holloszy, J.O. 1971. Adaptation of muscle to exercise: Increase in levels of palmityl CoA synthetase, carnitine palmityl-transferase, and palmityl CoA dehydrogenase and the capacity to oxidize fatty acids. *Journal of Clinical Investigation* 50: 2323–2329.

Montoye, H.J., and Faulkner, J.A. 1964. Determination of the optimum setting of an adjustable grip dynamometer. *Research Quarterly* 35: 29–36.

Moon, J.R., Tobkin, S.E., Costa, P.B., Smalls, M., Mieding, W.K., O'Kroy, J.A., Zoeller, R.F., and Stout, J.R. 2008. Validity of the Bod Pod for assessing body composition in athletic high school boys. *Journal of Strength and Conditioning Research* 22: 263-268.

Mooney, V., Kron, M., Rummerfield, P., and Holmes, B. 1995. The effect of workplace based strengthening on low back injury rates: A case study in the strip mining industry. *Journal of Occupational Rehabilitation* 5: 157-167.

Moore, M.A., and Hutton, R.S. 1980. Electromyographic investigation of muscle stretching techniques. *Medicine & Science in Sports & Exercise* 12: 322-329.

Moore, S.C. 2009. Waist versus weight—which matters more for mortality? *American Journal of Clinical Nutrition* 89: 1003-1004.

Morehouse, L.E. 1972. *Laboratory manual for physiology of exercise*. St. Louis: Mosby.

Moritani, T., and deVries, H.A. 1979. Neural factors versus hypertrophy in the time course of muscle strength gain. *American Journal of Physical Medicine* 58: 115–130.

Morris, N., Gass, G., Thompson, M., Bennett, G., Basic, D., and Morton H. 2002. Rate and amplitude of adaptation to intermittent and continuous exercise in older men. *Medicine & Science in Sports & Exercise* 34: 471-477.

Morrow, J.R., Jackson, A.S., Bradley, P.W., and Hartung, G.H. 1986. Accuracy of measured and predicted residual lung volume on body density measurement. *Medicine & Science in Sport & Exercise* 18: 647–652.

Muir, S.W., Berg, K., Chesworth, B., and Speechley, M. 2008. Use of the Berg Balance Scale for predicting multiple falls in community-dwelling elderly people: A prospective study. *Physical Therapy* 88: 449-459.

Muller, M.J., Bosy-Westphal, A., Klaus, S., Kreymann, G., Luhrmann, P.M., Neuhauser-Berthold, M., Noack, R.,

Pirke, K.M., Platte, P., Selberg, O., and Steiniger, J. 2004. World Health Organization equations have shortcomings for predicting resting energy expenditure in persons from a modern, affluent population: Generation of a new reference standard from a retrospective analysis of a German database of resting energy expenditure. *American Journal of Clinical Nutrition* 80: 1379-1390.

Munroe, R.A., and Romance, T.J. 1975. Use of the Leighton flexometer in the development of a short flexibility test battery. *American Corrective Therapy Journal* 29: 22.

Nader, G.A. 2006. Concurrent strength and endurance training: From molecules to man. *Medicine & Science in Sports & Exercise* 38: 1965-1970.

Nagle, F.S., Balke, B., and Naughton, J.P. 1965. Gradational step tests for assessing work capacity. *Journal of Applied Physiology* 20: 745–748.

Napolitano, M.A., Lewis, B.A., Whitely, J.A., and Marcus, B.H. 2010. Principles of health behavior change. In *ACSM's resource manual for guidelines for exercise testing and prescription,* 710-723. Philadelphia: Wolters Kluwer/Lippincott Williams & Wilkins.

Nashner, L.M. 1997. In *Handbook of balance function testing*, eds. G.P. Jacobson, C.W. Newman, and J.M. Kartush, 280-307. San Diego: Singular Publishing Group.

National Academy of Sciences. 2000. *Dietary reference intakes*. Washington, D.C.: National Academy Press.

National Cholesterol Education Program. 2001. Executive summary of the third report of the National Cholesterol Education Program (NCEP) Expert Panel on detection, evaluation, and treatment of high blood cholesterol in adults (Adult Treatment Panel III). *Journal of the American Medical Association* 285(19): 2486–2497.

National Institutes of Health and National Heart, Lung, and Blood Institute. 1998. Clinical guidelines on the identification, evaluation, and treatment of overweight and obesity in adults: The evidence report. *Obesity Research* 6 (Suppl. 2): S51–S209.

National Institutes of Health Consensus Development Panel. 1985. Health implications of obesity: National Institutes of Health Consensus development statement. *Annals of Internal Medicine* 103: 1073–1079.

National Osteoporosis Foundation. 2004. America's bone health: The state of osteoporosis and low bone mass. www.nof.org/advocacy/prevalence/.

National Osteoporosis Foundation. 2008. Osteoporosis fast facts. www.nof.org/osteoporosis/diseasefacts.

National Strength and Conditioning Association. 2008. *Essentials of strength training and conditioning,* 3rd ed. Champaign, IL: Human Kinetics.

Naughton, J., Balke, B., and Nagle, F. 1964. Refinement in methods of evaluation and physical conditioning before and after myocardial infarction. *American Journal of Cardiology* 14: 837.

Nelson, A.G., and Kokkonen, J. 2007. *Stretching anatomy*. Champaign, IL: Human Kinetics.

Nelson, M.E., and Folta, S.C. 2009. Further evidence for the benefits of walking. *American Journal of Clinical Nutrition* 89: 15-16.

Nelson, M.E., Rejeski, W.J., Blair, S.N., Duncan, P.W., Judge, J.O., King, A.C., Macera, C.A., and Castaneda-Sceppa, C. 2007. Physical activity and public health in older adults: Recommendations from the American College of Sports Medicine and the American Heart Association. *Medicine & Science in Sports & Exercise* 39(8): 1435-1445.

Ng, J.K., Kippers, V., Richardson, C.A., and Parnianpour, M. 2001. Range of motion and lordosis of the lumbar spine: Reliability of measurement and normative values. *Spine* 26: 53-60.

Ng, N. 1995. *Metcalc.* Champaign, IL: Human Kinetics.

Nichols, D.L., Sanborn, C.F., and Love, A.M. 2001. Resistance training and bone mineral density in adolescent females. *Journal of Pediatrics* 139: 494-499.

Nichols, J.F., Sherman, C.L., and Abbott, E. 2000. Treading is new and hot: 30 minutes meets the ACSM recommendations for cardiorespiratory fitness and caloric expenditure. *ACSM's Health & Fitness Journal* 4(2): 12–17.

Nicklas, B.J., Wang, X., You, T., Lyles, M.F., Demons, J., Easter, L., Berry, M.J., Lenchik, L., and Carr, J.J. 2009. Effect of exercise intensity on abdominal fat loss during calorie restriction in overweight and obese postmenopausal women: A randomized, controlled trial. *American Journal of Clinical Nutrition* 89: 1043-1052.

Nissen, S.L., and Sharp, R.L. 2003. Effect of dietary supplements on lean mass and gains with resistance training: A meta-analysis. *Journal of Applied Physiology* 94: 651-659.

Noakes, T.D. 2008. How did A V Hill understand the VO_2max and the "plateau phenomenon"? Still no clarity? *British Journal of Sports Medicine* 42: 574-580.

Noland, M., and Kearney, J.T. 1978. Anthropometric and densitometric responses of women to specific and general exercise. *Research Quarterly* 49: 322–328.

Norkin, C.C., and White, D.J. 1995. *Measurement of joint motion: A guide to goniometry.* Philadelphia: Davis.

Norris, C. 2000. *Back stability.* Champaign, IL: Human Kinetics.

Norris, R.A., Wilder, E., and Norton, J. 2008. The functional reach test in 3- to 5-year-old children without disabilities. *Pediatric Physical Therapy* 20: 47-52.

North American Spine Society. 2009. Exercise for a healthy back. www.spine.org/Pages/ConsumerHealth/Spine-HealthAndWellness/PreventBackPain.

Norton, K., Marfell-Jones, M., Whittingham, N., Kerr, D., Carter, L., Saddington, K., and Gore, C. 2000. Anthropometric assessment protocols. In *Physiological tests for elite athletes*, ed. C. Gore, 66–85. Champaign, IL: Human Kinetics.

Nunez, C., Kovera, A., Pietrobelli, A., Heshka, S., Horlick, M., Kehayias, J., Wang, Z., and Heymsfield, S. 1999. Body composition in children and adults by air displacement plethysmography. *European Journal of Clinical Nutrition* 53: 382–387.

O'Brien, E. 2003. Demise of the mercury sphygmomanometer and the dawning of a new era in blood pressure measurement. *Blood Pressure Monitoring* 8: 19-21.

O'Brien, E., Pickering, T., Asmar, R., Myers, M., Parati, G., Staessen, J., Mengden, T., Imai, Y., Waeber, B., and Palantini, P. 2002. Working group on blood pressure monitoring of the European Society of Hypertension International Protocol for validation of blood pressure measuring devices in adults. *Blood Pressure Monitoring* 7: 3-17.

O'Brien, E., Waeber, B., Parati, G., Staessen, J., and Myers, M.G. 2001. Blood pressure measuring devices: Recommendations of the European Society of Hypertension. *British Medical Journal* 322: 531- 536.

Ogden, C.L., Carroll, M.D., Curtin, L.R., McDowell, M.A., Tabak, C.J., and Flegal, K.M. 2006. Prevalence of overweight and obesity in the United States, 1999-2004. *Journal of the American Medical Association* 295: 1549-1555.

Ogden, C.L., Carroll, M.D., and Flegal, K.M. 2008. High body mass index for age among US children and adolescents, 2003-2006. *Journal of the American Medical Association* 299: 2401-2405.

Ohrvall, M., Berglund, L., and Vessby, B. 2000. Sagittal abdominal diameter compared with other anthropometric measurements in relation to cardiovascular risk. *International Journal of Obesity* 24: 497-501.

Oken, B.S., Zajdel, D., Kishiyama, S., Flegal, K., Dehen, C., Haas, M., Kraemer, D.F., Lawrence, J., and Leyva, J. 2006. Randomized, controlled, six-month trial of yoga in healthy seniors: Effects on cognition and quality of life. *Alternative Therapy in Health and Medicine* 12: 40-47.

Olmsted, L.C., Carcia, C.R., Hertel, J., and Schultz, S.J. 2002. Efficacy of the star excursion balance tests in detecting reach deficits in subjects with chronic ankle instability. *Journal of Athletic Training* 37: 501-506.

Olson, M.S., Williford, H.N., Blessing, D.L., and Greathouse, R. 1991. The cardiovascular and metabolic effects of bench stepping exercise in females. *Medicine & Science in Sports & Exercise* 23: 1311–1318.

Omboni, S., Riva, I., Giglio, I., Caldara, G., Groppelli, A., and Parati, G. 2007. Validation of the Omron M5-I, R5-I and HEM-907 automated blood pressure monitors in elderly individuals according to the International Protocol of the European Society of Hypertension. *Blood Pressure Monitoring* 12: 233-242.

Oppliger, R.A., Nielsen, D.H., and Vance, C.G. 1991. Wrestlers' minimal weight: Anthropometry, bioimpedance, and hydrostatic weighing compared. *Medicine & Science in Sports & Exercise* 23: 247–253.

Ornish, D. 2004. Was Dr Atkins right? *Journal of the American Medical Association* 104: 537-542.

Orr, R., Raymond, J., and Singh, M.F. 2008. Efficacy of progressive resistance training on balance performance in older adults. A systematic review of randomized controlled trials. *Sports Medicine* 38: 317-343.

Ortiz, O., Russell, M., Daley, T.L., Baumgartner, R.N., Waki, M., Lichtman, S., Wang, S., Pierson, R.N., and Heymsfield,

S.B. 1992. Differences in skeletal muscle and bone mineral mass between black and white females and their relevance to estimates of body composition. *American Journal of Clinical Nutrition* 55: 8–13.

Ostchega, Y., Prineas, R.J., Dillon, C., McDowell, M., and Carroll, M. 2004. Estimating equations and tables for adult mid-arm circumference based on measured height and weight: Data from the third National Health and Nutrition Examination Survey (NHANES III) and NHANES 1999-2000. *Blood Pressure Monitoring* 9: 123-131.

Page, P., and Ellenbecker, T. 2005. *Strength band training.* Champaign, IL: Human Kinetics.

Painter, J., Rah, J.H., and Lee, Y.K. 2002. Comparison of international food guide pictorial representations. *Journal of the American Dietetic Association* 102: 483-489.

Pajala, S., Era, P., Koskenvuo, M., Kaprio, J., Tormakangas, T., and Rantanen, T. 2008. Force platform balance measures as predictors of indoor and outdoor falls in community-dwelling women 63-76 years. *Journal of Gerontology* 63: 171-178.

Palatini, P., Dorigatti, F., Bonso, E., and Ragazzo, F. 2008. Validation of the Microlife BP W200-1 wrist device for blood pressure measurement. *Blood Pressure Monitoring* 13: 295-298.

Panotopoulos, G., Ruiz, J.C., Guy-Grand, B., and Basdevant, A. 2001. Dual x-ray absorptiometry, bioelectrical impedance, and near-infrared interactance in obese women. *Medicine & Science in Sports & Exercise* 33: 665-670.

Parker, S.B., Hurley, B.F., Hanlon, D.P., and Vaccaro, P. 1989. Failure of target heart rate to accurately monitor intensity during aerobic dance. *Medicine & Science in Sports & Exercise* 21: 230–234.

Partnership for Essential Nutrition. 2004. *The impact of the low-carb craze on attitudes about eating and weight loss: A national opinion survey conducted for the Partnership for Essential Nutrition.* http://www.essentialnutrition.org/survey.php.

Pate, R.R., Pratt, M., Blair, S.N., Haskell, W.L., Macera, C.A., Bouchard, C., Buchner, D., Ettinger, W., Heath, G.W., and King, A.C. 1995. Physical activity and public health: A recommendation from the Centers for Disease Control and Prevention and the American College of Sports Medicine. *Journal of the American Medical Association* 273: 402–407.

Patterson, P., Wiksten, D.L., Ray, L., Flanders, C., and Sanphy, D. 1996. The validity and reliability of the backsaver sit-and-reach test in middle school girls and boys. *Research Quarterly for Exercise and Sport* 67: 448–451.

Paulsen, G., Myklested, D., and Reestad, T. 2003. The influence of volume of exercise on early adaptations to strength training. *Journal of Strength and Conditioning Research* 17: 115-120.

Pavlou, K.N., Steffee, W.P., Lerman, R.H., and Burrows, B.A. 1985. Effects of dieting and exercise on lean body mass, oxygen uptake, and strength. *Medicine & Science in Sports & Exercise* 17: 466–471.

Payne, N., Gledhill, N., Kazmarzyk, P.T., Jamnik, V., and Keir, P.J. 2000. Canadian musculoskeletal fitness norms. *Canadian Journal of Applied Physiology* 25: 430–442.

Persinger, R., Foster, C., Gibson, M., Fater, D.C.W., and Porcari, J.P. 2004. Consistency of the talk test for exercise prescription. *Medicine & Science in Sports & Exercise* 36: 1632-1636.

Pescatello, L.S., Franklin, B.A., Fagard, R., Farquhar, W.B., Kelley, G.A, and Ray, C.A. 2004. American College of Sports Medicine position stand. Exercise and hypertension. *Medicine & Science in Sports & Exercise* 36: 533-553.

Peters, D., Fox, K., Armstrong, N., Sharpe, P., and Bell, M. 1992. Assessment of children's abdominal fat distribution by magnetic resonance imaging and anthropometry. *International Journal of Obesity* 16(Suppl. 2): S35 [abstract].

Petersen, T., Verstraete, D., Schultz, W., and Stray-Gundersen, J. 1993. Metabolic demands of step aerobics. *Medicine & Science in Sports & Exercise* 25: S79 [abstract].

Peterson, M.D., Rhea, M.R., and Alvar, B.A. 2004. Maximizing strength development in athletes: A meta-analysis to determine the dose-response relationship. *Journal of Strength and Conditioning Research* 18: 377-382.

Pickering, T.G., Hall, J.E., Appel, L.J., Falkner, B.E., Graves, J., Hill, M.N., Jones, D.W., Kurtz, T., Sheldon, G., and Rocella, E.J. 2005. Recommendations for blood pressure measurement in humans and experimental animals: Part 1: Blood pressure measurement in humans: A statement for professionals from the subcommittee of Professional and Public Education of the American Heart Council on High Blood Pressure Research. *Hypertension* 45(1): 142-161.

Pierce, P., and Herman, S. 2004. Obtaining, maintaining, and advancing your fitness certification. *Journal of Physical Education, Recreation and Dance* 75(7): 50-53.

Pietrobelli, A., Formica, C., Wang, Z., and Heymsfield, S.B. 1996. Dual-energy X-ray absorptiometry body composition model: Review of physical concepts. *American Journal of Physiology* 271: E941-E951.

Pi-Sunyer, F.X. 1999. Comorbidities of overweight and obesity: Current evidence and research issues. *Medicine & Science in Sports & Exercise* 31: S602–S608.

Pi-Sunyer, F.X. 2002. Glycemic index and disease. *American Journal of Clinical Nutrition* 76 (Suppl.): 290S-298S.

Plowman, S.A. 1992. Physical activity, physical fitness, and low-back pain. *Exercise and Sport Sciences Reviews* 20: 221–242.

Podsiadlo, D., and Richardson, S. 1991. The timed "up & go": A test of basic functional mobility of frail elderly persons. *Journal of the American Geriatrics Society* 39: 142-148.

Pollock, M.L. 1973. The quantification of endurance training programs. In *Exercise and Sport Sciences Reviews,* ed. J.H. Wilmore, 1: 155–188. New York: Academic Press.

Pollock, M.L., Bohannon, R.L., Cooper, K.H., Ayres, J.J., Ward, A., White, S.R., and Linnerud, A.C. 1976. A comparative analysis of four protocols for maximal treadmill stress testing. *American Heart Journal* 92: 39–46.

Pollock, M.L., Broida, J., and Kendrick, Z. 1972. Validity of the palpation technique of heart rate determination and its estimation of training heart rate. *Research Quarterly* 43: 77–81.

Pollock, M.L., Cureton, T.K., and Greninger, L. 1969. Effects of frequency of training on working capacity, cardiovascular function, and body composition of adult men. *Medicine and Science in Sports* 1: 70–74.

Pollock, M.L., Dimmick, J., Miller, H.S., Kendrick, Z., and Linnerud, A.C. 1975. Effects of mode of training on cardiovascular function and body composition of middle-aged men. *Medicine and Science in Sports* 7: 139–145.

Pollock, M.L., Foster, C., Schmidt, D., Hellman, C., Linnerud, A.C., and Ward, A. 1982. Comparative analysis of physiologic responses to three different maximal graded exercise test protocols in healthy women. *American Heart Journal* 103: 363–373.

Pollock, M.L., Gaesser, G.A., Butcher, J.D., Despres, J.P., Dishman, R.K., Franklin, B.A., and Garber, C.E. 1998. The recommended quantity and quality of exercise for developing and maintaining cardiorespiratory and muscular fitness, and flexibility in healthy adults. *Medicine & Science in Sports & Exercise* 30: 975–991.

Pollock, M.L., Garzarella, L., and Graves, J. 1992. Effects of isolated lumbar extension resistance training on BMD of the elderly. *Medicine & Science in Sports & Exercise* 24: S66 [abstract].

Pollock, M.L., Gettman, L., Milesis, C., Bah, M., Durstine, L., and Johnson, R. 1977. Effects of frequency and duration of training on attrition and incidence of injury. *Medicine and Science in Sports* 9: 31–36.

Pollock, M.L., and Jackson, A.S. 1984. Research progress in validation of clinical methods of assessing body composition. *Medicine & Science in Sports & Exercise* 16: 606–613.

Pollock, M.L., Miller, H.S., Janeway, R., Linnerud, A.C., Robertson, B., and Valentino, R. 1971. Effects of walking on body composition and cardiovascular function of middle-aged men. *Journal of Applied Physiology* 30: 126–130.

Pollock, M.L., Miller, H.S., Linnerud, A.C., and Cooper, K.H. 1975. Frequency of training as a determinant for improvement in cardiovascular function and body composition of middle-aged men. *Archives of Physical Medicine and Rehabilitation* 56: 141–145.

Pollock, M.L., Wilmore, J.H., and Fox, S.M. III. 1978. *Health and fitness through physical activity*. New York: Wiley.

Pondal, M., and del Ser, T. 2008. Normative data and determinants for the timed "up and go" test in a population-based sample of elderly individuals without gait disturbances. *Journal of Geriatric Physical Therapy* 31(2): 57-63.

Poortmans, J.R., and Francaux, M. 2000. Adverse effects of creatine supplementation: Fact or fiction? *Sports Medicine* 30: 155-170.

Pope R.P., Herbert, R.D., Kirwan, J.D., and Graham, B.J. 2000. A randomized trial of preexercise stretching for prevention of lower limb injury. *Medicine & Science in Sports & Exercise* 32: 271–277.

Porcari, J., Foster, C., and Schneider, P. 2000. Exercise response to elliptical trainers. *Fitness Management* 16(9): 50–53.

Porszasz, J., Casaburi, R., Somfay, A., Woodhouse, L.J., and Whipp, B.J. 2003. A treadmill ramp protocol using simultaneous changes in speed and grade. *Medicine & Science in Sports & Exercise* 35: 1596-1603.

Porter, D.E., Kirtland, K.A., Neet, M.J., Williams, J.E., and Ainsworth, B.E. 2004. Consideration for using a geographic information system to assess environmental supports for physical activity. *Preventing Chronic Disease: Public Health Research, Practice and Policy* 1(4): 1-6.

Porter, G.H. 1988. Case study evaluation for exercise prescription. In *Resource manual for guidelines for exercise testing and prescription*, ed. S.N. Blair, P. Painter, R.R. Pate, L.K. Smith, and C.B. Taylor, 248–255. Philadelphia: Lea & Febiger.

Powell, K.E., Thompson, P.D., Casperson, C.J., and Kendrick, J.S. 1987. Physical activity and the incidence of coronary heart disease. *Annual Review of Public Health* 8: 253–287.

President's Council on Physical Fitness and Sports. 1997. *The presidential physical fitness award program*. Washington, D.C.: author.

Prevalence of leisure-time physical activity among overweight adults—United States, 1998. 2000. *Morbidity and Mortality Weekly Report* 49(15), April 21.

Prineas, R.J., Ostchega, Y., Carroll, M., Dillon, C., and McDowell, M. 2007. US demographic trends in mid-arm circumference and recommended blood pressure cuffs for children and adolescents: Data from the National Health and Nutrition Examination Survey 1988-2004. *Blood Pressure Monitoring* 12(2): 75-80.

Prior, B.M., Cureton, K.J., Modlesky, C.M., Evans, E.M., Sloniger, M.A., Saunders, M., and Lewis, R.D. 1997. In vivo validation of whole body composition estimates from dual-energy X-ray absorptiometry. *Journal of Applied Physiology* 83: 623-630.

Prochaska, J.O., and DiClemente, C.C. 1982. Trans-theoretical therapy: Toward a more integrative model of change. *Psychotherapy: Theory, Research, and Practice* 19: 276–288.

Proske, U., and Morgan, D.L. 2001. Muscle damage from eccentric exercise: Mechanism, mechanical signs, adaptation, and clinical applications. *Journal of Physiology* 537: 333-345.

Province, M.A., Hadley, E.C., Hornbrook, M.C., Lipsitz, L.A., Miller, J.P., Mulrow, C.P., Ory, M.G., Sattin, R.W., Tinetti, M.E., and Wolf, S.L. 1995. The effects of exercise on falls in elderly patients. A preplanned meta-analysis of the FICSIT trials. Fraility and injuries: Cooperative studies of intervention techniques. *Journal of the American Medical Association* 273: 1341-1347.

Pruitt, L.A., Jackson, R.D., Bartels, R.L., and Lehnhard, H.J. 1992. Weight-training effects on bone mineral density in early postmenopausal women. *Journal of Bone Mineral Research* 7: 179–185.

Pruitt, L.A., Taaffe, D.R., and Marcus, R. 1995. Effects of a one-year high-intensity versus low-intensity resistance training program on bone mineral density in older women. *Journal of Bone Mineral Research* 10: 1788–1795.

Public Health Agency of Canada. 2009. Facts on current physical activity levels of Canadians. www.phac-aspc.gc.ca/pau-uap/paguide/back3e.html.

Quatrochi, J.A., Hicks, V.L., Heyward, V.H., Colville, B.C., Cook, K.L., Jenkins, K.A., and Wilson, W. 1992. Relationship of optical density and skinfold measurements: Effects of age and level of body fatness. *Research Quarterly for Exercise and Sport* 63: 402-409.

Rajaram, S., Weaver, C.M., Lyle, R.M., Sedlock, D.A., Martin, B., Templin, T.J., Beard, J.L., and Percival, S.S. 1995. Effects of long-term moderate exercise on iron status in young women. *Medicine & Science in Sports & Exercise* 27: 1105–1110.

Ratamess, N.A., Alvar, B.A., Evetoch, T.K., Housh, T.J., Kibler, W.B., Kraemer, W.J., and Triplett, N.T. 2009. ACSM position stand: Progression models in resistance training for healthy adults. *Medicine & Science in Sports & Exercise* 41: 687-708.

Ratamess, N.A., Kraemer, W.J., Volek, J.S., Rubin, M.R., Gomez, A.L., French, D.N., Sharman, M.J., McGuigan, M.M., Scheett, T., Hakkinen, K., Newton, R.U., and Dioguardi, F. 2003. The effects of amino acid supplementation on muscular performance during resistance training overreaching. *Journal of Strength and Conditioning Research* 17: 250-258.

Rawson, E.S., and Clarkson, P.M. 2003. Scientifically debatable: Is creatine worth its weight? *Gatorade Sport Science Exchange 91* 16(4): 1-13.

Rawson, E.S., Gunn, B., and Clarkson, P.M. 2001. The effects of creatine supplementation on exercise-induced muscle damage. *Journal of Strength and Conditioning Research* 15: 178-184.

Rebuffe-Scrive, M. 1985. Adipose tissue metabolism and fat distribution. In *Human body composition and fat distribution*, ed. N.G. Norgan, 212–217. Wageningen, Netherlands: Euronut.

Recalde, P.T., Foster, C., Skemp-Arlt, K.M., Fater, D.C.W., Neese, C.A., Dodge, C., and Porcari, J.P. 2002. The talk test as a simple marker of ventilatory threshold. *South African Journal of Sports Medicine* 8: 5-8.

Reese, N.B., and Bandy, W.D. 2003. Use of an inclinometer to measure flexibility of the iliotibial band using the Ober test and the modified Ober test: Differences in magnitude and reliability of measurements. *Journal of Orthopaedic and Sports Physical Therapy* 33: 326-330.

Reeves, R.A. 1995. Does this patient have hypertension? How to measure blood pressure. *Journal of the American Medical Association* 273: 1211–1218.

Reiman, M.P., and Manske, R.C. 2009. *Functional testing in human performance*. Champaign, IL: Human Kinetics.

Rhea, M.R., Alvar, B.A., Burkett, L.N., and Ball, S.D. 2003. A meta-analysis to determine the dose response for strength development. *Medicine & Science in Sports & Exercise* 35: 456-464.

Rhea, M.R., Ball, S.D., Phillips, W.T., and Burkett, L.N. 2002. A comparison of linear and daily undulating periodized programs with equated volume and intensity for strength. *Journal of Strength and Conditioning Research* 16: 250-255.

Rhea, M.R., Phillips, W.T., Burkett, L.N., Stone, W.J., Ball, S.D., Alvar, B.A., and Thomas, A.B. 2003. A comparison of linear and daily undulating periodized programs with equated volume and intensity for local muscular endurance. *Journal of Strength and Conditioning Research* 17: 82-87.

Richardson, C.R., Newton, T.L., Abraham, J.J., Sen, A., Jimbo, M., and Swartz, A.M. 2008. A meta-analysis of pedometer-based walking interventions and weight loss. *Annals of Family Medicine* 6: 69-77.

Riddle, D.L., and Stratford, P.W. 1999. Interpreting validity indexes for diagnostic tests: An illustration using the Berg balance test. *Physical Therapy* 79: 939-948.

Ridley, K., Ainsworth, B.E., and Olds, T.S. 2008. Development of a compendium of energy expenditures for youth. *International Journal of Behavioral Nutrition and Physical Activity* 5: 45-52.

Riebe, D., and Niggs, C. 1998. Setting the stage for healthy living. *ACSM's Health & Fitness Journal* 2(3): 11–15.

Rikli, R., Petray, C., and Baumgartner, T. 1992. The reliability of distance run tests for children in grades K-4. *Research Quarterly for Exercise and Sport* 63: 270–276.

Rikli, R.E., and Jones, C.J. 1999. Development and validation of a functional fitness test for community-residing older adults. *Journal of Aging and Physical Activity* 7: 127-159.

Rikli, R.E, and Jones, C.J. 2001. *Senior fitness test manual*. Champaign, IL: Human Kinetics.

Rixon, K.P., Rehor, P.R., and Bemben, M.G. 2006. Analysis of the assessment of caloric expenditure in four modes of aerobic dance. *Journal of Strength and Conditioning Research* 20: 593-596.

Roberts, J.M., and Wilson, K. 1999. Effect of stretching duration on active and passive range of motion in the lower extremity. *British Journal of Sports Medicine* 33: 259-263.

Robertson, R.J. 2004. *Perceived exertion for practitioners. Rating effort with the OMNI picture system*. Champaign, IL: Human Kinetics.

Robertson, R.J., Goss, F.L., Andreacci, J.L., Dube, J.J., Rutkowski, J.J., Frazee, K.M., Aaron, D.J., Metz, K.F., Kowallis, R.A., and Snee, B.M. 2005. Validation of the children's OMNI-resistance exercise scale of perceived exertion. *Medicine & Science in Sports & Exercise* 37: 819-826.

Robinson, R.H., and Gribble, P.A. 2008. Support for a reduction in the number of trials needed for the star excursion balance test. *Archives of Physical Medicine and Rehabilitation* 89: 364-370.

Roby, R.B. 1962. Effect of exercise on regional subcutaneous fat accumulations. *Research Quarterly* 33: 273–278.

Rochmis, P., and Blackburn, H. 1971. Exercise tests. A survey of procedures, safety and litigation experience in approximately 170,000 tests. *Journal of the American Medical Association* 217: 1061–1066.

Rockport Walking Institute. 1986. *Rockport fitness walking test*. Marlboro, MA: Author.

Rodd, D., Ho, L., and Enzler, D. 1999. Validity of Tanita TBF-515 bioelectrical impedance scale for estimating body fat in young adults. *Medicine & Science in Sports & Exercise* 31(Suppl.): S201 [abstract].

Rodgers, W.M., and Loitz, C.C. 2009. The role of motivation in behavior change: How do we encourage our clients to be active? *ACSM's Health & Fitness Journal* 13(1): 7-12.

Rodriguez, D.A., Brown, A.L., and Troped, P.J. 2005. Portable global positioning units to complement accelerometry-based physical activity monitors. *Medicine & Science in Sports & Exercise* 37 (Suppl.): S572-S581.

Roelants, M., Delecluse, C., Goris, M., and Verschueren, S. 2004. Effects of 24 weeks of whole body vibration training on body composition and muscle strength in untrained females. *International Journal of Sports Medicine* 25: 1-5.

Rogers, C.E., Larkey, L.K., and Keller, C. 2009. A review of clinical trials of tai chi and Qigong in older adults. *Western Journal of Nursing Research* 31: 245-279.

Rose, D.J. 2003. *Fall proof: A comprehensive balance and mobility training program.* Champaign, IL: Human Kinetics.

Ross, J., and Pate, R. 1987. The national children and youth fitness study II: A summary of findings. *Journal of Physical Education, Recreation and Dance* 58: 51–56.

Ross, R., and Janssen, I. 2001. Physical activity, total and regional obesity: Dose-response considerations. *Medicine & Science in Sports & Exercise* 33 (Suppl.): S521-S527.

Ross, W.D., and Marfell-Jones, M.J. 1991. Kinanthropometry. In *Physiological testing of the high-performance athlete,* ed. J.D. MacDougall, H.A. Wenger, and H.J. Green, 75–115, Champaign, IL: Human Kinetics.

Rossiter, H.B., Kowalchuk, J.M., and Whipp, B.J. 2006. A test to establish maximum O_2 uptake despite no plateau in the O_2 uptake response to ramp incremental exercise. *Journal of Applied Physiology* 100: 764-770.

Row, B.S., and Cavanagh, P.R. 2007. Reaching upward is more challenging to dynamic balance than reaching forward. *Clinical Biomechanics* 22: 155-164.

Rowlands, A.V., Marginson, V.F., and Lee, J. 2003. Chronic flexibility gains: Effect of isometric contraction duration during proprioceptive neuromuscular facilitation stretching techniques. *Research Quarterly for Exercise and Sport* 74: 47-51.

Roy, J.L.P., Smith, J.F., Bishop, P.A., Hallinan, C., Wang, M., and Hunter, G.R. 2004. Prediction of maximal $V.O_2$ from a submaximal StairMaster test in young women. *Journal of Strength and Conditioning Research* 18: 92-96.

Roza, A.M., and Shizgal, H.M. 1984. The Harris Benedict equation reevaluated: Resting energy requirements and the body cell mass. *American Journal of Clinical Nutrition.* 40: 168–182.

Rubin, C., Recker, R., Cullen, D., Ryaby, J., and McLeod, K. 1998. Prevention of bone loss in a post-menopausal population by low-level biomechanical intervention. *Bone* 23: S174 [abstract].

Rubini, E.C., Costa, A.L.L., and Gomes, P.S.C. 2007. The effects of stretching on strength performance. *Sports Medicine* 37: 213-224.

Runge, M., Rehfeld, G., and Resnicek, E. 2000. Balance training and exercise in geriatric patients. *Journal of Musculoskeletal and Neuronal Interactions* 1: 61-65.

Rush, E.C., Plank, L.D., Laulu, M.S., and Robinson, S.M. 1997. Prediction of percentage body fat from anthropometric measurements: Comparison of New Zealand European and Polynesian young women. *American Journal of Clinical Nutrition* 66: 2-7.

Sale, D. 1988. Neural adaptation to resistance training. *Medicine & Science in Sports & Exercise* 20: S135–S145.

Sale, D., MacDougall, J.D., Jacobs, I., and Garner, S. 1987. Interaction between concurrent strength and endurance training. *Journal of Applied Physiology* 68: 260–270.

Salem, J.G., Wang, M.Y., and Sigward, S. 2002. Measuring lower extremity strength in older adults: The stability of isokinetic versus 1RM measures. *Journal of Aging and Physical Activity* 10: 489-503.

Sallis, J.F., and Owen, N. 1999. *Physical activity and behavioral medicine.* Thousand Oaks, CA: Sage.

Samaha, F.F., Iqbal, N., Seshadri, P., Chicano, K.L., Daily, D.A., McGrory, J., Williams, T., Williams, M., Gracely, E.J., and Stern, L. 2003. A low-carbohydrate as compared with a low-fat diet in severe obesity. *New England Journal of Medicine* 348: 2074-2081.

Sands, W.A., McNeal, J.R., Stone, M.H., Russell, E.M., and Jemni, M. 2006. Flexibility enhancement with vibration: Acute and long-term. *Medicine & Science in Sports & Exercise* 38: 720-725.

Saris, W.H.M., Blair, S.N., van Baak, M.A., Eaton, S.B., Davies, P.S.W., Di Pietro, L., Fogelholm, M., Rissanen, A., Schoeller, D., Swinburn, B., Tremblay, A., Westerterp, K.R., and Wyatt, H. 2003. How much physical activity is enough to prevent unhealthy weight gain? Outcome of the IASO 1st Stock Conference and consensus statement. *Obesity Reviews* 4: 101-114.

Schade, M., Hellebrandt, F.A., Waterland, J.C., and Carns, M.L. 1962. Spot reducing in overweight college women: Its influence on fat distribution as determined by photography. *Research Quarterly* 33: 461–471.

Schaefer, E.J. 2002. Lipoproteins, nutrition, and heart disease. *American Journal of Clinical Nutrition* 75: 191-212.

Schlicht, J., Godin, J., and Camaione, D.C. 1999. How to help your client stick with an exercise program: Build self-efficacy to promote exercise adherence. *ACSM's Health & Fitness Journal* 3(6): 27–31.

Schmidt, P.K., and Carter, J.E.L. 1990. Static and dynamic differences among five types of skinfold calipers. *Human Biology* 62: 369-388.

Schot, P.K., Knutzen, K.M., Poole, S.M., and Mrotek, L.A. 2003. Sit-to-stand performance of older adults following strength training. *Research Quarterly for Exercise and Sport* 74: 1-8.

Schutte, A.E., Huisman, H.W., van Rooyen, J.M., Malan, N.T., and Schutte, R. 2004. Validation of the Finometer device for measurement of blood pressure in black women. *Journal of Human Hypertension* 18: 79-84.

Schutz, Y., and Herren, R. 2000. Assessment of speed of human locomotion using a differential satellite global positioning system. *Medicine & Science in Sports & Exercise* 32: 642-646.

Schwane, J.A., Johnson, S.R., Vandenakker, C.B., and Armstrong, R.B. 1983. Delayed-onset muscular soreness and plasma CPK and LDH activities after downhill running. *Medicine & Science in Sports & Exercise* 15: 51–56.

Scott, S. 2008. *ABLE bodies balance training.* Champaign, IL: Human Kinetics.

Segal, K.R., Van Loan, M., Fitzgerald, P.I., Hodgdon, J.A., and Van Itallie, T.B. 1988. Lean body mass estimation by bioelectrical impedance analysis: A four-site cross-validation study. *American Journal of Clinical Nutrition* 47: 7–14.

Sell, K., Lillie, T., and Taylor, J. 2008. Energy expenditure during physically interactive video game playing in male college students with different playing experience. *Journal of American College Health* 56: 505-511.

Seip, R., and Weltman, A. 1991. Validity of skinfold and girth based regression equations for the prediction of body composition in obese adults. *American Journal of Human Biology* 3: 91–95.

Sell, K.E., Verity, T.M., Worrell, T.W., Pease, B.J., and Wigglesworth, J. 1994. Two measurement techniques for assessing subtalar joint position: A reliability study. *Journal of Orthopaedic and Sports Physical Therapy* 19: 162–167.

Seshadri, P. 2004. A calorie by any name is still a calorie. *Archives of Internal Medicine* 164: 1702-1703.

Sharkey, B.J., and Gaskill, S.E. 2007. *Fitness and health,* 6th ed. Champaign, IL: Human Kinetics.

Shaw, B. 2009. *Beth Shaw's yogafit,* 2nd ed. Champaign, IL: Human Kinetics.

Shaw, C.E., McCully, K.K., and Posner, J.D. 1995. Injuries during the one repetition maximum assessment in the elderly. *Journal of Cardiopulmonary Rehabilitation* 15: 283-287.

Shaw, K., Gennat, H., O'Rourke, P., and Del Mar, C. 2006. Exercise for overweight or obesity. *Cochrane Database Systematic Reviews,* Issue 4, CD003817. DOI: 10.1002/14651858. CD003817.pub3.

Shephard, R.J. 1972. *Alive man: The physiology of physical activity.* Springfield, IL: Charles C Thomas.

Shephard, R.J. 1977. Do risks of exercise justify costly caution? *The Physician and Sportsmedicine* 5: 58–65.

Shigematsu, R., Okura, T., Nakagaichi, M., Tanaka, K., Sakai, T., Kitazumi, S., and Rantanen, T. 2008. Square-stepping exercise and fall risk factors in older adults: A single-blind, randomized controlled trial. *Journal of Gerontology* 63A: 76-82.

Shoenhair, C.L., and Wells, C.L. 1995. Women, physical activity, and coronary heart disease: A review. *Medicine, Exercise, Nutrition and Health* 4: 200–206.

Shrier, I. 1999. Stretching before exercise does not reduce the risk of local muscle injury: A critical review of the clinical and basic science literature. *Clinical Journal of Sport Medicine* 9: 221-227.

Shrier, I. 2000. Stretching before exercise: An evidence based approach. *British Journal of Sports Medicine* 34: 324-325.

Shrier, I., and Gossal, K. 2000. Myths and truths of stretching: Individualized recommendations for healthy muscles. *The Physician and Sportsmedicine* 28: 57-63.

Shubert, T.E., Schrodt, L.A., Mercer, V.S., Busby-Whitehead, J., and Giuliani, C.A. 2006. Are scores on balance screening tests associated with mobility in older adults? *Journal of Geriatric Physical Therapy* 29(1): 33-39.

Shumway-Cook, A., Baldwin, M., Polissar, N.L., and Gruber, W. 1997. Predicting the probability for falls in community-dwelling older adults. *Physical Therapy* 77: 812-819.

Shumway-Cook, A., Brauer, S., and Wollacott, M.H. 2000. Predicting the probability of falls in community-dwelling older adults using the timed up and go test. *Physical Therapy* 80: 896-904.

Shumway-Cook, A., and Horak, F.B. 1986. Assessing the influence of sensory interaction on balance. *Physical Therapy* 66: 1548-1550.

Shumway-Cook, A., and Woollacott, M.H. 1995. *Motor control: Theory and practical applications.* Baltimore: Williams & Wilkins.

Sinning, W. 1975. *Experiments and demonstrations in exercise physiology.* Philadelphia: Saunders.

Siri, W.E. 1961. Body composition from fluid space and density. In *Techniques for measuring body composition,* ed. J. Brozek and A. Henschel, 223–224. Washington, D.C.: National Academy of Sciences.

Sjodin, A.M., Forslund, A.H., Westerterp, K.R., Andersson, A.B., Forslund, J.M., and Hambraeus, L.M. 1996. The influence of physical activity on BMR. *Medicine & Science in Sports & Exercise* 28: 85–91.

Sjostrom, M., Lexell, J., Eriksson, A., and Taylor, C.C. 1992. Evidence of fiber hyperplasia in human skeletal muscles from healthy young men? *European Journal of Applied Physiology* 62: 301–304.

Skinner, J. 1993. *Exercise testing and exercise prescription for special cases.* Philadelphia: Lea & Febiger.

Slaughter, M.H., Lohman, T.G., Boileau, R.A., Horswill, C.A., Stillman, R.J., Van Loan, M.D., and Bemben, D.A. 1988. Skinfold equations for estimation of body fatness in children and youth. *Human Biology* 60: 709–723.

Smith, D.B., Johnson, G.O., Stout, J.R., Housh, T.J., Housh, D.J., and Evetovich, T.K. 1997. Validity of near-infrared interactance for estimating relative body fat in female high school gymnasts. *International Journal of Sports Medicine* 18: 531-537.

Smith, L.L. 1991. Acute inflammation: The underlying mechanism in delayed onset muscle soreness? *Medicine & Science in Sports & Exercise* 23: 542–551.

Smith, U., Hammerstein, J., Bjorntorp, P., and Kral, J.G. 1979. Regional differences and effect of weight reduction on human fat cell metabolism. *European Journal of Clinical Investigation* 9: 327–332.

Smutok, M.A., Skrinar, G.S., and Pandolf, K.B. 1980. Exercise intensity: Subjective regulation by perceived exertion. *Archives of Physical Medicine and Rehabilitation* 61: 569–574.

Smye, S.W., Sutcliffe, J., and Pitt, E. 1993. A comparison of four commercial systems used to measure whole-body electrical impedance. *Physiological Measurement* 14: 473-478.

Snijder, M.B., Kuyf, B.E., and Deurenberg, P. 1999. Effect of body build on the validity of predicted body fat from body mass index and bioelectrical impedance. *Annals of Nutrition and Metabolism* 43: 277- 285.

Spennewyn, K.C. 2008. Strength outcomes in fixed versus free-form resistance equipment. *Journal of Strength and Conditioning Research* 22(1): 75-81.

Springer, B.A., Marin, R., Cyhan, T., Roberts, H., and Gill, N.W. 2007. Normative values for the unipedal stance test with eyes open and closed. *Journal of Geriatric Physical Therapy* 30: 8-15.

Staron, R.S., Karapondo, D.L., Kraemer, W.J., Fry, A.C., Gordon, S.E., Falkel, J.E., Hagerman, F.C., and Hikida, R.S. 1994. Skeletal muscle adaptations during the early phase of heavy-resistance training in men and women. *Journal of Applied Physiology* 76: 1247-1255.

Stevens, J.A. 2006. Fatalities and injuries from falls among older adults—United States, 1993-2003 and 2001-2005. *Morbidity and Mortality Weekly Report* 55: 45.

Stolarczyk, L.M., Heyward, V.H., Hicks, V.L., and Baumgartner, R.N. 1994. Predictive accuracy of bioelectrical impedance in estimating body composition of Native American women. *American Journal of Clinical Nutrition* 59: 964-970.

Stone, M.H., Stone, M., and Sands, W.A. 2007. *Principles and practice of resistance training.* Champaign, IL: Human Kinetics.

Stout, J.R., Eckerson, J.M., Housh, T.J., and Johnson, G.O. 1994. Validity of methods for estimating percent body fat in black males. *Journal of Strength and Conditioning Research* 8: 243-246.

Stout, J.R., Eckerson, J.M., Housh, T.J., Johnson, G.O., and Betts, N.M. 1994. Validity of percent body fat estimations in males. *Medicine & Science in Sports & Exercise* 26: 632-636.

Stout, J.R., Housh, T.J., Eckerson, J.M., Johnson, G.O., and Betts, N.M. 1996. Validity of methods for estimating percent body fat in young women. *Journal of Strength and Conditioning Research* 10: 25-29.

Strath, S.J., Brage, S., and Ekelund, U. 2005. Integration of physiological and accelerometer data to improve physical activity assessment. *Medicine & Science in Sports & Exercise* 37 (Suppl.): S563-S571.

Sung, R.Y.T., Lau, P., Yu, C.W., Lam, P.K.W., and Nelson, E.A.S. 2001. Measurement of body fat using leg to leg bioimpedance. *Archives of Disease in Childhood* 85: 263-267.

Svendsen, O.L., Hassager, C., Bergmann, I., and Christiansen, C. 1992. Measurement of abdominal and intra-abdominal fat in postmenopausal women by dual energy X-ray absorptiometry and anthropometry: Comparison with computerized tomography. *International Journal of Obesity* 17: 45- 51.

Swain, D.P. 1999. V.O$_2$ reserve: A new method for exercise prescription. *ACSM's Health & Fitness Journal* 3(5): 10–14.

Swain, D.P., and Franklin, B.A. 2002. VO$_2$ reserve and the minimal intensity for improving cardiorespiratory fitness. *Medicine & Science in Sports & Exercise* 34: 152-157.

Swain, D.P., and Leutholtz, B.C. 1997. Heart rate reserve is equivalent to % VO$_2$reserve, not to VO$_2$max. *Medicine & Science in Sports & Exercise* 29: 410–414.

Swain, D.P., Leutholtz, B.C., King, M.E., Haas, L.A., and Branch, J.D. 1998. Relationship between % heart rate reserve and % VO$_2$reserve in treadmill exercise. *Medicine & Science in Sports & Exercise* 30: 318–321.

Swain, D.P., Parrott, J.A., Bennett, A.R., Branch, J.D., and Dowling, E.A. 2004. Validation of a new method for estimating VO$_2$max based on VO$_2$reserve. *Medicine & Science in Sports & Exercise* 36: 1421-1426.

Swank, A.M., Funk, D.C., Durham, M.P., and Roberts, S. 2003. Adding weights to stretching exercise increases passive range of motion for healthy elderly. *Journal of Strength and Conditioning Research* 17: 374-378.

Taaffe, D.R., Duret, C., Wheeler, S., and Marcus, R. 1999. Once-weekly resistance exercise improves muscle strength and neuromuscular performance in older adults. *Journal of the American Geriatrics Society* 47: 1208-1214.

Takeshima, N., Rogers, M.E., Watanabe, E., Brechue, W.F., Okada, A., Yamada, T., Islam, M.M., and Hayano, J. 2002. Water-based exercise improves health-related aspects of fitness in older women. *Medicine & Science in Sports & Exercise* 34: 544-551.

Takeshima, N., Rogers, N.L., Rogers, M.E., Islam, M.M., Koizumi, D., and Lee, S. 2007. Functional fitness gain varies in older adults depending on exercise mode. *Medicine & Science in Sports & Exercise* 39: 2036-2043.

Talag, T.S. 1973. Residual muscular soreness as influenced by concentric, eccentric, and static contractions. *Research Quarterly* 44: 458–469.

Tanaka, H., Monahan, K.D., and Seals, D.R. 2001. Age-predicted maximal heart rate revisited. *Journal of the American College of Cardiology* 37: 153-156.

Taylor, D.C., Dalton, J.D., Seaber, A.V., and Garrett, W.E. 1990. Viscoelastic properties of muscle-tendon units. The biomechanical effects of stretching. *American Journal of Sports Medicine* 18: 300-309.

Taylor, N.A.S., and Wilkinson, J.G. 1986. Exercise-induced skeletal muscle growth: Hypertrophy or hyperplasia? *Sports Medicine* 3: 190–200.

Taylor, W.D., George, J.D., Allsen, P.E., Vehrs, P.R., Hager, R.L., and Roberts, M.P. 2002. Estimation of VO$_2$max from a 1.5-mile endurance test. *Medicine & Science in Sports & Exercise* 35 (Suppl.): S257 [abstract].

Telford, R., Catchpole, E., Deakin, V., Hahn, A., and Plank, A. 1992. The effect of 7 to 8 months of vitamin/mineral supplementation on athletic performance. *International Journal of Sport Nutrition* 2: 135–153.

Terry, J.W., Tolson, H., Johnson, D.J., and Jessup, G.T. 1977. A work load selection procedure for the Åstrand-Ryhming test. *Journal of Sports Medicine and Physical Fitness* 17:

361–366.

Tesch, P.A. 1988. Skeletal muscle adaptations consequent to long-term heavy resistance exercise. *Medicine & Science in Sports & Exercise* 20: S132–S134.

Tesch, P.A. 1992. Short- and long-term histochemical and biochemical adaptations in muscle. In *Strength and power in sports. The encyclopaedia of sports medicine,* ed. P. Komi, 239–248. Oxford: Blackwell.

Thacker, S.B., Gilchrist, J., Stroup, D.F., and Kimsey, C.D. 2004. The impact of stretching on sports injury risk: A systematic review of the literature. *Medicine & Science in Sports & Exercise* 36: 371-378.

Thaler, M.S. 2010. *The only EKG book you'll ever need,* 6th ed. Philadelphia: Lippincott, Williams, & Wilkins.

Thomas, T.R., and Etheridge, G.L. 1980. Hydrostatic weighing at residual volume and functional residual capacity. *Journal of Applied Physiology* 49: 157–159.

Thomas, T.R., Ziogas, G., Smith, T., Zhang, Q., and Londeree, B.R. 1995. Physiological and perceived exertion responses to six modes of submaximal exercise. *Research Quarterly for Exercise and Sport* 66: 239–246.

Thompson, C.J., Cobb, K.M., and Blackwell, J. 2007. Functional training improves club head speed and functional fitness of older golfers. *Journal of Strength and Conditioning Research* 21(1): 131-137.

Thompson, J., Manore, M., and Thomas, J. 1996. Effects of diet and diet-plus-exercise programs on resting metabolic rate: A meta-analysis. *International Journal of Sport Nutrition* 6: 41–61.

Thompson, M., and Medley, A. 2007. Forward and lateral sitting functional reach in younger, middle-aged, and older adults. *Journal of Geriatric Physical Therapy* 30(2): 43-51.

Thompson, P.D. 1993. The safety of exercise testing and participation. In *ACSM's resource manual for guidelines for exercise testing and prescription,* ed. S.N. Blair, P. Painter, R. Pate, L.K. Smith, and C.B. Taylor, 361–370. Philadelphia: Lea & Febiger.

Thompson, W.R. 2008. Worldwide survey reveals fitness trends for 2009. *ACSM's Health & Fitness Journal* 12(6): 7-14.

Thomson, C.A., and Thompson, P.A. 2008. Healthy lifestyle and cancer prevention. *ACSM's Health & Fitness Journal* 12(3): 18-26.

Thorstensson, A., Hulten, B., vonDobeln, W., and Karlsson, J. 1976. Effect of strength training on enzyme activities and fibre characteristics in human skeletal muscle. *Acta Physiologica Scandinavica* 96: 392–398.

Thune, I., and Furberg, A-S. 2001. Physical activity and cancer risk: Dose-response and cancer, all sites and site-specific. *Medicine & Science in Sports & Exercise* 33 (Suppl.): S530-S550.

Timson, B.F., and Coffman, J.L. 1984. Body composition by hydrostatic weighing at total lung capacity and residual volume. *Medicine & Science in Sports & Exercise* 16: 411–414.

Tinetti, M.E. 1986. Performance-oriented assessment of mobility problems in elderly patients. *Journal of the American Geriatric Society* 34: 119-126.

Tinetti, M.E., Speechley, M., and Ginter, S.F. 1988. Risk factors for falls among elderly persons living in the community. *New England Journal of Medicine* 319(26): 1701-1707.

Tipton, C.M., Matthes, R.D., Maynard, J.A., and Carey, R.A. 1975. The influence of physical activity on ligaments and tendons. *Medicine and Science in Sports* 7: 165–175.

Tipton, K.D., Rasmussen, B.B., Miller, S.L., Wolfe, S.E., Owens-Stovall, S.K., Petrini, B.E., and Wolfe, R.R. 2001. Timing of amino acid-carbohydrate ingestion alters anabolic responose of muscle to resistance exercise. *American Journal of Physiology, Endocrinology and Metabolism* 281: E197-206.

Tipton, K.D., and Wolfe, R.R. 2004. Protein and amino acids for athletes. *Journal of Sports Science* 22: 65-79.

Topouchian, J.A., El Assaad, M.A., Orobinskaia, L.V., El Feghali, R.N., and Asmar, R.G. 2006. Validation of two automatic devices for self-measurement of blood pressure according to the International Protocol of the European Society of Hypertension: The Omron M6 (HEM-7001-E) and the Omron R7 (HEM 637-IT). *Blood Pressure Monitoring* 11: 165-171.

Torvinen, S., Kannus, P., Sievanen, H., Jarvinen, T.A.H., Pasanen, M., Kontulainen, S., Jarvinen, T.L.N., Jarvinen, M., Oja, P., and Vuori, I. 2002. Effect of four-month vertical whole body vibration on performance and balance. *Medicine & Science in Sports & Exercise* 34: 1523-1528.

Tothill, P., and Hannan, W.J. 2000. Comparisons between Hologic QDR 1000W, QDR 4500A, and Lunar Expert dual-energy X-ray absorptiometry scanners used for measuring total body bone and soft tissue. *Annals of the New York Academy of Sciences* 904: 63-71.

Town, G.P., Sol, N., and Sinning, W. 1980. The effect of rope skipping rate on energy expenditure of males and females. *Medicine & Science in Sports & Exercise* 12: 295–298.

Tran, Z.V., and Weltman, A. 1988. Predicting body composition of men from girth measurements. *Human Biology* 60: 167–175.

Tran, Z.V., and Weltman, A. 1989. Generalized equation for predicting body density of women from girth measurements. *Medicine & Science in Sports & Exercise* 21: 101–104.

Tremblay, M.S., and Willms, J.D. 2000. Secular trends in the body mass index of Canadian children. *Canadian Medical Association Journal* 163: 1429-1433. Published erratum in *Canadian Medical Association Journal* (2001) 164: 970.

Troiano, R.P., Berrigan, D., Dodd, K.W., Masse, L.C., Tilert, T., and McDowell, M. 2008. Physical activity in the United States measured by accelerometer. *Medicine & Science in Sports & Exercise* 40: 181-188.

Troped, P.J., Oliveira, M.S., Matthews, C.E., Cromley, E.K., Melly, S.J., and Craig, B.A. 2008. Prediction of activity mode with global positioning system and accelerometer data. *Medicine & Science in Sports & Exercise* 40: 972-978.

Trost, S.G., Owen, N., Bauman, A.E., Sallis, J.F., and Brown, W. 2002. Correlates of adults' participation in physical activity: Review and update. *Medicine & Science in Sports*

& Exercise 34: 1996-2001.

Tudor-Locke, C., Hatano, Y., Pangrazi, R.P., and Kang, M. 2008. Revisiting "How many steps are enough?" *Medicine & Science in Sports & Exercise* 40 (Suppl.): S537-S543.

Tudor-Locke, C., Sisson, S.B., Collova, T., Lee, S.M., and Swan, P.D. 2005. Pedometer-determined step count guidelines for classifying walking intensity in a young ostensibly healthy population. *Canadian Journal of Applied Physiology* 30: 666-676.

Tudor-Locke, C., Sisson, S.B., Lee, S.M., Craig, C.L., Plotnikoff, R., and Bauman, A. 2006. Evaluation of quality of commercial pedometers. *Canadian Journal of Public Health* 97: S10-S15.

Tudor-Locke, C., Williams, J.E., Reis, J.P., and Pluto, D. 2002. Utility of pedometers for assessing physical activity: Convergent validity. *Sports Medicine* 32: 795-808.

Turcato, E., Bosello, O., Francesco, V.D., Harris, T.B., Zoico, E., Bissoli, L., Fracassi, E., and Zamboni, M. 2000. Waist circumference and abdominal sagittal diameter as surrogates of body fat distribution in the elderly: Their relation with cardiovascular risk factors. *International Journal of Obesity* 24: 1005-1010.

Tyrrell, V.J., Richards, G., Hofman, P., Gillies, G.F., Robinson, E., and Cutfield, W.S. 2001. Foot-to-foot bioelectrical impedance analysis: A valuable tool for the measurement of body composition in children. *International Journal of Obesity* 25: 273-278.

U.S. Department of Health and Human Services. 1996. *Physical activity and health: A report of the Surgeon General—At a glance.* Atlanta: U.S. Department of Health and Human Services, Centers for Disease Control and Prevention, National Center for Chronic Disease Prevention and Health Promotion.

U.S. Department of Health and Human Services. 2000a. *Healthy people 2010—conference edition: Physical activity and fitness (22).* Atlanta: Author.

U.S. Department of Health and Human Services. 2000b. *Healthy people 2010: Understanding and improving health—overweight and obesity.* Washington, D.C.: U.S. Government Printing Office.

U.S. Department of Health and Human Services. 2004. *2005 Dietary Guidelines Advisory Committee report: Translating the science into dietary guidance.* Washington, D.C.: U.S. Government Printing Office.

U.S. Department of Health and Human Services. 2005a. *Dietary Guidelines for Americans 2005.* Executive Summary. www.health.gov/dietaryguidelines/dga2005/document/html/executivesummary.

U.S. Department of Health and Human Services. 2005b. MyPyramid. www.MyPyramid.com.

U.S. Department of Health and Human Services. 2007. *The Surgeon General's call to action to prevent overweight and obesity in children and adolescents.* Washington, DC: Author. http://www.surgeongeneral.gov/topics/obesity/calltoaction/fact_adolescents.html

U.S. Department of Health and Human Services. 2008. Physi-

cal activity guidelines for Americans. At-a-glance: A fact sheet for professionals. www.health.gov/paguidelines/factsheetprof.aspx.

Utter, A.C., Nieman, D.C., Mulford, G.J., Tobin, R., Schumm, S., McInnis, T., and Monk, J.R. 2005. Evaluation of leg-to-leg BIA in assessing body composition of high-school wrestlers. *Medicine & Science in Sports & Exercise* 37: 1395-1400.

Utter, A.C., Nieman, D.C., Ward, A.N., and Butterworth, D.E. 1999. Use of the leg-to-leg bioelectrical impedance method in assessing body-composition change in obese women. *American Journal of Clinical Nutrition* 69: 603-607.

Utter. A.C., Scott, J.R., Oppliger, R.A., Visich, P.S., Goss, F.L., Marks, B.L., Nieman, D.C., and Smith, B.W. 2001. A comparison of leg-to-leg bioelectrical impedance and skinfolds in assessing body fat in collegiate wrestlers. *Journal of Strength and Conditioning Research* 15: 157-160.

Vaisman, N., Corey, M., Rossi, M.F., Goldberg, E., and Pencharz, P. 1988. Changes in body composition during refeeding of patients with anorexia nervosa. *Journal of Pediatrics* 113: 925–929.

Vaisman, N., Rossi, M.F., Goldberg, E., Dibden, L.J., Wykes, L.J., and Pencharz, P.B. 1988. Energy expenditures and body composition in patients with anorexia nervosa. *Journal of Pediatrics* 113: 919–924.

Van Adrichem, J.A.M., and van der Korst, J.K. 1973. Assessment of flexibility of the lumbar spine: A pilot study in children and adolescents. *Scandinavian Journal of Rheumatology* 2: 87–91.

van den Beld, W.A., van der Sanden, G.A.C., Sengers, R.C.A., Verbeek, A.L.M., and Gabreels, F.J.M. 2006. Validity and reproducilibity of hand-held dynamometry in children aged 4-11 years. *Journal of Rehabilitation Medicine* 38: 57-64.

van der Kooy, K., Leenen, R., Seidell, J.C., Deurenberg, P., Droop, A., and Bakker, C.J.G. 1993. Waist-hip ratio is a poor predictor of changes in visceral fat. *American Journal of Clinical Nutrition* 57: 327-333.

Vanhelder, W.P., Radomski, M.W., and Goode, R.C. 1984. Growth hormone responses during intermittent weight lifting exercise in men. *European Journal of Applied Physiology* 53: 31–34.

Van Loan, M.D., and Mayclin, P.L. 1987. Bioelectrical impedance analysis: Is it a reliable estimator of lean body mass and total body water? *Human Biology* 59: 299–309.

Van Loan, M.D., and Mayclin, P.L. 1992. Body composition assessment: Dual-energy X-ray absorptiometry (DEXA) compared to reference methods. *European Journal of Clinical Nutrition* 46: 125–130.

Van Mechelen, W., Holbil, H., and Kemper, H.C. 1986. Validation of two running tests as estimates of maximal aerobic power in children. *European Journal of Applied Physiology and Occupational Physiology* 55: 503–506.

Vehrs, P.R., Drummond, M., Fellingham, D.K., and Brigham, G.W. 2002. Accuracy of five heart rate monitors during exercise. *Medicine & Science in Sports & Exercise* 34 (Suppl.): S272 [abstract].

Velasquez, K.S., and Wilmore, J.H. 1992. Changes in cardiorespiratory fitness and body composition after a 12-week bench step training program. *Medicine & Science in Sports & Exercise* 24: S78 [abstract].

Vera-Garcia, F.J., Grenier, S.G., and McGill, S.M. 2000. Abdominal muscle responses during curl-ups on both stable and labile surfaces. *Physical Therapy* 80: 564-569.

Verdijk, L.B., Jonkers, R.A.M., Glesson, B.G., Beelen, M., Meijer, K., Savelberg, H.H.C.M., Wodzig, W.K.W.H., Dendale, P., and van Loon, L.J.C. 2009. Protein supplementation before and after exercise does not further augment skeletal muscle hypertrophy after resistance training in elderly men. *American Journal of Clinical Nutrition* 89: 608-616.

Verhagen, E., van der Beek, A., Twisk, J., Bouter, L., Bahr, R., and Mechelen, W. 2004. The effect of a proprioceptive balance board training program for the prevention of ankle sprains: A prospective controlled trial. *American Journal of Sports Medicine* 32: 1385-1393.

Vescovi, J.D., Zimmerman, S.L., Miller, W.C., Hildebrandt, L., Hammer, R.L., and Fernhall, B. 2001. Evaluation of the Bod Pod for estimating percentage body fat in a heterogeneous group of adult humans. *European Journal of Applied Physiology* 85: 326-332.

Vincent, K.R., Braith, R.W., Feldman, R.A., Magyari, P.M., Cutler, R.B., Persin, S.A., Lennon, S.L., Gabr, A.H., and Lowenthal, D.T. 2002. Resistance exercise and physical performance in adults aged 60 to 83. *Journal of the American Geriatrics Society* 50: 1100-1107.

Voelker, S.A., Foster, C., Skemp-Arlt, K.M., Brice, G., and Backes, R. 2002. Relationship between the talk test and ventilatory threshold in cardiac patients. *Clinical Exercise Physiology* 4: 120-123.

Volek, J. 1999. Update: What we know about creatine. *ACSM's Health & Fitness Journal* 3(3): 27–33.

Volpe, S.L. 2009. Vitamin D and health: Do we need more than the current DRI?: Part 2. *ACSM's Health & Fitness Journal* 13(1): 33-34.

Wagner, D.R., and Heyward, V.H. 2001. Validity of two-component models of estimating body fat of Black men. *Journal of Applied Physiology* 90: 649-656.

Wagner, D.R., and Heyward, V.H. 2004. *Applied body composition assessment*. Champaign, IL: Human Kinetics.

Wagner, D., Heyward, V., and Gibson, A. 2000. Validation of air displacement plethysmography for assessing body composition. *Medicine & Science in Sports & Exercise* 32: 1339–1344.

Wallick, M.E., Porcari, J.P., Wallick, S.B., Berg, K.M., Brice, G.A., and Arimond, G.R. 1995. Physiological responses to in-line skating compared to treadmill running. *Medicine & Science in Sports & Exercise* 27: 242–248.

Wallin, D., Ekblom, B., Grahn, R., and Nordenborg, T. 1985. Improvement of muscle flexibility. A comparison between two techniques. *American Journal of Sports Medicine* 13: 263-268.

Wallman, H.W. 2001. Comparison of elderly nonfallers and fallers on performance measures of functional reach, sensory organization, and limits of stability. *Journal of Gerontology* 56: M589-M583.

Walts, C.T., Hanson, E.D., Delmonico, M.J., Yao, L., Wang, M.W., and Hurley, B.F. 2008. Do sex or race differences influence strength training effects on muscle or fat? *Medicine & Science in Sports & Exercise* 40: 669-676.

Wang, J., Thornton, J.C., Russell, M., Burastero, S., Heymsfield, S., and Pierson, R.N. 1994. Asians have lower body mass index (BMI) but higher percent body fat than do Whites: Comparison of anthropometric measurements. *American Journal of Clinical Nutrition* 60: 23-28.

Warburton, D.E.R., Sarkany, D., Johnson, M., Rhodes, R.E., Whitford, W., Esch, B.T.A., Scott, J.M., Wong, S.C., and Bredin, S.S.D. 2009. Metabolic requirements of interactive video game cycling. *Medicine & Science in Sports & Exercise* 41: 920-926.

Ward, D.S., Evenson, K.R., Vaugh, A., Rodgers, A.B., and Troiano, R.P. 2005. Accelerometer use in physical activity: Best practices and research recommendations. *Medicine & Science in Sports & Exercise* 37 (Suppl.): S582-S588.

Ward, R., and Anderson, G.S. 1998. Resilience of anthropometric data assembly strategies to imposed error. *Journal of Sports Sciences* 16: 755-759.

Ward, R., Rempel, R., and Anderson, G.S. 1999. Modeling dynamic skinfold compression. *American Journal of Human Biology* 11: 521–537.

Wathen, D. 1994a. Load assignment. In *Essentials of strength testing*, ed. T.R. Baechle, 435-446. Champaign, IL: Human Kinetics.

Wathen, D. 1994b. Periodization: Concepts and applications. In *Essentials of strength training and conditioning*, ed. T.R. Baechle, 459–472. Champaign, IL: Human Kinetics.

Watsford, M.L., Murphy, A.J., Spinks, W.L., and Walshe, A.D. 2003. Creatine supplementation and its effect on musculotendinous stiffness and performance. *Journal of Strength and Conditioning Research* 17: 26- 33.

Wattles, M.G. 2002. The dissection of exercise certifications. *Professionalization of Exercise Physiology*online 5(3): 1-13.

Weiss, E.C., Galuska, D.A., Khan, L.K., and Serdula, M.K. 2006. Weight-control practices among U.S. adults, 2001-2002. *American Journal of Preventive Medicine* 31: 18-24.

Weiss, L.W., Cureton, K.J., and Thompson, F.N. 1983. Comparison of serum testosterone and androstenedione responses to weight lifting in men and women. *European Journal of Applied Physiology* 50: 413–419.

Weits, T., Van der Beek, E.J., Wedel, M., and Ter Haar Romeny, B.M. 1988. Computed tomography measurement of abdominal fat deposition in relation to anthropometry. *International Journal of Obesity* 12: 217-225.

Weldon, S.M., and Hill, R.H. 2003. The efficacy of stretching for prevention of exercise-related injury: A systematic review of the literature. *Manual Therapy* 8: 141-150.

Weltman, A., Levine, S., Seip, R.L., and Tran, Z.V. 1988. Accurate assessment of body composition in obese females.

American Journal of Clinical Nutrition 48: 1179–1183.

Weltman, A., Seip, R.L., and Tran, Z.V. 1987. Practical assessment of body composition in adult obese males. *Human Biology* 59: 523–535.

Wessel, H.U., Strasburger, J.F., and Mitchell, B.M. 2001. New standards for Bruce treadmill protocol in children and adolescents. *Pediatric Exercise Science* 13: 392-401.

Whaley, M., Kaminsky, L., Dwyer, G., Getchell, L., and Norton, J. 1992. Predictors of over- and underachievement of age-predicted maximal heart rate. *Medicine & Science in Sports & Exercise* 24: 1173–1179.

Whitney, S.L., Poole, J.L., and Cass, S.P. 1998. A review of balance instruments for older adults. *American Journal of Occupational Therapy* 52: 666-671.

Willardson, J.M. 2008. A periodized approach for core training. *ACSM's Health & Fitness Journal* 12(1): 7-13.

Willett, W.C. 2001. *Eat, drink and be healthy: The Harvard Medical School guide to healthy eating.* New York: Simon & Schuster Adult Publishing.

Williams, D.M., Matthews, C.E., Rutt, C., Napolitano, M.A., and Marcus, B.H. 2008. Interventions to increase walking behavior. *Medicine & Science in Sports & Exercise* 40 (Suppl.): S567-S573.

Williams, D.P., Going, S.B., Massett, M.P., Lohman, T.G., Bare, L.A., and Hewitt, M.J. 1993. Aqueous and mineral fractions of the fat-free body and their relation to body fat estimates in men and women aged 49-82 years. In *Human body composition: In vivo methods, models and assessment*, ed. K.J. Ellis and J.D. Eastman, 109–113. New York: Plenum Press.

Williams, J.E., Wells, J.C., Wilson, C.M., Haroun, D., Lucas, A., and Fewtrell, M.S. 2006. Evaluation of Lunar Prodigy dual-energy X-ray absorptiometry for assessing body composition in healthy persons and patients by comparison with the criterion 4-component model. *American Journal of Clinical Nutrition* 83: 1047-1054.

Williams, M.H. 1992. *Nutrition for fitness and sport.* Dubuque, IA: Brown & Benchmark.

Williams, M.H. 1993. Nutritional supplements for strength trained athletes. *Sports Science Exchange* 6(6). Gatorade Sports Science Institute, Quaker Oats Co.

Williams, P.T. 2001. Physical fitness and activity as separate heart disease risk factors: A meta-analysis. *Medicine & Science in Sports & Exercise* 33: 754-761.

Williams, R., Binkley, J., Bloch, R., Goldsmith, C.H., and Minuk, T. 1993. Reliability of the modified-modified Schober and double inclinometer methods for measuring lumbar flexion and extension. *Physical Therapy* 73: 26–37.

Williford, H.N., Blessing, D.L., Barksdale, J.M., and Smith, F.H. 1988. The effects of aerobic dance training on serum lipids, lipoproteins, and cardiopulmonary function. *Journal of Sports Medicine and Physical Fitness* 28: 151–157.

Wilmore, J.H. 1974. Alterations in strength, body composition, and anthropometric measurements consequent to a 10-week weight training program. *Medicine and Science in Sports* 6: 133–138.

Wilmore, J.H., and Behnke, A.R. 1969. An anthropometric estimation of body density and lean body weight in young men. *Journal of Applied Physiology* 27: 25–31.

Wilmore, J.H., and Behnke, A.R. 1970. An anthropometric estimation of body density and lean body weight in young women. *American Journal of Clinical Nutrition* 23: 267–274.

Wilmore, J.H., Davis, J.A., O'Brien, R.S., Vodak, P.A., Walder, G.R., and Amsterdam, E.A. 1980. Physiological alterations consequent to 20-week conditioning programs of bicycling, tennis and jogging. *Medicine & Science in Sports & Exercise* 12: 1–9.

Wilmore, J.H., Frisancho, R.A., Gordon, C.C., Himes, J.H., Martin, A.D., Martorell, R., and Seefeldt, R.D. 1988. Body breadth equipment and measurement techniques. In *Anthropometric standardization reference manual*, ed. T.G. Lohman, A.F. Roche, and R. Martorell, 27–38. Champaign, IL: Human Kinetics.

Wilmore, J.H., Parr, R.B., Girandola, R.N., Ward, P., Vodak, P.A., Barstow, T.J., Pipes, T.V., Romero, G.T., and Leslie, P. 1978. Physiological alterations consequent to circuit weight training. *Medicine and Science in Sports* 10: 79–84.

Wilmore, J.H., Royce, J., Girandola, R.N., Katch, F.I., and Katch, V.L. 1970. Body composition changes with a 10-week program of jogging. *Medicine and Science in Sports* 2: 113–119.

Wilmoth, S.K. 1986. *Leading aerobic dance-exercise.* Champaign, IL: Human Kinetics.

Wilson, P.K., Winga, E.R., Edgett, J.W., and Gushiken, T.J. 1978. *Policies and procedures of a cardiac rehabilitation program—immediate to long term care.* Philadelphia: Lea & Febiger.

Withers, R.T., LaForgia, J., Pillans, R.K., Shipp, N.J., Chatterton, B.E., Schultz, C.G., and Leaney, F. 1998. Comparisons of two-, three-, and four-compartment models of body composition analysis in men and women. *Journal of Applied Physiology* 85: 238-245.

Witten, C. 1973. Construction of a submaximal cardiovascular step test for college females. *Research Quarterly* 44: 46–50.

Wolf, S., Barnhart, H., Kutner, N., McNeely, E., Coogler, C., and Xu, T. 1996. Reducing frailty and falls in older persons: An investigation of tai chi and computerized balance training. *Journal of the American Geriatric Society* 44: 489-497.

Wolf-Maier, K., Cooper, R.S., Banegas, J.R., Giampaoli, S., Hense, H.W., Joffres, M., Kastarinen, M., Poulter, N., Primatesta, P., Rodriquez-Artalego, F., Stegmayr, B., Thamm, N., Tuomilephto, J., Vanuzzo, D., and Vescio, F. 2003. Hypertension prevalence and blood pressure levels in 6 European countries, Canada, and the United States. *Journal of the American Medical Association* 289: 2363-2369.

Wolfe, B.L., LeMura, L.M., and Cole, P.J. 2004. Quantitative analysis of single- vs. multiple-set programs for resistance training. *Journal of Strength and Conditioning Research* 18: 35-47.

Wolfson, L., Whipple, R., Derby, C., Judge, J., King, M., Amerman, P., Schmidt, J., and Smyers, D. 1996. Balance and strength training in older adults: Intervention gains and tai chi maintenance. *Journal of the American Geriatric*

Society 44: 498-506.

Women's Exercise Research Center. 1998. Based on figures published by Brown, D.A., and Miller, W.C. 1998. Normative data for strength and flexibility of women throughout life. *European Journal of Applied Physiology* 78: 77–82.

Woodby-Brown, S., Berg, K., and Latin, R.W. 1993. Oxygen cost of aerobic bench stepping at three heights. *Journal of Strength and Conditioning Research* 7: 163–167.

World Health Organization (WHO). 1998. Obesity: Preventing and managing a global epidemic. *Report of a WHO Consultation on Obesity.* Geneva: Author.

World Health Organization. 2001. Global database on obesity and body mass index (BMI) in adults. http://www.who.int/nut/db_bmi.

World Health Organization. 2002a. Diabetes: The cost of diabetes. www.who.int/mediacentre/factsheets/fs236/en/print.html.

World Health Organization. 2002b. Reducing risks, promoting healthy life. *World Health Report 2002.* www.who.int/whr/2002/chapter4/en/index4.html.

World Health Organization. 2002c. Smoking statistics. www.wpro.who.int/public/press_release/press_view.asp?id=219.

World Health Organization. 2004. Cardiovascular disease: Prevention and control. www.who.int/dietphysicalactivity/publications/facts/cvd/en/.

World Health Organization. 2006. Obesity and overweight. Fact sheet no. 311. www.who.int/mediacentre/factsheets/fs311.

World Health Organization. 2007a. Cardiovascular diseases. Fact sheet no. 317. www.who.int/mediacentre/factsheets/fs317.

World Health Organization. 2007b. Prevalence of obesity by sex, adults aged 15 and over, latest available year, Europe. www.heartstats.org.

World Health Organization. 2008a. Cancer. Fact sheet no. 297. www.who.int/mediacentre/factsheets/fs297.

World Health Organization. 2008b. Diabetes. Fact sheet no. 312. www.who.int/mediacentre/factsheets/fs312.

Wosje, K.S., Knipstein, B.L., and Kalkwarf, H.J. 2006. Measurement error of DXA: Interpretation of fat and lean mass changes in obese and nonobese children. *Journal of Clinical Densitometry* 9: 335-340.

Wright, J.D., Kennedy-Stephenson, J., Wang, C.Y., McDowell, M.A., and Johnson, C.L. 2004. Trends in intake of energy and macronutrients—United States, 1971-2000. *Morbidity and Mortality Weekly Report* 53(4): 80-82.

Wu, G. 2002. Evaluation of the effectiveness of tai chi for improving balance and preventing falls in the older population—A review. *Journal of the American Geriatric Society* 50: 746-754.

Yamanoto, K. 2002. Omron Institute of Life Science [personal communication].

Yee, A.J., Fuerst, T., Salamone, L., Visser, M., Dockrell, M., Van Loan, M., and Kern, M. 2001. Calibration and validation of an air-displacement plethysmography method for estimating percentage body fat in an elderly population: A comparison among compartmental models. *American Journal of Clinical Nutrition* 74: 637-642.

Yee, S.Y., and Gallagher, D. 2008. Assessment methods in human body composition. *Current Opinion in Clinical Nutrition and Metabolic Care* 11: 566-572.

Yessis, M. 2003. Using free weights for stability training. *Fitness Management* 19(11): 26-28.

Yim-Chiplis, P.K., and Talbot, L.A. 2000. Defining and measuring balance in adults. *Biological Research for Nursing* 1(4): 321-331.

YMCA of the USA. 2002. *YMCA fitness testing and assessment manual.* 4th ed. Champaign, IL: Human Kinetics.

Yoke, M., and Kennedy, C. 2004. *Functional exercise progressions.* Monterey, CA: Healthy Learning.

Yoon, B.K., Kravitz, L., and Roberts, R. 2007. VO_2max, protocol duration, and the VO_2 plateau. *Medicine & Science in Sports & Exercise* 39: 1186-1192.

Zakeri, I., Adolph, A.L., Puyau, M.R., Vohra, F.A., and Butte, N.F. 2008. Application of cross-sectional time series modeling for the prediction of energy expenditure from heart rate and accelerometry. *Journal of Applied Physiology* 104: 1665-1673.

Zamboni, M., Turcato, E., Armellini, F., Kahn, H.S., Zivelonghi, A., Santana, H., Bergamo-Andreis, I.A., and Bosello, O. 1998. Sagittal abdominal diameter as a practical predictor of visceral fat. *International Journal of Obesity and Related Metabolic Disorders* 22: 655-660.

Zeni, A.I., Hoffman, M.D., and Clifford, P.S. 1996. Energy expenditure with indoor exercise machines. *Journal of the American Medical Association* 275: 1424–1427.

Zhu, S., Heshka, S., Wang, Z., Shen, W., Allison, D.B., Ross, R., and Heymsfield, S.B. 2004. Combination of BMI and waist circumference for identifying cardiovascular risk factors in whites. *Obesity Research* 12: 633-645.

Zhu, S., Heymsfield, S.B., Toyoshima, H., Wang, Z., Petrobelli, A., and Heshka, S. 2005. Race-ethnicity-specific waist circumference cutoffs for identifying cardiovascular disease risk factors. *American Journal of Clinical Nutrition* 81: 409-415.

Zhu, W. 2008. Promoting physical activity using technology. *President's Council on Physical Fitness and Sports Research Digest* 9(3): 1-8.

Zwiren, L., Freedson, P., Ward, A., Wilke, S., and Rippe, J. 1991. Estimation of $\dot{V}O_2$max: A comparative analysis of five exercise tests. *Research Quarterly for Exercise and Sport* 62: 73–78.

Index

Note: The italicized *f* and *t* following page numbers refer to figures and tables, respectively.

About the Author

Vivian H. Heyward, PhD, is a Regents professor emerita at the University of New Mexico where she has taught physical fitness assessment and exercise prescription courses for 26 years. In addition to the previous editions of this book, she has authored two editions of *Applied Body Composition Assessment* (Human Kinetics 1996, 2004) as well as numerous articles in research and professional journals dealing with various aspects of physical fitness assessment and exercise prescription.

Heyward has received many professional awards, including Distinguished Alumni Awards from the University of Illinois and the State University of New York at Cortland, and the SWACSM Recognition Award for distinguished professional service and achievement.

In her free time, she enjoys hiking, nature photography, and creative journaling. Heyward resides in Albuquerque, New Mexico.